THE GUIDE TO

The Handling of People

5TH EDITION

First published 1981
Second edition 1987
Third edition 1992
Reprinted January 1993 with amendments largely in Chapter 2
Fourth edition 1997
Reprinted February 1998 with revisions
Reprinted August 1998
Reprinted February 1999
Fifth edition 2005

Design by Jason Joseph Pelta and Ged Lennox
gedesign, Spring Cottage, Harley Wood, Nailsworth, Gloucestershire GL6 0LB
Tel: 01453 836860 Email: info@gedesign.org

Illustrations by Gemma Hastilow

Printed by HTT Managed Services Limited, 1b Park Square, Newton Chambers Road, Thorncliffe Park, Chapeltown, Sheffield S35 2PH
Tel: 0114 2203760 Fax: 0114 2203761

A catalogue record for this publication is available from the British Library
ISBN 0-9530582-9-8

Published by BackCare, the charity for healthier backs (registered as the National Back Pain Association), 16 Elmtree Road, Teddington, Middlesex, TW11 8ST
Tel: 0208 977 5474 Fax: 0208 943 5318 Website: www.backcare.org.uk

Forewords

BackCare

When the National Back Pain Association published the first edition of The Guide to the Handling of Patients in 1981, we had no idea that it would become the definitive handbook for all health professionals involved with moving and handling people.

Over the years handling training and equipment have become more sophisticated and there has been greater awareness of the risks of moving and handling tasks. Yet the Royal College of Nursing reported that in 2003 around 80,000 nurses sustained back injury due to lifting patients. And it's not just nurses who are affected. Without sufficient training and guidance, anyone who is responsible for lifting, moving or handling people in the course of their work, could risk damaging their back.

This new 5th edition is much more than a revision of the 4th edition. It covers new legislation and addresses the issues raised by recent legal cases; it includes the latest thinking on risk assessment, ergonomics and competence. Most importantly, the new edition incorporates the most recent evidence for safer handling of people. The practical chapters reference this evidence base and give objective scores for all the tasks described.

BackCare is very grateful for the enormous contributions that the Royal College of Nursing and the National Back Exchange have made to this book. Their expertise and commitment have ensured the high quality of this new publication. I would also like to express our gratitude to the sponsors of the Guide – the Department of Health and Arjo, a leading supplier of handling equipment and training.

Dr Michael McKiernan MB ChB FRCP FFOM
Chairman of Trustees

Department of Health

The joint Department of Health and Health and Safety Executive 'Back in Work' initiative is pleased to support the publication of this new 5th edition to The Guide to the Handling of People.

The national Back in Work campaign is aimed at everyone who works in the NHS whether in an acute hospital, the community or the local GP practice. This campaign aims to show that it is to the benefit of EVERYONE in the NHS to address the problem of work related sickness and injury and that NHS users will in turn benefit from healthier, happier staff who are fit for work.

In the NHS, manual handling accidents account for 40 per cent of all sickness absence. The cost to the NHS of manual handling accident related sickness absence is in the region of £400 million each year. Well motivated and productive people have to give up work because of pain and disabilty related to manual handling problems.

Compensation claims for manual handling accidents to staff are rising and the largest payment to a member of staff in the NHS so far is £800,000. Every NHS employee who retires early because of a back injury costs the NHS at least an extra £60,000.

This Guide offers an important tool in the campaign by showing how the risks to those lifting and moving people can be eliminated or minimised by good handling practice. The new Guide is essential reading for all those with a responsibility for handling people, whether directly or in training and managing others who do, to study BackCare's new guidance.

Julian Topping
Occupational Health & Safety Lead, NHS Employers

National Back Exchange

National Back Exchange is delighted to have been involved in the development of this new edition of The Guide to the Handling of People and to have been able to support BackCare in the development of this important publication. This edition marks the beginning of an exciting phase in the field of moving and handling, providing important steps to creating an evidence base for the handling transfers that are part of so many peoples' lives.

Some moving and handling decisions are easy, where everyone involved has found a workable safer solution. Sometimes however, handling decisions are more difficult to make and several perspectives need to be considered. It is important to empower both the person being assisted and the person performing the handling task to work together in partnership, with a shared respect and desire to care for the health of the other.

The practical chapters give the opportunity to base decisions on research and evidence collected by National Back Exchange members. As more research is undertaken and more evidence is collected this will aid the development of strategies to protect handlers and the people they assist.

This edition aims to make moving and handling safer for all involved and National Back Exchange looks forward to the positive impact the new publication will have in such an important area.

Carole Johnson
Former Chairman, National Back Exchange

Royal College of Nursing

There is no need for injury to be an occupational hazard. Hoists, sliding aids and other specialised equipment mean staff should no longer have to risk injury while doing their job. The Royal College of Nursing, together with BackCare (formerly the National Back Pain Association) has led the way in transforming the health care culture around safer manual handling of patients. The focus now is on delivering quality; safer care to patients, provided by staff whose own safety is well supported by safer handling policies and the physical resources to do the job.

Yet we still have work to do in ensuring that best practice applies in all health care settings. Nurses should have access to the right equipment for their patient's needs and training and support to use it properly. Yet manual handling continues to take its toll on nurses' health. One in four nurses have taken time off with a back injury sustained at work. For some it has meant the end of their nursing career.

The RCN Advisory Panel on Back Pain in Nurses has played a significant part in the drive to combat work related injuries in nursing. The RCN Code of Practice for Patient Handling, first published in 1996, sparked off a major debate on back injuries and prompted employers to take a hard look at their manual handling policies.

The RCN very much values its strong partnership with BackCare in supporting patient care through taking care of nursing staff. This latest edition is an invaluable tool to help put those policies into practice.

Beverly Malone
General Secretary of the Royal College of Nursing

Contributors

Editor

Jacqui Smith MSc MCSP SRP Cert OH

Jacqui Smith is a Consultant Occupational Physiotherapist with a Master's Degree in Ergonomics. She is a Director of Work Fit, an occupational physiotherapy, ergonomics and training company based in Yorkshire. A founder member of the National Back Exchange and Editor of The Column since August 2000, she is also a co-author of Guidance in Manual Handling for Chartered Physiotherapists (2002) and a contributor to the IPC and EBU. She is the Chairman of ACPOHE (The Association of Chartered Physiotherapists in Occupational Health and Ergonomics) and a past Editor of Occupational Health Physiotherapy journal. As an expert witness Jacqui has provided opinion in over 1200 cases for claimants, defendants and the HSE.

Editorial team

Nia Taylor MA ACMA

Nia Taylor, Chief Executive of BackCare, has been with the charity for 3 and a half years. She qualified as an accountant with an engineering firm and worked in various companies in the private and public sector. Before joining BackCare she worked at Charing Cross & Westminster Medical School and then (after merger) at Imperial College for 5 years.

Mandy Clift

Mandy is Marketing Manager for Arjo UK and Business Manager for Corpus, the Ergonomics Division of Arjo. Mandy is a member of the Royal College of Nursing Advisory Panel on Back Pain and has been closely involved in education programmes and seminars for healthcare professionals, specifiers and architects, as well as back injury prevention programmes in care homes and hospitals.

Emma Crumpton MSc (Ergs) BSc MCSP

Emma Crumpton is a freelance ergonomist with extensive experience in healthcare. Her recent work includes projects for HSE and RCN, the most relevant being the development of the RCN manual handling training guidance and competencies (see appendix 3).

Carol Bannister BA (Hons) RGN OHNC

Carol Bannister has worked for the Royal College of Nursing for the past nine years. She is the National Adviser to the RCN in occupational health which includes both policy and practice initiatives. She is also the Chair of the RCN Advisory Committee for Back Pain in Nurses and takes the lead on the RCN work aimed at reducing the incidence of manual handling risk to nurses. Carol is a coordinator within the Professional Nursing Department and has recently been working on RCN transformation projects including the redevelopment of the RCN website and the Professional Development Framework project.

Carol has been involved in the project group developing the RCN 'Working Well Initiative'. This aims to improve the health and well being of nurses as well as the environment in which they work. Campaign work includes violence to nurses, latex allergy and mental health and employment. In addition, she is the RCN Adviser to the RCN Society of Occupational Health Nursing, and the Federation of Occupational Health Nurses in the European Union (UK) Group.

Carole Johnson MCSP SRP Cert Ed
Former Chairman of National Back Exchange (1999 – 2004). Carol currently works as a freelance Back Care Adviser and is commissioned to provide training, audit, legal reports, analysis and solutions for simple and complex situations with children, young people and adults with disabilities within the community. Carol has spoken at seminars arranged by the Department of Health, National Audit Office, the Disabled Living Foundation and National Back Exchange and teaches on the Post Graduate Certificate Diploma Course for Back Care Advisers at Loughborough University.

Contributing authors

Michael Adams BSc PhD
Dr Michael Adams is a Senior Research Fellow in the Department of Anatomy at Bristol University. He is the author of approximately 90 research publications, most of which concern the mechanical properties of cadaveric spines and of articular cartilage, and the mechanisms of intervertebral disc degeneration. He is on the Editorial Boards of Spine and Clinical Biomechanics.

Pat Alexander MSc LPD PGCE MCSP MIOSH
Pat Alexander works as a Consultant Back Care Adviser, as well as teaching on several post and undergraduate courses. She is co-author of the 4th edition of the Guide to the Handling of Patients (1997/8), Evidence based patient handling (2003), Guidance in Manual Handling for Chartered Physiotherapists (2002) and contributor to the IPC. She has researched issues from manual handling in the community, the risks of neuro physiotherapy and the delegation of physiotherapy programmes to others. As an expert witness Pat has provided reports for the claimant, the defendant and the HSE.

Mike Betts LPD RGN
Mike Betts is Back Care Adviser for the Luton & Dunstable Hospital NHS Trust. He has held this post for 4 and a half years. Prior to this he was the Back Care Adviser for Greenwich Healthcare NHS Trust. Mike is currently studying for an MSc in Back Care Management at Loughborough University.

Patricia Dolan BSc PhD
Patricia Dolan is a Senior Lecturer in the Department of Anatomy at Bristol University. Following a doctorate in muscle physiology, and subsequent specialisation in spine biomechanics, her current research interests include the quantification of muscle forces acting on the musculoskeletal system and spine muscle dysfunction. She is on the Editorial Boards of European Spine Journal, Journal of Electromyography and Kinesiology, and Clinical Biomechanics.

Emma Crumpton MSc (Ergs) BSc MCSP
Freelance ergonomist.
(See above).

Mike Fray BSc (Hons) BHSc MCSP SRP
Mike Fray is Director of Handling Movement and Ergonomics Ltd. Mike has worked in the fields of ergonomics, rehabilitation and manual handling for 17 years and he is currently a Director of Handling, Movement and Ergonomics Ltd. He was co-author of Evidenced-based Patient Handling and the Derbyshire Inter Agency Group – A Code of Practice for children and adults and has published papers and presented at conferences. Through HME Ltd he is involved in giving advice and training services to healthcare, social care and educational providers and is the course tutor for the Postgraduate Programme in Back Care Management at Loughborough University offering certificate, diploma and Master's degree courses.

Jacqueline Hall MSc (Health Ergs) Msc (Health & Social Research)
Cert in Patient Handling & Moving NMA (Advanced)
NEBOSH Cert RNT RGN Cert Ed NNEB
Jacqui Hall is a Senior Lecturer and National Course Leader for the Diploma in Patient Handling, based at the University of Northumbria at Newcastle. She is a Registered Nurse who has specialised in this field following completion of research in Lifting with Learners, which was the area under investigation for her Masters Degree in Health and Social Research. Recently, she completed another research project for a further Master's Degree in Health Ergonomics at Surrey University, where her focus was on patient transfers between Paramedics and Accident and Emergency staff.

Sue Hignett PhD MSc MCSP MErgS EurErg
Dr Sue Hignett has worked in the healthcare industry for 20 years, with the last 10 years in Ergonomics. She is the Director of the Hospital Ergonomics and Patient Safety Unit (HEPSU), Dept of Human Sciences, Loughborough University, which currently holds research grants with NHS Estates, the Engineering and Physical Sciences Research Council and the Dept. of Health. Dr Hignett is the chair of the International Ergonomics Association Technical Committee on Hospital Ergonomics and co-chair of the European Panel on Patient Handling Ergonomics (EPPHE).

Carole Johnson MCSP SRP Cert Ed
Manual Handling Consultant
(See above).

Philippa Leggett MSc (Ergs) Dip Biomech PGC (MH) MCSP SRP
Philippa Leggett is a Freelance Manual Handling Consultant working from the North of England, where the majority of her work is in community care provision. She is a visiting lecturer in biomechanics and muscle mechanics for manual handling, nursing and physiotherapy courses at Northumbria University, and a member of the CSP external advisory panel on manual handling.

Michael Mandelstam
Michael Mandelstam worked at the Disabled Living Foundation, a national voluntary organisation, before moving to the Social Services Inspectorate at the Department of Health. Subsequent to this he has worked independently providing legal training and advice to local authorities, the NHS and voluntary organisations throughout the country. He has written a number of books on community care and related matters, including Manual Handling in Health and Social Care: an A to Z of law and practice (2002), and most recently Community Care Practice and the Law (3rd edition, February 2005).

Stephen May MA MCSP Dip MDT MSc
Stephen May qualified as a physiotherapist in 1990, and worked for many years in a musculoskeletal outpatient setting in primary care in the NHS. He completed an MSc in Health Services Research and Technology Assessment in 1998. He is the co-author, with Robin McKenzie, of The Human Extremities: Mechanical Diagnosis and Therapy (2000), and The Lumbar Spine: Mechanical Diagnosis and Therapy (2nd edition, 2003), and of several journal publications. In 2002 he become a Senior Lecturer in Physiotherapy at Sheffield Hallam University, Sheffield, UK.

Claire Mowbray LPD RGN
Claire Mowbray is a Back Care Specialist Nurse, Chiltern and South Bucks NHS Primary Care Trust. She has held this post for over ten years and covers acute, mental health, learning disabilities and primary care trusts. Claire is currently studying for an MSc in Back Care Management at Loughborough University.

Sheenagh Orchard RGN RNT CertEd (FE) DipNurs (Lond)
Sheenagh is currently an Independent Training Consultant and Trainer in the field of Manual Handling and Risk Assessment. Sheenagh works in all areas of the health care sector supporting staff in developing safe handling strategies and problem solving complex handling needs using Risk Assessment and evidence base as the framework.

In addition Sheenagh runs specialist moving and handling workshops, assists in the development of training resource materials, speaks at conferences and is an active member of the National Back Exchange, currently as chair of her local group and as Vice Chair of National Executive 1998 – 2001.

Christine Pennington BA (Hons) MSc
After graduating in 1986 with a first class BA (Hons) in Psychology and Statistics Christine Pennington spent several years undertaking social policy evaluations in the civil service and 'not for profit' sector before joining the NHS in 1994 as a research and development adviser and co-ordinator. During her time in the NHS she completed the Office for Public Management course 'Moving Up in the NHS'.

Since 1999 Christine has run a management consultancy, Rowanmast Ltd, providing project management and research expertise to the NHS and the Department of Health. Her recent MSc in Statistics and Management Science was awarded a distinction.

Howard Richmond
Deputy Director of Legal Services, Royal College of Nursing
Howard Richmond qualified as a solicitor in 1978. He has worked with the Legal Services Department of the RCN since September 1988 and became Deputy Director in November 1989. Howard has conducted many personal injury claims on behalf of RCN members, including significant manual handling cases.

Howard is a legal adviser to the RCN Advisory Panel on Back Pain in Nursing and in that capacity was involved in drafting the Codes of Practice for Manual Handling issued by the RCN in 1992, 1993, and 1996. He also contributed the chapters on legal professional matters in the 1992, 3rd edition and the 1997/8, 4th edition of The Guide to the Handling of Patients.

Sue Ruszala MSc MCSP Dip TP SRP
Manual Handling and Ergonomics Adviser, United Bristol Healthcare Trust
Sue Ruszala has 20 years experience with manual handling risk management in health and social care. She has contributed to working groups with the Health & Safety Advisory Committee, Chartered Society of Physiotherapy and Royal College of Nursing; and is a co-author for the systematic research review Evidence-based Patient Handling (Hignett et al, 2003) and The Guide to the Handling of Patients/People (1998/2005).

Sara Thomas Dip COT PGD SROT
Sara is an independent Occupational Therapy Consultant and freelance Back Care Adviser. Prior to this she was the Senior Movement Protocol Specialist for Corpus UK (The Ergonomics Division of Arjo). During 2003 to 2004 she was the Regional Officer (West) for the National Back Exchange. Sara has been involved with Occupational Back Care issues since 1994 when she was employed by Swansea County Council as a specialist risk assessor for home care until 1996 when she was employed by Neath and Port Talbot Social Services as a Back Care Adviser.

External reviewers

Ian Clancy Dip COT
Manual Handling Adviser(Community), Calderdale & Huddersfield NHS Trust

Christopher Donnison BA (Hons)
Solicitor, Douglas-Mann & Co

Alison Griffiths MSc, Dip COT
Occupational Therapist

Simon Love BA MCSP SRP
Manual Handling Consultant, LPS Training and Consultancy Ltd

Emily Millar RGN BSc (Hons) Dip Patient Handling and Moving PGCPSEd
Back Care Adviser, Homefirst Community Trust

Linda Rankin RGN BSc (Hons) Dip Patient Moving and Handling Teaching Cert
Back Care Adviser, Homefirst Community Trust

Glyn Smyth MSc MErgS MCSP SRP
Director, Work Fit Occupational Physiotherapy and Ergonomics Ltd

Jan Spencer DipCOT MSc
Manual Handling Adviser, Calderdale and Huddersfield NHS Trust

Elisabeth Thompson RGN DTSN BSc (Hons)
Manual Handling Adviser

Sara Wainman MA DipCOT PGCH SCE
Freelance Manual Handling Trainer

Sally Williams MRCVS
NBE Ambassador, formerly of HSE Health Services Unit

Members of the National Back Exchange evidence review panels

Review panel chairman
Carole Johnson

Data collection
Pat Alexander MSc LPD PGCE MCSP MIOSH
Philippa Leggett MSc (Ergs) Dip Biomech PGC (MH) MCSP SRP
Saintelia Douglas BA (Hons) Education Cert Ed FAETC RGN
Mary-Jayne Bosley RGN Cert Ed (F.E.)
Melanie Sturman RGN
Tina Ridgeway BA (OU) RTN RGN
Lesley Wonnacott RGN DipN BSc (Hons) LPD (Back Care Management)
Heather Collins BA (Hons) DipCOT

Data analysis
Emma Crumpton MSc (Ergs) BSc MCSP

Data recording
Mandy Clift
Sara Thomas

Administrative support
Pat Lee and **Sarah Meade**
of the National Back Exchange Administration Office

Editor's assistant

Pam Ball

Contents

Note

Throughout this text we have used the generic term "handler", to delineate the person encouraging, guiding, assisting or carrying out a handling task, and the term "person" to delineate the person who is being encouraged, guided, assisted or moved. The only exceptions are where a sentence is clearly referring to a patient or client in the context of the sentence or where it is a quote from an earlier reference source.

We have tried to avoid gender specific pronouns, except where such use has improved the clarity of the sentence or quote.

Disclaimer

The risks associated with lifting and handling tasks are complex and each situation must be judged on its own merits and it is unreasonable for readers simply to follow any aspects of the contents in the book without undertaking an adequate risk assessement which takes full account of individual circumstances.

The authors, the editor, editorial committee, collaborators and the publisher cannot accept responsibility for any consequences which might result from decisions made upon the basis of the advice given herein.

Introduction

by Jacqui Smith

This definitive text book is intended for all staff working in health and social care in the public and private sectors who may be involved directly or indirectly with the moving and handling of people. This includes line managers, budget holders, those who make decisions about meeting needs in social services, occupational health and safety staff and those involved in, and responsible for, devising, implementing and monitoring policy and safer systems of work that impinge on manual handling practice.

Importantly, this book is also intended for those people with health problems and disabilities, including children, and also family members/informal carers, who may need temporary or long term assistance with care, mobility or movement which involves manual handling, and who are affected by manual handling decisions – which will be most of us at some time in our lives.

It is also intended as a resource for back care advisers, manual handling trainers, including NVQ trainers, and the educators, in universities, of those working towards professional qualifications in health and social care. Manual handling, and manual handling decision making, are just as much core skills for healthcare professionals as any other area of their clinical practice, and as such, manual handling falls within professional practice guidelines for competence and safety.

No doubt this book will also be relied on by the legal profession and expert witnesses involved in person handling related personal injury litigation, as has each of the previous editions.

This edition is the fifth in a series of guides, the first four of which were produced in formal collaboration between BackCare (formerly the National Back Pain Association) and the Royal College of Nursing. In this new fifth edition, that collaboration has been extended to include the National Back Exchange. The publication is also supported by the joint Department of Health, and Health and Safety Executive 'Back in Work' initiative and sponsored by the Department of Health and by Arjo.

The first edition of this guide was published in 1981 and was aimed at nurse managers who were seen as potential agents for change in response to growing concerns about the prevalence of low back pain and injury in nurses. The thrust of the book related to prevention strategies including ergonomics, safety training, pre-employment medical screening and the management of back pain at work through early access to occupational health services and physiotherapy treatment. Interestingly, in the preface, the then President of the Royal College of Nursing, Marian Morgan, called for the nursing needs of every patient to be regularly assessed, that there should always be adequate numbers of nursing staff by day and by night, and that any special equipment identified during the assessment should be provided in ready to use condition. Sadly, the response to that publication by NHS employers was limited and involved mainly the provision of training of limited duration, variable content and usually on an ad hoc basis. It is also notable that, more than 25 years after it was first 'condemned', the controversial and hazardous Drag lift continues in custom and practice use in many settings and takes up much more copy and discussion in this edition than in the first.

Nevertheless, change did occur, albeit slowly, and the second and third editions each set updated standards in manual handling practice. Each was considered in turn to be a gold standard text and, on reflection, provide a historical record of 'where we were then' and of recommended good practice at the relevant time. Since its inception, the RCN Back Pain Panel has played a significant role in the drive to combat work related injuries in nurses. In 1988, of the Back Exchange, which became the National Back Exchange in 1994, and which provides a national forum for the exchange of information on back care to support all healthcare professionals who are working to reduce the high prevalence of occupational back pain in the health and social care sectors, has become an increasingly recognised and effective agent for change at national and at local level.

On 1 January 1993 a raft of new legislation was implemented, including the Management of Health and Safety at Work Regulations, which required that formal risk assessments should be undertaken by employers as part of their risk management systems. The requirement, in the Manual Handling Operations Regulations 1992, to avoid hazardous manual handling operations where reasonably practicable and assess those risks that could not, reasonably practicably be avoided did not immediately have a great impact on health and social care providers although they were welcomed, perhaps over optimistically, by those of us working in the field of person handling and injury prevention at that time.

The RCN took the professional lead in recognising the implications of the Regulations and load guidance for the 'lifting' of patients and set down the benchmark that no two nurses should lift a patient weighing more than 8 stones, even in ideal conditions, the natural conclusion being that the lifting of patients would have to cease altogether. Their revised Code of Practice for Patient Handling, produced in 1996, states *"manual handling may continue provided that it does not involve lifting most or all of the patient's weight"*.

However, it could be suggested that many individuals and organisations misinterpreted the extent of the requirement to avoid the manual handling of people, which led to increasingly prescriptive and proscriptive approaches to manual handling practice and the implementation of blanket 'no lifting' policies which failed to take adequate account of the social, care and handling needs of disabled people or of the full range of legislation impacting on manual handling decisions. A heated debate ensued between and within the healthcare professions and many conferences, presentations and papers discussed the issues of care 'versus' rehabilitation, and the apparent conflicts between manual handling legislation and the then 'new' Human Rights Act (1998). In 2002 the Chartered Society of Physiotherapy made its position clear in its Guidance in Manual Handling for Chartered Physiotherapists by stating that *"it is not always reasonably practicable to avoid manual handling in physiotherapy without abandoning the goal of patient rehabilitation"*. Similar ethics might be said to apply to meeting the social and care needs of disabled people and patients.

At the beginning of 2003, the High Court attempted to reconcile health and safety legislation with Human Rights and Community Care legislation in the landmark 'East Sussex' case by, in summary, enjoining the parties to adopt a balanced approach in which the family were to be fully involved in the risk assessment and decision making process. Those working in the health and social care sectors will recognise that the continuing high prevalence of musculoskeletal disorders in health and social care workers arises not from situations in which in depth manual handling risk assessments take account of both the person's and the handlers' needs, but rather, from the ongoing failure by many employers to implement safer systems of work which include adequate staffing, equipment, training, supervision, risk assessment, care planning, monitoring and review.

What is new about this 5th edition?

It is now seven years since the publication of the revised fourth edition of this guide and much has changed within healthcare and in the community. The relevant health and safety legislation has been variously updated, amended, extended and interpreted, and Human Rights legislation has focused attention back onto the needs of the disabled person – which is why we joined the care professions in the first place. Manual handling practice has also moved on as back care professionals have come together to develop and agree core principles for safer handling practice. In addition there is now a much greater range and availability of affordable manual handling aids and equipment.

This new edition is significantly extended and revised in both structure and content, particularly in the practical chapters. One major change is in the title with the use of the word 'people' instead of patient to acknowledge that the need for assistance with movement occurs in many settings. This is reinforced with the inclusion of an extensive new chapter on manual handling in social care. Also included is a very extensive chapter on the theory, practice and 'art' of risk assessment and risk management which takes full account of the 'human' aspects which are so often ignored.

Throughout all of the chapters herein the authors have quoted research evidence where it is available and this is also the case in practical chapters, the format for which is described in chapter 11. In addition to the work of the individual authors, most of the tasks described in each practical chapter were analysed by an evidence review panel consisting of volunteer members on the National Back Exchange, and the results of their work are set out at the end of each task. This is important because, as indicated above, this book is not intended to be prescriptive. A careful review of the evidence recorded will allow practitioners to make informed decisions relevant to a particular set of circumstances. There will inevitably be some differences between the approaches taken by trainers/practitioners/handlers to the tasks in these chapters. Some of these variations may be more, or less, hazardous to the handler or more, or less, comfortable for the person, or require more, or less, skill. It will however, be relatively simple in future for evidence to be gathered in relation to these alternatives and compared to that in this book. It is also the case that the particular prevailing circumstances, and the nature of the person, must be the key influence on the choice of method. It will not always be possible, or even desirable, to adopt a particular method for carrying out a task even though 'on paper' it might appear to be of a lower order of risk.

Readers must therefore be very clear that a review of a technique in this book, and consideration of the accompanying evidence, does not constitute a risk assessment, although certainly the information provided herein is a relevant factor to consider. The authors hope that the content of this edition will encourage practitioners to critically appraise and develop their own practice within a safer systems framework. In the absence of a systems approach, safer handling practice will not flourish.

Acknowledgements

I would like to express my personal thanks to the editorial committee, the contributing authors, external reviewers and others who have offered me wise counsel during the production of this 5th edition.

1 Legal and professional responsibilities

Howard Richmond
Deputy Director of Legal Services, Royal College of Nursing

1 Introduction

The law as it relates to the moving and handling of people has two obvious objectives; injury prevention and compensation for the injured handler. However, in a wider sense this law also operates in the context of meeting people's health and social care needs and of observing their human rights.

It therefore provides a framework within which "balanced decision making", as discussed further in chapter 2, can be developed. By such means it is possible to minimise, though never completely eliminate, both the risk of injuries to employees/practitioners and patients/ clients, and also the expense and management time involved in dealing with compensation claims. At the same time, it allows people's needs to be met and human rights to be respected. Indeed one can go further and say that "balanced practice" informed by compliance with the law set out in this chapter and in chapter 2 is essential if employers stand a chance of resisting litigation (whether related to personal injury, or to the meeting of health and social care needs or to human rights) – and of satisfying their insurers as well as the regulatory authorities.

Accident prevention is regulated by statute, principally in the form of the *Health and Safety at Work, Etc. Act, 1974 (HSWA 74)*, but also by various regulations, or Statutory Instruments, made under the authority of that Act. The term "Statute" includes primary legislation, Acts of Parliament, and delegated legislation, and regulations in the form of Statutory Instruments

Compensation for injury to the handler for accidents taking place on or before 31 December 1992, was only provided for by the common law, that is, law contained in previous decisions of the courts which assume the force of binding or persuasive precedent. For incidents taking place on or after 1 January 1993, various sets of regulations made under the authority of the HSWA 74 implementing the requirements set out in European Directives, principally the Manual Handling Operations Regulations (MHOR) 1992 became relevant both to the regulatory and the compensatory aspects of moving and handling.

2 Accident prevention by statute

Section 2(1), HSWA 74 imposes a duty on every employer:

... to ensure, so far as is reasonably practicable, the health, safety and welfare at work of all his employees.

The scope of the this general duty is further defined in section 2(2) of the *Health and Safety at Work, Etc. Act, 1974 HMSO* to include in particular, but only so far as is reasonably practicable:

- **a** The provision and maintenance of plant and work systems, that are safe and without health risks
- **b** Arrangements for ensuring safety and absence of health risks in the use, handling, storage and transport of articles and substances
- **c** Provision of information, instruction, training and supervision necessary to ensure health and safety
- **d** Maintenance of any place of work under the employer's control, and all means of access and egress from it in a condition that is safe and without health risks
- **e** Provision and maintenance of a working environment that is safe and without risks to health and adequate as regards facilities and arrangements for welfare at work.

Reasonably practicable

With regard to moving and handling of people, the most relevant requirements are contained in paragraphs:

- **a** plant and work systems, and
- **c** instruction and training

The employer's duty is not an absolute one. It is qualified by the important words "so far as is reasonably practicable".

An employer needs to comply with this duty only if the cost of providing, say, equipment or training is not grossly disproportionate to the benefit. Were the benefit to be minimal and the cost substantial, an employer might be relieved of complying with the duty (Edwards -*v*- National Coal Board)

Under Section 7, HSWA 74 the employee is under a corresponding duty to take reasonable care for his or her own health and safety and the health and safety of other people who may be affected by his or her acts or omissions, and to cooperate with the employer in performing the duties under the Act.

Where it is reasonably practicable to comply with one of these duties and the employer fails to do so, enforcement action can be taken by the Health and Safety Executive (HSE). HSE inspectors have a right of entry to conduct inspections and a power to serve Improvement Notices specifying particulars of the breach of health and safety law which has been contravened and specifying a time within which the breach should be remedied.

An example might be to require provision of suitable patient handling equipment in an orthopaedic ward with heavy, highly dependent patients, where there is no hoist available.

An HSE inspector has the additional power to serve a Prohibition Notice preventing activities being carried out if there is a risk of serious personal injury.

Failure to comply with improvement or prohibition notices, or commission of a breach of the general duties in Section 2(2)(a)-(e) in, or any regulations made under HSWA 74, can give rise to a criminal prosecution under the *Health and Safety at Work, Etc. Act, 1974 HMSO*.

On conviction:

- in the Crown Court the maximum penalties in the most serious cases are two years' imprisonment and an unlimited fine.

- in the Magistrates' Court, where most cases are heard, the maximum fine is £20,000, and where the conviction relates to failure to comply with prohibition or improvement notices, up to six months' imprisonment.

Corporate liability

Where an offence is committed by a corporate body (e.g. Limited Company or NHS Trust), senior managers or directors can also be made individually liable where the offence was committed with the consent or connivance of that manager or is attributable to that manager's neglect. Fines in excess of £100,000 have now become relatively commonplace in Health and Safety cases, and legal and management costs can easily exceed the amount of the fine.

3 Acccident prevention by regulation and guidance

As has already been mentioned the HSWA 74 is a general enabling Act which allows the Secretary of State to make regulations and the Health and Safety Commission (HSC) to issue codes of practice and guidance notes.

The Manual Handling Operations Regulations 1992, as amended by the Health and Safety Miscellaneous Amendments Regulations 2002, (MHOR) 1992 govern the moving and handling of people in the workplace.

The Management of Health and Safety at Work Regulations (MHSWR) 1999, the Provision and Use of Work Equipment Regulations (PUWER) 1992, the Workplace (Health, Safety and Welfare) Regulations (W(HSW)R) 1992 and the Lifting Operations and Lifting Equipment Regulations (LOLER) 1998 can also be relevant.

The purpose of these regulations is to translate into domestic law the UK's obligations under various European Community directives relevant to health and safety law. These directives are discussed more fully later in this chapter under the heading The 1992 European Directives.

As with accident prevention by statute, a breach of any provision in these regulations can ultimately lead to a prosecution being brought by the HSE.

Regulation 3(1) of the MHSWR 99 requires employers to make a suitable and sufficient assessment of all the risks to the health and safety of their employees while at work. When this general assessment indicates the possibility of risks to employees from the manual handling of loads, the provisions of regulation 4 of the MHOR 92 come into play.

Under regulation 4 the employer is required to follow a three stage procedure:

- first, to avoid manual handling operations involving a risk of injury (as identified in a general risk assessment carried out under the MHSWR), so far as is reasonably practicable;
- second, where hazardous manual handling operations cannot with reasonable practicability be avoided, to assess them, taking into account the task, the load, the working environment, and the individual capabilities of the handlers
- third, on the basis of the information supplied by the assessment, the employer must reduce the risk of injury to the lowest level that is reasonably practicable.

The assessment must be kept up to date, and the employee must be given a general indication of, where reasonably practicable, precise information on, the weight of the load. In most cases the cost of providing a reasonably up to date weight should not be grossly disproportionate. The assessment should be recorded and readily available.

The Manual Handling Operations Regulations 1992: HSE Guidance on the Regulations L23

The MHOR 92 are accompanied by HSE Guidance on the Regulations L23 which does not itself have the force of law. HSE inspectors can take it into account when considering whether there is compliance with the regulations. It is also of some persuasive value in civil claims, although judges may not necessarily follow what it says, since the wording of the regulations, and their interpretation in case law, take precedence. Guidance L23 was updated in *1998* and again, very recently, on 31 March 2004.

The Management of Health and Safety at Work Regulations 1999: code of practice.

The MHSWR 99 are accompanied by an Approved Code of Practice (ACoP) L21 which was revised in 2000. In any prosecution where it is proved that there has been a failure to observe a relevant provision in an ACoP, the defendant must show that the regulations are satisfied in some way other than by observing the ACoP.

Guidance on manual handling

The Health Services Advisory Committee to the Health and Safety Commission originally published guidance, "The Lifting of Patients in the Health Services", in 1984 and this was updated in its Guidance on Manual Handling of Loads in the Health Services 1992 and again in 1998.

This guidance can be taken into account by a court but only as assistance in considering whether there is evidence of a breach.

A suitable analogy might be with the Highway Code. A breach of the Highway Code might be evidence of an offence under the Road Traffic Acts or of negligence in civil law, but not conclusively.

There is also guidance of an unofficial nature; this volume itself, for instance; or the *Code of Practice for the Handling of Patients*, first issued by the Royal College of Nursing in *1982*, updated in *March 1993*, and then in *April 1996*.

The status of these documents is that of expert opinion albeit of a collective nature. Such opinion may be persuasive in that it represents the consensus of foremost experts in the field and, in the case of the Code of Practice, endorsed by the leading professional nursing organisation in the UK. However, such opinion is no more than potentially persuasive on any issue until accepted by a court, and it would be open to any defendant in court proceedings to bring expert evidence to seek to prove that the relevant regulations have been complied with in some other way.

These documents are not admissible in court proceedings on their own; they have to be drawn on and supported by an expert witness in each case, a point discussed in more detail in the following section on compensation.

4 Compensation for the injured handler

The employer's responsibility:
Section 47 HSWA 74 states that breach of the general duties in Section 2(2)(a)-(e) HSWA 74 does not give rise to civil liability, that is, that breach of these general duties does not entitle an employee to compensation for an injury alleged to have been caused by a person handling accident. However, this is a distinction without a difference in practice, since the common law places equivalent duties on the employer to take reasonable care for the safety of the employees and to carry out operations so as not to subject employees to unnecessary risk. This is a personal responsibility that cannot be delegated.

The modern authority for the employer's duty is set out in a House of Lords case called *Wilsons and Clyde Coal Limited -v- English 1938* AC 57 which requires that all employers provide and maintain, so far as is reasonable:

a a safe place of work with safe means of access and egress;
b safe appliances, equipment, and plant for doing work;
c a safe system for doing work;
d competent and safety conscious personnel.

This is an example of the Common Law in action. Well before Parliament had got around to legislating on health and safety the judges perceived an injustice and created a remedy by applying the general duty of care not to harm ones neighbour, as declared in the very first negligence case of *Donoghue -v- Stevenson 1932* AC 532 (the "snail in the ginger beer bottle" case), to the workplace.

In addition to the fourfold duty under the Clyde Coal case, the employer is responsible for negligence of the employees even if the employer is not at fault. This is known as vicarious liability, a legal principle that often causes confusion to lay people. It is discussed further, under Problem Areas, later in this chapter.

Claims for compensation for injury arising from patient handling accidents under the Common Law, are most often pursued on the basis of the employer's failure to provide a safe system of work, although a failure to provide equipment, a safe place of work, or competent fellow personnel can also be factors. The claimant has to prove that the employer has breached the duty in one of the above respects, and that this breach of duty caused the injury.

Each case is argued on its particular merits and expert evidence is required to prove what reasonably safe system of work could have avoided the accident and in what respects the employer fell short of that duty in the particular case before the court.

Previous editions of The Handling of Patients assisted courts to decide on the standard to be attained. For instance, in the case of *Edwards -v- Waltham Forest Health Authority (1989)* Mr. Justice Potts stated:

> "I have reached the conclusion that the standards set out in page 5 of The Handling of Patients, A Guide for Nurse Managers, and the measures to be adopted on bath transfers as described at page 35 (which provides that lifting a patient manually out of a bath should only be necessary in an emergency if a patient is taken ill or helpless and under no other circumstances) were well known in the nursing profession in April 1982. I am also satisfied upon the evidence that I have heard that those standards and measures were entirely proper and were the standards and measures that could and should have been adopted by all competent employers for their employees. I have to say that I am surprised that in this case, on the evidence, no responsible person at (the) hospital seems to have applied his or her mind to what is set out in this volume, and in particular to those parts mentioned".

It should not be assumed that The Handling of Patients sets the standard to be achieved in all circumstances. Although it embodies the opinion of several foremost experts in the field, its application to the facts of any particular case must be proved by an expert witness; a defendant could bring other experts to argue that in any particular set of circumstances the advice given was not appropriate or reasonable.

The very first court decision in a patient handling claim known to the author is that of

Williams -v- Gwent Health Authority (1982) where the defendant was held to be liable for having an unsafe system of work in allowing the drag lift to be used. Subsequent to that decision, and prior to the implementation of the MHOR 92 on 1 January 1993 claimants have recovered compensation where unsafe systems were found to be in place in the use of the orthodox lift *(Moore -v- Norfolk Health Authority – 1982)*, in respect of falling patients *(Bayley -v- Bloomsbury Health Authority – 1987)* in respect of a district nurse lifting a patient on her own *(Hammond -v- Cornwall and Isles of Scilly Health Authority – 1986)*, and in respect of the use of the Australian lift on a heavy patient where a hoist should have been used *(Munro -v- Plymouth Health Authority – 1991)*.

Further a health authority was found to be vicariously liable for the negligence of a co-lifter who failed to lift on the count of three, injuring the lifter taking the lead *(Page -v- Enfield and Haringey Health Authority – 1985)*.

Courts refused, however, to find breach of duty on the grounds of staff shortages alone *(Stewart -v- Highland Health Board – 1987)*.

Civil liability

As has been said at the start of this section on compensation, breach of the general duties in Section 2(2)(a)-(e) HSWA 74 does not give rise to civil liability. However, breaches of provisions in regulations made under HSWA 74 can give rise to civil liability for what is called breach of statutory duty, unless the regulations provide otherwise.

Regulation15 of the MHSWR 1999 (an updated and consolidated version of the original 1992 Regulations) originally stated that a breach of the duty imposed by those regulations did not confer a right of any action in any civil proceedings. However by virtue of Regulation 6 of *The Management of Health and Safety at Work and Fire Precautions (Workplace) (Amendment) Regulations 2003*, this bar was removed as from 27th October 2003. Accordingly, for accidents arising on or after that date, injured employees can now cite allegations of failures to comply with the MHSWR99 in compensation claims. This amendment was brought in belatedly out of concern that the original MHSWR 1992 did not comply with European Directives. The Health and Safety Commission suggests that there will be only a small increase in the number of civil claims for compensation as a result of this change, but that remains to be seen.

There never has been any such exclusion in the MHOR 92. This has meant that ever since implementation on 1st January 1993 any breach of any duty in regulation 4 setting out the assessment procedure can be invoked in a civil claim.

Regulation 4(1) (a) poses two questions that the employer must answer to determine whether it is under a duty to comply with the further duties in Regulation 4(1)(b)(i), (assessment), and 4(1)(b)(ii), (risk reduction). Firstly is there a risk of injury? and secondly, if so, is it reasonably practicable to avoid the manual handling operation? The answer to the first of these two questions about the risk of injury may already have been answered, at least in part, in carrying out the general assessment of all workplace risks under Regulation 3(1) of the MHSWR 99 referred to above. This is certainly the approach envisaged in paragraph 41 of the Guidance L23. The question is, in applying the Risk Assessment "Filter" set out in Appendix 3 referred to in paragraph 41 of the Guidance L23, how likely must that risk of injury be? The position has been clarified by the Court of Appeal in the case of *Koonjul v Thameslink Healthcare Services NHS Trust (2000).*

The claimant in that case was a care assistant working for the Trust at a residential home for children with special needs. She was making a bed designed for children suffering from conditions such as epilepsy. The bed was only 18 inches high and was pushed against the wall. In order to make the bed the claimant had to pull it away from the wall and it was while bending down to do this that she injured her back. The Court of Appeal held in answer to the first question in Regulation 4(1) (a) ("...is there a risk of injury?") that there was indeed a real risk of a foreseeable possibility of injury. The Court of Appeal went on to hold that, in applying Regulation 4, it was necessary to look at the particular manual handling operation in context. In this case the context was that of an everyday task which the claimant had been carrying out for a long time. She had also attended a moving and handling course and been trained how to bend down. Taking into account this particular context the Court answered the second question in 4(1)(a) ("... is it reasonably practicable to avoid the manual handling operation?") by holding that it was not reasonably practicable for the employer to avoid having low beds pushed against the wall because of the possibility of the children falling out. Further that, even if it had been possible to avoid that risk, it would not have been reasonably practicable for there to have been a precise assessment of the level of risk in carrying out each task, with a warning as to how that task should be carried out.

The very first application and interpretation of duties in Regulation 4(1)(b)(i), (assessment), and 4(1)(b)(ii), (risk reduction) was in the earlier Court of Appeal case of *Hawkes v London Borough of Southwark (1998).* The claimant Hawkes was an experienced carpenter who had worked for the defendant borough for many years and was used to working on his own. He had been asked by his supervisor to install doors in a block of flats. The doors were both large and heavy. The stairs were steep and narrow and there was no lift. The supervisor had himself installed the a same type of door in similar blocks of flats. The evidence at trial was that neither the claimant nor the supervisor had thought it to be a two man job, but that even if they had, there was no evidence that the help of a second man would have been found. In carrying a door up the stairs, the claimant fell and was injured. Although the defendant did not know about the MHOR 92 it denied that the task was one which carried a risk of injury.

The Court of Appeal here held that Regulation 4 applied, and that if a proper risk assessment had been carried out the clear conclusion would have been that this was a two man job. The evidence from Hawke's supervisor was that if he had carried out a risk assessment he would still have found the job to be a one man job. The County Court judge had accepted this argument, but the Court of Appeal considered that this hypothetical assessment made after the event would not have been "suitable and sufficient" in the words of Regulation 4(1)(b)(i). The defendants were liable because they had not reduced the risk to the lowest level practicable by employing a second man. There was no basis for contributory negligence on the part of the claimant because even if he had asked for help he would not, on the evidence, have received it. The Court of Appeal also confirmed that the definition of the words 'reasonably practicable' was as had been explained by *Asquith LJ in Edwards v National Coal Board (1949).*

Wells v West Hertfordshire Health Authority & Anor – High Court (2000) is a good example of a manual handling case in the healthcare context. Here the claimant was a midwife who suffered an exacerbation of a pre-existing back problem caused, she said, by her work in the delivery suite at the first defendant's hospital. The Judge accepted the claimant's evidence that she had informed her line managers that she had a history of back trouble, and that they should have referred her to occupational health for assessment. Because of this the judge held: that there was a foreseeable risk of injury to the claimant; that the defendants had breached their duty of care to the claimant by requiring her to work in the delivery suite in light of their knowledge of her back problems; and that they had failed to discharge their obligations under reg.4(1)(a) and 4(1)(b)(i) MHOR 92 by failing to assess the tasks involved in the delivery suite, and in particular the claimant's ability to perform them given her medical condition.

The case of Knott -*v*- Newham Healthcare NHS Trust [2002] EWHC 1992 is significant from the legal point of view on several counts, although tragically for the claimant who ended up very seriously injured. The claimant slipped slightly when getting out of the bath. The next day she awoke with severe back pain and was diagnosed as having suffered serious damage to intervertebral discs and neural damage. In other words, the onset of back pain did not occur after a particular incident at work .For just over two years prior to this incident the claimant had been working for the defendant Trust first, as a staff nurse, and then, as junior sister on an acute medical ward, where she cared for highly dependent patients. The judge accepted the claimant's evidence that there was only one hoist for use in two wards, and that this one hoist often did not work. Because of the lack of mechanical assistance the claimant would regularly use the drag lift to move heavy patients. The judge accepted expert evidence that the drag lift was an inherently unsafe method that carried with it a real risk of injury, as readers of previous editions of The Handling of Patients will know. Further, that the Defendant Trust, by requiring the claimant to carry out the lifting of patients without any of the appropriate equipment, assistance and training had, in breach of Reg.4 MHOR 92 operated an inadequate system for manually handling patients in that no real steps were taken to reduce the risk of injury to its employees to the lowest level reasonably practicable

Proving the injury

As well as proving the breach of duty itself, the claimant has to prove, with the assistance of expert medical evidence, that the breach of duty either caused, or materially contributed to, the injury sustained. Where there is only a single cause of the claimant's injury the so called "but for test" is applied; the question put to the medical experts is "... but for the breach of duty on the part of the defendant, would the claimant, on the balance of probabilities have suffered the injury?" Where there is more than one possible cause of an injury the question for the medical expert is".. did the breach of duty amount, on the balance of probabilities, to a material contribution to the injury?", "material" in this context meaning "more than negligible". The answers to these questions in the case of musculoskeletal injuries are by no means straight forward, for example, patient handlers can often be shown to have vulnerable backs, either resulting from naturally occurring degenerative changes, or from previous back injuries, or from the effects of cumulative strain from exposure to postural stresses and regular heavy lifting/handling. It can be a very difficult task to separate out the degree to which each of these factors contributes to the final onset of back pain, particularly in the absence of a specific identifiable accident. This is why it is difficult to obtain the evidence necessary to pursue a claim based on cumulative strain alone. In most cases one is considering the injury caused by a particular handling incident and the effect that incident may have in aggravating and/or accelerating existing injury, albeit symptom free, until that incident occurred.

Most people show signs of degenerative change in the spine, especially towards their middle years. There is no proven connection between the appearance of signs of degenerative change, and symptoms of pain. Consultants tend to rely upon their clinical experience and can come to greatly differing opinions as to the extent to which an accident has accelerated symptoms, say by two years as against 20 years in any one case. At the end of the period of acceleration the effects of the accident cease, so compensation for loss of past and future earnings, indeed all the considerations that influence the amount of compensation, crucially depend on the length of the period of acceleration. For example in the case of *Wells v West Hertfordshire Health Authority & Anor – High Court (2000)* referred to in the section above the judge found, on the basis of the medical evidence, that the claimant would, in any event, have suffered similar back symptoms within a period of two to three years of the incident. An award of £5,000 was made for the acceleration of pain, suffering and loss of amenity for two to three years, together with a further amount for loss of earnings and expenses for a period of two years.

These difficulties can further be illustrated by the case of *Knott -v- Newham NHS Trust [2002] EWHC 1992*, also referred to in the section above where, to repeat, onset of back pain first occurred when the claimant slipped slightly when getting out of the bath. Her pain was so serious that she had to have two operations despite which she was still left with considerable pain and discomfort, sleeping difficulties and an inability to have children. The defendant's medical evidence was that the claimant had exaggerated the amount of lifting she was required to do, and that her disc protrusion occurred spontaneously when she slipped getting out of the bath due to the natural progression of long standing degenerative disc disease. In stark contrast to this the claimant's medical experts considered that the natural degenerative deterioration of the claimant's lumbar spine was advanced by the process of lifting during her employment with the defendant ("cumulative strain" if you will) thereby increasing the likelihood of a disc protrusion and consequent neural damage. The judge was more convinced by the expert evidence advanced on behalf of the claimant and held that the defendants' breach of duty both in negligence, and under the MHOR92, caused or, materially contributed to the claimant's injury. That particular aspect of the judge's decision survived an appeal to the Court of Appeal.

There is no easy answer to these conflicts of medical evidence, although the fact that statistically the incidence of back pain peaks between the ages of 45 and 50 can provide good arguments against short acceleration periods in the case of younger claimants. For example, there would have to be fairly convincing evidence in support of a two year as against a 20 year acceleration period for a 25 year old claimant. These conflicts cause difficulties for all concerned, including the courts. The problem is caused by a lack of scientific knowledge. In the end it depends on what medical evidence the judge trying the case finds more convincing. In this respect the *Knott* case was decided on its own particular facts and should not be treated as a general precedent indicating that "cumulative strain" cases are necessarily any easier to win than they were before.

Another concept, which can cause confusion in personal injury claims, is that of "functional overlay", that is, exaggerated or inappropriate responses to injury. Functional overlay can be diagnosed by specific tests, which can be made while the person is being examined, and which are mainly intended to avoid unnecessary surgery. However, as long as the pain is shown to be genuine, even if overlaid by the claimant's over-sensitive personality or response to pain, compensation should not be affected.

The legal principle is that a defendant "must take a victim as it finds him (or her)", even if the claimant has an unduly vulnerable personality which the defendant did not know about or foresee. The House of Lords, in the case of Page -v- Smith (1995) held that a defendant is legally responsible as long as it could be reasonably foreseen that the conduct would expose the claimant to the risk of personal injury of some kind, whether physical or psychological. This principal was very usefully illustrated by the recent House of Lords case of *Christopher Simmons -v- British Steel PLC 2002 [2004] UKHL 20*. The claimant was awarded damages for physical injuries sustained in an accident at work. The way he had been treated caused him to be angry which itself caused an exacerbation of a pre-existing skin condition. The skin condition and the anger went on to cause a severe depression. Although the anger did not in itself attract compensation, because it was purely an emotional reaction and not a clinical condition, it provided a causal link between the original physical injury and the skin condition, and to the subsequent clinical condition of depression. Consequently the defendant was held liable to compensate the claimant for all these injuries both physical and psychological.

In many cases of soft tissue injury, no organic cause for pain can be discovered, even using up to date scanning techniques. There may be possible physical causes from scar tissue or changes in the nervous system causing chronic pain syndrome, which cannot be physically verified. Recent research by Matthew D. Lieberman Assistant Professor of Psychology at UCLA, has suggested that the brain registers physical and mental pain in much the same way [Science 10 October 2003] and that the way the brain feels pain is likely to be far more complicated than the traditional view that there is simply a direct causal link to tissue damage. Thus onward transmission of pain from the spinal cord is modified by impulses coming down from the brain, and culture, gender, beliefs about pain, and social context, can all modify how much pain a person feels [The Guardian Tuesday 14 October 2003] From the legal point of view, though, as long as the claimant's pain is considered to be genuine and caused, on the balance of probabilities, by the accident in question, the fact that it may be partly psychological in nature will not help the defendant.

The defendant will be relieved of legal responsibility only if it can be proved that the claimant is malingering, that is consciously inventing or exaggerating pain symptoms with a view to obtaining compensation. Such conduct is rare and is usually identified by covert video surveillance.

As a result of the interest generated by the case of *Walker -v- Northumberland County Council (1995)*, where a social worker recovered compensation for stress related illness caused by overwork, the door was opened to compensation claims for stress related illness alleged to have been caused by work. The HSE define "stress" as "the adverse reaction people have to excessive pressure or other types of demand placed on them". It emphasises that pressure in itself is not necessarily bad, since many people thrive on it, but that it is when pressure is experienced as excessive by an individual that ill health can result. In the case of *Sutherland -v- Hatton 2002* the Court of Appeal set out certain conditions, which had to be satisfied before a "stress" claim could succeed. These so called "propositions" only served to confirm that a claimant would find it very difficult to succeed with a "stress" claim. Those "propositions" have recently been approved by the House of Lords subject to minor amendments that slightly relax the criteria.

The relevance of stress here is that the heavy physical work involved in manual handling can be stressful, particularly where staffing levels are inadequate and the management approach required to comply with the MHOR 92 in not in place. Paragraph 14 of the *HSE Guidance on the Manual Handling Operations Regulations 1992 (as amended) L23* refers to the psychosocial risk factors relevant to the development of musculoskeletal injury such as "...high workloads, tight deadlines, and lack of control of the work and working methods". Even in the absence of specific injury the strong possibility of sustaining injury can itself be stressful.

A management response

Safer handling policies are suitable management responses to tackle manual handling related stress and ill-health, as well as reducing the incidence of musculoskeletal injury. Employers must identify any sources of occupational stress when making the risk assessment required by regulation 3 (1) of the MHSW 99, taking into account the HSE booklet *Tackling Stress at Work, a Guide for Employers (2001)*. The HSE are developing and piloting Managements Standards for tackling work related stress. Further up to date information can be found on the HSE website at www.hse.gov.uk/stress/manstandards.htm

Assessing damages and cash awards

Although the claimant in a civil claim has to prove negligence, by establishing on the balance of probabilities (i.e. more likely than not) that the breach of duty caused the injury, this is not an end in itself, it is only a means to an end – compensation. The aim of financial compensation is to put the claimant back into the position he or she would have been in if the accident had not happened. Where loss of earnings and extra expense are incurred, the arithmetic at least can be fairly straightforward. Lawyers call these items of financial loss "special damages".

Financial compensation for pain and suffering, restricted life style, or a destroyed career, whose path can only be guessed at, are more difficult and controversial. The trial judge has some discretion in assessing these so-called "general" damages within a framework of principles set down in previously decided cases. A good summary of the range of damages likely to be awarded for particular injuries is contained in the Guidelines for *The Assessment of General Damages in Personal Injury Cases* published by the Judicial Studies Board. Regularly updated, this slim paperback volume may be referred to in the courts and is useful to legal practitioners and lay people alike.

Awards for pain and suffering, and loss of amenity made by English courts are considered by many to be too low. Back injuries attract awards in the range of £1,000 to £20,000 in cases of injury categorised as minor or moderate. More severe cases where the victim suffers from continuing severe pain and discomfort, with aggravating features such as impaired sexual function, depression, and at the most serious end impotence or double incontinence, can merit awards from £20,000 up to about £87,500

However, where a handler's career is destroyed by the accident, awards can be greatly boosted by compensation for past and future loss of earnings. Angela Knott whose case has already been mentioned recovered a total of £420,000 [BBC News website at http://news.bbc.co.uk/1/hi/england/2333005.stm] The highest award made in a manual handling case known to the author is that of Karl Douglas who received an out of court settlement of £800,000 from Bexley and Greenwich Health Authority in 2000. [BBC News website at http://news.bbc.co.uk/1/hi/health/642381.stm] The legal costs associated with defending such claims can approach double the amount of the compensation paid.

In conclusion, although compensation claims are not intended to be punitive, the amounts that can be ordered to be paid are many times higher than any fines which might be levied under the HSWA 74, and in this regard compensation claims could be considered to have an indirect deterrent effect. The value of potential claims should therefore form part of the risk benefit calculation, which might lead employers to decide to allocate more resources to fulfil their duties under the MHOR 92.

Contributory negligence

Defendants routinely allege that claimants are partly to blame for their accidents; this is called contributory negligence. A finding of contributory negligence does not defeat the claim, but it does reduce the compensation. For example, a claimant found to be 25 per cent to blame would have the compensation reduced by 25 per cent. Experience shows that courts have been reluctant to make such findings in nurse patient handling cases.

Changes to Civil Litigation Procedures

Over the years there has been continuing concern about delays and cost in civil procedures, particularly personal injury claims. Lord Woolf's reports to the Lord Chancellor on the civil justice system in England and Wales, in June 1995 and July 1996, and implemented in the *Civil Procedure Rules 1998* brought about a revolution in civil procedures.

Of particular relevance to personal injury claims was the emphasis on greater court management of the proceedings by controlling the amount of legal work for which costs could be claimed so that it was proportional to the value or importance of the claim. There is an emphasis on the earliest possible disclosure of each party's case, initially in the form of a more detailed letter of claim and response thereto, and subject to the court so ordering, by requiring the exchange of all evidence to be disclosed before trial in the form of detailed witness statements and relevant documents. The purpose of this is that each party would know in detail the other parties' case at an earlier stage, whereas previously that would only be fully revealed at trial. This makes it easier for each party to decide whether to abandon, seek to settle, or fight a claim. For claims worth under £5,000 where the claim for damages for personal injury is at least £1,000 there is a fast track procedure with a date for trial being fixed at the outset, expert evidence being given on paper only, and fixed legal costs. Although these reforms may have shortened the time taken to conclude claims, they have not necessarily reduced and, indeed, may in some cases have increased costs.

The other significant change was to the funding of civil litigation. Under the *Access to Justice Act 1999* Legal Aid for personal injury claims was effectively abolished and replaced by Conditional Fee (or "no win no fee") Agreements. Solicitors are only paid their own charges if they win the case. If they lose they can only recover their disbursements (payments to third parties, for example to expert witnesses) from the client. To compensate solicitors for the risk of losing a proportion of their cases they can claim a success fee of up to 100% (but in practice somewhat less depending on the risk), from the losing Defendant who is usually an insurance company, or in the case of the National Health Service, the NHS Litigation Authority.

The effect of these changes to procedure and funding, while increasing access to the courts to claimants who would not have been eligible for legal aid or Trade Union assistance, has been to reduce the number of personal injury cases issued in the courts. Solicitors acting for claimants have every incentive to settle cases early and only to proceed to trial in cases that they are reasonably confident they will win.

Sick pay and other benefits

Although emphasis has been placed on compensation that can be recovered through bringing a civil action, it must be mentioned that compensation is available from other sources where an employee is incapable of working through sickness or accident. There may be an entitlement to sick pay from the employer, but only if this is provided for in the contract of employment. Employers also administer the Statutory Sick Pay ("SSP") Scheme, which provides benefits for the first 28 weeks of sickness. Incapacity Benefit may be available from the Department of Work and Pensions if there is no entitlement to SSP or the 28 week period has expired.

Industrial Injuries Disablement Benefit may also be available to those who have suffered disablement from a loss of physical or mental faculty caused by an industrial accident. However, benefit is only payable where the loss of faculty amounts to 14 per cent or more.

Of particular interest to National Health Service employees is the NHS Injury Benefits Scheme. Benefit is payable to all NHS employees, regardless of length of employment, who suffer an injury which can be shown to be wholly or mainly attributable to NHS employment. NHS Temporary Injury Allowance is for those absent temporarily through injury, and those whose employment is terminated. The aim is to compensate for reduction of earning ability caused by the injury and, depending on length of service and degree of reduction in earning ability, benefits can be awarded up to a maximum of 85 per cent of pre-injury pay, together with entitlement to a lump sum on termination of employment. Where compensation is recovered in a civil action, NHS Injury Benefit payments have to be repaid or adjusted. In this respect they can be considered to be payments on account of compensation although no fault need be proved. Although "no fault" eligibility for NHS Injury Benefit does, as has been said, require medical evidence that the injury is "wholly or mainly attributable" to NHS employment, the legal principles relating to causation discussed further above apply, and if benefit is initially refused, a three stage appeal procedure is available giving an opportunity for further and more detailed medical evidence and legal argument to be submitted.

The Compensation Recovery Unit of the Department of Work and Pensions requires repayment of certain social security benefits paid as a result of an accident, injury or disease where a compensation payment has been made. The duty to make that payment falls on the defendant/compensator who may reduce the amount of the damages by the amount of benefit the person has already received.

The scheme also covers the recovery of costs incurred by NHS hospitals for treatment of injuries from road traffic accidents.

5 Disability Discrimination Act 1995

To qualify as disabled under the *Disability Discrimination Act 1995* ("DDA 95"), a person must have a physical or mental impairment which adversely affects their ability to carry out normal day to day activities, and the adverse effect must be both substantial and long term. An adverse effect is long term if it has lasted, or is likely to *last*, at least 12 months, or, is likely to last for the rest of the life of the person that is affected. Express provision is made in the Act for recurring or fluctuating conditions. The DDA 95 applies to a person who had but no longer has a disability, as otherwise defined in the Act.

Many, if not most, persons suffering from chronic back pain should qualify as "disabled "for the purposes of the DDA 95. For instance in the case of *Law Hospital NHS Trust v Elizabeth Rush 8/2/2000* the applicant had been employed as a staff nurse by the respondent NHS Trust between 1976 and 1999. Following her dismissal it was denied by the respondent NHS Trust that she had been treated unfairly or discriminated against on grounds of disability.

The applicant had suffered a number of difficulties in her day-to-day activities due to back pain but was able to continue working. The Employment Appeal Tribunal confirmed, on an appeal from an Employment Tribunal on a preliminary issue, that the applicant was disabled because her impairment did have substantial adverse effects, and that the fact that she managed to continue in her job did not necessarily mean that she had no physical impairment.

It is also unlawful for an employer to discriminate against a disabled person in recruitment. More importantly, there is a duty on an employer to make reasonable adjustments to working arrangements that have an impact on disabled employees. Examples of steps that an employer may have to take include transferring a person to fill an existing vacancy, altering working hours, allowing an employee to be absent during working hours for rehabilitation assessment or treatment, and acquiring or modifying equipment. An employee who is dismissed as unfit for work as a result of back pain may have a case for unfair dismissal where the employer fails to consider adequately or at all what reasonable adjustments can be made to enable the employee to continue working.

6 Employment

An employee owes a duty to the employer to obey reasonable and lawful instructions and to act with reasonable care and skill. Thus a failure to perform as trained or instructed could render the employee liable to disciplinary proceedings and ultimately to dismissal. However, it is only a refusal to obey an employer's lawful instructions that can amount to misconduct leading to dismissal, for either refusal by an employee to do something which would be a breach of health and safety regulations, or a refusal to cooperate in the employer's breach, cannot amount to conduct that would justify dismissal.

Where the employer has complied fully with the health and safety obligations there are specific duties amplifying the general duty under Section 7 HSWA 74 under which the employee is under a duty to take reasonable care for his or her own health and safety, and for the health and safety of those who may be affected by his or her acts or omissions. In the context of moving and handling this applies both to the patient, and to fellow members of staff.

Regulation 1 of the MHSWR 99 requires an employee to use all work equipment and safety devices provided by the employer in accordance with the training and instruction which the employer is obliged to provide.

In relation to moving and handling, Regulation 5 of MHOR 92 obliges each employee, while at work, to make full and proper use of any system of work provided for the employee's use by the employer in complying with the duty to reduce the risk of injury to employees to the lowest level reasonably practicable, and where it is not reasonably practicable to avoid manual handling operations altogether.

This duty on the employee is an absolute duty. If injured, the employee would face a reduction in the compensation as a consequence of his or her contributory negligence to the extent that a court would consider just and equitable having regard to the employer's share in the responsibility for the damage. Further, such an employee's breach of the employer's instructions and procedures for safer handling could result in disciplinary proceedings.

Where the employer has complied with the obligations under the MHOR 92, there should be no problem for the employee. The problem arises when the employer has not complied with these obligations and the employee has to cope. Is the employee entitled to refuse to lift or handle in such circumstances? One can argue that an instruction to lift or handle in circumstances likely to cause injury where it is reasonably practicable to avoid that risk altogether, is an unlawful instruction entitling the employee to refuse. It is a brave employee who courts disciplinary proceedings, and proceedings in the industrial tribunal following dismissal, even if he or she is ultimately successful. Compensation is no substitute for a job. In any case, where patient well being is at stake, the transition to a safer handling policy has to be planned using the framework of law which puts obligations on employees and also provides them with some degree of protection.

Paragraph 49 of the revised 2004 guidance note L23 to the MHOR92 indicates that an assessment made at the last minute is unlikely to be "suitable and sufficient" as required by the regulations. Employers are asked, in consultation with employees, to use their experiences of the type of work being done, particularly in dealing with emergencies.

Where there is a lack of any proper system for implementing the MHOR 92 any request by an employer to carry out a manual handling task which carries the possible risk of injury could be said to the be "last minute" it could be argued that a request to carry out a manual handling task in such circumstances is an unlawful instruction.

There is a duty on all employees under Regulation 12 (2) MHSWR 99 to inform the employer of any work situation the employee reasonably considers to represent either a serious and immediate danger to health and safety, or a shortcoming in the employer's health and safety arrangements, as long as that situation arises out of that employee's own activity, and has not been previously reported to the employer. This is an absolute duty. Every employee should therefore be advised to remind his or her line manager if there is no safer handling policy in operation.

While not suggesting that the implementation of this absolute duty by the employee would bring sanctions from the employer, the employee has protection under Section 44 Employment Rights Act 1996. These provisions give employees the right not to suffer any detriment, which could be a failure to investigate safety concerns reported by that employee if a failure to do so impinged upon that employee, or be dismissed.

The protection is in the first instance granted to health and safety representatives, safety committee members, or other employees carrying out statutory or agreed health and safety functions. The protection is granted to employees where either there is no safety representative or safety committee, or it was not reasonably practicable to raise the concerns through such channels, and the employee used reasonable means to draw attention to work circumstances which the employee reasonably believed were harmful or potentially harmful to health and safety.

There are further rights granted to employees where they reasonably believe themselves to be in serious and imminent danger. In such circumstances the employee has a right to leave the work place or to take appropriate steps to protect him or herself. Such circumstances are rare in the context of handling.

An example known to the author from a personal communication is one in which staff on a ward refused, despite pressure from managers, to lift back into bed a 22 stone patient who had fallen on the floor. The staff summoned the manual handling assessor who called the fire brigade. It took eight firemen to move the patient back to bed safely. It is strongly arguable that the nurses were in serious and imminent danger and took appropriate steps to protect themselves by calling the fire brigade.

The Public Interest Disclosure Act 1998, which came in to force on 2 July 1999, gives protection to employees who make disclosures about health and safety and other matters of concern in the work place. The protections in Section 44 *Employment Rights Act 1996* for employees not to suffer detriment are also extended to the employee who makes disclosures, but only if made in compliance with the requirements of the Public Interest Disclosure Act 1998. This does not give the potential whistle blower licence to go straight to the media. Disclosures are only protected if made to the employer, a legal adviser and/or other prescribed bodies, including the Health and Safety Executive, as set out in the Public Interest Disclosure (Prescribed Persons) Order 1999 [SI 1999 No.1549]. http://www.hmso.gov.uk/si/si1999/19991549.htm

7 Human Rights Act 1998

The Human Rights Act 1998 (HRA 98), which came fully into force on 2 October 2000, incorporates into UK law most of the rights set out in the *European Convention on Human Rights (1950 as amended)*. Most relevant to health and personal injury law are

- Right to life (Article 2)
- Prohibition of torture, inhuman or degrading treatment or punishment (Article 3)
- Right to a fair trial (Article 6)
- Right to respect for private and family life (Article 8)

The UK has been a signatory to the European Convention for over 50 years but, prior to 2 October 2000, those who believed their rights have been violated had to take their case all the way to the European Court in Strasbourg. Those rights are now directly enforceable in UK Courts and tribunals are required to take account of the HRA '98 and to ensure that the development of the common law is compatible with the Convention rights taking into account previous European Court decisions. Already a significant body of "home grown" human rights case law has developed

All those involved in managing health and safety, particularly in the person handling field need to know about the case of R -*v*- (1) *East Sussex County Council ("ESCC")* (2) The Disability Rights Commission (Interested Party), ex parte A, B (by their litigation friend the Official Solicitor) X, Y [2003] EWHC 167 (Admin) (the "X,Y case") where the High Court, on an Application for Judicial Review, set out guidance on the principles to be considered by local authorities when drawing up policies on the manual lifting and moving by care workers of disabled people. The implications are considered further in chapter 2. Here the facts of the case and the decision are summarised.

A and B were two sisters in their twenties who suffered from profound physical and learning disabilities. They were looked after at home, which had been specially adapted and equipped for them, by their mother X, and stepfather Y. A and B suffered from greatly impaired mobility such that every movement, for instance getting out of bed and into a bath, required them to be lifted and moved by their carers. X and Y wanted A and B to be moved and lifted manually in many circumstances where the ESCC and the carers wished to use appropriate equipment for health and safety reasons. The High Court was asked by X and Y, with A and B being represented by the Official Solicitor, to consider whether ESCC's policy of not permitting carers to lift A and B manually was lawful taking in to consideration the MHOR92, and human rights and European law.

The judge stressed that he was only making findings concerned with the looking after of disabled persons in their own homes and in doing so held: that it was not reasonably practical to avoid manual handling of A and B altogether; that a manual handling policy that imposed a blanket proscription on all manual lifting, save in serious emergency, was likely to be unlawful; that the rights to human dignity and physical and psychological integrity derived form Articles 3 and 8 of the European Convention on Human rights required exceptional manual methods to be used where there is prolonged resistance or great and obvious distress. The judge did not criticise RCN Guidance but did observe that, as it focused primarily on nurses in hospitals, it was not relevant or safe in the context of this case. The judge also conceded that he was not qualified to carry out the assessment task himself, citing the Handling of Patients 4th edition as an indication of the expertise and competence required and emphasised that in striking the very difficult balance between the needs of A and B and the safety of the carers, the ESCC with expert assistance was the primary decision maker.

Another important case which, while not invoking human rights law, seeks somewhat to qualify the rights of the manual handler is Sussex *Ambulance NHS Trust v King [2002]* EWCA Civ 953 ("the Sussex Ambulance case"). Here the Court of Appeal held that the ambulance service owed a duty of care to patients, as well as to its employees, and that it was not liable for injuries sustained by an employee while carrying a patient using a hazardous method where, as the evidence was in this case, there was no practical alternative way of removing the patient from his home.

The claimant was injured in the course of his employment when, as one of a two man ambulance team, he answered a call to collect an elderly patient from his home and take him to hospital. The call was urgent, requiring a response within an hour, but was not an emergency. The two ambulance men were carrying the patient in a carry chair from an upstairs bedroom down a narrow and steep stairway with a bend in it. The other ambulance man lost his grip for a moment such that the claimant was left to bear its whole weight of the chair and patient for a brief moment, and as a result suffered injury. The claimant won his personal injury claim before the county court judge, who found that the employer was in breach of duty by failing to train its employees to give serious consideration to the alternative of using the fire brigade and by treating this option very much as one of last resort. The Court of Appeal was not convinced that calling the fire brigade would have been an appropriate measure, and that the Claimant had failed to show that his injuries would probably have been avoided by giving the fire brigade alternative more emphasis in training or more consideration on the day. More importantly, it held that, as well as owing the claimant the usual employer's duty of care under the common law rules of negligence, it also owed a duty of care to the members of the public who had called for assistance. In other words, the respective risks to the employee, and to the member of the public, had to be carefully balanced. In this case there was no evidence of anything that the employer could have done to prevent the risk to the claimant. In a private communication to the author it has been pointed out that there are now carry chairs on the market with built in stair climbers, which may well have provided a reasonably practicable alternative to the fire brigade option, and which could have reduced the risk of injury in this and similar cases. The Sussex Ambulance case lies behind the comments in paragraphs 32, 33 and 54 of the Revised HSE Guidance on the MHOR 92 (as amended) L23 Third Edition 2004. Paragraph 33 comments that the level of risk that an employer may ask an employee to accept may be higher when considering the health and safety of those in danger, although not to the extent of exposing employees to unacceptable risk of injury.

8 Professional conduct

Some professional people involved in moving and handling are subject to codes of conduct. Nurses are registered with, and accountable by statute to, the Nursing and Midwifery Council ("NMC"), formerly the United Kingdom Central Council for Nursing, Midwifery, and Health Visiting ("UKCC"). A nurse who refused to carry out what she considered was an unsafe lift was referred to the UKCC Professional Conduct Committee, but was found not guilty of professional misconduct defined as "conduct unbefitting a registered nurse" *(UKCC -v- Lalis Lillian Grant (Nursing Standard 18/2/89)**.

The UKCC, the predecessor to the NMC indicated that it would always look at any cases of refusal to lift on an individual basis, and stressed the importance of recording the reasons for making that decision. Although the most important consideration must be the patient's safety and well-being, this must not be at the expense of the nurse's health and safety. In most circumstances of this kind, it would be unlikely for the Professional Conduct Committee to find against a nurse (Nursing Times 10 April 1996, page 29).

Paragraph 1.5 of the Code of Professional Conduct published by the Nursing and Midwifery Council in April 2002 and which came into effect on 1 June 2002 provides that all nurses on the register must adhere to the laws of the country in which they are practising. It is therefore conceivable that a senior nurse with responsibility for standards of safety regarding moving and handling could be accountable to the nursing professional body as well as to the court. If a registered nurse was referred to the NMC for refusing to lift, a Professional Conduct Committee would now would take into account the developments in case law, in particular the Sussex Ambulance and A,B,X,Y cases, and the text of the new Code of Professional Conduct. However the balance to be struck is unlikely to be much differently expressed to that in the paragraph immediately above.

9 The European Directives

Important changes in health and safety law were originally brought about as a result of the completion of the single market in the then European Community now the European Union ("EU") on 31 December 1992.

The aim of the legislation was to harmonise health and safety standards throughout the EC so that undertakings operating in a country which might otherwise have lower health and safety standards, and consequently lower costs, do not have an unfair competitive advantage. This process is described in the jargon of bureaucracy as the creation of a "level playing field".

Authority for the legislation arises principally from Article 118a of the Treaty of Rome 1957 (amended by the Single European Act, 1987), which has the objective of harmonising health and safety standards in the EC and encouraging and maintaining improvements in those standards. Article 100a, which aims to remove technical barriers to trade, is also relevant.

The main instrument by which these aims are translated into domestic law is through the directive. A directive places obligations on a member state as to the result to be achieved by domestic legislation, but leaves open to each state the form and method of implementation as long as this is done within a stated time limit.

Regarding moving and handling, the relevant Directives are:

- *the Council Directive of 12 June 1989 (89/391/EEC)* on the introduction of measures to encourage improvements in the safety and health of workers at work, the so-called "Framework Directive" implemented by the MHSW 99, and
- the Council Directive of 29 May 1990 (90/269/EEC) on the minimum health and safety requirements for the manual handling of loads where there is a risk particularly of back injury to

workers the Manual Handling of Loads Directive implemented by the MHO Regulations 92.

10 Equipment

With increased use of equipment and other aids, it is appropriate to mention the employer's duties as regards work equipment. The common law duty and the general duty under the Health and Safety at Work Act are similar, namely, to provide and maintain work equipment in so far as is reasonably practicable. The employer can seek to ensure proper maintenance of and training for the use of equipment, but may not be able to avoid a hidden defect in its manufacture.

However, where an employee sustains personal injury because of a defect in equipment provided by the employer, and the defect is the fault of another party, for example, the manufacturer or maintenance contractor, the injury is still deemed to be attributable to the fault of the employer *(Employers Liability (Defective Equipment) Act, 1969)*. This means that the employer cannot defend a claim of negligence even though entirely blameless. The employer may have a claim against the third party, be it manufacturer or contractor, but is still primarily responsible for compensating the injured employee if the third party is proved or admitted to be negligent.

Alternatively, the injured employee may be able to claim compensation under Part I of the *Consumer Protection Act, 1987*. A product is defective if the safety of the product is "not such as persons generally are entitled to expect". There is an advantage here in that fault need not be shown. However, the employee can only claim against the employer if the manufacturer cannot be identified.

Work equipment is now regulated under the *Provision and Use of Work Equipment Regulations 1992 (PUWE Regulations 92)* which implement a EU directive of 30 November 1989 concerning the minimal health and safety requirements for the use of work equipment by workers (89/655/EEC).

The regulations came into force on 1 January 1993 for all work equipment first provided after 1 January 1993 and for all work equipment, whenever provided, by 1 January 1997. The duty falling on the employer, which is an absolute duty, is to ensure that work equipment is so constructed or adapted as to be suitable for the purpose for which it is used.

An employee bringing a claim for injury caused by using unsuitable work equipment will be able to rely on this strict duty. Work equipment must not only be suitable when first introduced, but must be maintained in an efficient state, in efficient working order, and in good repair. Paragraph 70 of the guidance note to this regulation emphasises that "efficient" relates to how the condition of the equipment might affect health and safety and is not concerned with productivity. The absolute duty to maintain is linked to a duty to keep any maintenance log up to date.

There are also absolute duties to provide employees with adequate health and safety information, and where appropriate, written instructions. Those instructions should include any foreseeable abnormal situation and any conclusions to be drawn from experience in using the equipment. For example, any problems in using a hoist should be noted in writing by some means attached to the hoist.

Every employer is under an absolute duty to ensure that all persons who use work equipment have received adequate training for the purposes of health and safety, including any risks that may be entailed in using it, and the precautions to be taken. Breach of any or all of these duties can be invoked where injury is the consequence.

The employer is also under a duty to consult with safety representatives in good time concerning the introduction of new technologies into the work place. This would apply to much of the equipment involved in safer patient handling.

The Lifting Operations and Lifting Equipment Regulations (LOLER) 1998 [SI 1998 No. 2307] imposed further very detailed duties on employers from 5th December 1998.

- First there are requirements to ensure strength and stability of lifting equipment, and specifically as regards person lifting equipment, to ensure that a person using it will not be crushed, trapped, struck, or fall from it.

- Second, there is a requirement to ensure that lifting equipment is positioned or installed in such a way as to reduce to as low as is reasonably practicable the risk of the lifting equipment or a load striking a person and that it is otherwise safe.

- Third, employers must ensure that machinery and accessories for lifting loads are clearly marked to indicate their safe working loads, and that lifting equipment that is designed for lifting persons is appropriately and clearly marked to this effect.

- Fourth, the employer must ensure that every lifting operation involving lifting equipment is properly planned by a competent person; appropriately supervised; and carried out in a safe manner.

- Fifth, employers must ensure that before lifting equipment is put into service for the first time it is thoroughly examined for any defect unless it has not been used before and has an EU declaration of conformity, and that where the safety of lifting equipment depends on the installation conditions, it is thoroughly examined before being put into service for the first time or before being put into service at a new location to ensure that it has been installed correctly and is safe to operate.

- Sixth, that any lifting equipment or accessory for lifting persons which is exposed to conditions causing deterioration liable to result in dangerous situations is thoroughly examined by a competent person every 6 months (or less, as imposed by the competent person) to ensure that health and safety conditions are maintained and that any deterioration can be detected and remedied in good time. Lifting equipment not falling into the above category must be examined at least every 12 months by a competent person who will specify when the next thorough examination is to be carried out. The person making that thorough examination must notify the employer forthwith of any defect in the lifting equipment which in his opinion is or could become a danger to persons; and, as soon as is practicable thereafter make a report of that thorough examination in writing to the employer, and to any person from whom the lifting equipment has been hired or leased. Where there is in his opinion a defect in the lifting equipment involving an existing or imminent risk of serious personal injury that person must also, as soon as is practicable, send a copy of the report to the relevant enforcing authority.

These are detailed obligations, which in most cases are absolute duties, that is, those to which there is no defence in the event of a breach. Employees, or, for that matter patients injured by hoists that are defective, or improperly serviced or used will probably find an allegation to back their claim somewhere among these regulations.

11 The work place

Emphasis on the suitable equipment required to introduce a safer patient handling policy should not detract from the importance of a safer work place. Schedule 1, paragraph 3 to the MHOR92 concerning the factors to which the employer must have regard, and the questions which must be considered in carrying out manual handling assessments, emphasises the importance of the working environment.

The *Workplace (Health, Safety and Welfare) Regulations 1992* (W(HSWR)) 1992 came into full effect on 1 January 1996 after three years during which they applied only to new, extended or modified work places. There are provisions requiring:

- adequate ventilation (Regulation 6) a reasonable temperature (at least 16 degrees Centigrade) with sufficient thermometers to monitor it (Regulation 7)
- suitable and sufficient lighting (Regulation 8)
- every room must have sufficient floor area, height and space for the purposes of health and safety (Regulation 10)
- workstations (which arguably can include beds) should be arranged so that they are at a suitable height and can be reached without undue bending or stretching (Regulation 11).

Slipping and tripping accidents are a significant risk in the health services, second only to lifting accidents. In some lifting accidents there is an element of slipping. Under Regulation 12 W(HSW)R 92 relating to the condition of floors and traffic routes, there is an absolute duty from 1 January 1996 to ensure that every floor in a work place is suitable for its purpose, and in particular should have no hole, slope, or be uneven or slippery, so as to expose any person to a risk to their health and safety. Further, every floor shall be kept free from obstructions or any article or substance that may cause a person to slip, trip or fall.

This duty is subject to the qualification "so far as is reasonably practicable", so an employer can seek to defend a claim by arguing that the cost of complying with this duty was grossly disproportionate to the risk.

The EC directive giving rise to these regulations imposes a stricter duty. It remains to be seen whether the English courts will find that the stricter duty in the directive should be preferred to the qualified duty in the regulations. Precedent suggests that they will.

12 Problem areas

Concern is often expressed in two particular areas:

- the legal responsibilities of the handling trainer towards the student handler
- the duty of the employer where a member of the lifting team is not an employee but an agency worker who's training or competence is unknown

The legal responsibilities of the person handling trainer

The person handling trainer owes a duty to provide proper instruction and supervision to trainees, so far as is reasonable, and the more inexperienced the trainees, the greater is that duty. In the case of *Beattie -v- West Dorset Health Authority (1990)* the claimant was injured during a training session. She and a co-trainee, who was seven and a half inches taller than her, were practising the use of the Cradle or Orthodox lift. Another trainee weighing ten and a half stones acted as the patient. The court held that the trainer was negligent in pairing the plaintiff with a totally inexperienced and significantly taller partner without instructing that partner in how to compensate for the height difference, and in failing to intervene to prevent them from practising a hazardous lift.

Where the trainer is acting in the course of employment, the employer must meet any claim by providing legal representation, satisfying any court judgment, or paying any compensation which may be agreed between the parties. The employer's obligation stems from the doctrine of vicarious liability mentioned above. It applies regardless of whether the employer is negligent by, for instance, failing to train the trainer fully. The employee trainer is always wise to ensure that the precise scope of training duties is set out in writing in the contract of employment or job description.

The doctrine of vicarious liability applies only to events taking place in the course of employment and not to acts committed by employees who are, in the delightful phraseology used by the courts "off on a frolic of their own".

Where the handling trainer is not an employee but an independent contractor, the employer's duty to provide a safe system for training in the moving and handling of patients, so far as is reasonable, remains. The employer can delegate the performance of the duties to provide a safe system, but never the responsibility. The employer can discharge responsibility by taking reasonable care in the selection of independent contractors. In future, the scope of this duty may be significantly tightened by the impact of Article 5.2 of the Framework Directive which provides that where the employer enlists competent external services or persons to comply with the employer's obligations under the directive, this shall not "discharge him from his responsibilities in this area".

Agency workers

This leads to the situation of the agency worker contracted to form part of a moving and handling team. It is arguable that the employer must take reasonable steps to ensure that any outside contractor has been trained and assessed as competent in moving and handling patients, and that failure to do so is in breach of duty to the employees who may be injured as a result of that contractor's handling error. However, the combined effects of Articles 5.2 and 5.4 of the Framework Directive would suggest that employers might be legally responsible for the failures of outside contractors, regardless of fault, in most circumstances.

If the agency worker is injured, her position is at first sight less favourable than that of the employee. This is because the duties under Regulation 4 of the MHO Regulations are expressed as those of the employer towards the employee. Non-employees who are injured can invoke the general law of negligence, which in theory imposes duties less onerous than those imposed by the MHOR.

The courts have appreciated the trend towards self employment but will not allow that trend to assist employers in avoiding their health and safety obligations. In the case of a skilled person, the question is: whose business is it to be responsible for that person's health and safety – is the agency nurse carrying out her own business or that of the contractor? Agency nurses are indistinguishable from their full time employed colleagues, apart from being self employed for income tax purposes, being required, for instance, to observe ward routines and procedures. They are almost certain to be treated as employees and to be owed the duties under the MHO Regulations *(Lane -v-* Shire Roofing (Oxford) Ltd [1995]) IRLR).

Disclaimers

Occasionally health care providers attempt to limit their legal responsibilities for injury to their employees by the use of exclusion clauses or disclaimers. An example would be an attempt to relieve the employer or handing trainer from any responsibility for injury caused to the employee or another party by asking the employee to sign a disclaimer along the following lines:

At the conclusion of this training I was competent to handle manually as taught. Accordingly, I disclaim any responsibility on my place of work or trainer for any subsequent injury.

Where an employee might make a claim for personal injury despite having signed a disclaimer of this kind, the disclaimer would be rendered ineffective by Section 2 (1) of the Unfair Contract Terms Act 1977 which provides that a contract term or notice cannot restrict any person's legal responsibility for death or personal injury resulting from his or her negligence.

Where third parties may make a claim for personal injury against an employee who had signed a disclaimer, the employer is not relieved from the legal responsibility for the negligence of the employee, under the doctrine of vicarious liability. This means that the employer must meet any claim against an employee where that employee is acting in the course of employment, and this rule operates regardless of any fault on the part of the employer. An employer may also be legally responsible for the negligence of self employed persons acting under the employer's control. *The Employer's Liability (Compulsory Insurance) Act 1969* requires employers, with some exceptions, to take out insurance to cover claims by their own employees, and it is a criminal offence to fail to do so. The exceptions include public bodies such as NHS trusts and local authorities who will have sufficient resources to meet claims from their own funds.

More generally, English courts have always been reluctant to attach legal responsibility to authors whose negligent misstatements have allegedly caused loss to readers who have relied on them. To be able to sue for financial loss alleged to have been caused by wrong advice, a person has to show that the adviser knew that the advice would be relied upon, and that it was reasonable in all the circumstances to rely on such advice. Where there is a close relationship between the parties, and the recipient of the advice is an individual or a small identifiable group, for instance between an occupational health nurse as consultant and the nurses employed by a NHS trust, it is more likely that legal responsibility will arise. Any disclaimer of legal responsibility in a contract would not be effective unless it passed the "reasonableness" test in the Unfair Contract Terms Act 1977. In an ordinary contract for the supply of professional services it would be difficult to justify an exclusion of liability for negligence. Indemnity insurance for the self employed professional concerned is therefore a must.

References

Statutes

Access to Justice Act 1999 HMSO Website www.hmso.gov.uk/ acts/acts1999/19990022.htm#aofs
Consumer Protection Act, 1987 HMSO
Disability Discrimination Act 1995 HMSO Website www. legislation.hmso.gov .uk/acts/acts 1995/Ukpga_19950050_en_1.htm
Employer's Liability (Compulsory Insurance) Act 1969 HMSO
Employers Liability (Defective Equipment) Act, 1969 HMSO
Employment Rights Act 1996 HMSO Website www.hmso.gov.uk/ acts/acts1996/1996018.htm#aofs
Health and Safety at Work, Etc. Act, 1974 HMSO
Human Rights Act 1998 HMSO Website www.legislation.hmso.gov.uk/acts/a cts1998/19980042.htm
Treaty of Rome 1957 (amended by the Single European Act, 1987) Website europa.eu.int/abc/treaties_en.htm
Public Interest Disclosure Act 1998 HMSO Website www.legislation.hmso.gov.uk/acts/a cts1998/ 19980023.htm
Unfair Contract Terms Act 1977 HMSO

Regulations

Civil Procedure Rules 1998 (as amended)
Council Directive of 12 June 1989 (89/391/EEC) on the introduction of measures to encourage improvements in the safety and health of workers at work "the Framework Directive" europe.osha.eu.int/ legislation/directives/leg2.php3?cat_id=1.1&ctab=cat_a
Council Directive of 29 May 1990 (90/269/EEC) on the minimum health and safety requirements for the manual handling of loads where there is a risk particularly of back injury to workers "the Manual Handling of Loads Directive" europa.eu.int/smartapi/cgi/sga_doc?smartapi!celexapi!prod!CELEXnumdoc&lg=EN&numdoc=31990L0269&model=guichett
Council directive of 30 November 1989 concerning the minimal health and safety requirements for the use of work equipment by workers (89/655/EEC) http://europa.eu.int/ smartapi/cgi/sga_doc?smartapi!celexapi!prod!CELEXnumdoc&lg=EN&numdoc=31989L0654&model=guichett.
Health and Safety (Miscellaneous Amendments) Regulations 2002. [S.I.2002 No. 2174] www.hmso.gov.uk/si/si2002/20022174.htm
Lifting Operations and Lifting Equipment Regulations 1998. [S I

1998 No. 2307] www.legislation. hmso.gov.uk/si/si1998/19982307. htm.

Management of Health and Safety at Work Regulations 1999 [S.I.1999 No. 3242] www.legislation. hmso. gov.uk/si/si1999/19993242.htm

Management of Health and Safety at Work and Fire Precautions (Workplace) (Amendment) Regulations 2003 [S.I.2003 No. 2457] www.legislation.hmso.gov.uk/si/si2003/20032457.htm

Manual Handling Operations Regulations 1992 [S. I. 1992 No. 2793] www.legislation.hmso. gov.uk/si/si1992/Uksi_19922793_en_1.htm

Provision and Use of Work Equipment Regulations 1992 [S. I. 1992 No. 2932] www.legislation.hmso. gov.uk/si/si1992/Uksi_19922932_en_1.htm

Public Interest Disclosure (Prescribed Persons) Order 1999 [SI 1999 No.1549]. www.hmso.gov.uk/ si/si1999/19991549.htm

Workplace (Health, Safety and Welfare) Regulations 1992 [S. I. 1992 No.3004] www.legislation. hmso. gov.uk/si/si1992/Uksi_19923004_en_1.htm

Guidance

Code of Practice for the Handling of Patients, Royal College of Nursing , April 1996 www.rcn.org.uk/ publications/pdf/code-practice-patient-handling.pdf

Nursing and Midwifery Council Code of Professional Conduct April 2002 www.nmc-uk.org/nmc/main/ publications/codeOfProfessional Conduct.pdf

"Management of Health and Safety at Work". Management of Health and Safety at Work Regulations 1999 Approved Code of Practice L21 revised 2000

Health Services Advisory Committee to the Health and Safety Commission Guidance Manual Handling of Loads in the Health Services 1998

HSE booklet "Tackling Stress at Work, a Guide for Employers" (2001)

"Manual Handling" Manual Handling Operations Regulations (as amended) Guidance on Regulations L23 – Third Edition 2004

The Highway Code: www.highway code.gov.uk/00.shtml

Cases

Bayley -v- Bloomsbury Health Authority (1987) – Unreported

Beattie -v- West Dorset Health Authority (1990) – Unreported

Christopher Simmons -v- British Steel PLC [2004] UKHL 20 www. parliament.the-stationery-office. co.uk/ pa/ld200304/ldjudgmt/jd040429/simmon-1.htm

Donoghue -v- Stevenson [1932] AC 532 www.scottishlawreports. org.uk/resources/keycases/dvs/donoghue-v-stevenson-report.html

Edwards -v- National Coal Board [1949] All ER 743

Edwards -v- Waltham Forest Health Authority (1989) – Unreported

Hammond -v- Cornwall and Isles of Scilly Health Authority – Unreported

Hawkes -v- London Borough of Southwark [1998] EWCA Civ 310 www.bailii.org/cgi-bin/ markup. cgi? doc=/ew/cases/EWCA/Civ/1998/310.html.

Knott -v- Newham Healthcare NHS Trust [2002] EWHC 2002 www.bailii .org/cgi-bin/markup. cgi?doc=/ew/ cases/EWHC/QB/2002/2091.html

Knott -v- Newham Healthcare NHS Trust [2003] EWCA Civ 771 www. bailii.org/cgi-bin/markup.cgi?doc=/ ew/cases/EWCA/Civ/2003/771.html

Koonjul -v- Thameslink Healthcare Services NHS Trust [2000] PIQR

Law Hospital NHS Trust v Elizabeth Rush 8/2/2000 [2001] ScotCS 149

British and Irish Legal Information Institute www.bailii.org/cgi-bin/markup. cgi?doc=/scot/cases/ ScotCS/2001/149.html

Lane -v- Shire Roofing (Oxford) Ltd [1995] IRLR

Moore -v- Norfolk Health Authority – Unreported

Munro -v- Plymouth Health Authority – Unreported

Page -v- Enfield and Haringey Health Authority – Unreported

Page -v- Smith [1995] 2 All ER 736

Stewart -v- Highland Health Board (1987) – Unreported

Sussex Ambulance NHS Trust v King [2002] EWCA Civ 953 www. bailii. org/cgi-bin/markup.cgi? doc=/ew/ cases/EWCA/Civ/2002/953.html

Sutherland -v- Hatton [2002] EWCA Civ 76 www.bailii.org/ew/cases/ EWCA/Civ/2002/76.html

and Barber –v- Somerset County Council [2004] UKHL 13 www.bailii.org/cgi-bin/ markup.cgi?doc=/uk/cases/UKHL/2004/13.htm

R v (1) East Sussex County Council ("ESCC") (2) The Disability Rights Commission (Interested Party), ex parte A, B (by their litigation friend the Official Solicitor) X, Y [2003] EWHC 167 (Admin) www. bailii.org/cgi-bin/markup.cgi?doc=/ew/cases/EWHC/Admin/2003/167.html

United Kingdom Central Council for Nursing Midwifery & Health Visiting (UKCC) -v- Lalis Lillian Grant (Nursing Standard 18 February 1989)

Walker -v- Northumberland County Council [1995] All ER 737000

Williams -v- Gwent Health Authority (1982) – Unreported

Wilsons and Clyde Coal Limited -v- English [1938] AC 57

Wells -v- West Hertfordshire Health Authority & Anor – High Court (2000) – Unreported

Useful summaries of most of the cases shown above and marked as "Unreported" can be found in "Manual Handling in Health and Social Care – an A to Z of Law and Practice" Michael Mandelstam 2002.

Articles

"Aaarrgghhhh!" Luisa Dillner The Guardian October 14 2003 www.guardian.co.uk/health/story/0,,1062339,00.html

"Back pain nurse Angela Knott awarded £420,000". Wednesday, 16 October, 2002 [BBC News website at news.bbc.co.uk/1/hi/england/2333005.stm]

"Nurse Karl Douglas wins £800,000 for back injury". Tuesday, 15 February, 2000. [BBC News website at www. news.bbc.co.uk/1/hi/health/642381.stm]

Books

The Guidelines for the Assessment of General Damages in Personal Injury Cases 6th Edition Oxford University Press 2002 : ISBN 0-19-925795-7

Access to Justice Interim Report to the Lord Chancellor on the civil justice system in England and Wales Lord Woolfe June 1995 www.dca.gov.uk/ civil/interfr.htm

Access to Justice – Final Report Lord Woolfe July 1996 www.dca. gov.uk/civil/final/contents.htm

2

Manual handling in social care: law, practice and balanced decision making

Michael Mandelstam
Independent legal consultant and trainer

1 Introduction

This chapter focuses on the relevant law underlying decisions and practices relating to manual handling in social care, and to the work of local social services authorities and the care providers with whom those authorities contract [1].

This relevant legal framework is extensive and serves to emphasise that, legally, manual handling decisions taken by local authorities are about a great deal more than the *Manual Handling Operations Regulations 1992*, the avoidance of accidents to staff and personal injury litigation.

In order to make this framework accessible to the reader, the chapter is divided into various areas of law. Each area is broadly summarised and illustrated with everyday examples.

Balanced decision making

The overall theme of the chapter is the legal requirement on local authorities to achieve a measure of balanced decision-making in the context of manual handling. Essentially this means balancing the safety (and human rights) of paid staff with the assessed needs and human rights of service users.

At the beginning of 2003, the High Court attempted, in a lengthy and complex judgment, to reconcile health and safety at work legislation with community care legislation and human rights legislation. The judgment emphasised repeatedly the need to strike a balance, whilst recognising that this would not always be easy *(A&B, X&Y v East Sussex County Council)*.

The legal framework includes social services (community care and children's legislation), housing, human rights, disability discrimination, and health and safety work legislation – not to mention the law of negligence, contract law and regulatory legislation. This legislation, diverse in type and purpose, has to be welded together when local authority social service departments take decisions.

Achieving the type of balance referred to in the *East Sussex* case can be elusive. In practice, it would appear that staff frequently either put themselves, or are placed by their employer, at excessive and unnecessary risk. Alternatively they are directed to take such extreme precaution that the welfare of service users can suffer, their assessed needs may not be met – and sometimes their human rights may be breached. Either way the balance is not achieved; the court stated that neither disabled people's rights nor paid carer's rights should override the other.

The requirement of balanced decision making is one that both legally, and as good professional practice, applies not only to local social services authorities but also to the NHS – when it assessed need and delivers services under the NHS Act 1977 and is similarly subject to human rights, disability discrimination, and health and safety at work legislation.

Conflicts of view

Sometimes local authority staff and managers feel that it is all very well for the courts to talk about balanced decision-making, but that everyday reality gets in the way. Clearly, there will from time to time be tensions involving the needs and rights of service users, and the safety of staff.

Some of these tensions may be difficult or on occasion impossible to resolve fully. Equally however, manual handling advisers frequently point out that with sufficient expertise devoted to assessment, the delivery of services and to negotiation, many apparently intractable problems can be overcome.

Example: hoist breakdown and human rights

When hoists break down in people's homes, staff within one particular local authority are anxious because they feel there is a potential conflict between their own safety and the human rights and assessed needs of service users. Under current arrangements, the repair or replacement time for malfunctioning or broken hoists can sometimes be as long as 48 hours or more. An apparent dilemma arises as to whether service users – who pose a high manual handling risk to staff – should be left in bed during this period, even if this would be to their significant detriment. Alternatively, should staff get them out of bed manually even high risk? The local authority finds a simple solution; it places a new contract for the repair of hoists that guarantees, in case of urgency, a four-hour response time.

Example: improving practice

A local authority recognises that balanced decision making requires competent risk assessment and risk management. In order to achieve this, it employs two manual handling advisers, puts in place enhanced basic training for its care staff, provides specialist training for its occupational therapists, and imposes more demanding contractual conditions on independent care providers to ensure the competence of their staff.

---

1 The term local authority (or local social services authority) is used throughout for the sake of brevity. However, unless otherwise stated, it should be understood to refer also to local authority social work departments in Scotland and to health and social services trusts in Northern Ireland.

Such possible tensions will be in evidence throughout the chapter. For example, in relation to direct payments and health and safety (section 2.8.1), taking reasonably practicable steps under health and safety at work legislation to safeguard employees' safety whilst still meeting the needs of service users (section 6.1.1), and conflicting risk assessments between assessors and providers (section 8).

2 Social services legislation

Logically community care legislation is the place to start because it is here that assessment of people's needs by local authorities begins. It is the community care legislation that brings a local authority into contact with an individual.

When local authority social services departments take decisions in respect of individual service users, those decisions are closely hedged around by community care legislation. This contrasts with comparable decision-making in the NHS, which is more loosely governed by legislation.

Duty of assessment

Under s.47 of the *NHS and Community Care Act 1990*, which applies to England and Wales, a person is entitled to an assessment of his or her needs, if it appears that he or she may be in need of community care services. Section 47 is largely concerned with adults. It is not an absolute duty but the courts have held that it is nevertheless a strong one[2].

In the case of a disabled person, the local authority must anyway make a decision about the person's needs under the terms of s.4 of the *Disabled Persons (Services, Consultation and Representation) Act 1986*. This decision in turn relates to services under s.2 of the *Chronically Sick and Disabled Persons Act 1970* (see below).

Having carried out an assessment, a local authority must then decide whether the person's assessed needs call for the provision of services by the authority. Not all needs will necessarily be judged to call for services; it is only assessed, so called 'eligible', needs that will trigger service provision. An eligible need is a need that is assessed to come above, rather than below, the threshold that local authorities set in order to determine eligibility for service provision.

Risks to independence

In England and Wales, guidance has been issued by the Department of Health and the National Assembly for Wales stating that local authorities must assess need in terms of risk to people' s independence. The guidance refers to "fair access to care" in its title (LAC (2002)13, NAFWC 9/02)[3].

The guidance states that local authorities should evaluate risks to a person's independence by focusing on a) autonomy and freedom to make choices; b) health and safety including freedom from harm, abuse and neglect, housing and community safety; c) ability to manage personal and other daily routines; d) involvement in family and wider community life, including leisure, hobbies, unpaid and paid work, learning and volunteering. The reader will appreciate that all these aspects of people's lives may have manual handling ramifications, not just in respect of living in the home but also of accessing and participating in the community.

To assist with this evaluation, local authorities have been told that they should consider whether any such risks to a person's independence are critical, substantial, moderate or low. The guidance then states that authorities should set a threshold, above which needs will be eligible for service provision, and below which they will not. Local authorities have not been told where to set the threshold. It appears that many have set it either between substantial and moderate or between moderate and low. The guidance applies only to social services provided for adults.

The guidance goes onto to provide indicators to assist in the categorisation of these levels of risk to independence. A glance at the indicators makes it clear that assessment should be about far more than physical risk. Certainly, under the critical category, reference is made to threat to life, significant health problems, little or no choice and control over vital aspects of the immediate environment, serious abuse or neglect, and vital personal care or domestic routines. But beyond such issues, reference in the critical category is made also to vital involvement in work or education or learning, vital social support systems and relationships, vital family and other social roles and responsibilities.

Example: critical risk to independence, home and work

A local authority assesses a range of different needs that a disabled person has. Of these a number relate to how he is going to transfer from place to place and thus they raise potential manual handling issues. They concern not just the home environment, but also his ability to go out to work each day. Therefore, amongst other things, the local authority assesses that there is a critical risk to his vital involvement in work.

Guidance on what has been called a 'single assessment' for older people, referring to joint assessments by local authorities and the NHS, has been issued in England, Wales and Scotland. Like the guidance on fair access to care, it too emphasises the importance of ensuring that assessments focus on the views and perceptions of service users (HSC 2002/001; NAFWC 9/02; CCD 8/2001)

---

2 Section 47 of the 1990 Act covers England and Wales. The equivalent provision in Scotland covering individual assessment lies in s.12A of *the Social Work (Scotland) Act 1968*. In Northern Ireland there is no equivalent, individual duty of assessment in the legislation. However, the duty to take a decision in the case of a disabled person under s.4 of the *Disabled Persons (Services, Consultation and Representation) Act 1986* applies across England, Wales and Scotland. In Northern Ireland, the equivalent duty is to be found in s.4 of the *Disabled Persons (Northern Ireland) Act 1989*.

3 Guidance on 'fair access to care' has not been issued in Scotland and Northern Ireland, but the principles of assessment are anyway similar. First, this is because the lawfulness of the application of a threshold of eligibility was established not by the English and Welsh guidance but by the law courts in a House of Lords judicial review case applicable throughout the United Kingdom (*R v Gloucestershire CC, ex p Barry*).
Second, other existing guidance in Scotland and Northern Ireland anyway refers to the importance of factors such as people's independence and choice over how they live (CCD 8/2001; DH/SO 1991; DHSS 1991). It should be noted that list of risk related indicators in the Welsh guidance is very similar, but not identical, to that in the English guidance.

Assessment of need: relevant factors and manual handling

Apart from the plentiful guidance issued by central government about assessment, the law courts have themselves identified on a number of occasions the factors that must be taken into account if community care assessments are to be lawful.

These factors have included, for instance, psychological issues *(R v Avon CC, ex p M)*, cultural and language issues *(R (Khana) v Southwark LBC)*, medical factors *(R v Birmingham CC, ex p Killigrew)*, people's preferences *(R v North Yorkshire CC, ex p Hargreaves)*, social, recreational and leisure needs *(R v Haringey LBC, ex p Norton)*. All these different types of factor may bear on manual handling related issues.

In another case, specifically about manual handling, the court stated that the local authority would have to take account of the emotional, psychological and social impact on two women of the different methods, including hoisting, of effecting physical transfers. This would be in terms of their wishes, feelings, reluctance, fear, refusal, dignity, integrity and quality of life *(A&B, X&Y v East Sussex County Council)*.

A local authority therefore has to take into account all the factors relevant to an individual case when reaching its decision. But that final decision does, in law, rest with the local authority. For example, taking account of a person's preferences is one thing, following them in every case quite another. Neither community care legislation nor the *Human Rights Act 1998* simply obliges a local authority to provide exactly what a person wants in every case.

Individual need and blanket policies

This very requirement to consider individual needs and situations underlay the judgment in the East Sussex case. The court stated that blanket 'no lifting' policies would be likely to be unlawful; as would policies that necessarily prohibited lifting a) unless life and limb were at risk or b) if equipment could be used to effect a transfer. Essentially this was because such policies would pre-judge the outcome of assessments. This point of view was nothing new; the Health and Safety Executive had already warned against such policies (HSE 2002).

Community care services

Community care assessments are conducted in order to decide whether a person has a need for community care services. Various services are referred to in the legislation covering local authority social services. They include care homes, a wide range of domiciliary care services, community activities, day services, respite care, adult placement schemes and so on – all with potential manual handling implications.

Residential accommodation

Local authorities place people in residential accommodation under the *National Assistance Act 1948* (covering England and Wales), *Social Work (Scotland) Act 1968* or the *Health and Personal Social Services (Northern Ireland) Order 1972.*

Case example: manual handling in a care home

One local government ombudsman investigation concerned a situation in which the local authority paid a higher than usual fee to a care home. This was to cover the extra personal assistance, including manual handling, that one of the residents required (*Redbridge LBC 1998*).

The ombudsman's investigation in the above case revealed that the arrangements ultimately went badly wrong. However, it serves as a general reminder that local authorities should assess and state in residents' care plans significant manual handling related needs. In this case there was medical evidence that hoist use, or the alternative of staying in bed for long periods, would be detrimental to the resident.

The case illustrated also the potential problems of leaving too much of the decision-making about manual handling to care homes, which, in some instances, might fail to strike the balance between staff safety and the assessed needs of their residents. One reason for this could be that the care home might simply not have the expertise to assess more complex manual handling related issues.

Example: manual handling and care plans

In one local authority, occupational therapists become concerned because people being placed in care homes have their care plans drawn up by social workers, who generally have little expertise in manual handling. Occupational therapists have no involvement. They are particularly concerned because certain service users are rapidly losing physical function when they are placed in care homes – precisely because they do not receive manual handling assistance to transfer and to walk. Instead they are routinely hoisted and pushed in wheelchairs, even when manual handling assistance would not pose unacceptable risks to properly trained and supervised care staff.

This contrasts with care plans for people who are supported in their own homes, who have therapist input in respect of manual handling matters. The dangers of care home residents' needs consequently being overlooked are pointed out to senior managers, who agree that practice must change – so that manual handling issues are in future properly considered for care home residents as well as for people in their own homes.

Non-residential services

Under s. 2 of the *Chronically Sick and Disabled Persons Act 1970 (CSDPA)*, a local authority has a duty to provide various non-residential services, in order to meet the assessed, eligible needs of disabled people [4].

Services that could involve manual handling issues include practical assistance in the home, recreational facilities, lectures, games, outings, taking advantage of educational facilities available to a person, works of adaptation to the home and additional facilities for greater safety, comfort or convenience and holidays.

Case example: services in the community

In one protracted legal dispute, it was being argued on behalf of two service users with profound physical and learning disabilities that they must have access to swimming, horse riding and shopping trips.

The local authority countered that the manual handling risks to paid carers were too great (*A&B, X&Y v East Sussex County Council*).

4 Section 2 of the *CSDPA 1970* applies directly in England and Wales, and in Scotland by virtue of the *Chronically Sick and Disabled Persons (Scotland) Act 1972*. In Northern Ireland, the equivalent of s.2 of the1970 Act is to be found in s.2 of the *Chronically Sick and Disabled Persons (Northern Ireland) Act 1978*. Therefore, for brevity, reference is made below only to s.2 of the *CSDPA 1970* but can be taken to apply across the United Kingdom.

Absolute duty to meet assessed, eligible needs

The courts have ruled that, at least under some community care legislation, an absolute duty is imposed on a local authority to meet assessed, eligible needs without undue delay. An eligible need means a need that has been assessed as coming over the threshold of eligibility that the local authority has set.

One piece of legislation to which this rule has been held to apply is s.2 of the *Chronically Sick and Disabled Persons Act 1970*, already referred to above *(R v Gloucestershire CC, ex p Barry)*. Other legislation so governed, for example, covering residential accommodation includes s.21 of the *National Assistance Act 1948 (R v Sefton MBC, ex p Help the Aged; R v Royal Borough of Kensington and Chelsea, exp Kujtim)*.

Meeting a need cost effectively

Once a duty to meet a need has been incurred, the need must be met one way or another. If more than one way of meeting it exists, the local authority may offer the cheapest option, so long as that option does genuinely meet the need and is compliant with other relevant legislation such as the *Human Rights Act 1998*.

However, met the need must be, even if the only way of doing so is relatively costly. A lack of resources would be no legal defence *(R v Gloucestershire CC, exp Barry; R v East Sussex CC, ex p Tandy; R v Royal Borough of Kensington & Chelsea, exp Kujtim; R v Lancashire CC, ex p RADAR)*.

Example: duty to provide personal assistance rather than a hoist

Following a serious car accident, a person is continuing a process of rehabilitation in his own home. He needs to build up strength over a period of time. Provision of a hoist and one assistant would be cheaper than providing two personal assistants each day to help transfer him.

However, hoist use has been assessed as not meeting the person's needs and indeed it would be a threat to his independence. He can reliably take some of his own weight on transfers. This is essential for the rehabilitation process. Hoist use is not necessitated by risk to staff, since the risk, if properly managed, has been assessed as low under the *Manual Handling Operations Regulations 1992*. In such circumstances, the hoist is unlikely to be a lawful way of meeting the man's assessed community care needs. The local authority would instead have to supply the two personal assistants, albeit at greater cost.

Thus, a local authority is not legally obliged to meet a need by means of an option that involves an unacceptable level of risk to staff; but it is obliged to seek to find an option that meets an assessed need without such a degree of risk, even if this means greater expenditure.

Withdrawing or changing services

Generally speaking, it is likely to be lawful for a local authority to change, reduce or withdraw services in the following circumstances.

First a reassessment would have to take place *(R v Gloucestershire CC, ex p Mahfood)*. Second, a reduction in service could only be justified if:

a the person's needs had likewise reduced or changed,
b the same needs could be met in a different way,
c the local authority's threshold of eligibility for services (see above) had risen,
d there was explicit or implicit (e.g. through unreasonable behaviour) refusal of service by the person.

Absent these factors, and a reduction in service is generally likely to be unlawful even if manual handling requirements have made a care package more expensive that hitherto.

Case example: manual handling assessment and reducing a person's services

Following a manual handling assessment of a woman with multiple sclerosis, a local authority provides two personal assistants instead of one, but halves the amount of assistance provided. The local authority does not show that this reduction equated to a change in the woman's assessed, eligible needs, to a change in the eligibility criteria, or to meeting her needs in a different way. The judge is therefore concerned that the decision was totally resource led and strikes down the assessment decision as unlawful (*R v Birmingham CC, ex p Killigrew*).

Furthermore, even where a reduction may be legally justifiable, both the courts *(R v Gloucestershire CC, ex p RADAR)* and central government guidance in England and Wales have urged caution in deciding whether, or how, to withdraw services from people (LAC (2002)13, NAFWC 9/02).

Case example: withdrawing manual handling services

A woman with Alzheimer's Disease was doubly incontinent, completely immobile and required assistance from carers three times a day, seven days a week. She had received manual handling assistance in the past, but this now represented an increasing risk to staff. For this reason, the social services department then reportedly stated that unless her husband agreed to have a hoist installed, the carers would be withdrawn. This was after carers refused to lift her manually.

The husband then attempted to kill both himself and his wife by leading a hose from the exhaust of his car into the bedroom; however, a neighbour heard the car engine running, saw the hose and intervened. The husband had left a note blaming a social worker and the owner of a private care company, stating that those evil people had deemed that services should be withdrawn and his wife left unattended

His wife died a month later in a care home from an unrelated chest infection; on release from hospital he was arrested and charged with attempted murder. He pleaded guilty. The judge sentenced him to a year's probation but also criticised the Crown Prosecution Service for bringing the case at all, stating that it was not in the public interest to have done so (*R v Bouldstridge*).

Children

Disabled children's needs are in large part assessed under s.2 of the *Chronically Sick and Disabled Persons Act 1970)* and s.17 of the *Children Act 1989* (in England and Wales).

On request by a disabled child's informal carer (including parents), a local authority has a duty to decide whether the child's needs call for the provision of services under the *CSDPA 1970*. This duty is contained in s.4 of the *Disabled Persons (Services, Consultation and Representation) Act 1986* for England, Wales and Scotland - and in s.4 of the *Disabled Persons (Northern Ireland) Act 1989* in relation to the *CSDP(NI)A 1978*. Examples of services from the 1970 Act have already been given above.

Under s.17 of the *Children Act 1989*, there is a general duty to safeguard and promote the welfare of children in need. The duty is wide in scope, and provision of services in relation to manual handling issues could come under it. In addition, it covers not just disabled children but also other children whose health or development is at risk. It also allows for the provision of accommoda-tion, something that cannot be provided under s.2 of the 1970 Act, and which might bear on manual handling issues. Furthermore, services can be provided under s.17 not just to a child in need, but also to any member of his or her family[5].

Nevertheless, s.17 is a relatively weak duty; enforcement of it for an individual child is generally very difficult *(R (On application of G) v Barnet LBC)*. This compares with the relatively strong duty under s.2 of the *Chronically Sick and Disabled Persons Act 1970* (e.g. *R v Bexley LBC, ex p B)*.

Looked after children

Under s.22 of the *Children Act 1989* for England and Wales, local authorities also have a specific duty to safeguard and promote the welfare of any child they are looking after. A looked after child is a child in the local authority's care or provided with accommodation arranged by the local authority (including foster placements).

The equivalent duties in Scotland are under s.17 of the *Children (Scotland) Act 1995*, and in Northern Ireland under a.27 of the *Children (Northern Ireland) Order 1995*.

In the case of a disabled child for whom the local authority is providing accommodation under the *Children Act 1989*, the authority must, so far as is reasonably practicable, secure that the accommodation is not unsuitable to the child's particular needs (s.23). In Northern Ireland, the equivalent duty is under a.27 of the *Children (Northern Ireland) Order 1995*. This could of course bear on manual handling related issues.

Further, in respect of local authority foster parents, regulations in England for example, stipulate that the fostering service provider (local authority or inde-pendent agency) must ensure that each child is provided with the individual support, aids and equipment which he or she may require due to health needs or disability; and that the foster parents are provided with training, advice, infor-mation and support (SI 2002/57,rr.15, 17). Self evidently, such obligations could bear on manual handling issues; a failure to heed could lead to manual handling related personal injury litiga-tion *(Beasley v Buckinghamshire CC)*.

Carers

In addition to assessing a disabled person, local authorities have various duties in respect of informal carers[6]. These duties are highly relevant, given the physical and mental stresses on informal carers involved in manual handling. There has been a perception that informal carers are not always supported and assisted in relation to manual handling by statutory bodies such as local authorities and the NHS. This can compare unfavourably with those organisations' concern about their own staff (Marriott 2003) and lead to injury (Henwood 1998).

Generally, informal carers who are providing regular and substantial care, and who request it, are entitled to a local authority assessment of their ability to care. In addition (except in Scotland), the local authority has a duty to decide whether the assessed needs of the carer call for services, and whether to provide those services.

Example: advice and training for informal carers

By way of a carer's service, a local authority offers information, advice and training service for informal carers engaged on manual handling tasks.

It is also notable that guidance issued, for example, by central government in England and Wales on the *Carers and Disabled Children Act 2000* urges that assessment should be sensitive to both the physical and psy-chological impact of caring on individual carers (DH 2001;NAW 2001).

Even if a carer refuses an assessment, the local authority still has a duty to 'have regard' to his or her ability to care under s.8 of the *Disabled Persons (Services, Consultation and Representa-tion) Act 1986* (England, Scotland and Wales) and s.8 of the *Disabled Persons (Northern Ireland) Act 1989*. In Scotland, there is an additional duty, when assessing a service user, to take account of the views of the carer so far as is reasonably practicable (s.12A *Social Work (Scotland) Act 1968)*.

Direct payments

A direct payment means that instead of itself arranging a service, the local authority gives service users a reason-able amount of money to enable them to purchase non-residential services or equipment themselves. Some people might receive direct payments to purchase personal assistance and equipment that involves manual handling.

Example: purchasing manual handling assistance to get to work

A person is assisted each day with getting out, and going back, to bed. Manual handling with various items of assistive equipment is required. However, the local authority cannot provide the service before 9am, which is the time the person needs to be at work. She therefore suggests that the local authority provide her with a direct payment, so that she can purchase personal assistance on terms to suit her needs better.

Certain conditions must be satisfied. The person must consent to the direct payment; that is both have the ability to consent and also want the payment. He or she must also have the ability to manage the payment, with or without

5 The equivalent duty in Scotland lies in s.22 of the *Children (Scotland) Act 1995*, and in Northern Ireland within a.18 of the *Children (Northern Ireland) Order 1995*. Under schedule 2 of the *Children Act 1989* (England and Wales), there is a further general (and therefore in principle weak) duty to provide services to minimise the effect of their disabilities on disabled children in general in the area. The equivalent duty in Northern Ireland is contained in schedule 2 of the *Children (Northern Ireland) Order 1995*. The comparable duty in Scotland appears to be of the stronger variety, since it refers to minimising the effect on 'any child' (rather than on children in general) (*Children (Scotland) Act 1995, s.23)*.

6 These duties come under the *Carers (Recognition and Services) Act 1995 and under the Carers and Disabled Children 2000* (England and Wales). In Scotland, the pro-visions are similar (but not the same) under s.12AA of the *Social Work (Scotland) Act 1968* and under s.24 of the *Children (Scotland) Act 1968*. In Northern Ireland, similar provisions are to be found in the *Carers and Direct Payments (Northern Ireland) Act 2002*, and articles 17A and 18A of the *Children (Northern Ireland) Order 1995*. Guidance has been issued in Scotland (CCD 2/2003) and Northern Ireland (DHSSPS 2003) also.

assistance. The service in question must meet the assessed need. There are a number of exclusions relating to some people who come under certain mental health and criminal justice legislation[7].

The legislation does not permit direct payments to be made in respect of NHS or housing services. If the conditions are met, then in England, Scotland and Northern Ireland there is a duty to make a direct payment. At the time of writing (April 2004), in Wales, there is only a power to make a payment, but this is expected to become a duty in the future.

Where a person clearly lacks capacity to consent or to manage the payment with or without assistance, a direct payment cannot be made to the person. However, there are ways around this. In Scotland, guardians or welfare attorneys with the appropriate powers under the *Adults with Incapacity (Scotland) Act 2000* are able to receive direct payments. Elsewhere in the United Kingdom it may be possible to make 'indirect' or 'third party' payments, which do not come under the direct payments legislation. This became clear during the course of a manual handling dispute:

Case example: manual handling and user independent trust

One legal case concerned two women with profound physical and learning disabilities cared for by their parents at home. The local authority and parents engaged in an extended dispute about manual handling for the two women. It was accepted by all involved that direct payments would not be possible because of the two women's inability to consent or to manage the payment with or without assistance.

However, the judge stated that it would be possible for a 'user independent trust', in the form of a registered company, to be formed. The local authority could make payments (sometimes referred to as 'indirect' or third party payments) to the trust, which in turn would purchase personal assistance including manual handling assistance. The arrangements would lie not under direct payments legislation but under s.30 of the *National Assistance Act 1948 (A&B, X&Y v East Sussex County Council)*.

7 In England, people eligible for direct payments are all community care service users aged 18 or over, disabled children aged 16 or 17 years, carers aged 16 or over, parents of disabled children, disabled parents of children in need (*Health and Social Care Act 2001, s.17A Children Act 1989*). In Northern Ireland the position is the same under the *Carers and Direct Payments (Northern Ireland) Act 2002* and a.18C of the *Children (Northern Ireland) Order 1995*.

Scotland and Wales are working toward including the same groups but have not yet reached that point. In Scotland, carers will anyway not be included, since here carers are not potentially eligible for services directly in their own right as in the rest of the United Kingdom.

In Wales, at the time of writing, the relevant legislation is the *Community Care (Direct Payments) Act 1996* but will in future be the *Health and Social Care Act 2001*. In Scotland, direct payments come under s.12B of the *Social Work (Scotland) Act 1968*.

Direct payments, health and safety, manual handling

The purpose of direct payments is to give people greater choice and control over their own lives. Nevertheless, local authorities still remain statutorily responsible in the sense that direct payments are made following assessment of need, and must then be used to meet that need. This situation may result in a degree of tension in some circumstances.

For instance, a dilemma may arise if a disabled person chooses to use the money in such a way as to give rise to serious health and safety concerns on the part of the local authority. If the local authority takes a 'hands-off' approach it may be concerned about litigation in respect of any accident that occurs – even if the recipient has, as a condition of the direct payment, taken out insurance. Yet, an excessively 'hands-on' or interventionist approach would risk undermining the whole purpose of direct payments.

Guidance issued in England states that recipients should be given information about health and safety and also the results of any risk assessment carried out by competent staff on behalf of the local authority. In addition, recipients should be encouraged to develop strategies on lifting. However, the guidance clearly states that: "As a general principle, local councils should avoid laying down health and safety policies for individual direct payment recipients" (DH 2003).

This Department of Health policy appears to advocate what could be termed a 'hands-off' approach. However, in case of accident involving negligence, it is unclear whether the courts would necessarily approve such an approach, or would instead tend to hold a local authority liable for not intervening in situations of high risk. From a legal (as distinct from a policy) point of view at least, the term 'general principle' contained in the guidance might be better interpreted to mean that at least in some circumstances local authorities should consider intervening if serious health and safety risks are seen to arise.

Example: excessive risk and intervention?

A local authority care manager visits to review a direct payments package. She finds that the personal assistant employed by the direct payment recipient is regularly carrying the latter up and down the garden path. They have fallen on more than one occasion. She suggests that this is, on any view, a high-risk activity and therefore not acceptable. The direct payment recipient disagrees and maintains that it is up to her as employer to organise her assistance. The care manager ponders how to intervene, in order to try to find a compromise.

Example: finding a direct payment solution

A disabled person wishes to be transferred manually, rather than mechanically with equipment, in his own home and in the community. However, on the basis of an individual risk assessment, the manual handling protocols developed by the local authority rule this out. The man asks for a direct payment as a way around the problem.

After much negotiation, the local authority agrees not to impose directly its manual handling protocols as a condition of the direct payment. The disabled person in turn agrees to go to an independent living agency that specialises in setting up independent living packages for disabled people. This solution reassures the local authority because the agency is experienced in personal assistance and manual handling issues. The disabled person is likewise reassured because the agency has a good reputation in respect of independent living.

Community equipment services

Equipment plays a key role in manual handling. The ready availability of appropriate types of equipment is essential both to the meeting of people's needs and to staff safety. Indeed, sometimes the right type of equipment can resolve conflicts of view between local authority and service user.

Nevertheless, community equipment services have long been recognised as a confused area of provision. They have generally been characterised by poor organisation and funding, resulting in delay, non-provision and considerable dispute between local authorities and the NHS about where responsibility for certain types of equipment lies (see generally Audit Commission 2000).

Example: manual handling, hoists and beds

Disputes sometimes arise about mobile hoists or special beds (e.g. profiling beds) to be used in people's homes. Local authorities may refuse to provide them, but the NHS only provide them if district nurses are in attendance. In such circumstances, the problem for the service user requiring such a hoist or bed without district nurse attendance is obvious. Even where there are jointly run community equipment stores, such a problem may still persist in terms of which staff can or can't authorise certain types of equipment – where such authorisation is linked to respective budget contributions from the local authority and the NHS.

The solution to such disputes is of course not to conduct endless arguments about what constitutes health, social care (or housing) equipment. Such arguments are often fruitless, since so much equipment falls into a grey area of being arguably either health or social care. Indeed, legally, it would almost certainly be a futile task attempting to get the courts to rule on such matters.

The answer would appear in part to be flexible joint working between local authorities and the NHS. To this end, Department of Health policy in England has been directed to improving these services (HSC 2001/008).

3 Housing legislation: home adaptations

Adapting the environment is sometimes a way of solving mobility and manual handling issues in the home. Under the *Housing Grants, Construction and Regeneration Act 1996*, local housing authorities in England and Wales have a strong duty to award mandatory disabled facilities grants if certain conditions are met[8].

Grant applications must be approved if the adaptation is in respect of access to, and use of, various parts and facilities within the dwelling. In addition, the adaptation must be regarded as necessary and appropriate (e.g. in respect of meeting community care needs or of independence) and as reasonable and practicable in relation to the age and condition of the dwelling. A means test also applies. Of course if equipment could meet the relevant needs of a person, then an adaptation will not be 'necessary and appropriate'.

The Act itself, as well as guidance issued by central government, is clear that not only private sector owner occupiers and tenants are eligible to apply for grants, but so too are council tenants and tenants of registered social landlords. Unfortunately, some housing authorities neither recognise this eligibility across all these housing sectors, nor do they adhere to the time scales set in legislation for processing grant applications. The consequences of not carrying out adaptations in timely fashion can have drastic manual handling consequences for disabled people and their informal carers.

Case example: manual handling implications of delay in home adaptations

An elderly man with chronic arthritis and Parkinson's disease requested help with adaptations. The request took several years to deal with. During this time, apart from distress, worry and inconvenience, the demands made on his wife were enormous. The husband was embarrassed and frustrated. Three years after the initial request, the wife was usually alone with her husband all day, having to get him up, dress him the stairs, and help him on the stairs. His prostate problems meant that she needed to help him up and down more often – and when he fell, he often pulled her down with him. The local government ombudsman found maladministration (*Barking and Dagenham 1998*, case 97/A/0337).

Sometimes an adaptation does not come within the remit of the disabled facilities grants legislation. Alternatively, the means test may affect some people unduly harshly because it can, by law, take no account of outgoings. In such circumstances, local social services authorities may have a duty to assist under s.2 of the *Chronically Sick and Disabled Persons Act 1970*.

Lastly, local housing authorities in England and Wales have a wide discretion to assist with adaptations outside of the disabled facilities grants system, as well as to assist people to move house where this is the preferred solution. Such assistance can be given under the terms of the *Regulatory Reform (Housing Assistance) (England and Wales) Order 2002*.

4 Human rights legislation

In October 2000, the *Human Rights Act 1998* came into force. It acted as the vehicle for bringing into United Kingdom law the *European Convention on Human Rights*. The Act and Convention apply to public bodies, such as local authorities, NHS Trusts and central government departments – but not directly to independent care providers. This means that local authority decision-making in respect of manual handling must comply not just with relevant domestic legislation, but also with the articles of the Convention.

A number of Convention articles are relevant to local social services authorities in general. In respect of manual handling issues, the courts have to date referred to three in particular. These concern the right to life (article 2), the right not to be subjected to inhuman or degrading treatment (article 3) and the right to respect for home, private and family life (article 8).

8 Mandatory disabled facilities grants are also available under the *Housing Order (Northern Ireland) 2003* in Northern Ireland, where in addition power remains to give discretionary disabled facilities grants for a person's welfare, accommodation or employment. In Scotland, there is a duty to provide (access to) standard amenities, and a power to carry out other adaptations for a disabled person, under the *Housing (Scotland) Act 1987*. As in England and Wales, a duty to assist with adaptations may also arise under s.2 of the *Chronically Sick and Disabled Persons Act 1970* in Scotland or s.2 of the *Chronically Sick and Disabled Persons (Northern Ireland)* Act 1978 in Northern Ireland.

Case example: blanket policies on manual handling
In relation to human rights, the courts have ruled that certain types of manual handling policy are likely to be unlawful in the context of community care. These were 'no lifting'; no lifting unless life or limb were at risk; and no lifting if equipment could physically effect the transfer (*A&B, X&Y v East Sussex CC*).

Case example: leaving people to perish
Leaving disabled people as a matter of manual handling related policy or protocol to drown in the bath or perish in a fire could engage article 2 and the right to life (*A&B,X&Y v East Sussex CC*).

Case example: degrading treatment of a disabled prisoner
A severely physically disabled person was sent to prison for contempt of court, for failing to disclose her assets in a debt case. In the police cell she was unable to use the bed and had to sleep in her wheelchair where she became very cold. When she reached the prison hospital, she could not use the toilet herself, the female duty officer could not manage to move her alone, and male prison officers had to assist. The European Court found that to detain a severely disabled person in conditions where she is dangerously cold, risks developing pressure sores because her bed is too hard or unreachable, and is unable to go to the toilet or keep clean without the greatest difficulty, constituted degrading treatment contrary to article 3. Damages of £4,500 were awarded (*Price v United Kingdom*).

Case example: leaving people in degrading circumstances
If manual handling policies or protocols were to mean that care staff would leave disabled people for hours sitting in their own bodily waste or on the lavatory, article 3 might be engaged – i.e. the right not to be subjected to inhuman or degrading treatment (*A&B, X&Y v East Sussex County Council*).

Case example: physical and psychological integrity of a disabled person
Article 8 (right to respect for home, private and family life) has been held to include the physical and psychological integrity of disabled people, both within and without the home. Thus in a manual handling dispute, involving two women with severe physical and learning disabilities, it applied both to issues such as the dignity surrounding hoisting and transfers within the home – and to their participation in the life of the community, including recreational and cultural activities.

However, the judge pointed out that paid carers, too, had rights relating to integrity and dignity under article 8. He also emphasised that hoisting was not inherently degrading, but that whether it was or not would depend on all the circumstances of the particular situation (*A&B, X&Y v East Sussex County Council*).

Case example: leaving a disabled person dependent and humiliated
A local authority social services department assessed a need of suitable accommodation and adaptations for a 48-year old disabled woman (who had suffered a stroke) living with her family and six children. Two years later nothing had happened; the family was not eligible for assistance from the housing department, and social services had not acted.

As a consequence, the woman could not reach the lavatory and soiled herself several times a day, had no privacy, could not go out of the house, could not go upstairs, and could not go anywhere without her husband's assistance. She had to share a cramped living room with her husband and two youngest children; the other children had to go through that room in order to go upstairs. Her husband's health was at risk; his back problem deteriorated from manual handling. She felt frustrated and humiliated because she was unable to do anything for her family and was totally dependent on them.

The judge concluded that although some people would regard the above conditions as degrading, particularly in relation to the incontinence, he did not believe they crossed the threshold posed by article 3 of the Convention, although the matter was finely balanced. However, he did find a breach of article 8 (*R v Enfield London Borough Council, ex p Bernard*).

On the courts' current interpretation of 'public body', the Act and Convention do not apply directly, for example, to independent care providers of care homes or of domiciliary services. Nevertheless, it would be open to local authorities to require care providers, as a matter of contract, to adhere to human rights in respect of manual handling or any issues (*R v Leonard Cheshire Foundation, ex p Heather*). And, in any case, if a local authority knew, or should reasonably have known, that a care provider with whom it had contracted was acting contrary to human rights, the courts might find that authority to be in breach of the Act.

5 Disability discrimination

Under the *Disability Discrimination Act 1995* (DDA), which applies to the whole of the United Kingdom, providers of goods and services to the public must not discriminate against disabled people. Local authorities are providers of goods and services to the public. So too are independent care providers, since unlike the *Human Rights Act 1998*, the DDA is not confined to public bodies. The Act also applies to the provision of education in schools, and in further and higher education.

Discrimination occurs when such a provider treats a disabled person less favourably and unjustifiably for a reason relating to his or her disability. This would be in respect of not providing a service or of the terms or standards on which the service is provided. In order to establish that treatment was less favourable, the comparison can be made between the disabled person and either a non-disabled person or a disabled person with a different type of disability.

Alternatively, discrimination occurs when a provider fails to take reasonable steps, with the result that it is unreasonably difficult or impossible for a disabled person to use a service.

Nevertheless, even if less favourable treatment does occur, or reasonable steps are not taken, the Act allows for justification if certain grounds can be made out. One of those grounds relates to health and safety. This justification relies on the provider of services being of the opinion that the ground applies and that it is reasonable in all the circumstances for it to hold that opinion.

The reader will appreciate that the lessons to be learnt from the following example, illustrating the importance of proper risk assessment, could easily be applied to a comparable situation involving manual handling.

Case example: risk assessment

A school prevented a 14-year old boy with diabetes going on a water sports holiday with the school. This was on the basis of an episode of hypo-glycaemia on a previous school trip, and his alleged irresponsible management of his own condition. A health and safety justification for this less favourable treatment was put forward.

The court rejected this on the basis that the "initial decision was fatally flawed in the manner in which it was taken and thereafter the school adopted a defensive stance and simply confirmed the decision. There was no involvement of [the boy] or his parents in the decision-making process, the matters held against him were never put to him for an explanation and there was no serious attempt at a risk assessment taking into account the nature of the holiday and the medical realities. A climate of blame was used to justify a decision that would avoid a repeat of the earlier frightening incident. The belief that exclusion was justified could not be said to be based on a reasonably held opinion that it was necessary in order not endanger [the pupil's] health or safety" (*White v Clitheroe Royal Grammar School*).

To date, the 1995 Act seems not to have featured significantly in any court cases involving manual handling. For example the case of *A&B, X&Y v East Sussex CC*, already referred to, focused on human rights rather than disability discrimination, although the Disability Rights Commission did involve itself in the case. Even so, guidance published by the Health and Safety Executive does state that blanket no lifting policies run the risk of breaching the DDA (HSE 2002).

Nevertheless it can be seen from the example immediately above *(White v Clitheroe Royal Grammar School)* that if people are treated less favourably on manual handling related grounds, then any health and safety justification must be soundly supported by genuine, and not token, risk assessment.

6 Health and safety at work legislation

Health and safety at work legislation is central to decisions about manual handling and clearly applies to local authority social services functions, as well as to independent care providers. However, perhaps not so obviously, the relevant provisions are not limited to the *Manual Handling Operations Regulations 1992* (MHOR 1992).

In addition, the relevant legislation is not restricted in scope to employees alone. It applies as well, both explicitly and implicitly, to non-employees, including service users and informal carers[9].

Reasonable practicability

Of pivotal importance to an understanding of the health and safety at work legislation outlined below is the term 'reasonably practicable'. This term governs key duties relating to manual handling.

The traditional test of reasonable practicability used by the courts has arisen from cases involving risk to employees. The approach has been to weigh up the level of risk to employees against the cost of doing something about it in terms of resources, staff, time and effort. If the cost involved would be clearly disproportionate to the risk, then it might not be reasonably practicable to eliminate or reduce the risk.

Case example: balancing risk against resources

A local authority carpenter was carrying doors weighing 72 pounds up the stairs of a block of flats. He sustained an injury. The Court of Appeal accepted that the risk of manual handling injury appeared from the evidence to have been relatively low. However, providing him that day with an assistant would not have been a disproportionate drain on the resources of an employer the size of the local authority. The local authority was therefore found to be in breach of the MHOR 1992 (*Hawkes v Southwark LBC*).

9 Reference is made in the following paragraphs to the *Health and Safety at Work Act 1974, Management of Health and Safety at Work Regulations 1999, Manual Handling Operations Regulations 1992, Lifting Operations and Lifting Equipment Regulations 1998* and the *Provision and Use of Work Equipment Regulations 1998*. All these apply to England, Scotland and Wales.
The equivalent provisions covering Northern Ireland are: *Health and Safety at Work Order (Northern Ireland) 1978, Management of Health and Safety at Work Regulations (Northern Ireland) 1999, Manual Handling Operations Regulations (Northern Ireland) 1992, Lifting Operation and Lifting Equipment Regulations (Northern Ireland) 1999, Provision and Use of Work Equipment Regulations (Northern Ireland) 1999*).
For the sake of brevity, these equivalent Northern Ireland references are not given in the following paragraphs but should be taken to apply unless otherwise stated.

Reasonable practicability: benefit or utility

In a number of recent cases involving public services, the courts have referred to another element that must be taken into account when deciding how far it is reasonably practicable to reduce risk to employees. This element is, namely, the benefit or utility of the activity in question to the relevant member(s) of the public. The courts are in effect pointing out that the test of reasonable practicability can only be made sense of, if the relevant public service context is taken into account.

Case example: community care services

A dispute arose between a local authority and the parents of two women with profound physical and learning disabilities. The parents were generally opposed to the use of hoists within the home and wished their daughters to be manually handled. They also wished their daughters to get out and participate in the community, particularly in respect of swimming, shopping and horse-riding. The local authority felt unable to agree to the wishes of the parents, because of what it perceived to be the high manual handling risks to staff.

The court held in effect that, when considering what was reasonably practicable to protect employees under the *MHOR 1992*, the local authority had also to consider the assessed community care needs of the women and their human rights. This would involve balanced decision-making. It would not mean that the rights of disabled people should override those of paid carers; nor would it mean that those of paid carers should override those of disabled people. Nevertheless, it might mean that in certain circumstances paid carers might have to work at higher, but not unacceptable, levels of risk – depending on the needs, and threat to the human rights, of a disabled person (*A&B, X&Y v East Sussex County Council*).

Case example: NHS care assistant

A care assistant in an NHS residential home for disabled children allegedly sustained an injury through pulling out and making beds that were low and stood against the wall. The Court of Appeal accepted in principle that certain features of the beds, though potentially increasing the risk for staff, might be justifiable in relation to the needs of the children (*Koonjul v Thameslink NHS Health Care Trust*).

Case example: ambulance service

The ambulance service was called to collect a man from his home and take him to hospital. It was an urgent call, requiring a response within an hour, but not an emergency. The man lived in a cottage, and was upstairs in a bedroom, reached by a steep, narrow staircase with a bend in it. The two ambulance men started to carry the man down the stairs in a carry chair. One of the ambulance men momentarily relaxed his grip on the front of the chair; the other ambulance man briefly had to bear the whole weight, and suffered injuries to his thumb, back and knees.

The injured ambulance man brought a personal injury case, arguing that he should have been trained to give serious consideration to the alternative of using the fire brigade to remove the man through a window with a crane – and that the ambulance service wrongly treated use of the fire brigade as an absolute last resort.

The Court of Appeal rejected the ambulance man's argument, partly on the basis that public service workers sometimes have to work at higher, thought not unacceptable, levels of risk. The court also pointed out that, in determining whether to call for the fire brigade to effect quite a drastic form of removal, various relevant factors had to be taken account of. These included distress to the patient and reaction of the carers (*King v Sussex Ambulance Service*).

Such a judicial approach is arguably entirely consonant with Health and Safety Executive guidance, which points out that reasonable practicability does not necessarily entail that all risk be removed. Otherwise there would, for instance, be no adequate fire brigade (HSE 2004). In other words risk assessment must be performed in context. The Health and Safety Commission has stated that within the health services, certain situations and activities will sometimes inevitably involve higher risk. One such activity would be rehabilitation (HSC 1998). This approach is further argued in guidance on manual handling issued by the Chartered Society of Physiotherapy (CSP 2002).

In the community care context, this benefit or utility as part of the reasonable practicability equation is, legally, supplied by people's assessed need and human rights under community care and human rights legislation respectively.

Duty to employees

Various duties are imposed on employers in respect of employees.

Health and Safety at Work Act 1974

Under s.2 of the *Health and Safety at Work Act 1974*, employers have a duty to safeguard the health, safety and welfare of their employees at work, as far as is reasonably practicable.

The overall duty includes the provision and maintenance of safe systems of work together with instruction, information, training and supervision. It also covers safe use, handling, transport and storage of equipment, as well as a safe working environment. All this has to be achieved in so far as it reasonably practicable to do so. Clearly, these duties are generally relevant to manual handling, notwithstanding the more specific regulations outlined immediately below.

Duty to employees: Management of Health and Safety at Work Regulations 1999

Under the *Management of Health and Safety at Work Regulations 1999*, employers have various duties. These include the duty to assess risks to the health and safety of their employees at work, in order to identify risks relating to other, relevant health and safety at work legislation such as the *Manual Handling Operations Regulations 1992.*

In addition a range of other duties are contained in the 1999 regulations, including the provision of information and training to employees. Employers must also cooperate and coordinate activities in a workplace shared with other employers or self-employed people in order to ensure compliance with relevant health and safety requirements. They are also obliged in a shared workplace to provide health and safety information to other employers or to self-employed people working in the employer's undertaking. These duties could apply to manual handling situations.

Example: shared workplace

A disabled person is receiving a complex care package in her own home. This includes various items of equipment for assisting with transfers and involves regular input from NHS district nurses, social services care staff, and care assistants from an independent care provider. The care package therefore involves three employers in a shared workplace (the person's home). Unnecessary risk may arise if communication is poor and relevant information is not shared about, for instance, changes in the service user's abilities. Likewise if it is unclear, for example, as to who is responsible for the maintenance of any manual handling equipment being used.

Duty to employees: Manual Handling Operations Regulations 1992 (MHOR 1992)

Under the *MHOR 1992*, employers must take various steps. As far as is reasonably practicable, they must avoid the need for their employees to undertake manual handling involving a risk of injury. The assessment that identifies such risk generally in the first place takes place under the 1999 regulations (see immediately above).

If it is not reasonably practicable for an employer to avoid the risk of injury to its employees, then it must carry out a suitable and sufficient assessment, and take appropriate steps to reduce the risk to the lowest level reasonably practicable. If reasonably practicable it must also provide precise information on the weight, and heaviest side of, the 'load'.

The employer must have regard to the physical suitability of an employee to carry out the tasks together with clothing, footwear and other personal effects being carried. It must also have regard to any relevant risk assessment under r.3 of the 1999 regulations and whether an employee has been identified by that assessment as coming within a group of employees particularly at risk. It must have regard to the results of any health surveillance carried out under r.6 of the 1999 Regulations.

Example: managing and reducing a higher risk

A woman living in her own home is assessed as posing a higher risk to the local authority carers who will need to transfer her each day from bed to wheelchair, wheelchair to bath etc. Some of these transfers will need to be achieved by hoist and some by transfer board. The assessment also shows that failure to get the woman up and about by means of these transfers will have a detrimental effect on her physically, medically and psychologically.

It is therefore decided that she will be cared for by a named team of carers, who will be specially trained and supervised for the first two weeks of their involvement. A special sling is used. Some of the transfer activity involves kneeling. It is known that some carers working for the local authority have difficulty kneeling and so those carers are specifically excluded from the team.

Both the 1999 regulations (see above) and the *MHOR 1992* impose a duty on employers to review the risk assessment if there is reason to believe that it is no longer valid or if there has been significant change in the situation. The employer must then make any changes required.

Case example: maintaining risk assessments and care plans

In one negligence case, the risks posed by a woman who was assisted to walk at a day hospital had increased. This had, correctly, been recorded in her notes. However, the physiotherapist had not taken correspondingly greater precautions, and this had resulted in injury to an occupational therapy assistant. The NHS Trust was held liable for the injury (*Stainton v Chorley and South Ribble NHS Trust*).

Duties of employees

The *Health and Safety at Work Act 1974* (s.7) imposes a duty on an employee to take reasonable care of his or her own health and safety and also that of other people who may be affected by the employee's acts or failure to act. Under the *MHOR 1992*, an employee must make full and proper use of any system of work provided in relation to the reduction of risk under the *MHOR 1992*. And under the *Management of Health and Safety at Work Regulations 1999*, employees must use equipment in accordance with any training provided and with instructions provided by the employer.

Self-employed people

Under s.3 of the *Health and Safety at Work Act 1974*, self-employed people have a duty to conduct their undertaking in such a way as to ensure that, as far as reasonably practicable, other people who may be affected are not exposed to risk to their health and safety. In addition, the duties imposed on employers, as outlined above in both the *Management of Health and Safety at Work Regulations 1999* and the *MHOR 1992*, apply also to self-employed people.

Duties to non-employees

As already explained, employers must take account of non-employees such as service users when deciding what is reasonably practicable in order to safeguard employees. However, there are in addition explicit duties owed toward non-employees.

Under s.3 of the 1974 Act, an employer must conduct its undertaking in such a way as to ensure, so far as is reasonably practicable, that non-employees who may be affected are not exposed to risks to their health and safety. In addition, under r.3 of the *Management of Health and Safety at Work Regulations 1999*, there is a duty to carry out a suitable and sufficient assessment of the risks to the health and safety of non-employees arising from, or connected with, the employer's undertaking.

The term non-employee is wide in scope. Non-employees of a local authority include, for example, community care service users, informal carers, NHS staff, employees of independent care providers, self employed people providing a service to the local authority.

Case example: poor contracting

A local authority contracts out provision of its domiciliary community care services to a local independent care provider. However, the authority is in a financial crisis. It allocates inadequate funding to the contract. It also fails to check on the safety record of the contractor in question and to monitor the performance of the contract.

Poor practice and unsafe working flourish, leading to two serious accidents to the care provider's staff. The Health and Safety Executive considers whether to prosecute both the care provider and the local authority under respectively sections 2 and 3 of the *Health and Safety at Work Act 1974*.

For a comparable actual case, see: *HSE v London Borough of Barnet 1997*,which did involve manual handling: the contractor provided a refuse collection service.

Duties in respect of maintaining and reviewing manual handling equipment

Under *the Lifting Operations and Lifting Equipment Regulations 1998*, employers have various duties in respect of lifting equipment being used at work, including thorough examination. Under the *Provision and Use of Work Regulations 1998*, employers have various duties in respect of all equipment used at work, including lifting equipment. These duties include a strict obligation to maintain work equipment in an efficient state, efficient working order and in good repair.

When equipment (for lifting or otherwise) is used only by service users or informal carers, these two sets of regulations do not apply, because it would not be classed as work equipment. However, a duty to maintain equipment to a comparable standard would still arise under s.3 of the *Health and Safety at Work Act 1974* and r.3 of the *Management of Health and Safety at Work Regulations 1999* – both of which contain duties toward non-employees (see above, and see HSE 2002).

7 Common law of negligence

The law of negligence is for the most part 'common law' and is therefore to be found not in legislation but in the decisions of the law courts. It concerns harm (physical but sometimes psychological and in some circumstances financial) suffered. The claimant has to show that a duty of care was owed by the person who allegedly caused the harm, that the duty was breached by a careless action or omission, and that the breach directly caused the harm complained of. In the manual handling context, the law of negligence is likely to be used in two main ways.

First, non-employees who have suffered harm are not able to use health and safety at work legislation to bring a civil law claim for compensation. This is notwithstanding that they are in principle protected by s.3 of the *Health and Safety at Work Act 1974* and by r.3 of the *Management of the Health and Safety at Work Regulations 1999*. Therefore such claimants have to use the law of negligence.

Second, although employees can make use of some health and safety at work legislation (e.g. the *MHOR 1992*) to bring a civil compensation claim, they may nevertheless bring the claim in negligence as well. This would be just in case the claim were to fail under health and safety at work legislation. Although it is unlikely that a claim will succeed in negligence but fail under the *MHOR 1992*, this did occur in one Scottish case *(Fraser v Greater Glasgow Health Board)*.

Case example: injured social worker
In 1989, a social worker aged 30 visited a service user at home who weighed 15 stone. She found him lying half out of bed, with a neighbour there (who happened to be a nurse). The nurse guided the social worker in moving him; the latter felt something give in her lower back. She had received no training in lifting techniques. The case succeeded in the County Court, because it was reasonably foreseeable that she might be confronted with emergency situations. Although the situation was unusual, she should have been warned not to lift in such circumstances. Even if a long training course was not warranted, the risks of lifting should have been brought to her notice. There was no contributory negligence. She was eventually awarded over £200,000 damages (*Colclough v Staffordshire CC*).

Local authorities may owe a duty of care, too, to service users or to foster carers:

Case example: dropping a woman or providing a defective bed
A woman with disseminated sclerosis sought damages for negligence against the local authority. Her claim relating to the adequacy of the home help provided failed because it related to a statutory duty (involving policy, priorities, resources etc). However, the court noted that a claim in negligence might have been possible if, for instance, the home help had dropped the woman and injured her, or if the bed provided by the local authority had been defective, collapsed and caused injury (*Wyatt v Hillingdon LBC*).

Case example: foster carer
A woman had been acting as a paid foster carer to a handicapped teenage boy, placed with her by the council. She claimed that she had suffered a back injury when trying to catch, lift, save or restrain him. She argued that she should have been provided with a hoist or other lifting equipment earlier than she was; that the local authority failed properly to assess the placement; and that had it done so, it would not have placed such a heavy and disabled child with her. This was in the light of her complete lack of experience in caring for children with such a disability. She also claimed that she should have been trained in lifting techniques and should have been warned of the risks of the work. The local authority denied that it had a duty of care at all to her, let alone that it had acted without due care. The court found that it did owe a duty of care, and that a further hearing should take place to decide whether this duty had been breached through carelessness (*Beasley v Buckinghamshire CC*).

8 Contracting with the independent sector

Since community care was formally introduced in April 1993, local authorities have made increasing use of independent care providers to deliver community care services on local authorities' behalf. Nevertheless, overall, it is the local authority that retains statutory responsibility for meeting a person's community assessed care needs and for ensuring that a person's care plan is adhered to. As already outlined above, it is also clear that local authorities retain health and safety at work responsibilities even when services have been contracted out.

If local authorities are to fulfil these various legal responsibilities, then they have to pay serious attention to contracting. This should include matters such as the tendering process, allocating sufficient money to contracts, terms and conditions within the contract, penalty clauses, monitoring and review of contract performance.

Even if a contract does not specify particular matters, local authorities and care providers should bear in mind that there is an implied – even if not explicitly written – term in every contract for services, that the service will be delivered with reasonable care and skill *(Supply of Goods and Services Act 1982)*. Furthermore, there is nothing to stop a local authority setting contractual terms that exceed the 'care standards' associated with regulatory legislation such as the *Care Standards Act 2000* and the *Regulation of Care Scotland) Act 2001* (see e.g. *R v Cleveland CC, ex p Cleveland Care Homes Association)*.

Nevertheless, it sees that local authorities are sometimes tempted to take an 'out of sight out of mind' approach to the contracting out of services. However, as the following examples show, the consequences of such an approach can in some circumstances result in breach of health and safety law, in the failure of the local authority to perform its statutory duty to meet people's assessed community care needs, in breach of contract by care providers and in a wastage of public money.

Case example: contracting failure leads to health and safety at work breach
Failure in the contracting process, may lead to breaches of s.3 of the *Health and Safety at Work Act 1974* in respect of a local authority's duty to service users and to the staff of contracted providers (see example referred to above in section 6.5: *Health and Safety Executive v London Borough of Barnet*).

In the following manual handling related case, the local ombudsman found maladministration because, hedged in by restrictive limitations imposed by care providers, the local authority failed to understand its obligation to meet a service user's manual handling related needs.

Case example: local authority preventing itself from meeting a person's needs
A local authority had a list of approved home care providers; it would not go outside of this list. However, a particular approved provider could not provide the two carers that a risk assessment had identified as required to meet the assessed need of a woman to be hoisted in and out of bed. The provider had at first stated that it would not take on situations requiring two carers (because of the logistical difficulty of coordinating their whereabouts during the day); it later corrected this by stating that it would 'double up' its own carers, but would on no account work have its carers double up with carers from another agency.

By rigidly refusing to go outside of its approved provider list to enable 'spot purchasing', and by also anyway imposing a

£360.00 weekly limit on how much it would spend, the local authority was found to have 'fettered its discretion' and failed in its duty to meet a person's assessed need. The ombudsman pointed out that in the final analysis it was the needs of individuals that should have determined the council's response and not its contractual arrangements (*Cambridgeshire CC 2002*).

The following example likewise illustrates the typical sort of pressure that builds up on both local authority and care provider.

Example: conflicting manual handling risk assessments in the community

A local authority assesses that assistive manual handling is required for a person living in his own home. It concludes that the risks involved are relatively low and that there should be no problem for care agency staff. According to the contract specification, the agency is meant to ensure, through training and supervision, a certain level of competence amongst its staff. However, the agency now carries out its own risk assessment and demands that the local authority provide a hoist. It refuses to allow its carers to assist the person to transfer manually. Otherwise, it will withdraw provision of care altogether. The agency takes this stance because it knows its staff to be insufficiently competent and therefore at greater risk of injury.

The legal consequence of this is that the local authority will be in danger of breaching its duty to meet the person's needs. It has to find a way around the problem. This could be by way of persuading the care provider to change its mind and find competent staff, or going to another provider. In addition, the care provider risks being in breach of contract to take on reasonable care packages from the local authority, as well as to have competent staff.

Unnecessary expenditure, by local authority or service user, may also result from over simple rules imposed by care providers:

Example: blanket policy imposed by care provider

A care provider tries to impose a two-pronged policy to the effect that if any service user requires assistance with a transfer, then a hoist must be used and two paid staff must always be present. The local authority rejects this, since it takes account neither of the individual need of the service user, nor of the level of risk to staff. It could also result in unnecessary expenditure (where the risk does not demand two staff) by the local authority or by service users who have been assessed as able to pay for home care services.

The next example, concerning informal carers, again points to the need to avoid excessively rigid rules.

Example: blanket policy working with informal carers

A care agency states that its staff will not work with informal carers unless in every case the informal carer goes on a formal training course. The local authority resists this demand as excessive and not related to levels of risk in individual situations. While some informal carers may welcome such training, the authority argues that it will not be needed, appropriate or desired in every case. For instance, individual instruction and demonstration of manual handling tasks in the home may be perfectly adequate to manage risk in many cases; and some informal carers may anyway be unable or unwilling – for good reason – compulsorily to attend such training.

The following case illustrates just how complex matters can become and how deep disputes can run.

Case example: care home, manual handling dispute

A local authority places a man in a residential home and pays an extra amount, to cover additional personal assistance for him. This includes manual handling by way of assisted transfers. The care home manager subsequently refuses to provide such assistance and insists instead that the man use a hoist. The manager argues that two carers have been injured while manually handling the man; he argues that they were in fact injured when assisting other residents.

The manager supports his position with a risk assessment, which does not accord with that of the local authority.

The man refuses to be hoisted. The manager tells him he will have to stay in bed. His elderly parents begin to visit to provide their son with the personal assistance he needs. The man contacts his social worker, who tells him that he will have to stay in bed if he refuses to use a hoist. This is despite the fact that there is medical evidence that both hoist use and staying in bed will be detrimental.

The subsequent local government ombudsman investigation concluded that there was convincing evidence that the man could safely be given assisted transfers. He also found that the local authority had been in breach of its duty to meet the man's assessed needs. In addition, he pointed out that by continuing to pay an extra contractual amount of money to the home, for a service not being provided, the local authority was wasting public money (Redbridge LBC 1998).

The above examples have concerned the independent sector; it should be pointed out however that very similar tensions, between assessed need and actual care provision, can occur also in the case of local authority 'in-house' care services that also sometimes impose over restrictive rules concerning the tasks they are prepared to undertake.

9 National regulatory legislation

Registration and inspection of care providers takes place under the *Care Standards Act 2000* and is carried out in England by the Commission for Social Care Inspection (CSCI) and the Healthcare Commission. These two bodies replaced the National Care Standards Commission in April 2004. In Wales, the Care Standards Inspectorate for Wales is the responsible body. In Scotland, the Commission for the Regulation of Care is responsible under the *Regulation of Care (Scotland) Act 2001*. In Northern Ireland, the Regulation and Improvement Authority will in future be the responsible body under the *Health and Personal Social Services (Quality and Improvement and Regulation) (Northern Ireland) Order 2003*.

For the purpose of registration and inspection, various standards must be taken account of, although they do not have the force of law. In England, standards have been produced covering, for example, care homes for older people, care homes for younger adults, adult placements, domiciliary care children's homes, fostering services, residential special schools etc. Manual handling is in places referred to explicitly and in detail; for example, the standards on domiciliary care in England make a number of references in standard 12 (DH 2003a).

Example: domiciliary care national minimum standards

Standard 12 is entitled risk assessment. Under this standard, for instance, the registered person must ensure that a trained and qualified person undertakes risk assessment. A separate 'moving and handling' risk assessment must be undertaken by a member of staff trained for the purpose. A comprehensive plan to manage manual handling (and other) risks must be drawn up in consultation with the service user, his or her relatives or representatives. This must be included in the service user's plan and be kept in the person's home for staff to refer to. A copy should also be kept in the service user's personal file kept in the agency. The risk management plan should be implemented and reviewed annually or more frequently if necessary.

Only staff that are both trained to undertake risk assessments and competent to provide the care should be assigned to emergency situations. Two people fully trained in up to date manual handling techniques and in equipment use should always be involved in the provision of care when the need is identified from the manual handling risk assessment. The name and contact number of the organisation responsible for providing and maintaining any equipment under health and safety at work regulations should be recorded on the risk assessment.

The registered manager must ensure that manual handling equipment is in a safe condition to use, that inspections by manufacturers have taken place on time and if necessary reminds the organisation providing the equipment that a maintenance check is due.

Registration and inspection activity could in principle have a considerable impact on manual handling practices. However, much may depend on the local knowledge and particular interests of individual registration and inspection teams.

Example: varying inspection practices

In one locality, an inspection team diligently looks for a balanced approach to manual handling policy and practice in domiciliary care.

However, in another locality, the registration and inspection team applauds the blanket policies of domiciliary care providers (which include 'no lift' and 'two carer always present' policies), apparently unaware of the potential legal, professional and indeed financial objections. This approach appears to be based on a misunderstanding of the national minimum standards, which do indeed state that two people should always be involved - but only where 'the need is identified' by a risk assessment.

10 Discussion and conclusion

Discussion

This chapter has set out the legal underpinning for the taking of balanced decisions in social care, involving weighing up the safety of staff against the needs and rights of service users in the context of manual handling.

Nevertheless, concerns have been expressed that the courts' emphasis on such balanced decision making, in the light of human rights, could lead to a significant increase in manual handling injury to staff in social care – as well as in health care (e.g. Griffith, Stevens 2004).

At first sight, there would appear to be some logic underpinning such concerns, insofar as the courts have confirmed that in some circumstances higher risks may have to be entertained in order that a public service be provided. A further, potentially unattractive consequence is that if a higher risk has been properly assessed and managed, but injury still occurs, the employee may fail to win his or her personal injury litigation (e.g. *King v Sussex Ambulance Service)*.

However, this view needs to be considered more carefully.

- First, the courts have referred to the requirement to observe *both* the safety of paid staff, and the needs and rights of service users – and that neither set of rights overrides the other.

- Second, the courts have not perversely demanded that paid staff must undertake higher risks and suffer injury merely for the sake of it. They have simply referred to the importance of not overlooking the assessed needs and human rights of service users. With sufficient thought, assessment and negotiation, those needs and rights can often be observed precisely without undue risk to staff of injury.

- Third, the courts have referred to higher risks sometimes being taken by staff, but emphasised that this should not involve 'unacceptable' risks. For instance, in the *East Sussex* case, the judge stated quite clearly that in the case of hazardous lifts in the home, manual handling would be the exception. Health and Safety Executive guidance likewise states that unsafe work practices are not acceptable (HSE 2002).

- Fourth, a trawl through manual handling case law in health and social care over the past fifteen years or so (Mandelstam 2002), would seem to reveal that the main reason for manual handling injury is not due to the taking of well managed, higher risk. It is instead due, whether in the presence of higher or lower risk, to the absence of proper risk management – in terms of adequate allocation of resources, expertise, assessments, care plans, staffing, training, information, supervision and equipment etc. The gulf between properly managed and unmanaged risk is vast; indeed, it is clearly arguable that higher risk well managed will ultimately pose a lower risk of injury than lower risk poorly managed.

- Fifth, there may be a temptation for some organisations (and individual professionals), which are failing to assess and to manage risk competently, irrationally to blame human rights for consequent injuries to staff. The temptation should be resisted; to blame such failure on human rights is seriously mistaken and is a red herring.

Two relatively recent examples of legal cases, resulting in high compensation payments, illustrate the point. They both involved nurses who provided care for highly dependent people in hospital. Serious injury was caused in the one case due to absent or defective hoists, and a system of work that tolerated routine use of a lifting technique (the 'drag lift) well known to be unsafe *(Knott v Newham Healthcare NHS Trust)*. In the other case, the injury arose from an absence of adjustable height beds, and an ill maintained wheelchair *(Commons v Queen's Medical Centre)*. Legally, neither case had anything to do with the nurses taking higher risks because of people's human rights – but everything to do with basic organisational failure to manage risk.

- Sixth, a balanced approach is likely to make it more difficult for local authorities (and care providers) to execute the short cuts that result in poor risk management (and all that it entails: see point 4 immediately above).

    One such shortcut comes in the form of blanket policies that overlook the individual assessed needs of service users and sometimes breach their human rights. Driven typically by administrative convenience and financial constraint, these policies purport to protect staff that are poorly trained and supervised, and so are genuinely unable to assess and to manage even relatively straightforward and lower levels of risk. However, the policies are unacceptable, because they are operated and tolerated to the detriment of service users. In such circumstances, staff too may suffer detriment because, when confronted with risk (low or high, expected or unexpected), they are not equipped to identify, assess and manage it.

- Lastly, the courts' concern that blanket policies should not be applied, and that the needs and human rights of service users must be weighed in the balance as well as staff safety, is no more than basic good professional practice. Debate about human rights may have highlighted this, but good professional practice and existing law demanded such an approach even before the advent of the Human Rights Act.

    A balanced approach based on individual assessment means those professionals carrying out manual handling assessments and drawing up care plans may sometimes have to make difficult decisions. Answers will not always be black and white and 'served up on a plate'. Instead, informed, professional judgement has to be exercised in individual cases and has to be justifiable in terms of documented evidence, reasoning and conclusions.

Conclusion

This chapter has shown the breadth of legislation applying to manual handling related decisions in social care contexts. In order to comply with this legislation, the requirement of balanced decision-making is an inevitability. 'Tunnel vision', whether employed in respect of staff safety or the rights of service users simply will not do.

Acknowledgements

I would like to thank the many people with whom I have had discussions about the issues covered in this chapter over the last few years. Amongst these are Jacqui Smith (editor of The Column), Pippa Archibald (Southampton City Council), Norma Richardson (Disabled Living), Sue Smith (Hammersmith and Fulham Council) and Alison Cooke (Surrey County Council). Clearly any errors or infelicities are my own.

References

Cases

A&B, X&Y v East Sussex County Council [2003] EWHC 167 (Admin), High Court.

Barking and Dagenham London Borough Council (1998). Commission for Local Administration in England. Case 97/A/0337.

Beasley v Buckinghamshire County Council [1997] PIQR P473, High Court.

Cambridgeshire County Council (2002). Commission for Local Administration in England. Case 01/B/00305.

Colclough v Staffordshire County Council [1994] CL 94/2283, County Court, on liability; and (1997), High Court, unreported, see: Zindani 1998, p.189).

Commons v Queen's Medical Centre Nottingham University Hospital NHS Trust (2001, County Court, unreported).

Fraser v Greater Glasgow Health Board (1996) Rep LR 58, Court of Session, Scotland.

Hawkes v Southwark London Borough Council (1998), unreported, Court of Appeal.

HSE v Barnet London Borough Council (1997, unreported, Crown Court).

King v Sussex Ambulance NHS Trust [2002] EWCA Civ 935, Court of Appeal.

Knott v Newham Healthcare NHS Trust [2002] EWHC 2091, High Court.

Koonjul v Thameslink NHS Health Care Trust [2000] PIQR P123, Court of Appeal.

Price v United Kingdom (2001) 34 EHRR 1285, European Court of Human Rights.

R(Khana) v Southwark London Borough Council [2001] EWCA Civ 999, Court of Appeal.

R (On the application of G) v Barnet London Borough Council [2003] UKHL 57

R v Avon County Council, ex p M [1999] 2 CCLR 185, High Court.

R v Bexley LBC, ex p B [1995] 1 CLYB 3225, High Court..

R v Birmingham City Council, ex p Killigrew [2000] 3 CCLR 109, High Court.

R v Bouldstridge (reported in Kelso P (2000). 'He only wanted to end his wife's pain. He ended up court, at 84'. The Guardian, 7th June 2000, p.1).

R v Cleveland County Council, ex p Cleveland Care Homes Association [1993] 158 LgRevR 641, High Court.

R v Enfield London Borough Council, ex p Bernard [2002] EWHC 2282 (Admin), High Court.

R v Gloucestershire County Council, ex p Barry [1997] 2 All ER 1, House of Lords.

R v Gloucestershire County Council, ex p Mahfood (1995) 160 LGRR 321, High Court.

R v Gloucestershire County Council, ex p RADAR [1996] COD 253, High Court.

R v Haringey London Borough Council, ex p Norton [1998] 1 CCLR 168, High Court.

R v Lancashire County Council, ex p RADAR [1996] 4 All ER 422, Court of Appeal.

R v Leonard Cheshire Foundation, ex p Heather [2002] EWCA Civ 366, Court of Appeal.

R v North Yorkshire County Council, ex p Hargreaves [1994] 26 BMLR 121, High Court.

R v Kensington and Chelsea Royal Borough, ex p Kujti m [1999] 2 CCLR 341, Court of Appeal.

R v Sefton Metropolitan Borough Council, ex p Help the Aged [1997] 3 FCR 573, Court of Appeal.

Redbridge London Borough Council 1998. Commission for Local Administration in England, case

95/C/1472 and 95/C/2543.
Stainton v Chorley and South Ribble NHS Trust (1998), unreported, High Court.
White v Clitheroe Royal Grammar School (2002), Preston County Court.
Wyatt v Hillingdon London Borough Council [1978] 76 LGR 727, Court of Appeal.

Other references

Audit Commission (2000). Fully equipped: the provision of equipment to older or disabled people by the NHS and social services in England and Wales. London: Audit Commission.
CCD 8/2001. Single shared assessment of community care needs. Edinburgh: Scottish Executive.
CCD 2/2003. Community Care and Health (Scotland) Act 2002: new statutory rights for carers: guidance. Edinburgh: Scottish Executive.
CSP (2002). Chartered Society of Physiotherapy. Guidance on manual handling for chartered physiotherapists. London: CSP, p.11.
DH (2001). Department of Health. Carers and people with parental responsibility for disabled children. London: DH.
DH (2003). Department of Health. Direct payments guidance. London: DH.
DH (2003a). Department of Health. Domiciliary care: national minimum standards: regulations. London: DH.
DH/SO (1991). Department of Health; Scottish Office. Care management and assessment: practitioners' guide. London: DH, SO.
DHSS (1991). Department of Health and Social Services (Northern Ireland). Care management: guidance on assessment and the provision of community care. Belfast: DHSS.
DHSSPS (2003). Carers and Direct Payments Act (Northern Ireland) 2002: guidance. Belfast: Department of Health and Social Services and Public Safety.
Griffith R, Stevens M (2004). Manual handling and the lawfulness of no-lift policies. Nursing Standard; vol.18, no.21, 4-10 February 2004.
Henwood M (1998). Ignored and invisible? Carers' experience of the NHS. London: Carers National Association.
HSC (1998). Health and Safety Commission. Manual handling in the health services. Sudbury: HSC, p.43.
HSC 2001/008; LAC (2001)13. Community equipment services. London: Department of Health.
HSC 2002/001; LAC(2002)1. Guidance on the single assessment for older people. London: Department of Health.
HSE (2004). Health and Safety Executive. Manual handling: Manual Handling Operations Regulations 1992: guidance on regulations. Sudbury: HSE, p.8.
HSE (2002). Health and Safety Executive. Handling home care: achieving safe, efficient and positive outcomes for care workers and clients. Sudbury: HSE, p.3.
LAC(2002)13. Fair access to care services: guidance on eligibility criteria for adult social care. London: Department of Health.
Mandelstam M (2002). Manual handling in health and social care: an A-Z of law and practice. London: Jessica Kingsley Publishers.
Marriott H (2003). The selfish pig's guide to caring. Clifton-upon-Teme: Polperro Heritage Press.
NAFWC 9/02. Health and social care for adults: creating a unified and fair system for assessing and managing care. Cardiff: Welsh Assembly.
NAFW (2001). Carers and Disabled Children Act 2000: guidance. Cardiff. National Assembly for Wales.
SI 2002/57. Fostering Services Regulations 2002.
Zindani G (1998). Manual handling: law and litigation. London: CLT Professional Publishing.

3 Creating change

Mike Fray BSc (Hons) BHSc MCSP SRP
Director: Handling Movement and Ergonomics Ltd

1 Introduction

Organisational change is a complex and well researched area. It is the aim of this chapter to explain the processes of change management and discuss the behaviour that may be seen in the organisation, and people, in the changing situation. The discussion will show that in many situations the process of change is not given enough attention, and guidance will be given to the areas where change management may need to be used and suggest some of the strategies that may be appropriate. Examples will be given of how and where they have been implemented successfully.

For the most part the development of safe systems of work, in the moving and handling field, have been focused on the physical improvements in the workplace. Large-scale improvements have been seen through the application of ergonomics and risk management to handling problems. Successful interventions that reduce the risk to handlers from moving people are seen in the workplace in:

- The provision of improved equipment, e.g. the development of better hoists and slings.
- Changes in the work methods and routines, e.g. replacing lifting with sliding in bed to trolley transfers or promoting a person's independence.
- Improved knowledge and skills, through improved training and information.

All of these intervention strategies are unlikely to impact on safer practice if the organisation does not accept them into its normal practice. The problems with these situations are that in addition to the technical information, risk assessments and safer systems, the improvements in practice can only be seen if the carers and staff undergo a level of behavioural change. When investigating change there is a fine line between organisational change and individual's changes in behaviour. All organisations are made up of groups of individuals and one type of change cannot occur without the other.

As an example of how the change process can be difficult to implement we need only examine the issues of the 'Underarm Drag Lift' of moving a person from sitting to standing. The 1987 version of the *Guide to The Handling of Patients (RCN/NBPA, 1987)* specifically suggested that a series of activities called underarm drag lifts should be avoided because they were deemed to be hazardous to both handlers and the person being moved. Many years on, after hours of training, information and supervised practice, the underarm drag lifts continue to be a concern for the moving and handling fraternity as they are still seen in practise. The use of underarm drag lifts is a particularly intriguing situation. If you ask care staff about the practice they will usually acknowledge the known hazards and yet they continue to use the technique. Such are the complexities of human behaviour and the change process (see also chapter 9).

2 Theories of change management

From the plethora of published material on the issues of change management there are many models that might seem to be applicable to the areas of handling in health and social care. The aim of this section is to explore a few models of the change process and give examples of how and why they may help anyone who wishes to change behaviour within their own workplace. In his book *"The Theory and Practice of Change Management" John Hayes (2002)* states, 'Change is often managed less effectively than it might be because those responsible for managing it fail to attend to some of the critical aspects of the change process'. It is the key stages of the change process that are described here.

One widely recognised model of change is that described by *Lewin (1947, 1951)*. Lewin's model suggests that there are three key stages to any change.

- Unfreeze or unlock from the existing level of behaviour.
- Change the behaviour or move to a new level
- Refreeze the behaviour at the new level.

Re-examining the continued use of the underarm drag lift in current practice, using Lewin's model it could be argued that although much effort has been made to create a new modified behaviour, the workforce never unlearned the original behaviour. Therefore they will always revert to their previous learned activity whenever the change motivation is weak.

Lewin's model can be applied to almost all change situations to analyse the successes and failures of the change process. The model was expanded by *Lippet, Watson, Westley, (1958)* who suggested that the moving phase could itself, be divided into three distinct stages:

- The clarification or diagnosis of the problem
- The examination of the alternatives and establishing the plan of action for change
- The transformation of intentions into actions to bring about change

These additions create a clear process that is applicable to the situations of the care handling environment.

These stages can also be seen in the underarm drag lift scenario.

External change

For most care organisations the original information to change the practice and remove the underarm drag lift came from external sources. E.g. RCN, HSE. Direction given from outside the organisation or change group is sometimes seen as unhelpful or a burden to the group.

Recognition

The staff using the technique had little knowledge regarding the dangers of the underarm drag lift technique and consequently did not perceive that there was indeed a problem to be resolved. *Lewin (1951)* stated that one of the key facts in this phase is dissatisfaction with the current behaviour, which obviously did not occur with the underarm drag lift and change was not sought.

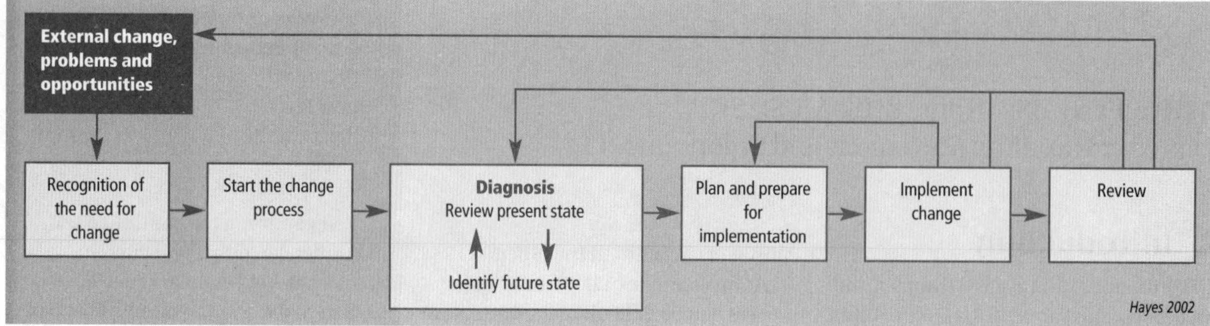

Start of the process

The point where the need for change becomes a desire to change is accepted as the pivotal point. In the example, the stimulus for change was initiated from the RCN, external to the organisations. The care organisations were not involved in the process to decide on change and consequently there was not a clear starting point when the need for change became a desire to change.

Diagnosis

If the desire to change has been accepted, it is important to examine the present state and consider what the future behaviour will be. Information needs to be gathered to examine what was wrong with the initial behaviour and how things need to be improved. This diagnosis phase allows an appropriate plan to be developed to facilitate the change.

When considering the removal of the underarm drag lift from current practice this stage may not have occurred. Even in areas that had the recognition and desire they may have had little knowledge of the alternatives and the equipment that was available. In many care organisations there may have been no alternatives available to enable the carers to move clients more safely. Without the physical options and a good change environment the group are always likely to revert back to the initial behaviour.

Plan and prepare for Implementation

In respect of manual handling situations there are two aspects of planning for change. One is the physical and systems based issues, e.g. the risk assessment, the equipment, the change in method or technique. The second is to plan the change method, how are the group going to be introduced to this new system.

It is simply not enough to say, "The underarm drag lift is dangerous, stop doing it". If it were that simple, it would not be seen in current practice.

Review

Review is often understood as being a retrospective measure of whether the change has occurred. In reality a continuous input of motivation is required to keep the change process moving. This would account for one of the reasons that training, in isolation, provides weak change outcomes. It is a one shot process and little is built into the monitoring and review phase. Even annual update training is likely to prove ineffective, as there will be sufficient time between sessions to revert to the original practice.

It is important when attempting to put the change process in place, that all of the appropriate stages are given due consideration. There must be a strategy for change and the methods of implementation clearly thought through before the process begins. Such strategies need not be set in tablets of stone, flexibility during any given change situation may well facilitate the process.

Even with a well planned approach there will always be certain elements of our organisational structures that may show resistance to the change process. It is important to appreciate why people resist change in order to counteract those barriers. *Kotter and Schlesinger (1979)* identified four key reasons for resisting change:

- **Self interest.** People resist change if they perceive that they may lose out in some way. This could be as simple as loss of power or input in decision-making. There are many individuals that simply resent being told what to do. Similarly, staff often consider that their own approach is the best. An example of this could be the statement " I've done this for years and I don't have a back problem".

- **Misunderstanding and lack of trust.** Unlikely though it may seem, efforts to create safer working systems can be negatively received, and responses such as 'if we use hoists it becomes impersonal', or 'now with all this equipment they will ask us to do more or work on our own' have been heard in the workplace.

- **Different assessments or expectations.** There are often different perceptions of the change process from the people involved. If we examine the purchasing of a new hoist for a small care home; the manager of the home needs to see some improvements in the delivery of care, the Back Care Advisor wishes to improve practice and reduce the risks of injury, the handlers need the equipment to be quicker, easier and safer to use.

This conflict is seen when the benefits of the change are too biased to one side or the other. If the change is seen to benefit the management structure and add further work for the staff the there is likely to be little co-operation with the process.

- **Low tolerance for change.** In some work areas people simply demonstrate a low tolerance for change. It should be clear to anyone working in the fields of health and social care that they need to be able to work in a changing structure. As such they should have a high tolerance for change. However, many exhibit signs of change fatigue due to the constant pattern of change in these rapidly developing areas. It is sometimes noted that staff consider that change is for change's sake and that there is little benefit to the staff or the people receiving care.

These signals of resistance to change are best identified in the personal behaviours of the change group. *Fink et al (1971)* suggested that there is in all organisations some energy that wishes to maintain the status quo and some energy that is willing to change. The authors created an identifiable transition cycle that an individual may follow through the change process. The energy levels that are available to support the change process vary with each stage in any group or organisation. At any given time, depending upon where an individual is in the process, they can be supporting or fighting the change. *John Adams et al (1976)* described an extension of Fink's cycle. This shows seven stages of behaviour related to the change process:

- **Awareness/shock.** Often the news of change comes unannounced. This creates a state of anxiety in the individual. This almost seems to paralyse the individual and they show little sign of moving towards the new behaviour. It is important to prepare people for change to reduce the time spent in this phase.

- **Denial.** This stage is sometimes called defensive retreat. The individual will work hard to avoid the change and will cling on to the previous behaviours. Resistance to change is at its highest at this point and the change manager needs to use all his/her powers of negotiation to help the individual through.

- **Depression.** At the end of the denial stage the individual has to face up to the situation that the change is necessary or it is going to happen whether they like it or not. The feelings of depression are usually associated with the realisation that the change is out of their control.

- **Letting go/acceptance of reality.** The realisation that the change is necessary is characterised by the letting go of the previous behaviours. It is sometimes described as a loss to the individual and a period of mourning is sometimes observed. This stage is where the individual is most vulnerable and therefore has the greatest emotional need. The change manager will need to support staff closely through this phase to encourage them through to the next phase.

- **Testing.** As the individual understands the change is necessary there comes an evaluation phase where trial and error behaviour or testing out new behaviours is observed. This forms part of the 'on the job' practice and skill learning phase. This is a positive energy phase and the individual is really working towards the new task.

- **Consolidation.** The completion of the changing behaviour stage. The individual has moved to the new behaviour, which has begun to be the normal behaviour. In some processes there is very little consolidation, this can lead to poor understanding of the behaviour, which may in time allow the old behaviour to reappear. It is especially important at this stage to reinforce the behaviour by reward and compliment or by completing closure on the old behaviour.

- **Internalisation/reflection and learning.** The final stage of the change within the individual. The full understanding of the new behaviour has been achieved. At this phase the individual can appreciate how the new situation has improved the work situation and that the previous actions were not as effective. A changed individual with good behavioural consolidation is very useful to allow the conversion of others within a group of workers.

In community healthcare and social services work there are many examples of safer working practices not being adopted because of problems in the change process. The conflicts and extremes of personal behaviour can be seen in situations where a care package has not been to the liking of an individual or family group. This is readily noted when a person does not wish a hoist to be introduced. The care package suggests that a hoist should be used following a risk assessment based on the handling and care needs. The person sees no benefit from the change as their family carers are lifting them at present. If the change is imposed they feel disempowered, they feel as if they are in a situation that is out of their control and their response is one of anger and resentment. In these situations the process rarely gets out of the recognition phase and the change is never started. The people in the change group would clearly be in the shock/denial or depression behaviour patterns as they consider that the change is being forced upon them.

The development of these conflict situations can lead to difficult court cases. Once a major point of conflict has been created it takes a large amount of effort to retrieve the situation and it may never be completely resolved. The change management literature would suggest that some time spent considering the change process may well be beneficial.

3 Managing the change

It is the domain of the Back Care Advisor, manager or Health and Safety Advisor to create and facilitate change within the work area. Due to the developments in both technology and knowledge within the field there are usually good physical solutions available for most care handling situations e.g. provision of equipment or changes in methods. In order to effect a successful change from existing behaviour to the new improved method, there are a number of strategies that may help. In describing the behaviours that are seen with resistance to change *Kotter and Schlesinger (1979)* also described the strategies that may help facilitate a more successful change. The change agent will need to consider which of these is suitable and at which stage in the process to apply them.

Education and persuasion

One of the most frequently used ways of minimising the resistance to change is to educate people about the need to change. Many styles of information and education may be used to invigorate the individual or organisation towards change. Although education is useful at all stages of the process it is particularly important in the recognition phase. Handlers and people alike are comfortable with 'we've always done it this way' and making them aware that change is needed is a key step.

These are some approaches that may help persuade people that changes are needed in handling practice and to assist the process.

a *The Legal Argument.* The use of legislation as a tool for change has mixed effect. Some people respond well and appreciate the benefits of being protected at work, others see health and safety legislation as a distant set of rules from government. If people can grasp the level of empowerment that the legislation grants the individual, then it can be a most powerful tool. Educating or empowering people so that they can say no to hazardous activities is however, sometimes difficult in the face of emotional pressure from others in the care environment, e.g. patients, service users, family or peers. Recent legal cases have raised the profile of some Human Rights issues in the care handling world. All handlers and people receiving care should have a working knowledge of the Human Rights issues and an understanding of how they balance with each other. A key part of the legal argument strategy is that all involved understand the process of risk assessment and balanced decision making (see chapter 2).

b *The Ethical Argument.* The ethical argument that no one should be injured when they go to work is also a useful tool for raising the awareness of hazards in the workplace. There are many sources of injury data for all the areas involved in care handling, both local and national. People respond better to information that is related to them, therefore, where possible, quote cases in their local area. Research a case that relates to your change group and use it to your advantage. e.g. 'Fred in the next unit hurt his back doing this very activity and has been off for a month' or we 'have retired some staff due to back trouble and this is their story.'

c *The Financial Argument.* The cost of implementing change is a common barrier to change at management or board level. All involved in the change process in manual handling will know that the implementation of change usually involves some investment of money or time or both. When considering proposals to management for investment it is important that the financial argument is well considered. A cost benefit analysis should clarify that there will be tangible benefits to the organisation implementing the change.

The largest cost for most care organisations is staff time and consequently any reductions in sickness absence should be factored into the argument. These cost benefits can also be argued in terms of time, as safer handling systems and practice are more efficient and therefore save time. There may also be other organisational benefits that can be drawn into the argument: improvements in the quality of care, patient satisfaction and reduced length of stay through the provision of appropriate rehabilitation.

It cannot be stressed highly enough that if the change in behaviour requires financial investment then it must be secured for the change to be successful. How many safer handling training sessions include information on equipment that is not available in all areas of the workplace?

d *The Evidence Argument.* The application of ergonomics to problems related to assisting people to move is a powerful tool to support change. Knowledge gained from biomechanics, work physiology, psychology and the measurements of anthropometry can all be used in the design of a user-centred solution that reduces the risks to all handlers and people involved with movement activities. Though the evidence surrounding the manual handling in health and social care settings is not extensive, there is some evidence to create a good argument for encouraging changes in practice. *Hignett et al (2003)* contains a systematic manual handling literature review and can be used easily to support changes in the workplace. This work has been further developed in the practical chapters (11-18) of this publication.

e *Professional Standards.* All professional bodies and organisations that support handlers in health and social care set out professional guidance and information that assists the development of safer systems for moving and handling. e.g. NBE, RCN, CSP, COT, Unison, etc. It may be appropriate to be familiar with the national and professional guidance to support the change process.

Participation and involvement

It is essential that staff, carers and those receiving care are involved in the decisions surrounding the change process. Involvement in the choice of practice will give at least a part ownership and helps the process to succeed. Several styles of participation in this process have proved successful:

a Participative workshops will aid in the realisation of hazards in the workplace. They can be used to show that the old practice is difficult or hard. Comparison with a new method should show them the new is better than the old. Confirmation can be improved with collecting factual information on the task. An example of this could be seen when introducing slide sheets to an area. Demonstrate sliding with and without slide sheets. Ask the carers to compare one to another, and then reinforce the message by measuring the forces needed to complete the tasks with a force meter. It is important to ensure that the new methods do not hinder the workers e.g. does it take more time, need more staff, will the carers have easy access to the new equipment?

b In some situations a good facilitator can adopt a problem solving approach with a group. A problem is set to the group, and with the aid of the facilitator the group work out a suitable solution. This approach may be a high risk strategy, as a skilled facilitator is needed to aid the process to the appropriate conclusion.

c Another useful participative approach is to include carers, staff and users in the process of equipment evaluation. In this situation the aim is to achieve the thought that 'we helped choose this equipment so we know it's the best thing for us to use'. The evaluation and trialling of equipment is a useful tool when trying to overcome the barriers of introducing equipment into a home care package when resistance is seen (see 'user trials' in chapter 4).

Facilitation and support

If negative feelings towards the change process are evident then it is usually important to consider the empathetic and sympathetic approach of facilitation and support to the individuals. This can be provided in a range of ways:

a Training is usually seen as a good start to improve the level of support in the change process. This does need to include a caring approach to the learner and not be dictatorial. Good quality training can bring the change group together and support individuals that may be struggling with the process. Cohesiveness of the change group can lead to a much stronger compliance and longer lasting consolidation of new behaviour due to peer review and direction.

b Many change agents are confronted with the statement 'you don't know what it's like out in the real world'. Co-working is one way to overcome these issues. Spending time in the care environment will demonstrate to both the change agent and the carers that the process works and is complimentary to the care environment.

c Supervision can also help with the process and support people through a period of change and all aspects of the counselling and guidance mechanisms can be used.

Skilled facilitators are an excellent addition to any workforce and will assist the change process. As stated previously the willingness to spend time preparing the change process as well as the factual content of the change is key. It is appropriate to ask the question, "what support or assistance will be needed if the change does not go smoothly?" A good facilitator will have a range of methods to help the individuals or groups through the difficult periods.

Negotiation and agreement

As part of the acceptance of the new methods and behaviours, there are likely to be some issues that will be difficult for the group to agree. It may be appropriate at this time to offer negotiation to assist conclusion. The process of negotiation may have to include some of the 'letting go' stage from both the change manager and the individual, or group, in the change process. It is important to appreciate when pursuing change that both sides of the process need to have tangible benefits. Change is often resisted, as the group perceive that 'it's just another thing they want us to do.' If there is give and take within the process there may be a better acceptance of the change. Once the negotiation has been completed there may be the need for formal or informal agreements to be created to confirm the decisions and statements made. These will form part of the monitoring and consolidation phase to keep reminding the group of the change arrangements.

An example of these formal agreements are sometimes seen when a person is returning to work following an injury (see chapter 7). Job restrictions and conditions are designed to support a safe and effective return, and all interested parties must sign up to the contract to ensure undue pressure is not placed on any individual or group.

One less formal method of negotiation is to try and achieve a consensus decision from a particular group. Consensus decisions are notably difficult to achieve in technical data areas but there have been good examples of this method in the field of manual handling. For example, the Derbyshire Inter-Agency Group Code of Practice, *(Fray et al 2001)*, the Buckinghamshire Moving and Handling Protocol, *(Douglas and Mowbray 2001)* and the *All Wales NHS Manual Handling Training Passport and Information Scheme (2003)*. Although reaching a consensus can be very difficult and fraught with the emotions of the change process, the realisation and format of the group decision does lead to very good consolidation within the formative group.

Manipulation and co-option

If a change process is not working smoothly a change manager may choose a more subversive method to manipulate people to agree. The power of creating systems that are, duty bound, to be followed is not unusual. One strategy that is often seen in this area is that of co-opting. The change facilitator co-opts someone into the system who is challenged and possibly rewarded to assist the change process. This may be an internal or external appointment and can be very effective. Questions are sometimes raised about the group dynamic, as it can be perceived that the group has been hijacked by another influence. There are also the emotions of the person brought in as they often feel like an outsider to the group. If the change was dependent on the infiltration of this key individual the lasting effects of the change may be poor as they may leave the group soon after the change and not facilitate the consolidation phase.

Implicit or explicit coercion

The final strategy for creating change is down to the creation of a power situation where the change manager has the ability to create a need in the group by either offering to give or remove something of value. It would be positive to think that the rewards of not having accidents and injuries in a workplace would be sufficient but is very unlikely. Rewards for performance or punishment for poor performance may hold the key in some change situations.

Some care organisations have been able to consider the disciplinary approach to change behaviour, in particular in areas where clearly defined procedures are documented. It would always be suggested as a last resort, but possibly an important step to take to show how important the compliance with the new behaviour is.

If reward or punishment is the driving force behind the change there is always the possibility of the change reverting to the initial behaviour once the coercion has been removed.

Review and monitoring

The process of review and monitoring in most intervention based areas is accepted as being a physical measure of how well the new behaviour is being adopted. When considering the change process, review needs to be a constant and forever evolving process that assists the group to comply with the new behaviour. All of the methods outlined above can be part of the process for moving the change forward. Ultimately there may be a stage where the group have reached an acceptably high level of consolidation and the new behaviour has become the normal behavioural response. Even when these situations are evident it is important that the change manager continues to evaluate performance to prevent the behaviour reverting back to the initial situation.

4 Conclusion

The skills, knowledge and experience of the individuals whose responsibility is to bring about change in manual handling practice in any organisation, group or individual are varied and complex. They will require a working knowledge of health and safety, and care legislation and how it relates to their workplace. They also require a good knowledge of ergonomics and have the ability to devise solutions to the wide variety of workplace problems. They must be expert communicators for the purpose of training and collecting information from all the interested parties and be familiar with the vast range of equipment that is available in the market place (for further definition of the Back Care Advisor role, *NBE 2001, 2003*). All this knowledge and skill may however come to little if the process of managing change is not taken into account.

The change process can be applied to both individuals or to groups or to whole organisations. The intricacies of people's response to stimuli make the path to change difficult and full of barriers and pitfalls. Adequate preparation and planning of the process, involvement at all stages of the interested parties and the appropriate level of empathy, support and encouragement throughout the process does however increase the potential for successful change.

Robson and Beary (1995) indicate that the skills associated with the facilitation and management of the change process are more necessary in today's workplace than ever. People's rising expectations of work, their need for personal development and a reluctance to be treated en masse means that an individual approach to change management is more and more likely to be needed. It is therefore important to spend time on creating a good environment for change as well as designing the physical nature of the safer system of work.

The role of the Back Care Advisor is relatively new in terms of the health and social care workplace. The discussion in this chapter has shown that change management is an essential skill for the Back Care Advisor. This role is one of strategic importance within these organisations and should be recognised by senior management to enable the Back Care Advisor to utilise the change process to facilitate improvements in practice and help reduce the prevelence and effects of accidents and injuries at work.

References

Adams J, Hayes J and Hopson B (1976). Transitions: Understanding and Managing Personal Change, London: Martin Robertson

All Wales NHS Manual Handling Training Passport and Information Scheme (2003) www.wales.nhs.uk/documents/NHS_manual_handling_passpor.pdf

Douglas S, Mowbray C (2001). 'Buckinghamshire Inter-Agency Moving and Handling Protocol'. The Column August 2001, NBE.

Fink SL, Beak J, Taddeo K (1971). 'Organisational Crisis and Change', Journal of Applied Behavioural Science, 7(1) pp.15–37

Fray M et al (2001). Care Handling for People in Hospital, Community and Educational Settings. A Code of Practice. DIAG

Hayes J (2002). The Theory and Practice of Change Management. Palgrave, Hampshire UK

Hignett S, Crumpton E, Ruszala S, Alexander P, Fray M, Fletcher B, Evidence Based Patient Handling. – Tasks, Equipment and Interventions. London: Routledge.

Kotter JP, Schlesinger LA (1979). 'Choosing Strategies For Change', Harvard Business Review, March/April in Hayes J (2002). The Theory and Practice of Change Management. Palgrave, Hampshire UK

Lewin K (1947). Frontiers in Group Dynamics, Human Relations, 1, pp5–41

Lewin K (1951). Field Theory in Social Science, New York, Harper and Row.

Lippet R, Watson J, Westley B (1958). The Theory of Planned Change, New York: Harcourt, Brace, Jovanovich

NBE, 2002. Essential Back-Up. 2nd Edition. NBE

NBE, 2001. Parameters of Person Specification for Back Care Advisor. www.nationalbackexchange.org.uk/index_files/pdf/trainer

Robson M, Beary C (1995). Facilitating, Gower, Hampshire, England

RCN/NBPA (1987). The Guide to the Handling of Patients. 2nd Edition. RCN/NBPA

4

Ergonomics in health and social care

Sue Hignett PhD MSc MCSP MErgS EurErg
Director, HEPSU, Loughborough University

1 Introduction

This chapter presents an overview of ergonomics in health and social care. It gives examples of a wide range of patient handling activities and shows how ergonomics can be used to reduce the risk of musculoskeletal disorders (MSDs).

A broad outline of Ergonomics is given to identify the two central principles of:

- Design, for products, systems and interventions
- Change, relating to organisational systems and interventions.

There are sections giving information about epidemiology, task analysis, postural analysis, participatory ergonomics, user trials and case studies to illustrate how ergonomics methods have been applied in health and social care.

2 Ergonomics

Ergonomics is the '*scientific discipline concerned with the understanding of interactions among humans and other elements of a system, and the profession that applies theoretical principles, data and methods to design in order to optimise human well-being and overall system performance*' *(IEA, 2000)*. It is useful to summarise ergonomics practice in the two following objectives *(Sanders and McCormick, 1993)*:

1. To enhance the effectiveness and efficiency with which work and other activities are carried out.
2. To enhance certain desirable human values, including improved safety, reduced fatigue and stress, increased comfort, increased job satisfaction and improved quality of life.

There are various models which have been used to illustrate the theory and practice of ergonomics. Figure 4.1a gives a model which is commonly used to show the theoretical background, drawing on physical dimensions (e.g. anthropometry, biomechanics, engineering and physiology), cognitive dimensions (psychology) and organisational dimensions (management studies, sociology). In contrast figure 4.1b proposes a model to represent the interactions at an individual level (micro), group level (meso) and organisational level (macro). These three levels can be clearly seen in the example for office design in figure 4.2.

Figure 4.1. Models of ergonomics (*Hignett and Wilson 2004*)

a 1980's

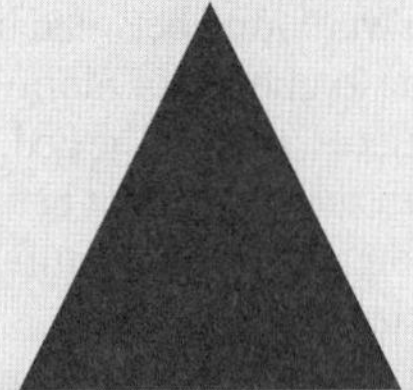

b 2000's

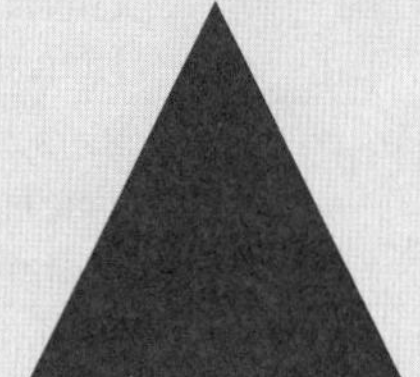

> **Figure 4.2**. Example of multi-level application of ergonomics for office design (*Hignett 2001a*)
>
> The micro level intervention is represented by modifications to a single physical work station or working pattern for one person to address an individual problem.
>
> At the meso level all the employees in the office might be involved in a group intervention looking at the work flow and interactions between individuals as well as other groups of workers (physical work movements in the office).
>
> At the macro level the systems of the organisation impinging on the office design would be considered including working patterns (hot desking, flexible working) as well as communication channels for introducing change. There may be issues relating to product design, specifying products from preferred or single suppliers, and resources.

In practise there are two key elements which define ergonomics, these are design *(Helander, 1997)* and change *(Caccamise, 1995)*. The design element is used in all projects to a greater or lesser extent whereby a product design may be evaluated and recommendations made or an organisational system (e.g. risk management) may be designed. The change element is more applicable at a systems level when an intervention programme is being implemented. The aim is to achieve a change in the working practices, attitudes, behaviours etc. There are ergonomic methods which can be used operationally to assist with the implementation of new systems as well as for evaluation, e.g. participatory ergonomics.

In order to address a range of dimensions the ergonomics practitioner will almost always use multiple methods, often mixing qualitative and quantitative, in order to gain as much information as possible about the complex systems of human interactions.

3 Epidemiology of back problems in nursing

Pheasant summarised epidemiological issues about back problems in nurses in the previous edition of this publication

(1998). He defined epidemiology as the branch of medical science which deals with the statistics of disease by identifying the risk factors which are statistically associated with the onset and development of diseases. He suggested that back problems were difficult to study epidemiologically for a number of reasons.

1 Back problems have a diverse pathophysiology; the back can go wrong in a number of different ways.
2 Back problems have multifactorial aetiology: a person may be at risk for a number of different reasons. Some of these risk factors are external to the individual concerned – most importantly the nature of their work. Others are specific to an individual – for example relating to the person's lifestyle, physical make-up and genetic endowment.
3 Back problems have a diverse natural history. Many episodes are short lived but they may be precursors of something worse to come. There is a danger that the results of surveys based on the self reporting of symptoms may be swamped by these relatively trivial episodes – and the risk factors which are associated with more serious problems may be hidden.
(See also chapters 5 and 8).

There have been various epidemiological studies studying back pain in nurses *(Stubbs et al, 1983; Seccombe and Ball, 1992; Smedley et al, 1995)*. These have all found that the incidence and prevalence are significantly higher than in comparison with the general population.

Over a 5 year period (1996/7-2000/1) over 61,100 healthcare workers suffered an injury reportable to the Health and Safety Executive (HSE) under the *Reporting of Injuries, Diseases and Dangerous Occurrences Regulations (RIDDOR) 1995* (www.hse.gov.healthservices/index.htm).

The rate of over 3-day injuries in the health services sector fell by 5% in 2002/03 to 9,551 from 10,077 in 2001/02. However 53% (5,027 of 9,551) of the over 3-day injuries were as a result of handling accidents. This compared with 17% due to slips or trips and 14% as a result of physical assault *(HSE, 2003)*.

The National Audit Office (NAO, 2003) compared the level of accidents and sickness absence in the NHS with a previous report in 1996. They found that the overall proportion of accidents due to moving and handling had increased from 17% to 18% whereas a decrease was reported for needle stick/sharps incidents and for slips and trips. The major reason for staff absence in the NHS is sickness at an average rate of 4.9% compared with an average of 3.7% for other public sector organisations. When looking at the implementation of risk management policies the NAO found that only 12% of Trusts included risk assessment in induction training and that there were often different reporting routes to the Trust Board for clinical and non-clinical risks.

More recently *Eriksen et al (2004)* looked at the predictors of low back pain in a group of 4266 Norwegian nurses' aides in a prospective study over 15 months. They found that, after a wide range of adjustments, low back pain symptoms were predicted by:

- Frequent positioning of patients in bed.
- Perceived lack of support from immediate superior.
- Perceived lack of pleasant and relaxing culture in the work unit.

These findings agree with *Smedley et al (1995)* where a significant association was found between back pain and the frequency of manually moving patients around the bed, manual transferring patient between bed and chair, and manual lifting patients from the floor.

Engkvist (2004) also attempted to identify predicting factors with a prospective (13 month) study with 127 nurses in Australia. Cluster analysis revealed five well-defined clusters but the majority of accidents occurred during patient transfer in the bed or to/from the bed. Engkvist found a number of contributing factors including a lack of transfer devices and a reluctance to use transfer devices. *Kneafsey (2000)* explored occupational socialisation in relation to patient handling activities, suggesting that manual handling could be viewed 'as an area of ritualistic practice'. By this she means that the methods of transferring patients have been developed over time and that manual techniques (rather than the use of equipment) may be the established norm of behaviour. So students and new staff may be socialised into a culture where patient handling is badly managed and change can only be introduced if the implementation strategy is aimed at the staff members who set the norms of behaviour. This may be the ward managers and senior nursing staff but may also be nursing aides and auxiliaries who carry out many of the care handling activities.

4 Task analysis

Task analysis is the study of what an operator (or team of operators) is required to do in terms of actions and/or cognitive processes to achieve a system goal *(Kirwan and Ainsworth, 1992)*. It includes many methods which can be used to document and display information. This provides a 'blue print' of human involvements in a system which is used to build a clear and detailed picture of the system. Kirwan and Ainsworth (1992) describe task analysis in terms of five steps with associated methods as shown in Table 4.1. More detail about the individual methods can be found in *Kirwan and Ainsworth (1992)* and *Wilson and Corlett (1995)*. As with most ergonomics

Table 4.1. Task analysis stages and methods

Data collection	Critical Incident Technique, Questionnaires, Structured interviews, Verbal Protocol Analysis (VPA), Activity Sampling.
Task Description	Hierarchical Task Analysis (HTA), Link Analysis, Time line analysis, charting and networks, Operational sequence diagrams.
Simulation	Walk-throughs, Mock-ups, computer modelling, table top analysis.
Behaviour assessment	Event Trees, Fault Trees, Hazard and Operability analysis (HAZOP), Failure mode and effects analysis (FMEA)
Evaluation	Checklists, Interface Surveys

analyses it would be rare to only use one method, generally a combination of data are used which have been collected from interviews, observations, document analysis and experiments.

The outputs from a task analysis can include information about the allocation of function (between human and machine), person specification (knowledge and skills required to perform the task), job organisation (and staff needed to achieve the task goals), the interface design and finally a quality assurance of the performance of the task by providing a benchmark against which the task can be evaluated. An example of Link Analysis is shown in the case study section to look at the layout of the equipment in the passenger saloon of an accident and emergency ambulance.

5 Postural analysis

Postural analysis provides a description of the posture with respect to (a) the spatial arrangement of individual body sections and (b) an assessment of the posture tolerability *(Colombini and Occhipinti, 1985)*. Postures are considered to be tolerable when they do not involve feelings of short-term discomfort or cause long-term MSDs. There are many ways to collect information on posture but the assessor should always report their findings in the context of a full ergonomics assessment as posture is only one component of human interactions.

There are a number of postural analysis tools and more information about the range can be found in Wilson and *Corlett (1995)*. The methods described below are all used mostly for field data collection.

RULA

Rapid Upper Limb Assessment (RULA) was developed by Lynn McAtamney and Nigel Corlett at the Institute for Occupational Ergonomics, University of Nottingham *(McAtamney and Corlett, 1993)*. It is a quick survey method which can be used as part of a ergonomic workplace assessment where musculoskeletal disorders involving the upper limbs are reported. RULA assesses biomechanical and postural loading on the neck, shoulders and upper limbs and was designed to assess predominantly sedentary work. It allocates scores based on the position of groups of body parts with additional scores for force/load and muscle activity. The final RULA score is a relative rather than an absolute score and gives an indication of the risk level on a four-point action category scale from action category (AC) 1, where the posture is acceptable, through to AC4 where investigation and changes are needed immediately.

REBA

Rapid Entire Body Assessment (REBA) is a whole body assessment tool. It was initially designed to provide a pen-and-paper postural analysis tool to be used in the field by direct observations or with photographic stills/video *(Hignett and McAtamney, 2000)*. A full version of REBA is included as Appendix 1 at the end of this publication.

REBA was developed to assess the type of unpredictable working postures found in health care and other service industries and was validated using examples from the electricity, health-care and manufacturing industries. Data are collected about the body posture, forces used, type of movement or action, repetition and coupling. A final REBA score is generated giving an indication the level of musculoskeletal risk and urgency with which action should be taken on a five point action category scale of 0-4 from no action required (AC0) through to action necessary now (AC4). The AC reflects the magnitude and severity of exposure and recommends the priority for the control measures. The method was designed to evaluate tasks where postures are dynamic, static or where gross changes in position occur. In particular REBA was designed to:

- Provide a postural analysis system sensitive to musculoskeletal risks in a variety of occupational tasks.
- Divide the body into segments which are coded individually with reference to movement planes.
- Provide a scoring system for muscle activity caused by static, dynamic, rapid changing or unstable postures.
- Reflect that coupling is important in the handling of loads but may not always be via the hands.
- Give an action level with an indication of urgency.
- Require minimal equipment.

Borg Scale (physiological method)

The Borg Scale or scale of rated perceived exertion (RPE) provides a linear scale to reflect the curvi-linear relationship between the intensity of a physical stimuli and human perception of the intensity *(Borg, 1985, Kilbom, 1990)*. The scale steps (6-20) are adjusted so that they relate to the heart rate divided by 10 (figure 4.3). The scale is presented to the participant with the endpoints (6 and 20) defined and they are asked to rate their activity. *Kilbom (1990)* recommends that RPE scales should be used cautiously for industrial applications as there have been suggestions that the ratings are not only influenced by the overall perception of exertion but also by previous experience and the motivation of subjects, whereby highly motivated subjects tend to underestimate their exertion.

Figure 4.3. Borg's RPE scale:

6	No Exertion At All
7	Extremely Light
8	
9	Very Light
10	
11	Light
12	
13	Somewhat Hard
14	
15	Hard (Heavy)
16	
17	Very Hard
18	
19	Extremely Hard
20	Maximal Exertion

6 Participatory ergonomics

Participatory Ergonomics can be very simply described as an umbrella a concept involving the use of participative techniques and various forms of participation in the workplace *(Vink and Wilson, 2003, Hignett, Wilson, and Morris, (2005))*. The degree of employee participation can range from a top-down approach with information flowing from management to workers on plans for action; gathering of information and experience from workers; consultation where workers can make suggestions and present points of view; negotiations in formalised committees; through to joint decision making in agreement between involved parties *(Dachler and Wilpert, 1978; Haines et al. 2002)*.

The participative techniques can include *(Haines and Wilson, 1998)*:

1 Problem analysis e.g. link analysis, activity analysis.
2 Creativity stimulation and idea generation e.g. round robin questionnaire, world map.
3 Idea generation and concept development e.g. design decision group, focus group.
4 Concept evaluation e.g. layout modelling and mock-ups, checklists.
5 Preparation and support e.g. team formation and building.

The practicality of tools is important as the educational background of the participants may vary, so it may be useful to start with a hands-on exercise e.g. simulations or mock-ups, and then progress into problem solving, from idea generation and concept evaluation, ending in an action proposal with a recommendation for implementation *(Kuorinka, 1997)*.

Hignett (2003) reported on a systematic review looking at the range of interventions used to reduce musculoskeletal injuries associated with patient handling tasks. It was found that, although a number of intervention strategies were successful, the best results were obtained when multi-factor intervention strategies included worker participation. The most successful strategies involved changes in work organisation, working practices and the design of the working environment. One example of a participatory ergonomics intervention programme in a UK hospital was evaluated by the HSE. The intervention used a range of ergonomics methods to tackle MSD problems in all staff groups *(Hignett, 2001b)* and was evaluated to have made a saving in excess of £3.6 million over three years (www.hse.gov.uk /healthservices/casestudies/ nottingham.htm).

7 User trials

Many of us will have made comments about both domestic products as well as the equipment we use in the work place and often feel that we can suggest design improvements. User trials provide a systematic framework to collect data from a range of user populations about different aspects of a product so that the design can be reviewed and improved. They are used to answer one or more specific questions about the effectiveness of a product *(Wilson and Corlett, 1995)*. It is useful for designers to test their ideas and prototypes to find out how future users might operate it, whether they will understand the intended way of operation and if they are likely to perform the manipulations required for correct functioning *(Roozenburg and Eekels, 1995)*. There are more examples of comparative testing, e.g. the Consumers Association (http://www.which.net/), than prototype and developmental testing due to commercial confidentiality.

The NHS is the largest purchaser of medical equipment in the UK. Although the NHS Purchasing and Supply Agency (http://www.pasa.doh.gov.uk/) does include as one of its aims the 'development and improvement of the provision of comparative information on the purchasing and supply performance of the NHS' their advice seems to be directed more towards comparative cost than functionality or usability. The Medical and Healthcare Products Regulatory Agency (MHRA) publishes product evaluations on a wide range of topics. These include mobile hoists and slings *(A3, 1993: A10, 1994; MH2, 2000)*, moving and transferring equipment *(A19, 1996)*, handling equipment for moving dependent people in bed *(A23, 1997)*, portable bath lifts *(MH1, 1998)* and electrically powered profiling beds *(MH4/MHRA 03038, 2003)*. Information about these publications, together with descriptions of how to plan and carry out user trials for moving and handling equipment, can be found at http://www.medical-devices.gov.uk.

8 Examples of ergonomics in health and social care

Social Care

Alexander (2003) evaluated a risk management programme for community nurses with respect to the nursing managers' ability to implement the recommendations for risk reduction. The risk reduction recommendations included provision of hoists, increasing staffing levels, addressing space constraints, tackling difficulties identified with both patients and carers (including sudden changes in clinical condition). She found that the managers perceived that an increased awareness through education would be the main factor in reducing sickness absence for back and neck pain whereas the staff believed that provision of equipment would be the main factor. A significant relationship was found with respect to the implementation of risk reduction recommendations. There was also a reduction in sickness absence from 28% to 9% in the implementation group over 12 months.

Home Care

Sitzman and Bloswick (2002) referred to the repealed OSHA Ergonomics Program Standard (http://www.osha.gov/SLTC/ergonomics/index.html) suggesting that ergonomics could be applied to a range of risk activities associated with the provision of home care e.g. moving clients, carrying nursing bags and driving. This included basic screening tools and detailed ergonomic guidelines and information.

Owen and Skalitsky Staehler (2003) looked at nursing activities in patient homes to identify the tasks perceived to be the most physically stressful. They found that the nurses rated lifting a patient up in bed as the most stressful (using rated perceived exertion) with body mechanics listed as the most frequent contributor due to bending, reaching, twisting, lifting and enduring static postures. They also collected stress reduction ideas from the nursing aides including environmental factors (e.g. adjustable beds, assistive devices for lifting and transferring patients), policy changes (e.g. permit more than one aide for visits with heavy and difficult patients) and patient factors (e.g. have patient help more).

Disability services

Ore (2003) reported on an analysis of approximately 2700 manual handling injuries among disability services workers in an Australian state government agency between 1997 and 2000. These workers support clients living in small group homes (about 5 in a house) who require varying levels of

Figure 4.4. Space needed to use a mobile hoist for a Chair-to-Bed transfer showing:

4.4a the experimental layout

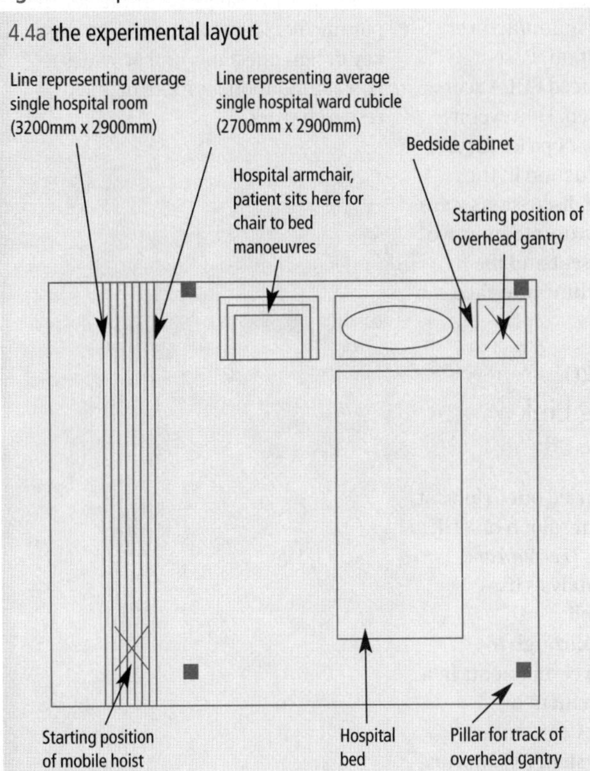

4.4b the average route (*Keen, 2004*)

support. The client group included people with an intellectual disability, autism, neurological disability and acquired brain injury and most are involved in rehabilitation programmes. Nearly half of the workers injuries were associated with providing support, for example assisting unsteady clients into the bath and shower; dressing clients; assisting clients into and out of bed; holding clients during epileptic seizures and preventing clients from falling out the bus. He suggests that ergonomic interventions could include providing sufficient space in the bathing areas to minimise awkward postures, redesigning the client rooms, toilets, beds, wheelchairs and recommending appropriate transfer devices.

Space to operate hoists – the hospital bed space

Health Building Notes were developed by NHS Estates in the 1980s to assist architects plan sufficient space for clinical activities but there were limitations identified in the process by *Stanton (1983)* with respect to the inclusion of user data. *Keen (2004)* carried out a project in the Hospital Ergonomics and Patient Safety Unit at Loughborough University to investigate how much space was needed to operate hoists in a single bed area.

Keen compared a mobile hoist and an overhead gantry hoist by videoing two patient handling transfers: (1) bed-chair and (2) floor-bed. The data were analysed to measure the space required for each task as shown in figure 4.4. The layout of the experimental room (mock-up) is shown in figure 4.4a, with floor guidelines to give a range of bed space dimensions from 2.7m wide (recommended cubicle bed width for hoist use, *HBN, 1995)* to 3.2m wide (recommended single room width, *HBN, 1995)*. Additional lines were added for the analysis to enable the average route (figure 4.4b) to be measured.

The minimum width of the bed space needed to operate a mobile hoist was found to be 3.6m. This is a considerable increase on the initially recommended 2.5m (HBN, 1986) and indicates a need for task analysis in the design of hospital bed spaces. This needs to be investigated further in more detailed research.

Ultrasonography

Ultrasonography is used for general investigations of soft tissues as well as specific diagnostic tests in a range of clinical specialities, for example gynaecology, obstetrics, cardiology, vascular and paediatrics. Sonography has been available as a diagnostic tool since 1942 and was recognised as a separate profession in 1974 *(Ransom, 2002)*. Sonographers use a hand-held transducer which is applied to the area needing investigation, linked to a scanning machine, which relays the images collected by the transducer. It typically involves a static posture to maintain the arm in a fixed position (unsupported abduction) while pressing the transducer against the patient (figure 4.5). The layout of the workplace may vary according to the preferences of the mother and sonographer. The

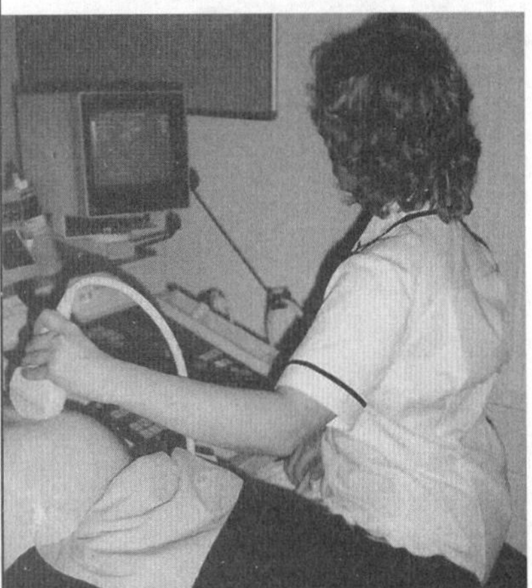

Figure 4.5. Obstetric sonography

mother may wish to view the monitor during the scan and the sonographer may prefer use their dominant hand for either the transducer or the scanning machine controls.

Russo et al (2002) reported on a survey in British Columbia, finding that the majority of sonographers (91%) had work-related musculoskeletal problems. They collected data about the work environment and corporate culture, schedule, tasks, and equipment to look for associations with physical symptoms. Factors included the number of hours scanning, static and awkward postures, and psychosocial factors, including social support (co-worker, supervisor and senior management) and decision-making with respect to planning the workload and taking breaks.

A problem was identified by ultra-sonographers in a Cardiology Department when they were performing cardiac scans. The patient lies on their left-hand-side and the sonographer reaches over the patient's chest to place the transducer on the left-hand-side of the chest. Initially the plinth was not designed to accommodate the sonographer so they either stood or perched on the edge of it in an awkward twisted position (figure 4.6). As the work required both upper limbs to carry out fine motor activities a high level of concentration was required so a slumped posture was often observed as the sonographer concentrated on the (1) visual display, (2) machine controls, and (3) transducer placement. On initial assessment using RULA a score of 7 was recorded which placed this posture in AC 4, indicating that immediate investigation and change was required.

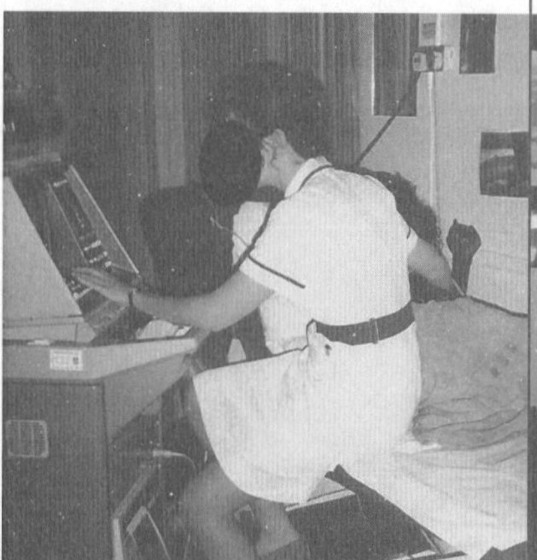

Figure 4.6. Cardiac ultrasonography (*Hignett 2004*)

RULA Score = 7, Action Category = 4 (Investigate and change immediately)

A modified plinth was designed in collaboration with the manufacturer with a cut-out seat section. Post implementation a reduced RULA score of 6 (AC 3) was recorded. However it was felt that there was scope for further improvement (and reduction in the RULA score) so further discussions were held with the manufacturer to improve both the design of the seat and the plinth ultrasound machine interface.

Ambulance design: an example using Link Analysis

A link analysis was carried out to look at the layout of the patient saloon of a UK emergency ambulance *(Ferreira and Hignett, 2005)*. Link analysis uses spatial diagrams and relies on observation or a walk-through to establish links between components in a system. A link is a movement of attentional gaze or physical contact between parts of the system *(Kirwan and Ainsworth, 1992)*. From this analysis it was possible to identify that the preferred working position (seat B, figure 4.7b) resulted in the paramedic having to perch on the edge of the seat in order to reach the patient. The attendant seat (seat A, figure 4.7b) was rarely used except in clinically critical situations (e.g. cardiac arrest) so the paramedic was working without seat belt protection and not as the manufacturer had designed the task for this vehicle. There are multiple design implications from these findings. These include the location of equipment, placement of doors (bulkhead versus side door) and safety restraints for the paramedic. This student project raises key design questions and provides a good foundation for more detailed research work.

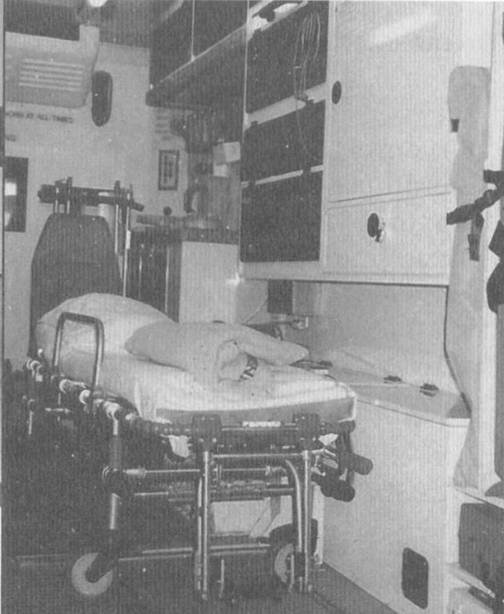

Figure 4.7a. Interior layout of ambulance

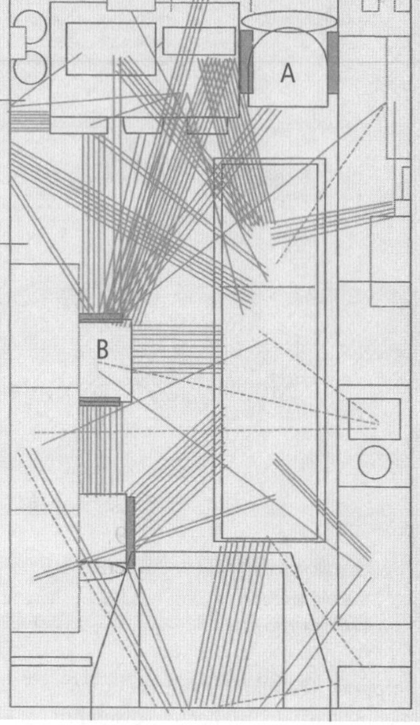

Figure 4.7b. Link Analysis diagram (*Hignett 2004*)

9 Summary

A range of examples have been given to illustrate how ergonomics methods and tools have been used to assist in the design and evaluation and the investigation and modification of health and social care tasks. Most are related to musculoskeletal risks but ergonomics methods are also used in a wide range of other areas for example, military, manufacturing, consumer product design, human computer interaction, process and transport control, health and safety, human error analysis, pollution and waste management. There is a growing body of ergonomics research in health and social care in the area of patient safety and it is important that the interaction between patient and carer safety is made clear. Both need to be addressed to improve the system rather than changing one element at the cost of the other.

References

Alexander P (2003). Community Care nurses. In Hignett S et al (2003). Evidence-based patient handling. Tasks, equipment and interventions. London: Routledge.

Borg G (1985). An Introduction to Borg's RPE-Scale. Ithaca, NY: Movement Publications.

Caccamise DJ (1995). Implementation of a team approach to nuclear critically safety: The use of participatory methods in macro-ergonomics. International Journal of Industrial Ergonomics. 15, 397-409.

Colombini D and Occhipinti E (1985). Posture Analysis. Ergonomics. 28, 1, 275-285

Dachler HP and Wilpert B (1978). Conceptual dimensions and boundaries of participation in organisations: a critical evaluation. Administrative Science Quarterly. 23, 1-39.

Engkvist IL (2004). The accident process preceding back injuries among Australian nurses. Safety Science. 42, 221-235

Eriksen W, Bruusgaard D and Knardahl S (2004). Work factors as predictors of intense or disabling low back pain; a prospective study of nurses' aides. Occupational and Environmental Medicine. 61, 398-404

Ferreira J and Hignett S (2005). Reviewing Ambulance Design for clinical Efficiency and Paramedic Safety. Applied Ergonomics (in press)

Haines HM, Wilson JR, Vink P and Koningsveld E (2002). Validating a framework for participatory ergonomics. Ergonomics. 45, 4, 309-327

Haines HM and Wilson JR (1998). Development of a framework for participatory ergonomics. Contract Research Report 174/1998, Health and Safety Executive. London: HSE Books

HBN (1986). Health Building Note No. 40 Common Activity Spaces: Vol. 2, Treatment Areas. London: HMSO, Dept. of Health.

HBN (1995). Health Building Note No. 40. Common Activity Spaces. Vol. 2. Treatment Areas. London: The Stationary Office. ISBN 0113221851

Helander MH (1997). The Human Factors Profession. Chapter 1. In Salvendy G (Ed.) Handbook of Human Factors and Ergonomics. (2nd Ed.) New York: John Wiley and Sons.

Hignett S (1998). Ergonomics: Chapter 13 in Pitt-Brooke J, Reid H, Lockwood J and Kerr K. Rehabilitation of Movement. Theoretical Basis of Clinical Practice. London: WB Saunders Co. Ltd., ISBN 0 7020 2157 1. 458-494

Hignett S (2001a). Using Qualitative Methodology in Ergonomics: theoretical background and practical examples. Ph.D. thesis, University of Nottingham.

Hignett S (2001b). Embedding ergonomics in hospital culture: top-down and bottom-up strategies. Applied Ergonomics. 32, 61-69

Hignett S (2003). Intervention strategies to reduce musculoskeletal injuries associated with handling patients: A systematic review. Occupational and Environmental Medicine. Vol 60, no 9, e6 (electronic paper). http://wwwoccenvmed.com/cgi/content/full/60/9/e6

Hignett S (2005). Physical Ergonomics in Healthcare. In Carayon, P. (Ed.) Handbook of Human Factors and Ergonomics in Health Care and Patient Safety. Mahwah, NJ: Lawrence Erlbaum Associates, Inc. (in press).

Hignett S and McAtamney L (2000). Rapid Entire Body Assessment (REBA). Applied Ergonomics, 31, 201-205

Hignett S and McAtamney L (2005). REBA and RULA: Whole Body and Upper Limb Rapid Assessment Tools. In Karwowski, W. and Marras, W.S. (Eds.) The Occupational Ergonomics Handbook. (2nd Ed.) Boca Raton, Fl: CRC Press.

Hignett S, Wilson JR and Morris W (2005). Finding Ergonomics Solutions – Participatory Approaches. Occupational Medicine. (in press)

Hignett S and Wilson JR (2004). The role for qualitative methodology in ergonomics: A case study to explore theoretical issues. Theoretical Issues in Ergonomics Science. November-December. Vol 5, No 6, 473 - 493

HSE (2003). Health and Safety Statistics Highlights. www.hse.gov.uk/statistics/overall/hssh0203.pdf. Accessed 8 June 2004.

IEA (2000). International Ergonomics Association, Triennial Report. (Santa Monica, CA: IEA Press). 5.

Keen E (2004). Investigation into space allocation when using a mobile hoist and overhead gantry hoist. B.Sc. Dissertation. Loughborough University.

Kilbom Å (1990). Measurement and assessment of dynamic work. In Wilson JR and Corlett EN (Eds.) Evaluation of Human Work. A practical ergonomics methodology. (1st Ed.) London: Taylor and Francis

Kirwan B and Ainsworth LK (1992). A Guide to Task Analysis. London: Taylor and Francis.

Kneafsey R (2000). The effect of occupational socialization on nurses' patient handling practices. Journal of Clinical Nursing. 9, 585-593.

Kuorinka I (1997). Tools and means of implementing participatory ergonomics. International Journal of Industrial Ergonomics. 19, 267-270.

McAtamney L and Corlett EN (1993). RULA: a survey method for the investigation of WRULD. Applied Ergonomics. 24, 2, 91-99

National Audit Office (2003). A Safer Place to Work. Improving the management of health and safety risks to staff in NHS Trusts. London: National Audit Office. ISBN : 0102921431

Ore T (2003). Manual handling injury in a disability services setting. Applied Ergonomics. 34, 89-94

Owen BD and Skalitsky Staehler K (2003). Decreasing Back Stress in Home Care. Home Healthcare Nurse. 21, 3, 180-186

Pheasant S (1998). Back Injury in Nurses – Ergonomics and Epidemiology. In Lloyd, Fletcher B, Holmes D, Tarling C and Tracy M (1998, revised) The Guide to the Handling of Patients. (4th Edition) National Back Pain Association/Royal College of Nursing.

Ransom E (2002). The causes of musculoskeletal injury among sonographers in the UK. Society of Radiographers, 207 Providence Square, Mill Street, London. SE1 2EW

Roozenburg NFM and Eekels J (1995). Product Design: Fundamentals and Methods. Chichester: John Wiley and Sons Ltd.

Russo A, Murphy C, Lessoway V and Berkowitz J (2002). The prevalence of musculoskeletal symptoms among British Columbia sonographers. Applied Ergonomics. 33, 385-393

Sanders MS and McCormick EJ (1992). Human Factors in Engineering and

Design (2nd Ed.). New York: McGraw-Hill, Inc.
Seccombe I and Ball J (1992). Back injured nurses: a profile. A discussion paper for the Royal College of Nursing. London: Institute of Manpower Studies.
Sitzman K and Bloswick D (2002). Creative Use of Ergonomics Principles in Home Care. Home Healthcare Nurse. 20, 2, 98-103
Smedley J, Egger P, Cooper C and Coggon D (1995). Manual handling activities and the risk of low back pain in nurses. Occupational and Environmental Medicine. 52, 160-163
Stanton G (1983). The development of ergonomics data for health building design guidance. Ergonomics. 30, 2, 359-366
Stubbs DA, Buckle PW, Hudson MP, Rivers PM and Worringham CJ (1983). Back pain in nursing profession: Epidemiology and pilot methodology. Ergonomics. 26, 8, 755-765
Vink P and Wilson JR (2003). Participatory Ergonomics. Proceedings of the XVth Triennial Congress of the International Ergonomics Association and The 7th Joint conference of the Ergonomics Society of Korea/Japan Ergonomics Society. 'Ergonomics in the Digital Age'. August 24-29, 2003. Seoul, Korea
Wilson JR and Corlett EN (1995). Evaluation of Human Work. A practical ergonomics methodology (2nd Ed.) London: Taylor and Francis.

5

Biomechanics of low back pain

Michael A Adams BSc PhD
Senior Research Fellow
Patricia Dolan BSc PhD
Senior Lecturer
Department of Anatomy, University of Bristol

Summary

- Severe back pain usually arises from intervertebral discs, apophyseal joints and sacroiliac joints
- Discs are most easily damaged by heavy lifting, and apophyseal joints and sacroiliac joints by asymmetrical spinal loading, including twisting
- Tissue damage can occur by injury, or by fatigue failure during repetitive loading
- Links between tissue damage and pain are complicated by stress shielding and pain sensitisation
- Tissues can be predisposed to damage by virtue of genes, age, nutritional compromise, and fatigue
- Degenerative changes in spinal tissues rapidly *follow* structural damage
- "Functional pathology" can explain pain arising from undamaged tissues
- Psychosocial factors influence all aspects of pain behaviour, including responses to treatment.

Pain-provocation studies suggest that the most common origin of *severe and chronic* back pain is the posterior part of the intervertebral disc, and the longitudinal ligament that adheres to it. The apophyseal joints and sacroiliac joints are painful in substantial minorities of patients.

Pain can be caused by mechanical failure, and the most common mechanisms are as follows: ligaments of the neural arch are most easily damaged ("sprained") by forward bending movements; the apophyseal joint surfaces by twisting and backwards bending; the vertebral body by compression; and the disc by awkward bending and compression, or following compressive damage to the vertebral body. Mechanical failure can occur during a single application of load, simulating some incident such as a stumble or fall, or by the process of accumulating "fatigue failure" in which the forces remain relatively low but are applied many times. Links between tissue damage and back pain are complicated by stress-shielding and pain sensitisation phenomena. Tissues can be weakened (and so predisposed to damage) by virtue of genetic inheritance, age, nutritional compromise, and prior fatigue loading. Biological (cell-mediated) degeneration rapidly *follows* structural failure, although in some cases may precede it.

Pain can arise in the absence of structural failure if high stress concentrations are generated within innervated tissues. Such "functional pathology" may possibly result from abnormal muscle activity and from excessively lordotic or flexed postures, especially if they are held for long periods.

Psychosocial factors such as depressive tendencies and dissatisfaction with work can influence all aspects of pain behaviour, including responses to treatment.

In conclusion, current evidence suggests that mechanical loading plays a central role in the aetiology of most people's back pain. This applies even if the patient appears psychologically disturbed, reports no history of trauma, or shows evidence of biological (cell mediated) degenerative changes in spinal tissues.

1 Introduction

Back pain is the most frequent medical cause of work absence in the U.K., and although it may sometimes be used as a convenient excuse for taking time off, there can be little doubt that many people have real and severe problems. But how much of the blame for back pain can really be attributed to mechanical loading of the spine in activities such as person handling?

Psychosocial factors greatly affect the success or failure of treatment, especially in chronic back pain or when compensation claims are involved *(Yang, King 1984)* . They are important to employers too, because return to work is influenced by attitudes to the workplace and work colleagues. However, in patients who are well motivated at the outset, unhappiness and litigation may simply represent normal human reactions to persisting pain and ineffective treatment.

Specific diseases such as ankylosing spondylitis can cause back pain, but only in a minority of patients. More usually the onset of pain is related to some incident involving mechanical loading of the back. However, a simple "injury" model of back pain is no longer considered to be adequate *(Yang, King 1984)* , because the associated incident is often trivial, and in many patients pain can be difficult to explain in terms of any identifiable spinal pathology. This may be because factors such as genetic inheritance can render some tissues more vulnerable to damage than others, and because pain-sensitisation and stress-shielding phenomena can obscure the relationship between pathology and pain.

The purpose of the present chapter is to review the recent research literature concerning the role of psychological, biological, and mechanical factors in the aetiology of back pain. This should place the role of mechanical loading in a wider context, and should complement other chapters of the book that concentrate on ergonomics considerations in person handling.

The information is divided into six main sections.

- Section 2 tackles the problem of where back pain comes from by considering the relevant anatomy, together with evidence from pain-provocation and pain-blocking studies.
- Section 3 reviews the epidemiological evidence that indicates who develops back pain, and in so doing suggests *why* they do.
- Section 4 introduces spinal mechanics and considers how high mechanical loading might cause injury or fatigue ("wear and tear")

damage to spinal tissues.

- Section 5 is an account of how spinal tissues can be rendered vulnerable to mechanical damage by factors such as age and genetic inheritance.
- Section 6 describes how living tissues respond biologically to mechanical damage, and suggests how these responses may mask the essentially mechanical origin of degenerative changes within them.
- Section 7 considers how "functional pathology" might generate painful stress concentrations in spinal tissues without injuring them.
- Section 8, as a final discussion, attempts to pull together the various topics to present a concise account of the biomechanics of back pain.

2 Anatomical basis of low back pain

The lumbar spine

The lumbar spine includes the five lowest vertebrae. This is a particularly mobile region of the spine, and is also subjected to the highest forces, so it is not surprising that it is the region most likely to be damaged and painful. Each vertebra has a chunky "vertebral body" which is the main weight bearing structure, and a "neural arch" which is a bony arch protecting the spinal cord. Various "processes" attached to the neural arch act as levers so that muscles can move the spine about.

Adjacent vertebral bodies are separated by a pad of cartilage called an "intervertebral disc" which consists of a central region of soft hydrated material (the "nucleus pulposus") surrounded by tough concentric rings of tough gristly cartilage (the "annulus fibrosus") as shown in Figure 5.1. Intervertebral discs allow the spine a certain amount of flexibility, and they also play a minor role in shock absorption. Many middle-aged discs show various signs of structural disruption, including "slipped disc", and there are strong associations between certain forms of disc disruption and back pain.

Adjacent vertebrae are also linked by ligaments (tough fibrous bands which prevent excessive movement) and by a pair of "apophyseal joints", which are small sliding joints the size of a fingernail. These joints stabilise the spine and protect the discs from

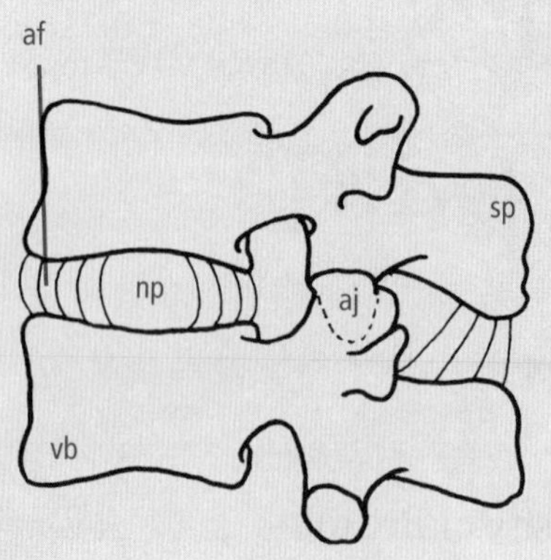

Figure 5.1. Side view of two lumbar vertebrae, posterior on the right. The weight bearing vertebral bodies (vb) are separated by an intervertebral disc, which comprises a soft *nucleus pulposus* (np) surrounded by the tough *annulus fibrosus* (af). Small *apophyseal joints* (aj) increase stability. The spinous processes (sp) can be felt by running a finger down someone's back.

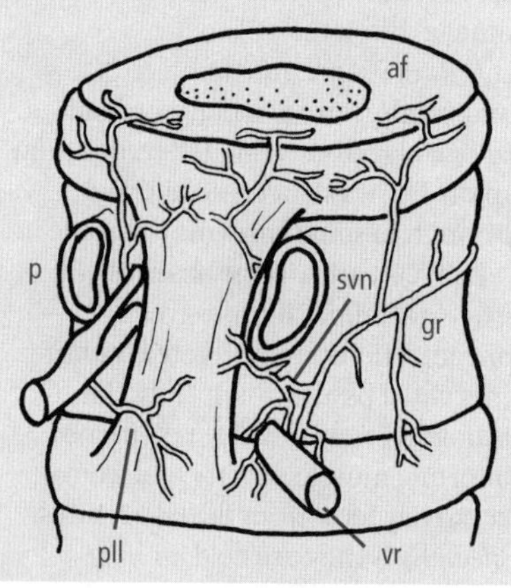

Figure 5.2. Oblique posterior view of the lumbar spine showing the sinuvertebral nerve (svn), which supplies the annulus fibrosus (af) of the intervertebral disc and the posterior longitudinal ligament (pll). The neural arch has been cut away at the pedicles (p). The sinuvertebral nerve is a mixed nerve containing fibres from the grey rami communicantes (gr) and the ventral ramus (vr) of the spinal nerve. Adapted from (1).

excessive movements, especially twisting and bending. Apophyseal joints of people aged over 40 often show signs of osteoarthritis, including cartilage thinning and marginal osteophytes.

The innervation of spinal tissues

The nerve supply to most spinal structures is uncontroversial. However, the innervation of intervertebral discs and longitudinal ligaments has been hotly debated, with negative findings being taken at face value, or attributed to technical failure. According to the widely accepted account of *Bogduk (1997)*, a mixed autonomic and somatic nerve, the sinuvertebral nerve, supplies the posterior and posterolateral annulus fibrosus, and the posterior longitudinal ligament (Figure 5.2). Within healthy discs, free nerve endings of various types have been identified, but only in the outermost few millimetres of the annulus fibrosus. Nerve endings and capillaries can grow in to the centre of degenerated discs *(Freemont, Peacock, Goupille et al. (1997)*, probably because they no longer exhibit the high internal pressure that keeps nerves and blood vessels out of the central regions of normal discs (see left).

Pain provocation and pain blocking studies

In a large-scale pain provocation study on 193 patients awaiting surgery for herniated ("slipped") disc or spinal stenosis, local anaesthesia was applied progressively to the skin, fascia, ligaments, muscles, apophyseal joints, nerve roots, annulus fibrosus and vertebral endplates *(Lu, Hutton, Gharpuray 1996)*. Before each structure was anaesthetised, it was stimulated, either electrically or mechanically. Patients' leg pain could be reproduced only from an inflamed or compressed nerve root, and it was always removed by injecting local anaesthetic beneath the nerve sleeve at the site of compression. The posterior annulus was "exquisitely tender" in one third of patients, "moderately tender" in another third, and insensitive in the rest. Back pain produced from the annulus was often similar to that suffered pre-operatively, and the gentle nature of the probing required to elicit this pain provides evidence for the phenomenon of "pain sensitisation", which is considered below. The posterior longitudinal ligament and vertebral body end plate were frequently painful, but it was difficult to stimulate them independently of the annulus. The facet joint capsule produced some sharp, localised pain in approximately 30% of patients, but the ligaments, fascia and muscles were relatively insensitive. Discogenic pain was further established by *Schwarzer, Aprill, Bogduk (1995)* and related to structural disruption of the tissues.

The same group also established the importance of the apophyseal joints in producing low back pain *(Snook, Webster, McGorry et al. 1998)*. They injected local anaesthetic into several facet joints in each patient, and reported some pain relief in 47% of patients. However, when the procedure was repeated approximately two weeks later, only 15% of all patients reported consistent relief of pain from the same joint on both occasions. The authors concluded that the apophyseal joints are frequently a cause of pain, but questioned the existence of a specific "facet syndrome". The relationship between pain and osteoarthritic changes in the apophyseal joints remains unclear, but the very high incidence of the latter in elderly people suggests that they are frequently asymptomatic.

The sacroiliac joints also have been investigated using pain-provocation and pain blocking techniques *(Schwarzer, Aprill, Derby et al. 1994)*. Of 43 patients with chronic low back pain below the level of L5-S1, 40% experienced exact reproduction of their pain when the sacroiliac joints were injected with X-ray contrast medium, and 30% gained relief from their pain when lignocaine was injected.

Muscles and ligaments are probably the origin of many cases of acute back pain that clear up after a few weeks, although there is little evidence to support this widely held belief. Indirect involvement of back muscles in acute and chronic back pain is considered below.

3 Epidemiology of low back pain

The greatest known risk factors for back disorders are mostly mechanical, such as awkward and repetitive manual handling tasks *(Melrose, Ghosh, Taylor et al. 1992)* and exposure to vibrations *(Porter, Adams, Hutton 1989)*. Related pathology is also strongly dependent on mechanical loading: for example, bending and lifting weights in excess of 25 lb more than 25 times per day makes you up to six times as likely to develop a prolapsed disc *(Kerttula, Serlo, Tervonen et al. 2000)*. It is important to realise, however, that the body can eventually adapt to mechanical loading by becoming stronger (see section 6, below) and that a strong back will be less vulnerable to accidental injury. For this reason, epidemiological surveys probably underestimate the tendency for vigorous manual work to cause short-term fatigue damage to "unadapted" backs. It is also worth noting that epidemiological studies which *quantify* spinal loading tend to report closer associations between loading and back pain than do studies which rely on self-attested reports of "job heaviness" *(Ferguson, Marras 1997)*. The outcome measure in epidemiological surveys should not be simple "back pain" because most of the population report such pain, and it is impossible to identify risk factors for conditions that affect everyone. Psychosocial factors are particularly good at predicting relatively trivial back pain whereas mechanical factors are more closely involved with back pain involving medical attention or time off work *(Adams, Mannion, Dolan 1999)*.

The majority of people in high-risk occupations remain unaffected by severe back pain, suggesting that personal risk factors predispose certain individuals to back problems while sparing others. Some of these are already known: a long back and a heavy body are associated with increased risk of a herniated disc *(Heliovara 1987)* and for obvious reasons: these individuals are lifting on longer lever arms, and moving an increased bodyweight around. People with a poor range of movement in the lumbar spine *(Mannion, Dolan 1999)* and those with easily fatigued back muscles *(Adams, Mannion, Dolan, Adams 1996)* are also at increased risk of first-time back pain, although the effects are small. Poor spinal mobility leads to increased bending stresses acting on the lumbar discs and ligaments *(Dolan, Adams 1993)*, and fatigued back muscles are less able to protect the back from excessive bending during repetitive lifting movements *(Dolan, Adams 1998)*. Genetic risk factors, and the effects of ageing, are considered in Section 5 (below).

Psychosocial risk factors such depressive tendencies, or negative feelings about work colleagues, are also important in the aetiology of back pain *(Yang, King 1984)*. However, the available evidence suggests that they help to explain how people *behave* in response to their back pain, rather than how they get it in the first place, and measured psychosocial factors (between them) explain only 2-3% of reports of first-time back pain *(Mannion, Kaser, Weber et al. 2000)*. In this context, back pain "behaviour" includes the decision to report symptoms as "back pain", to take time off work, to respond (or not) to treatment, and to allow the pain to affect normal living.

4 Mechanical damage to the lumber spine

Mechanical properties of the spine

The apophyseal joints resist forces that act perpendicular to their broad articular surfaces. Thus, they severely limit the range of axial rotation and resist forward shearing movements of the lower lumbar spine. Little of the spinal compressive force normally falls on the apophyseal joints unless the discs are narrowed by degenerative changes, in which case the neural arch can resist more compression than the adjacent discs *(Pollintine, Dolan, Tobias et al. 2004)*. The apophyseal joints'

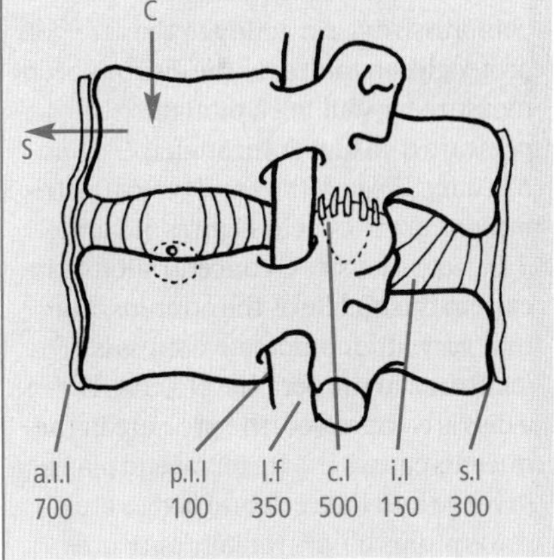

Figure 5.3. A spinal motion segment as in Figure 1, showing the intervertebral ligaments and their typical tensile strength (in Newtons, where 9.81 N = 1 kg). a.l.l.=anterior longitudinal ligament, p.l.l.=posterior longitudinal ligament, l.f.=ligamentum flavum, c.l.=capsular ligaments, i.l.=interspinous ligament, s.l.=supraspinous ligament. Compressive forces (C) act down the long axis of the spine, perpendicular to the mid-plane of the discs. The shear force (S) moves a vertebra forwards or backwards relative to the one below. The centre of rotation for forwards or backwards bending normally lies within the region shown by the dashed circle.

resistance to compression comes from the articular surfaces, and from extra-articular impingement of the inferior facet on the lamina below *(Adams, Bogduk, Burton, Dolan 2002)*.

Intervertebral ligaments have strengths ranging from about 100N for the posterior longitudinal ligament to about 1kN or more for the apophyseal joint capsular ligaments (Figure 5.3). They resist bending movements of the spine, particularly forward bending. Tension generated in posterior intervertebral ligaments during flexion acts to compress the intervertebral discs, so that the intra-discal pressure increases by 100% or more in full flexion, even for the same applied compressive force *(Adams, Bogduk, Burton, Dolan 2002)*.

Intervertebral discs behave like hydraulic "cushions" between adjacent vertebrae (Figure 5.4). The nucleus pulposus has a high water content and behaves like a pressurised fluid. The inner annulus also behaves like a fluid despite its regular lamellar structure *(Adams, McNally, Dolan 1996)* but the outer annulus is a fibrous solid that acts as a tensile "skin" for the rest of the disc, resisting bending and torsional movements. The distribution of compressive stress acting in the proteoglycan matrix of the disc has been measured by pulling a miniature pressure transducer through it *(Adams, McNally, Dolan 1996)* and typical distributions are shown in Figures 5.5 and 5.6. Note that stress concentrations can exist in the middle of the annulus, and that very little compressive stress is measured in the peripheral 3mm. When a disc is compressed, the pressure in the nucleus causes the vertebral end plates to bulge into the vertebral bodies and the annulus bulges radially outwards *(Brinckmann, Grootenboer 1991)*.

Injury mechanisms

The *vertebral body* is the "weak link" of the spine and is the first structure to fail in compression *(Adams, Bogduk, Burton, Dolan 2002)*. Its compressive strength depends greatly on the sex, age and body mass of the individual. Damage is mostly located in the end plate, or in the trabeculae just behind it *(Adams Freeman, Morrison et al. 2000)*, and is presumably caused by the nucleus pulposus of the adjacent disc bulging into the vertebra. If the spine is compressed while moderately flexed, as it often is in manual handling *(Dolan, Earley, Adams 1994)*, then failure can occur in the anterior margins of the vertebral body to create an anterior "wedge fracture". This is a typical form of injury in old osteoporotic spines, where it can lead to a humpback deformity. Advanced disc degeneration can pre-dispose to vertebral wedge fractures because narrowed degenerated discs can cause the anterior regions of the vertebral body to be "stress-shielded" (and therefore weakened) during normal erect standing postures, but heavily loaded whenever the spine is flexed *(Pope 1989)*.

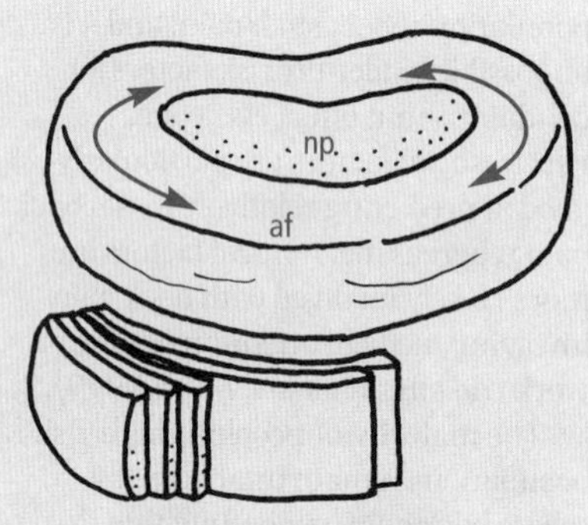

Figure 5.4. When an intervertebral disc is compressed, the hydrostatic pressure in the nucleus pulposus (np) is raised, and this creates tensile "hoop" stresses in the annulus fibrosus (af). (Inset) The annulus consists of concentric lamellae with alternating fibre angles. Note that some lamellae are discontinuous.

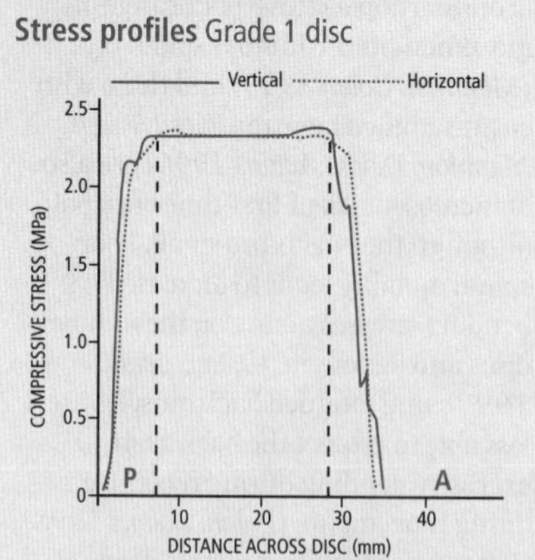

Figure 5.5. Distribution of horizontal and vertical compressive stress along the mid-sagittal plane of a typical non-degenerated "grade 1" intervertebral disc. The disc was subjected to 2kN of compressive loading when the measurements were taken. The central section, in which stress does not vary with direction or location, indicates a region of hydrostatic pressure. Adapted from (Adams, Bogduk, Burton, Dolan 2002).

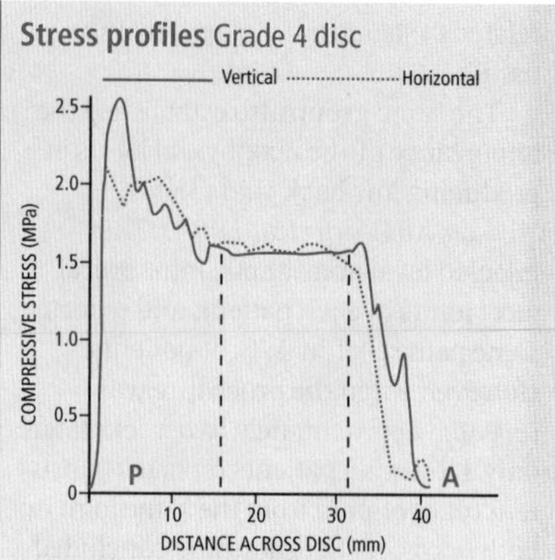

Figure 5.6. Pressure profiles (as in Figure 5.5) for a degenerated "grade 4" disc. Degenerative changes reduce the size of any hydrostatic region, and increase the size of stress peaks in the annulus, especially the posterior annulus.

Fractures of the *pars interarticularis* similar to those seen in spondylolysis can be caused by forces acting on the inferior articular processes *(Green, Allvey, Adams 1994)*. Gravity causes the lower lumbar vertebrae to move forwards and down relative to the vertebra below and this bends the inferior facets backwards about the pars interarticularis. Lumbar extension movements also bend the inferior articular processes backwards, whereas lumbar flexion tensions the apophyseal joint ligaments and bends the inferior processes forwards *(Green, Allvey, Adams 1994)*. Alternating forward and backwards bending movements would create large stress-reversals in the pars and may eventually cause fatigue failure within the bone. This may explain why spondylolysis is so common among sportsmen who frequently flex and extend their lumbar spine. Backwards bending movements generate high stress concentrations in the inferior margins of the apophyseal joint surfaces, *(Adams, Bogduk, Burton, Dolan 2002)* especially after sustained ("creep") loading which reduces the water content and height of the intervertebral discs (see below). Severe (pathological) disc narrowing greatly increases loading of the neural arch *(Pollintine, Dolan, Tobias et al. 2004)*, and may cause the tips of the inferior facets to impinge on the lamina below. There is no articular cartilage on the very tip of the inferior facet, so any extra-articular impingement may be painful. Axial rotation of the lumbar spine compresses the apophyseal joints on one side of the body, and excessive movement may damage the cartilage or subchondral bone of these joints *(Adams, Bogduk, Burton, Dolan 2002)*. Damage to the apophyseal joint surfaces, either in bending or torsion, may lead eventually to osteoarthritic changes, as in other synovial joints.

The intervertebral ligaments that span adjacent neural arches provide most of the spine's resistance to flexion, with the remainder coming from the disc. In hyperflexion, the first structure to sustain damage is the interspinous ligament *(Adams, Bogduk, Burton, Dolan 2002)* so it is not surprising that this ligament is often found damaged in cadaveric spines. Further flexion is required to damage the apophyseal joint capsular ligaments, and still more to injure the disc. If lateral flexion is combined with anterior flexion, then the contra-lateral capsular ligament will be put to an additional stretch and might be damaged before the interspinous ligament. The visco-elastic nature of ligaments and discs increases their resistance to stretching during rapid movements, whereas sustained flexion reduces the spine's resistance to bending by 40% in just five minutes *(Adams, Dolan 1996)*, due mainly to "stress relaxation" in the spinal ligaments. Thus, rapid bending movements are more likely to injure the discs and ligaments, and sustained stooping may reduce ligamentous protection of the discs during subsequent activity. The interspinous ligament may be damaged in hyperextension by being squashed between opposing spinous processes. Usually the apophyseal joints or disc would be damaged first, but this depends on individual details of anatomy such as the spacing of the spinous processes *(Adams, Bogduk, Burton, Dolan 2002)*. Hyperextension movements bend the inferior articular processes backwards about the pars interarticularis: the facet tip may then damage the posterior margins of the apophyseal joint capsule.

Intervertebral discs are not damaged directly by compressive loading of the spine: compressive failure always affects the adjacent vertebral bodies. Torsional loading normally damages the lumbar apophyseal joints first *(Adams, Bogduk, Burton, Dolan 2002)*,

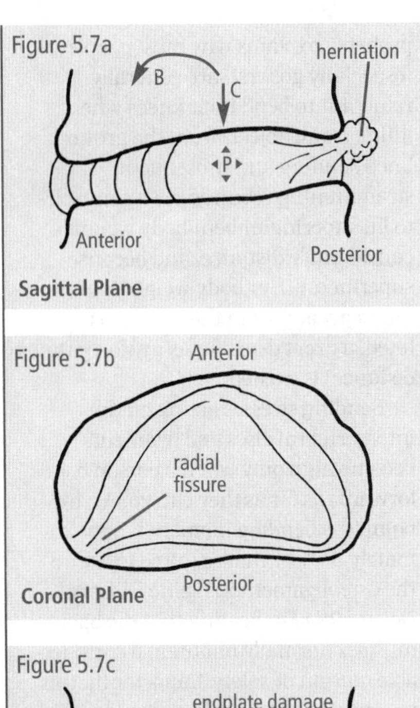

Figure 5.7. Types of structural disruption commonly seen in lumbar intervertebral discs. (Top) Posterior herniation of nucleus pulposus ("slipped disc") can occur when a disc is subjected to compression C, at the same time as bending B, which stretches and thins the posterior annulus. (Middle) Radial fissures can grow into the postero-lateral corners of lumbar discs in response to repetitive loading in bending and compression. (Lower) A damaged end plate depressurises the nucleus and can lead to internal disruption of the annulus.

but if these are removed, torsion can cause the lamellae of the annulus to separate circumferentially. Hyperflexion injury to an isolated disc, unprotected by the ligaments or apophyseal joints, occurs in the outer posterior annulus. The only loading conditions known to cause discs to prolapse *in vitro* in ways similar to those seen *in vivo* involve a combination of compression, lateral bending and forward bending *(Adams, Hutton 1982)*. Bending stretches and thins the postero-lateral annulus *(Adams, Hutton 1982)* while compression raises the hydrostatic pressure in the nucleus (Figure 5.7a). In cadaver experiments, prolapse can occur in a single loading cycle if the motion segment is flexed several degrees beyond its normal range of motion, so that the interspinous ligament is over-stretched *(Adams, Hutton 1982)* or if the compressive force is extremely high *(Adams, Freeman, Morrison et al. 2000)*. Prolapse occurs more readily when the discs are fully hydrated (as they would be in the early morning in living people) and when the forces are applied rapidly *(Mannion, Connolly, Wood et al. 1997)* and *(Adams, Hutton 1985)*. Repetitive application of a moderate compressive force to a fully flexed motion segment causes some non-degenerated discs to prolapse by the gradual formation of a radial fissure which allows soft nucleus pulposus material to migrate into the postero-lateral corners *(Adams, Hutton 1985)* (Figure 5.7b). Adding torsion to bending and compression makes prolapse easier. Discs that prolapse most readily are from the lower lumbar spine of cadavers aged less than 50 years, which show little sign of degeneration *(Adams, Hutton 1982)*. Severely degenerated discs cannot be made to prolapse, presumably because the nucleus is too fibrous to exert a hydrostatic pressure on the annulus *(Adams, McNally, Dolan 1996)*. Some spine surgeons suggest that only degenerated discs can prolapse, but this view is no longer compatible with biomechanics research, and it probably arose because severe degenerative changes occur *after* prolapse, and before surgery, for reasons discussed in Section 6 below. Severe backwards bending and compression can cause discs to prolapse anteriorly, but this is a rare occurrence in life.

Structural failure of the disc often involves inwards buckling of the annulus (Figure 5.7c), rather than outwards prolapse of nuclear material. Internal derangements could be caused by previous minor injuries to adjacent vertebral bodies, because such injuries decompress the nucleus and generate high concentrations of compressive stress in the annulus *(Adams, Freeman, Morrison et al. 2000)*. Subsequent repetitive loading can then cause the inner lamellae to collapse into the nucleus. This mechanism is supported by the finding that vertebral damage in young teenagers is followed several years later by signs of disc degeneration *(Klaber Moffett, Hughes, Griffiths 1993)*.

Spinal loading during manual handling

The above evidence supports the common sense notion that intervertebral discs and ligaments are most easily damaged by high loading in combined bending and compression. During manual handling, the spine is compressed by tensile forces acting in the back muscles as they attempt to raise the upper body and weight into the upright position (Figure 5.8). The back muscles act close to the "pivot point" within the discs, so they need to generate high forces to lift even modest weights. Moderate flexion of the lumbar spine (i.e. flattening the lumbar lordosis) tensions the lumbodorsal fascia so that it is able to assist the back muscles in generating an extensor moment. This is useful, because the fascia acts on a longer lever arm than the back muscles, and so generates a smaller compressive "penalty" on the spine for a given extensor moment *(Dolan, Mannion, Adams 1994)*. A tensioned fascia also absorbs "strain energy" during spinal flexion (rather like a stretched spring) and then releases it later, reducing the metabolic cost of lifting. A desire to save energy probably explains why most people (especially golfers!) are generally reluctant to bend their knees when lifting small objects from the ground: knee bending and subsequent straightening requires the leg muscles to lift superincumbent body weight a considerable distance, and because superincumbent body weight is often much greater than the object to be lifted, a great deal of energy (force times distance) is wasted.

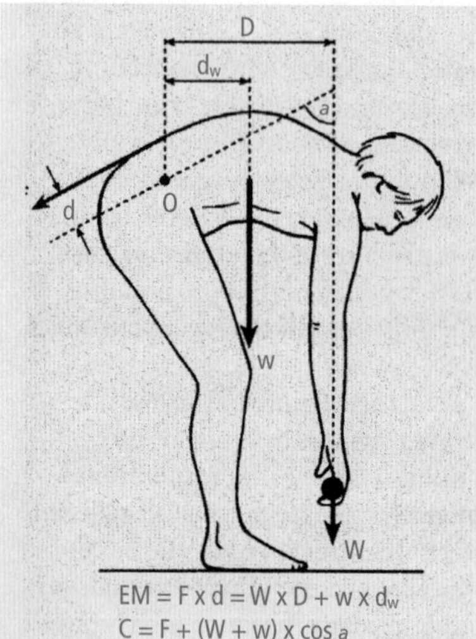

Figure 5.8. When a person stoops to lift an object, their back muscles must develop an extensor moment (EM) to lift the weight (W) and superincumbent body weight (w). Typical lever arms of the back muscles (d) are much smaller than the lever arms of the weights (D and dw) so the back muscle tension (F) is much greater than W or w. Therefore, the spinal compressive force (C) is mostly due to muscle tension. Adapted from *Adams MA, Bogduk N, Burton K, Dolan P* (2002).

Bending stresses acting on the intervertebral discs and ligaments become high only when a person bends forwards as far as they can go. At this point, the bending moment is approximately 35% of that required to injure the osteoligamentous spine *(Adams, Dolan 1991)* indicating that the back muscles normally maintain a considerable margin of safety. Importantly, this margin of safety can be reduced if the back muscles become fatigued *(Dolan, Adams 1998)* or if the spinal reflexes become desensitised by repeated or sustained bending *(Solovieva, Lohiniva, Leino-Arjas et al. 2002)*. Backwards bending of the spine has not been examined closely *in vivo*, but cadaveric experiments show that it can generate high stress concentrations in the posterior regions of lumbar discs, and in the neural arch *(Adams, Bogduk, Burton, Dolan 2002* and *Adams, May, Freeman et al. 2000)*.

Compressive and bending stresses acting on the lumbar spine during manual handling have been measured in a large group of healthy men and women *(Dolan Earley, Adams 1994)*. The peak compressive force is minimised by lifting slowly, with the object as close to the body as possible. Peak bending moment is minimised by bending the knees, and ensuring the object to be lifted is close to, but not between, the feet. Twisting round increases both compression and bending.

Detailed advice on person handling is given elsewhere in this book, but certain general principles arise directly from these biomechanical studies.

- Firstly, the person should be as close to the handler as possible, and should not be lifted quickly
- Secondly, the handler 's lower back should be moderately flexed (flattened) to tension the lumbodorsal fascia, but not so flexed that high bending stresses are thrown on to the intervertebral discs and ligaments. This can be achieved by bending the knees and attempting to maintain a lordosis *(Adams, Bogduk, Burton, Dolan 2002)*, so that the lumbar spine is flexed approximately 80% of the range between erect standing (0%) and full flexion (100%). Some lumbar flexion is unavoidable: when challenged to lift a weight from the floor while maintaining a full lumbar lordosis, a group of healthy subjects were obliged to flex their lumbar spine by 58% on average *(Dolan, Mannion, Adams 1994)*.
- A third principle in person handling is that the lifter should try to avoid prolonged effort, especially in a stooped position, because this can reduce back muscle protection of the underlying spine.

Tissue damage and back pain

The increasing availability of MRI during the last 10 years has revealed variable links between tissue pathology and back pain. Most types of spinal pathology, including disc degeneration and prolapse, can be seen in a moderately high proportion of people who have never suffered from significant back pain *(Boos, Rieder, Schade et al. 1995)* and *(Jensen, Brant-Zawadzki, Obuchowski et al. 1994)*. As discussed above, this has lead to greater understanding of psychosocial influences on back pain behaviour. Unfortunately, it has also encouraged some investigators to denigrate the importance of tissue changes in the generation of back pain itself, and this is a mistake. The MRI studies just cited also showed that certain *structural* features of disc degeneration, such as herniation or radial fissures, are more common in those with back pain. A more recent study showed that the risk of severe back pain is increased by 120% – 460% if MRI scans reveal evidence of structural changes in discs, such as narrowing and annular tears, especially when those changes are associated with increased exposure to mechanical loading *(Videman, Leppavuori, Kaprio et al. 1998)*. Schmorl's nodes also are associated with back pain, although they can also occur in asymptomatic people *(Hamanishi, Kawabata, Yosii et al. 1994)*.

It is instructive to turn the usual question around and ask: "why do some people manage to escape back pain even though they have severe spinal pathology?" This is a major current research concern, and two explanations can be offered already. Firstly, damaged tissues resist loading less, and tend to be stress-shielded by adjacent healthy tissues. For example, a collapse of disc height can lead to nearly all of the spinal compressive force being resisted by the neural arch, so that the damaged disc tissues are largely unloaded *(Pollintine, Dolan, Tobias et al. 2004)*. Secondly, pain-sensitisation phenomena appear to be involved in discogenic pain *(Chen, Cavanaugh, Song et al. 2004* and *Pollintine, Przybyla, Dolan et al. 2004)*, and they probably depend on exactly how near any displaced nucleus pulposus tissue can get to nerve endings in the outer annulus fibrosus and nerve root.

5 Factors that predispose spinal tissues to mechanical damage

Ageing

Ageing causes progressive changes in spinal tissues, particularly in biochemical composition. With increasing age, the intervertebral discs lose proteoglycans and hence water, especially from the nucleus pulposus *(Antoniou, Steffen, Nelson et al. 1996)*. This reduces nucleus pressure, causing the annulus to bulge like a flat tyre *(Brinckmann, Greetenboer 1991)* and to resist high concentrations of compressive stress *Adams, McMillan, Green et al. 1996)* and *(Adams, McNally, Dolan 1996)*. The annulus generally loses height with age, but overall disc height can appear to be normal if the nucleus bulges further into the vertebral bodies. Disc height loss increases apophyseal joint load bearing *(Pollintine, Przybyla, Dolan et al. 2004)*, and reduces the X-sectional area of the intervertebral foramen. Collagen fibres within discs, articular cartilage and ligaments become more cross-linked with age. Some of the cross-linking involves glucose compounds, and they can lead to the tissues becoming yellow-brown in colour, stiffer, and more vulnerable to injury *(DeGroot, Verzijl, Wenting-Van Wijk et al. 2004)*. Vertebrae steadily lose bone mineral with advancing age, especially after the menopause in women, and this reduces their strength to such an extent that fracture can occur during the activities of daily living *(Olmarker, Blomquist, Stromberg et al. 1995)*. Age also tends to decrease the number and metabolic rate of cells that maintain the integrity of the extracellular matrix *(Antoniou, Steffen, Nelson et al. 1996)*. For all of these reasons, age weakens the spine and makes it more vulnerable to mechanical loading.

Genetic inheritance

Epidemiological studies on twins have shown that genetic inheritance can explain (in a statistical sense) approximately 70% of intervertebral disc degeneration *(Schwarzer, Aprill, Derby et al. 1995)*, and a slightly lesser proportion of back pain. Osteoarthritis and osteoporosis also depend heavily on genetic inheritance. The hunt is on to find the genes responsible, and those discovered to date mostly relate to the strength of the extracellular matrix: for example, genes for collagen and vitamin D receptors *(Stokes, Wilder, Frymoyer et al. 1981)* and *(Videman, Nurminen, Troup 1990)*. Other defective genes may possibly hinder cell metabolism, affect mechanical characteristics such as internal lever arms, or impair motor control in such a manner that the risk of injuries is increased.

Nutritional compromise

As the largest avascular structures in the body, the lumbar intervertebral discs have a precarious supply of nutrients. Cells deprived of oxygen become less metabolically active, and create an acidic environment that further impairs cellular metabolism, while cells deprived of glucose can die *(Horner, Urban 2001)*. Nutritional compromise probably explains why factors that impair metabolite transport, such as smoking cigarettes, or an impermeable vertebral endplate, are associated with disc degeneration *(Battie, Videman, Gill et al. 1991)*.

Prior fatigue loading

Failure occurs at lower loads if they are applied repetitively, so that microscopic cracks can multiply within the tissues. Typically, the compressive strength of vertebrae and the tensile strength of annulus fibrosus are reduced by approximately 50% if 5,000 loading cycles are applied *(Adams, Bogduk, Burton, Dolan 2002)*. Compressive fatigue damage to vertebrae is probably a common event in life, because micro-fractures and healing trabeculae are found in most cadaveric vertebral bodies, particularly in the vertically orientated trabeculae behind the endplate *(Videman, Battie, Gibbons et al. 2003)*. Fatigue damage may accumulate rapidly in the end plate if the spine is exposed to mechanical vibrations *(Porter, Adams, Hutton 1989)*.

6 Biological consequences of mechanical loading

Adaptive remodelling *versus* fatigue failure

Physical exercise strengthens muscles, whereas disuse weakens them. Most of the forces acting on the spine come from the musculature *(Dolan, Earley, Adams 1994)*, and skeletal tissues adapt to increased or decreased forces by becoming stiffer and stronger, or softer and weaker. For example, the racquet arm of professional tennis players contains 30% more bone mineral than the other arm, and elite weight lifters have very dense and strong vertebrae. Manual labourers are more likely to have osteophytes (bony spurs) around the margins of their vertebral bodies, which could represent an adaptive response to increase the load-bearing area of the vertebra and hence reduce compressive stress *(Waddell 1998)*. Intervertebral discs probably respond in similar fashion, but this is difficult to demonstrate in animal experiments because disc metabolic activity is so slow that the adaptive remodelling response may be masked by the accumulation of fatigue damage within the disc. Physically active people do have stronger discs and vertebrae, but disc strength appears to increase less, or less rapidly, than vertebral strength *(Sambrook, MacGregor, Spector 1999)*. In this way an abrupt increase in physical workload could lead to disc injuries as disc strength lags behind that of the adjacent vertebrae and muscles *(Adams, Dolan 1997)*. Such a rate-dependent process may explain why the abrupt application of severe mechanical loading causes degenerative changes in the intervertebral discs of small animals without harming the vertebrae *(Kuslich, Ulstom,Michael 1991)*.

Most epidemiological studies consider populations of *survivors*: people who presumably have developed strong backs after many years of hard work. Such studies fail to account for people who injure their backs soon after starting an arduous job, in the period when the discs are still "catching up" with strengthening muscles and bones. This interpretation is supported by the high number of back injuries sustained by young nurses during their first year on the wards *(Kroeber, Unglaub, Wang et al. 2002)*.

Response to structural failure

Adaptive remodelling is a normal reversible process which should not be confused with the degenerative changes which variably affect ageing spines, and which are associated with gross structural failure within specific tissues. (The word "degenerative" implies progressive *deleterious* changes, and it should not be used to include the inevitable chronological changes, which characterise growth and development.) Damaged collagen fibres in ligaments and in the annulus fibrosus deteriorate markedly, probably because loss of tension predisposes them to enzymatic attack *(Hsieh, Lotz 2004)*. Damaged vertebrae heal, but the original shape is not normally regained. Injured intervertebral discs show little sign of true healing *(Myers, Wilson 1997)*, probably because collagen synthesis within the avascular disc is so slow. Structural changes in the annulus therefore become increasingly common with increasing age. The discs of rabbits, sheep and pigs degenerate rapidly following scalpel "injuries" to the annulus or vertebral endplate *(Kawchuk, Kaigle, Holm et al. 2001)* and *(Myers, Wilson 1997)*. Annulus defects are filled with fibrous tissue, but fissures can progress until the mechanical integrity of the disc is eventually destroyed. An even more rapid "degenerative" response occurs when displaced nucleus pulposus is allowed to swell unopposed in surrounding fluid for several hours: swelling allows proteoglycan loss and gross tissue shrinking during the following few days *(Dolan, Adams, Hutton 1987)*. In life, therefore, disc prolapse would cause rapid physicochemical changes in the displaced tissue, which might give an illusion of a slowly developing condition. This would be followed by long-term structural and biochemical changes in the remaining disc. Degenerative changes are usually observed in prolapsed disc material removed at surgery, encouraging spinal surgeons to assume that degenerative changes must necessarily *precede* disc prolapse. This may possibly be true in some individuals, but the weight of scientific evidence suggests that cell-mediated degeneration *follows* the mechanical disruption of spinal tissues.

Gross structural failure probably represents a crucial "point of no return" in the process of disc degeneration, because it permanently impairs disc function. Typically, the nucleus becomes decompressed and high stress concentrations appear within the annulus *(Adams, Freeman, Morrison et al. 2000)*. The former would inhibit cell metabolism in the nucleus *(Ishihara, McNally, Urban et al. 1996)*, and the latter would promote enzymatic degradation of the annulus *(Handa, Ishihara, Ohshima et al. 1997)*. In this way, cell activity is unable to restore disc integrity and function – indeed, it would tend to make them worse. As a result, the disc enters a progressive degenerative spiral, rather than responding to restore the status quo as in adaptive remodelling.

7 Functional pathology

Posture and stress concentrations in the spine

A cadaveric lumbar spine shows a natural lordotic curvature of about 40° in the sagittal plane when cut free from all muscle attachments (Figure 5.9). In the upright standing posture, this lordosis is increased by about 13-15°, whereas upright sitting reduces it by 20-35° so that the lumbar spine becomes straight *(Adams, Bogduk, Burton, Dolan 2002)*. The relative merits of "lordotic" and "flat back" postures are summarised in Table 5.1. High stress concentrations in the posterior annulus and apophyseal joints may explain the dull backache experienced by many following prolonged (lordotic) standing. It seems that lordotic posture has been advocated in the past because it reduces the hydrostatic pressure in the nucleus pulposus. However, this apparent benefit is lost when the compressive force rises to high levels, and it occurs at low loads only because the load is transferred from the nucleus pulposus to the posterior annulus fibrosus and apophyseal joints, which are less able to resist it *(Adams,May, Freeman et al. 2000)*.

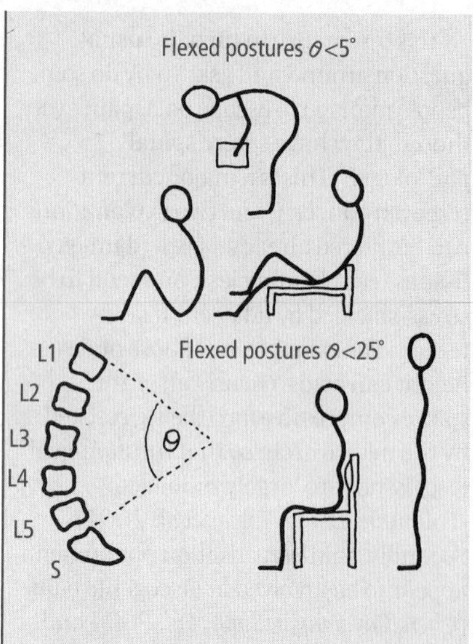

Figure 5.9. The orientation of the lumbar vertebral bodies in the sagittal plane can be defined by the lumbar curvature (è). This angle increases in erect postures such as upright standing, and decreases, or is reversed, in flexed postures.

The effect of sustained and repetitive loading on spinal mechanics

During the first few hours of each day, physical activity drives water from the intervertebral discs and reduces their volume by approximately 20% *(Botsford, Esses, Ogilvie-Harris 1994)*. Changes are reversed following a night's rest, giving rise to a diurnal variation in human stature of about 15–25 mm. In the laboratory, reducing the water content of discs by sustained loading causes them to bulge radially outwards, like a "flat tyre", and potentially painful concentrations of compressive stress appear within the posterior annulus *(Adams, McMillan, Green et al. 1996)*. Diurnal disc height loss affects the mechanical properties of the whole spine (Figure 5.10). It increases vertical loading of the apophyseal joints, slackens the intervertebral ligaments so that they resist bending movements less, and reduces the discs' susceptibility to prolapse *(Adams, Bogduk, Burton, Dolan 2002* and *Adams, Dolan, Hutton et al.*

Table 5.1

A comparison of the effects of moderately flexed and lordotic postures on the lumbar spine. Reproduced from *Adams, Bogduk, Burton and Dolan 2002* with permission.

	Advantages of moderately flexed postures:
1	even distribution of stress in the intervertebral discs
2	increased supply of metabolites to vulnerable regions of discs
3	reduced loading of the apophyseal joints
4	increased volume of intervertebral foramen and spinal canal
5	lumbodorsal fascia is able to resist lumbar flexion
	Advantages of lordotic postures:
1	reduced pressure in the nucleus pulposus
2	reduced compressive stresses in the anterior annulus
3	apophyseal joints contribute to spinal compressive strength
4	improved shock absorption during locomotion
5	spinal stretch reflexes preserved

1990). Diurnal changes in spinal mechanics can be readily appreciated by trying to touch your toes just before going to bed, and then trying again during the first few minutes after getting up, when it will be more difficult. Although there appear to be no epidemiological studies concerning diurnal variations in the onset of back pain, there is clinical evidence that forwards bending and lifting movements should be avoided during the first few hours of the day *(Solomonow, Baratta, Zhou et al. 2003)*.

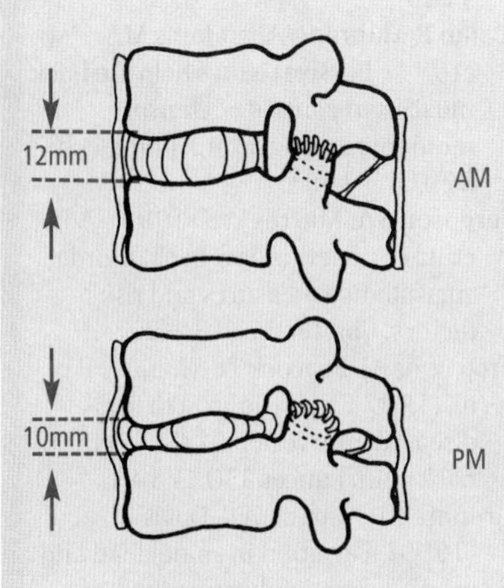

Figure 5.10. Motion segments in the sagittal plane (anterior on the left) showing the consequences of a 2mm diurnal change in intervertebral disc height. Late in the day (PM), the dehydrated disc is narrowed, and the apophyseal joints become load bearing. The ligaments and annulus fibrosus gain some "slack" and the spine resists bending movements less.

Muscle dysfunction and chronic back pain

Back pain may lead to abnormal muscle function, which in turn may lead on to recurrent or chronic problems in muscle and underlying tissues. For example, pain may inhibit normal spinal movements, causing muscle atrophy, a reduction in joint mobility, a loss of the flexion-relaxation phenomenon, and a shift in back muscle fibre type from fast-twitch to slow-twitch *(Marras, Lavender, Leurgans et al. 1993)*. The back muscles are required to protect the underlying spine from excessive bending, but this protection is reduced by poor spinal mobility *(Adams, Mannion, Dolan 1999* and *Dolan, Adams 1993)* and may be reduced if the muscles become weaker and slower *(Dolan, Adams 1998)*. Also, sustained or repetitive bending movements can inhibit the normal spinal reflexes that protect the underlying spine *(Solovieva, Lohiniva, Leino-Arjas et al. 2002)*. Finally, unilateral pain may cause an imbalance in muscle activity leading to asymmetry in spinal posture and movement *(Adams, Bogduk, Burton, Dolan 2002)*. As discussed above, small changes in lumbar curvature can lead to high and potentially painful stress concentrations in the discs and apophyseal joints.

Spinal movements and low back pain

Spinal movement patterns have been used to distinguish between "normal" and "back pain" populations. People with back pain tend to move their backs less, and more slowly, presumably because vigorous full-range movements exacerbate their pain. Also, they sometimes show abnormal "coupling" of movements in different planes *(Vernon-Roberts, Pirie 1973)*. However, there is no evidence that abnormal movement patterns *cause* back pain, and the variability found in normal pain-free people makes it difficult to assign any individual patient to a specific diagnostic group on the basis of spinal movements. The fact that experienced weight lifters employ more variable muscle recruitment patterns than novice lifters *(Granata, Marras, davis et al. 1999)* argues against the importance of specific muscle recruitment patterns during manual handling.

8 Discussion

This chapter attempts to explain the role played by mechanical loading in the aetiology of back pain. The evidence considered above shows that mechanical loading is not necessarily harmful at all: indeed it tends to make the spine stronger and more resistant to injury. However, when loading becomes excessively severe or repetitive for a given individual, then injury or fatigue failure can occur. The most vulnerable structure appears to be the vertebral body endplate, but discs, ligaments and apophyseal joints can also be injured by the various combinations of compression, bending, and torsion that are applied to the spine during manual handling. Disrupted tissues resist loading abnormally, and animal models show that cell-mediated degenerative changes then occur in the tissues. Pain can follow pathological changes, but the relationship between the two is complicated by pain-sensitisation phenomena, and by the fact that injured tissues are often "stress-shielded" by adjacent healthy tissues. Pain may occur in the absence of pathology if certain postural habits cause stress concentrations to be generated within innervated tissues. Psychosocial factors can explain relatively trivial symptoms, and frequently exert an important influence on all aspects of back pain *behaviour*, including work absence and response to treatment.

The major thrust of recent research has been to explain why some backs are more vulnerable than others to the effects of mechanical loading. Genetic inheritance has a direct and major influence on the strength of spinal tissues, and probably also on cell-mediated repair processes. In addition, advancing age causes inexorable biochemical changes which further weaken certain tissues, and the combined effects of ageing and fatigue loading can cause microdamage to accumulate in tissues such as the intervertebral discs which have a slow metabolic rate. Finally, the transportation of metabolites into the lumbar intervertebral discs is so precarious that any disruption (perhaps arising from smoking cigarettes, or injury to a vertebral endplate) can probably lead to cell death and tissue weakening. Perhaps the best way to avoid back pain (apart from changing one's parents!) is to ensure that spinal tissues are strengthened slowly and continuously during early life so that they have an improved ability to survive the repetitive loading and unpredictable incidents associated with manual handling. Correct handling technique and sensible manual handling regulations should ensure that tissue tolerances are exceeded only in the most vulnerable backs.

Correspondence should be sent to:
Dr. M.A. Adams, University of Bristol, Department of Anatomy, Southwell Street, Bristol BS2 8EJ, U.K.

Tel. 0117 9288363
Fax. 0117 9254794
Email: M.A.Adams@bris.ac.uk

Acknowledgements
Some of the text, and many of the ideas, are adapted from a book of the same name.

References

Adams MA, Bogduk N, Burton K, Dolan P (2002). The Biomechanics of Back Pain, Churchill Livingstone, Edinburgh, U.K.

Adams MA, Dolan P (1991). A technique for quantifying the bending moment acting on the lumbar spine in vivo. J Biomech 24(2): 117-26.

Adams MA, Dolan P (1996). Time dependent changes in the lumbar spine's resistance to bending. Clin Biomech 11 194-200.

Adams MA, Dolan P (1997). Could sudden increases in physical activity cause intervertebral disc degeneration? Lancet 350 734-735.

Adams MA, Dolan P, Hutton WC et al. (1990). Diurnal changes in spinal mechanics and their clinical significance. J Bone Jt Surg 72B 266-70.

Adams MA, Freeman BJC, Morrison HP et al. (2000). Mechanical initiation of intervertebral disc degeneration. Spine 25 1625-36.

Adams MA, Hutton WC (1982). Prolapsed intervertebral disc: a hyperflexion injury. Spine 7 184-191.

Adams MA, Hutton WC (1985). Gradual disc prolapse. Spine 10 524-531.

Adams MA, Mannion AF, Dolan P (1999). Personal risk factors for first-time low back pain. Spine 24 2497-2505.

Adams MA, May S, Freeman BJC et al. (2000). The effects of backwards bending on lumbar intervertebral discs: relevance to physical therapy treatments for low back pain. Spine 25 431-7.

Adams MA, McMillan DW, Green TP et al. (1996). Sustained loading generates stress concentrations in lumbar intervertebral discs. Spine 21 434-8.

Adams MA, McNally DS, Dolan P (1996). Stress distributions inside intervertebral discs: the effects of age and degeneration. J Bone Joint Surg 78B 965-72.

Antoniou J, Steffen T, Nelson F et al. (1996). The human lumbar intervertebral disc: evidence for changes in the biosynthesis and denaturation of the extracellular matrix with growth, maturation, ageing, and degeneration. J Clin Invest 98:996-1003.

Battie MC, Videman T, Gill K et al. (1991). Smoking and lumbar intervertebral disc degeneration: an MRI study of identical twins. Spine 16(9): 1015-21.

Bogduk N (1997). Clinical Anatomy of the Lumbar Spine and Sacrum. 3rd Edition. Churchill Livingstone, Edinburgh, U.K.

Boos N, Rieder R, Schade V et al. (1995). The diagnostic accuracy of MRI, Work perception,, and psychosocial factors in identifying symptomatic disc herniations. Spine 20 2613-25.

Botsford DJ, Esses SI, Ogilvie-Harris DJ (1994). In-vivo diurnal variation in intervertebral disc volume and morphology. Spine 19 935-940.

Brinckmann P, Grootenboer H (1991). Change of disc height, radial disc bulge and intradiscal pressure from discectomy: an in-vitro investigation on human lumbar discs. Spine 16 641-6.

Chen C, Cavanaugh JM, Song Z et al. (2004). Effects of nucleus pulposus on nerve root neural activity, mechanosensitivity, axonal morphology, and sodium channel expression. Spine 29:17-25.

DeGroot J, Verzijl N, Wenting-Van Wijk MJ et al. (2004). Accumulation of advanced glycation end products as a molecular mechanism for aging as a risk factor in osteoarthritis. Arthritis Rheum 50(4): 1207-15.

Dolan P, Adams MA (1993). Influence of lumbar and hip mobility on the bending stresses acting on the lumbar spine. Clin Biomech 8 185-192.

Dolan P, Adams MA, Hutton WC (1987). The short-term effects of chymopapain on intervertebral discs. J Bone Jt Surg 69-B 422-428.

Dolan P, Adams MA (1998). Repetitive lifting tasks fatigue the back muscles and increase the bending moment acting on the lumbar spine. J Biomech 31(8): 713-21.

Dolan P, Earley M, Adams MA (1994). Bending and compressive stresses acting on the lumbar spine during lifting activities. J Biomech 27 1237-1248.

Dolan P, Mannion AF, Adams MA (1994). Passive tissues help the back muscles to generate extensor moments during lifting. J Biomech 27 1077-1085.

Ferguson SA, Marras WS (1997). A literature review of low back disorder surveillance measures and risk factors. Clin Biomech 12: 211-26.

Freemont AJ, Peacock TE, Goupille P et al. (1997). Nerve ingrowth into diseased intervertebral disc in chronic back pain. Lancet 350:178-81.

Granata KP, Marras WS, Davis KG et al. (1999). Variation in spinal load and trunk dynamics during repeated lifting exertions. Clin Biomech 14(6): 367-75.

Green TP, Allvey JC, Adams MA (1994). Spondylolysis: bending of the inferior articular processes of lumbar vertebrae during simulated spinal movements. Spine 19 2683-91.

Hamanishi C, Kawabata T, Yosii T et al. (1994). Schmorl's nodes on MRI: their incidence and clinical

relevance. Spine 19 4 450-53.
Handa T, Ishihara H, Ohshima H et al. (1997). Effects of hydrostatic pressure on matrix synthesis and matrix metalloproteinase production in the human lumbar intervertebral disc. Spine 22 1085-1091.
Heliovara M (1987). Body height, obesity and risk of herniated lumbar intervertebral disc. Spine 12 469-72.
Horner HA, Urban JP (2001). Effect of nutrient supply on the viability of cells from the nucleus pulposus of the intervertebral disc. Spine 26: 2543-9.
Hsieh AH, Lotz JC (2004). Role of annular tension in maintaining lamellar architecture in vivo. Presented to the 50th meeting of the Orthopaedic Research Society, San Francisco, February 2004.
Ishihara H, McNally DS, Urban JP et al. (1996). Effects of hydrostatic pressure on matrix synthesis in different regions of the intervertebral disk. J Appl Physiol 80: 839-46.
Jensen MC, Brant-Zawadzki MN, Obuchowski N et al. (1994). Magnetic resonance imaging of the lumbar spine in people without back pain. N Engl J Med 331(2): 69-73.
Kawchuk GN, Kaigle AM, Holm SH et al. (2001). The diagnostic performance of vertebral displacement measurements derived from ultrasonic indentation in an in vivo model of degenerative disc disease. Spine 26(12): 1348-55.
Kelsey JL, Githens PB, White AA et al. (1984). An epidemiologic study of lifting and twisting on the job and risk for acute prolapsed lumbar intervertebral disc. J Orthop Res 2 61-66.
Kerttula LI, Serlo WS, Tervonen OA et al. (2000). Post-traumatic findings of the spine after earlier vertebral fracture in young patients: clinical and MRI study. Spine 25: 1104-8.
Klaber Moffett JA, Hughes GI, Griffiths P (1993). A longitudinal study of low back pain in student nurses. International Journal of Nursing Studies 30 197-212.
Kroeber MW, Unglaub F, Wang H et al. (2002). New in vivo animal model to create intervertebral disc degeneration and to investigate the effects of therapeutic strategies to stimulate disc regeneration. Spine 27: 2684-90.
Kuslich SD, Ulstrom CL, Michael C (1991). The tissue origin of low back pain and sciatica. Orthop Clin N Amer 22 181-7.
Lu YM, Hutton WC, Gharpuray VM (1996). Do bending, twisting, and diurnal fluid changes in the disc affect the propensity to prolapse? A viscoelastic finite element model. Spine 21(22): 2570-9.
Mannion AF, Connolly B, Wood K et al. (1997). The use of surface EMG power spectral analysis in the evaluation of back muscle function. J Rehabil Res Dev 34(4): 427-39.
Mannion, AF, Dolan P, Adams MA (1996). Psychological questionnaires: do "abnormal" scores precede or follow first-time low back pain? Spine 21(22): 2603-11.
Mannion AF, Kaser L, Weber E et al. (2000). Influence of age and duration of symptoms on fibre type distribution and size of the back muscles in chronic low back pain patients. Eur Spine J 9(4): 273-81.
Marras WS, Lavender SA, Leurgans SE et al. (1993). The role of dynamic three-dimensional trunk motion in occupationally related low back disorders. Spine 18 617-28.
Melrose JP, Ghosh P, Taylor TK et al. (1992). A longitudinal study of the matrix changes induced in the intervertebral disc by surgical damage to the annulus fibrosus. J Orthop Res 10 665-76.
Myers ER, Wilson SE (1997). Biomechanics of osteoporosis and vertebral fracture. Spine 22 (24S) 25-31.
Olmarker K, Blomquist J, Stromberg J et al. (1995). Inflammatogenic properties of nucleus pulposus. Spine 20 665-9.
Pollintine P, Przybyla AS, Dolan P et al. (2004). Neural arch load bearing in old and degenerated spines. J Biomech 37:197-204.
Pollintine P, Dolan P, Tobias JH et al. (2004). Intervertebral disc degeneration can lead to "stress shielding" of the anterior vertebral body: a cause of osteoporotic vertebral fracture? Spine 29(7): 774-82.
Pope MH (1989). Risk indicators in low back pain. Annals of Medicine 21 387-392.
Porter RW, Adams MA, Hutton WC (1989). Physical activity and the strength of the lumbar spine. Spine 14 2 201-3.
Sambrook PN, MacGregor AJ, Spector TD (1999). Genetic influences on cervical and lumbar disc degeneration. Arthritis & Rheumatism 42 366-72.
Schwarzer AC, Aprill CN, Derby R et al. (1995). The prevalence and clinical features of internal disc disruption in patients with chronic low back pain. Spine 20 1878-83.
Schwarzer AC, Aprill CN, Bogduk N (1995). The sacroiliac joints in chronic low back pain. Spine 20 31-7.
Schwarzer AC, Aprill CN, Derby R et al. (1994). Clinical features of patients with pain stemming from the lumbar zygapophyseal joints. Spine 19 1132-37.
Snook SH, Webster BS, McGorry RW et al. (1998). The reduction of chronic non-specific low back pain through the control of early morning lumbar flexion. A randomised controlled trial. Spine 23(23): 2601-7.
Solomonow M, Baratta RV, Zhou BH et al (2003). Muscular dysfunction elicited by creep of lumbar viscoelastic tissue. J Electromyogr Kinesiol 13:381-96. (C)
Solovieva S, Lohiniva J, Leino-Arjas P et al. 2002. COL9A3 gene polymorphism and obesity in intervertebral disc degeneration of the lumbar spine: evidence of gene-environment interaction. Spine 27: 2691-6.
Stokes IAF, Wilder DG, Frymoyer JW et al. (1981). Assessment of patients with low-back pain by biplanar radiographic measurement of intervertebral motion. Spine 6 (3) 233-240.
Vernon-Roberts B, Pirie CJ (1973). Healing trabecular microfractures in the bodies of lumbar vertebrae. Ann Rheum Dis 32(5): 406-12.
Videman T, Battie MC, Gibbons LE et al. (2003). Associations between back pain history and lumbar MRI findings. Spine 28:582-8.
Videman T, Leppavuori J, Kaprio J et al. (1998). Iatragenic polymorphisms of the vitamin D receptor gene associated with intervertebral disc degeneration. Spine 23 2477-85.
Videman T, Nurminen M, Troup JDG (1990). Lumbar spinal pathology in cadaveric material in relation to history of back pain, occupation and physical loading. Spine 15 8 728-40.
Waddell G. (1998). The back pain revolution. Edinburgh, Churchill Livingstone.
Yang KH, King AI (1984). Mechanism of facet load transmission as a hypothesis for low back pain. Spine 9 557-565.

6 Mechanics and human movement

Philippa Leggett
MSc(Ergs) DipBiomech PGC(MH) MCSP SRP
Freelance manual handling consultant

Summary

In order to understand how humans move themselves and others, this chapter will look at four areas:

- The principles of mechanics – force, gravity, friction, stability, pressure, stress, strain, elasticity and leverage.
- How humans develop and move using these mechanical principles.
- How biomechanics allows mathematical calculation of forces during movement and the limitations of using them.
- Examples of how these calculations can be used in manual handling situations.

At the conclusion, the reader should understand the basis of mechanics, the importance of biomechanical principles in human movement, and how to structure a simplistic mathematical evaluation and analysis of a moving task.

1 Introduction

The Manual Handling Operations Regulations 1992 require that workers are not exposed needlessly to "hazardous manual handling". High mechanical loading is a well-known major factor in back pain (see chapter 4), and many approaches to manual handling are based on numerical parameters; the NIOSH lifting equation, for instance, is widely used to calculate the limitations of load handling for humans (*Waters et al. 1993*).

In order to determine how these forces are calculated, principles of *mechanics* are applied. Sir Isaac Newton (1643–1727), followed on from the work done by Copernicus and Galileo and developed the theory of gravity, plus the laws of motion, which dictate how objects move on this planet. Einstein (1879–1955) postulated his theory of (space-time) relativity based on Newton's principles, and Hawking (1942–present day) is responsible for the mathematical theory linking gravity with quantum mechanics and the "unified theory" of the universe. In April 2004, the Gravity-B satellite began to generate data telling how the Earth distorts space, which will prove or disprove Einstein's theory.

Anatomy was poorly explored in Newton's day but nowadays it is known how the human body functions in great detail, and all the mechanical principles such as gravity, pressure, friction, hydrodynamics, and elasticity apply somewhere within its internal functions. Humans are tailor-made to respond and react to the physical forces generated by life on Earth, and *biomechanics* is the study of mechanics applied to living tissue.

2 Principles of mechanics

Force

Newton's laws deal with the relationship between time, distance and mass.

- *Mass* is an inherent property of all objects and is expressed in *kilograms (kg)*
- *Time* is expressed in *seconds (s)*
- *Distance* is expressed in *metres (m)*

Newton's laws of motion

1. **Law of inertia.** An object at rest will stay at rest, and an object in motion will stay in motion, unless it is acted on by an external force. *Inertia* is a resting state of an object; to move that object, a force greater than the *inertial force* has to be produced (*see below*).
2. **Law of acceleration.** There is a constant relationship between mass, acceleration and force. (*see below*)
3. **Law of interaction.** Every action (*force*) has an equal and opposite reaction (*force*). Forces occur in pairs; movement occurs when the overall force action is unbalanced.

Mechanics is the study of the applications and effects of *forces*. Force is an invisible concept which is a product of *mass* and *acceleration*:

$$F = ma$$

In homage to their "discoverer", units of force are expressed in *Newtons (N)*.

Acceleration is not the same concept as *velocity:*

- *Velocity* (often referred to as *speed*) is measurement of *distance* through *time* and is therefore expressed as *metres per second (m/s)*
- *Acceleration* is measurement of *velocity* increasing through time, so is therefore *metres per second per second (m/s/s,* usually expressed *m/s^2)*

Gravity

Everything on Earth undergoes a powerful acceleration towards the planet's centre, which is *gravity.* It is a *constant* due to the curvature of the Earth, and from Newton's calculations (allegedly begun by an apple falling on his head) this acceleration is:

$$9.81\ m/s^2$$

(Often in biomechanical calculation this figure is "rounded up" to **$10\ m/s^2$** but care must be taken to avoid too much approximation, as this obviously adds a large percentage of error. "Rounding up" should always be acknowledged.)

Every mass possesses a *centre of gravity*, which occupies a position within the three dimensions according to the object's mass distribution.

So if an object has a *mass* of 60kg, it exerts a force created solely by gravity of

$$F = ma \quad 60(9.81) = 588.6N$$

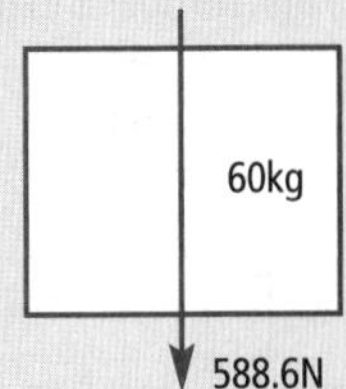

This is the object's *inertial force* (Newton's first law) and it is being resisted by an opposing force from the resting surface (Newton's third law), which "cancels it out".

In order for this to occur, the forces must be acting in opposite directions:

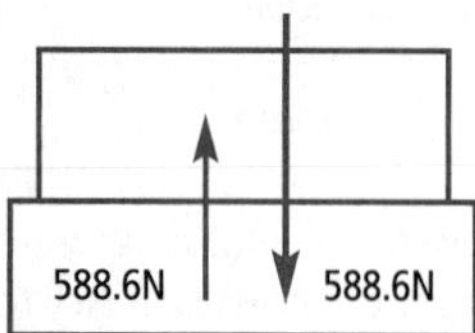

The *net* or *resultant* force is therefore zero, and the object will remain in this position indefinitely, until some force alters the status quo. This state of zero net force is called *equilibrium* and is expressed:

$$\Sigma F = 0$$

that is, the *summation* (Σ) of forces acting on this object is zero.

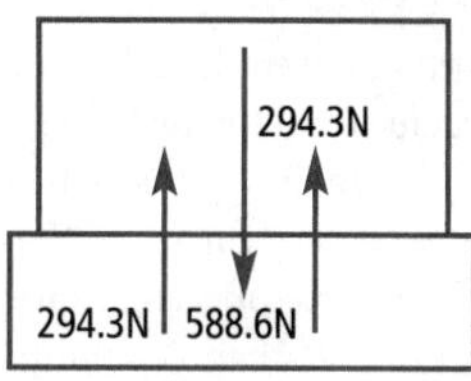

The forces acting upon this object are represented by arrows, which show the:

- Magnitude
- Direction
- Point of application of the forces involved

This is very important, as it affects the overall outcome of the applied force. Forces acting in the same direction may be summated and forces acting in opposite directions will be subtracted. Overall, if there is a *net* (resultant) force from these calculations, one of three things will happen to the object:

- Movement of the object in the direction of the net force
- A *tendency* for the object to move in the force direction, or
- Deformation of the object

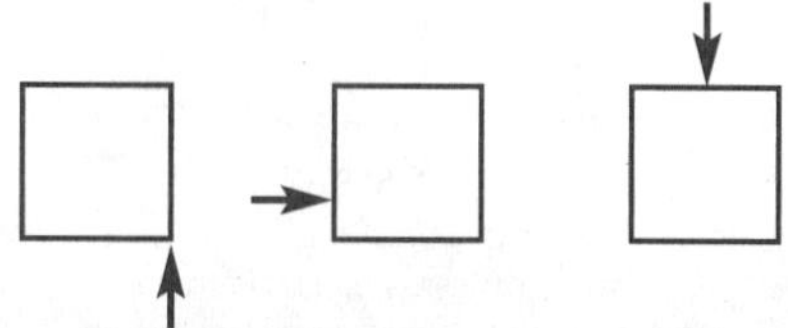

The first box will tilt to the left, the second will slide to the right, and the third will deform at the top. Obviously, if the magnitude of the net applied force is not greater than the inertial force of the object, it will not move, although a tendency will have been created. The object may deform, which may change its shape permanently or temporarily, dependent upon the *elastic limit* of the material. Once force has been created, it has to have an effect, even though sometimes the effect is not easily visible.

In order to perform complex calculations, a *force diagram* may be used.

Some forces are a known constant dependent upon the material they apply to, for instance, *friction* and *stress*.

Friction

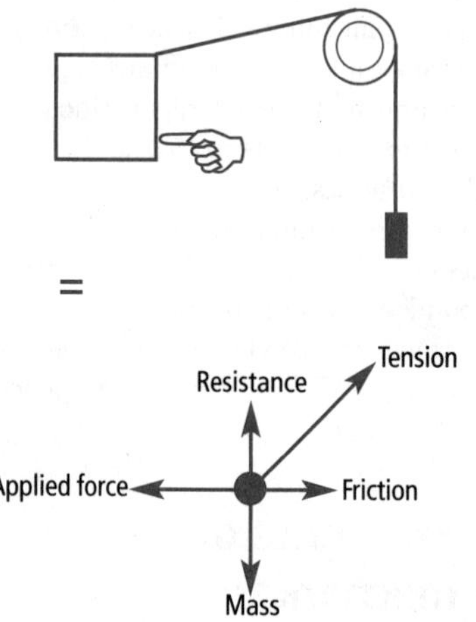

Friction is a resistant force which holds surfaces together; every surface material has a known *friction co-efficient* which is a constant, indicating the level of resistance the material offers to horizontal movement. Obviously this adds to the *inertial force* of an object to be overcome before movement can happen, and friction is often responsible for an object's deceleration. To date, Newton's concept of "perpetual motion" (first law) has never been achieved due to the effects of friction, which applies to gases and liquids as well as solids.

Stress and strain

Hooke's law states that when external force (*stress*) is applied to a solid, the material responds by a linear elongation of its molecular structure. This departure from resting shape (*deformation*) has a magnitude (*strain*) which is directly proportional to the magnitude of stress.

This is a definition of the *elasticity* of a substance, and every substance has a specific resistance to deformation known as *Young's modulus*; those with a high resistance are "stiff". Eventually the stress will exceed the material's *elastic limit* where molecular deformation is permanent, and the material will assume new dimensions (becoming *plastic*) before failing completely. In some materials, the plastic state is much more prolonged than others.

The *tensile strength* of a material is the maximum of *tensile stress* that it can absorb before it enters the plastic state.

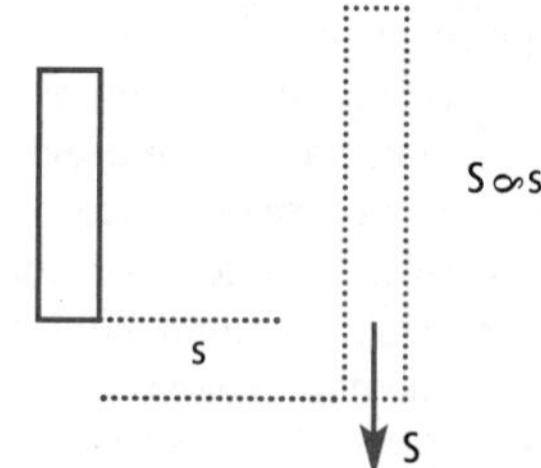

Stability

If the *line of gravity* (which runs through the centre of gravity) falls within an object's base, then that object is *stable* i.e. balanced. (*Base* is contact with a supporting surface-not necessarily the floor.) Once an object's line of gravity falls outside its base, then the object will begin to *topple* and fall under gravitational influence.

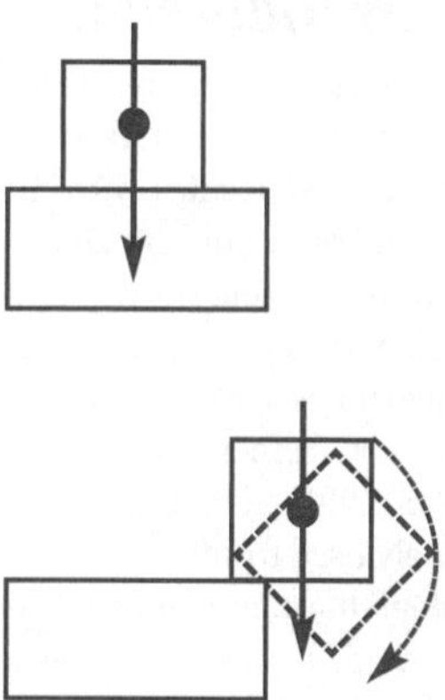

Pressure

Pressure is the product of *force* and *unit area*, therefore units of pressure are expressed in Newtons per square metre or $\mathbf{N/m^2}$. However, pressure is more generally expressed in *Pascals (P)* again after their "discoverer".

A force of 100N may induce

different pressure levels dependent upon the unit area:

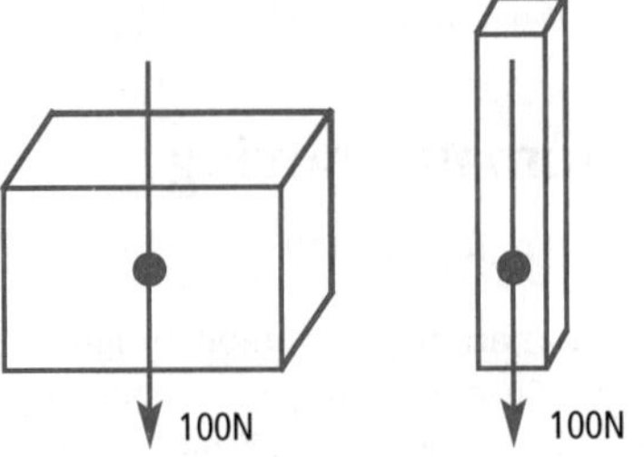

$\frac{100N}{1.0m^2} = 100P$ $\frac{100N}{0.2m^2} = 500P$

Leverage

A lever is a solid object that is used to transfer force over its distance. It can be used to increase the applied force, make a mass move in a different direction from the applied force, or move through a greater distance. The movement that occurs will be rotational (i.e. through an arc, or part of a circle) around a fixed *axis* or *fulcrum*. There are three "orders" or "classes" of lever, which vary the effect upon the applied force depending upon the arrangement of the components:

First order levers are where the axis lies between the "applied force" (FA) and "resistant force" (FR):

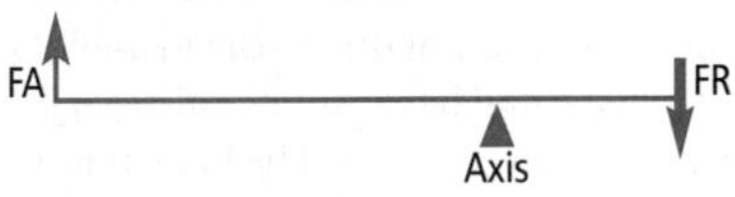

Second order levers are where the resistant force lies between the applied force and the axis:

Both these orders of levers confer *mechanical advantage* (MA), which means that the magnitude of the applied force will move a force greater than itself, especially if the resistant force is close to the axis.

The ratio of mechanical advantage can be calculated:

$$MA = \frac{\text{Resistant force}}{\text{Applied force}} \quad N$$

for instance, if the load's mass was **60kg** that would present (approx.) **600N** and the applied force was **20kg** that would present (approx.) **200N**

So

$$\frac{600N}{200N} = 3:1$$

This in turn means that in order to move the 60kg mass by applying only 20kg, the distance from the applied force to the axis must be **x 3** that of the distance between the resistant force and the axis.

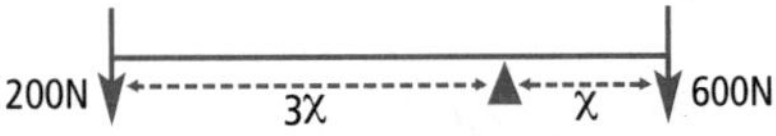

Third order levers do *not* confer mechanical advantage; in this system the applied force lies between the axis and the resistant force:

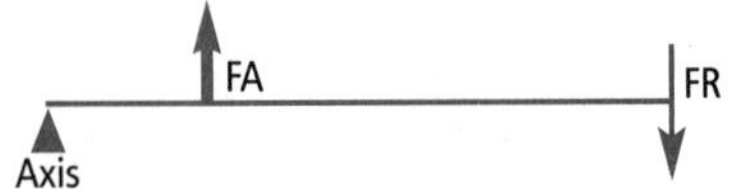

Third order levers mean that the applied force cannot now be less than the resistant force, but what the applied force now confers is movement of the resistant force through a *greater distance*. This increases the *velocity ratio*:

$$VR = \frac{\text{Distance moved by applied force}}{\text{Distance moved by resistant force}} \quad \text{metres}$$

By applying a force over a third order lever, the effect on the resistant force will be to move it a greater distance through an arc around the axis at greater velocity. Consider this example:

The axis of movement is the end of the flag in the ground; the soldiers are applying force at a short distance from the axis, and as a result, the end of the flag is moving from the ground describing a much larger arc than the end they are pushing. Consider also the amount of force they are having to apply and the fact that this is an example of a *concurrent* force system-all the pushing (and pulling) is in the same direction, so it *summates.*

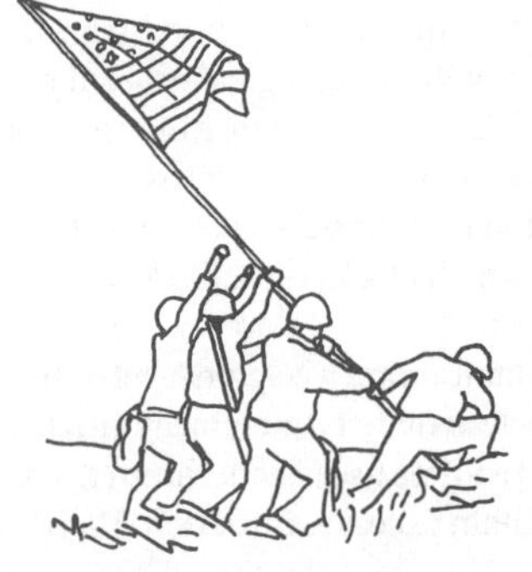

The overall combination of force (**N**) over a distance (**m**) means that expressions of leverage-which are called *moments-* are expressed in *Newton metres (**Nm**)* and moments are created by force-or a force vector-acting over the length of a lever arm (or *moment arm*) and having an application point that lies at 90° to the lever arm-*perpendicularly.* This will be considered later in the chapter.

3 Biomechanics

Human development

Like many animals, humans are born small and feeble, and are incapable of independent movement for some weeks. Being at the top of the food chain enables them to concentrate on learning and interpreting the world around them before having to stand and walk. Having a small body mass with a relatively large head, babies learn to control head movement initially via "head on neck" reflexes (*Green et al. 1995*).

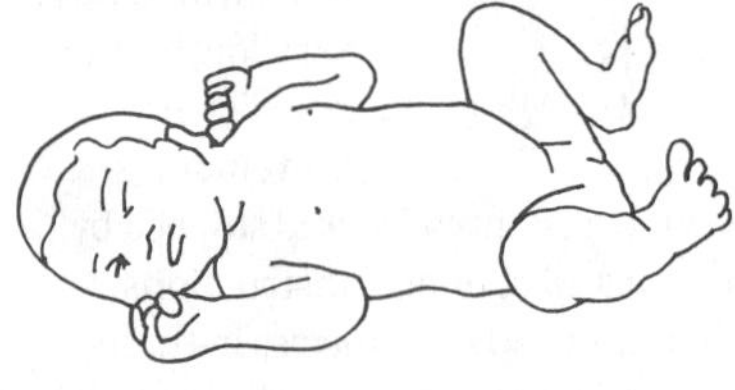

Once these are established, the baby is able to initiate body movement by using head movement, via "head on body" reflexes; once the head turns, the body follows behind. This reflex stays through into adult life and the head continues to *initiate* whole body movement (*Hollands et al. 2001*). Movement *patterns* are learned and retained by constant repetition, allowing the neuromuscular system to "practice" the smooth controlled movements required of the muscles, joints, and ligaments in complex and varied configurations.

Following on from head control, babies have to learn thoracic control in order to move their arms, and trunk control in order to sit up. Unsurprisingly, they learn these complicated manouevres in a stable supported position, lying down and then progressing to sitting up.

Finally they are ready to learn pelvic control, which will allow them to stand upright and eventually walk.

3 Structure of the body

The human body is structured with an internal framework made of bone, composed of hollow systems akin to reinforced concrete, which combine strength with low density to make them light but with a high tensile strength (*Buckwalter & Cooper 1987, Smit et al. 1997*). The skeleton is jointed to allow strength and flexibility to co-exist in the system, especially in the spine. Rigidity is achieved when the joints are "close-packed" with their surfaces congruent (*Kapandji 1974*).

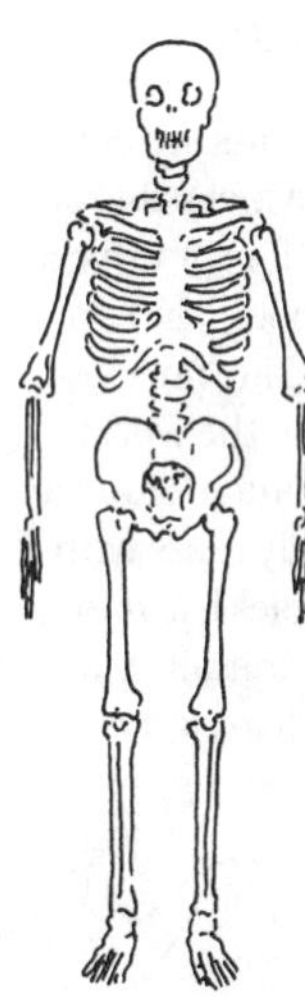

Muscles are the most "elastic" structures, able to absorb external forces within themselves as energy, and release it when required. Ligaments, cartilage and collagen also have elastic properties. Synovial joints contain synovial fluid, which has a very low friction co-efficient. Movement is produced, controlled and stopped by neural and chemical instructions operating pairs of muscles in three planes about the axes of the joints. The circulatory and respiratory systems are constructed to work with atmospheric and hydrostatic pressures.

The central mass of the body-head, thorax and abdomen-contains the important life systems; attached to the thorax is one pair of light mobile limbs and attached to the pelvis is a pair of heavy weight-bearing limbs. The hip and shoulder joints, although of the same model, differ in their construct to illustrate this difference in function, with the hip joint being tightly packed and surrounded by large powerful muscles and ligaments. The shoulder joint by contrast, is very loosely held in place by small, relatively weak tendons and ligaments, and is therefore easily dislocated by external forces (*Robertson et al. 2003, van der Helm 1994*).

Everything in the body is structured to cope with and respond to gravitational forces, which is why it becomes physiologically necessary to have an artificial "gravity" field available for long term space dwellers in Mir station.

Biomechanical structure

In the adult, the proportions of the body have not only grown but changed. The head is still large, but the pelvic area now outweighs it, Head, thorax and abdomen contain first and second class lever systems, giving these segments power. The limbs are arranged with their mass decreasing distally and using third class levers to allow segmental velocity.

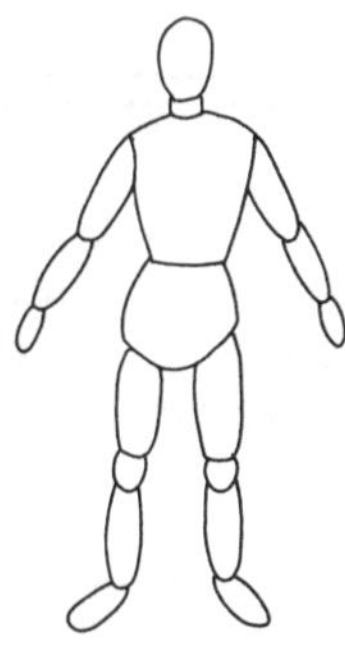

Most of the large muscle groups attach centrally, often in a convergent force system which increases the muscle pull in all three planes of movement, e.g. deltoid. In the distal limbs, a third class leverage system ensures that when biceps contracts in the arm, the hand describes a high-velocity arc ten times greater than that of the length of the muscle contraction.

Velocity is also enhanced by *tone*, which is an inherent muscle property. It

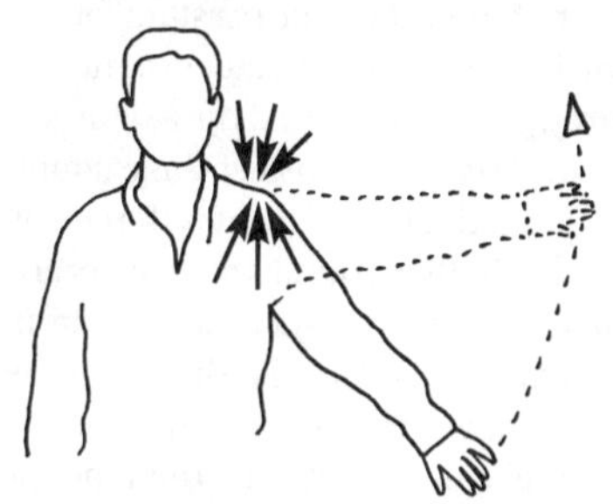

is the "readiness" of muscle tissue to respond to any stimulus, and within humans there is a continuum of tonic maintenance. Whatever the baseline level, humans who are apprehensive will increase tonic level via adrenaline, ready for quick action if necessary. In people with neurological problems, e.g. hemiplegia, this increase may manifest as *spasm*, which is one extreme end of the tonic continuum (*Pisano et al. 1996*) and which blocks rather than enhances movement.

Maintaining a certain level of higher muscle activity is necessarily fatiguing, as it requires use of muscle energy to maintain excess contraction. High tension also mechanically inhibits full circulation to the muscles involved (*Bonde-Petersen et al. 1975*).

4 Humans moving

Humans in standing

Small humans begin to stand upright and learn to control balance in standing on two feet, in other words, on a small base. This is complicated and requires a lot of practice, but as with everything else, children learn by copying adults and by "trial and error". Instability in humans is compensated for by increasing the base and getting support. Toddlers do this by spreading their feet and hanging on to furniture and other

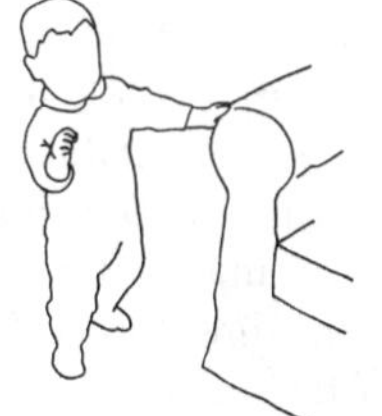

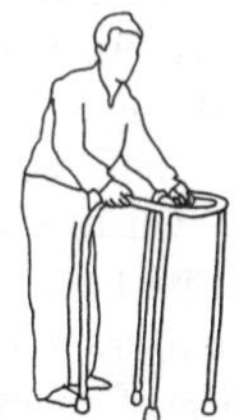

people, for example, older humans do this by adding an artificial base and hanging on to furniture and other people.

Once upright standing has been achieved, it is a position which lends itself to movement due to the instability of such a small base, but it is also very mechanically efficient. The body has a centre of gravity that is constantly altering; as with other living creatures, humans can alter their dimensions at will. The centre is to be found in the dimensional centre of the occupied space, that is, in the centre of the height, width, and depth:

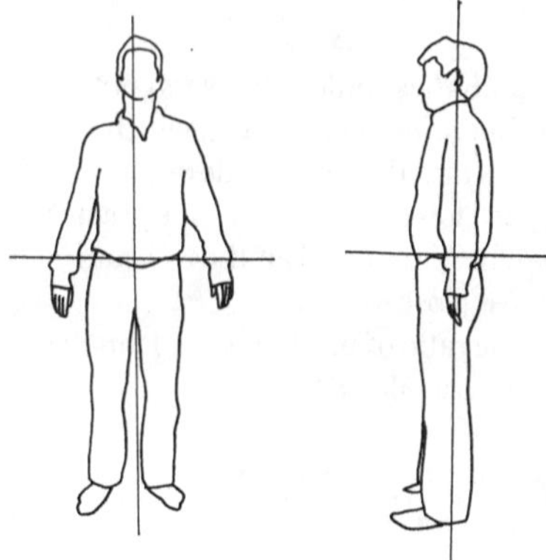

In standing, there should be an equal number of joint axes on either side of the centre of all three planes; this means the lever distances of the major muscle groups from the line of gravity are very small and this upright position, if maintained "correctly", requires low energy to maintain because of its approximation to mechanical equilibrium.

The rigidity of the spine ensures weight-bearing capability and effectively resists the compressive force created by gravity. In standing, the centre is to be found "inside" the pelvis around the first and second sacral level, which makes control of the pelvis paramount for standing, walking and sitting.

Humans walking

Having mastered the art of standing and balancing on two feet, young growing children must now move on to balancing on one foot, in order to learn to walk. Gait is extremely complicated in terms of movement patterning and control, and it requires a vast level of "fine tuning" and co-ordination. Moments created about the hip by the forces of heel strike during gait are in three planes, tending to take the hip into adduction, flexion and external rotation. The arrangement of the gluteal muscles ensures that these moments are simultaneously resisted to allow smooth co-ordinated movement at the hip.

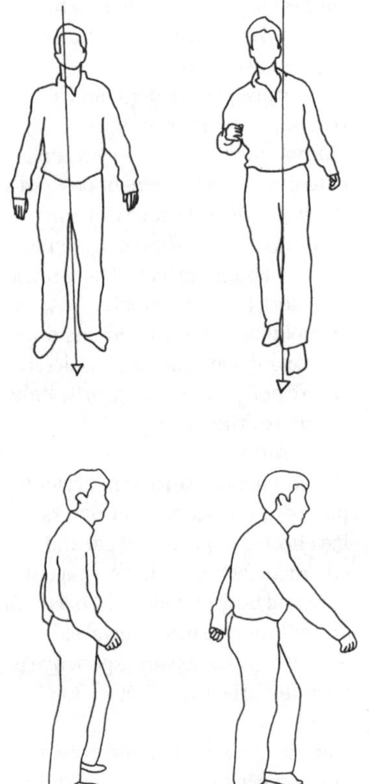

There is little wonder that it takes young children about four or five years to perform complex movements such as going downstairs one foot at a time (*Brenière & Brit 1998*), and that gait is the first pattern to be lost if anything goes wrong either at the command (brain) or execution (musculoskeletal) end of the system. People who have problems may be able to stand, but without pelvic control they will be unable to walk or maintain a standing position.

Humans sitting to standing

In sitting, the base area is now greater, which increases stability, and the centre lies just over the thighs. In order to move from sitting, a person has to at least bring their abdomen over their thighs, i.e. lean forward and bring weight over the centre. If the abdominal muscles are weak or compromised, such as by age, pregnancy or surgery, weight can be brought forwards by moving the pelvis. (It is worth noting that if this cannot be achieved by pelvic movement, effective standing is unlikely.) If it can be achieved, moving forwards makes the person more unstable (and therefore ready to move) by making their supporting base smaller:

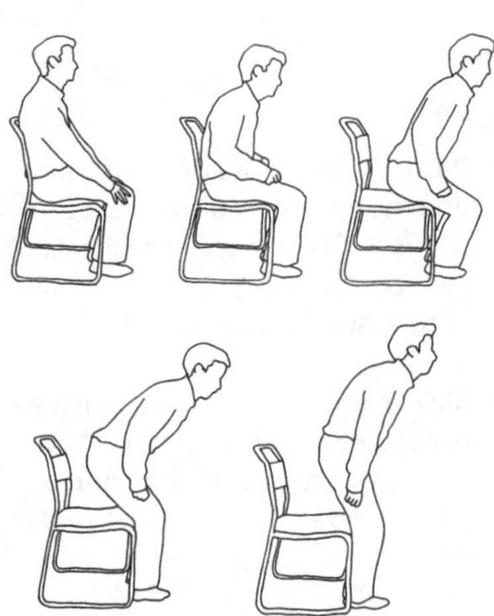

As they stand, their feet are flat and they will then move from the pelvis, pushing their hips forward and their knees out over their feet before extending the knees and pushing down with the arms on the chair seat, if applicable. The higher the seat, the greater pull can be exerted by the quadriceps to assist in pulling the body mass forward. In order to gain momentum for the muscle energy required for this effort, many people find "rocking" helpful.

During the movement they will "unlock" the pelvis to allow it to rotate anteriorly and form the lumbar lordosis in standing. Lifting the head upwards assists the thorax to come forwards and upwards to complete this "unlocking" procedure. The base they move into may be widened by a walking frame.

Humans turning over in bed

In flat lying, the centre of gravity is in the same position as standing, as the planes have been transposed through 90°. In order to move the body, the trunk must be moved, and movement is either initiated from the shoulder girdle, which controls the thorax, or from the pelvis, which controls the abdomen. Humans with a greater body mass have to have enough muscle power to overcome their inertial force, which is often a problem with very heavy people. The provision of something to pull on (e.g. a Bedlever) will assist people in turning themselves, as will sliding sheets to reduce the friction element.

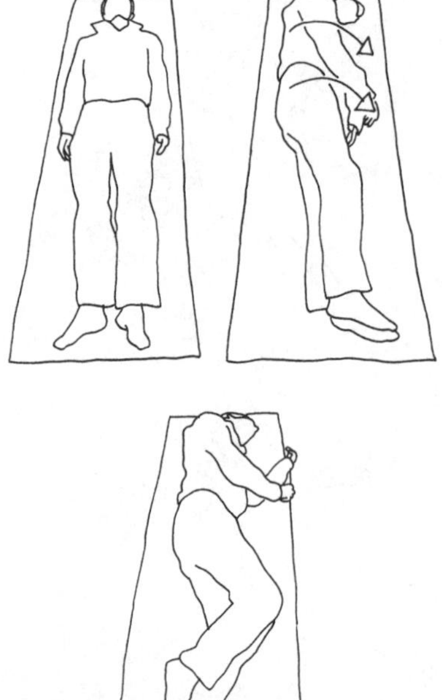

Humans in a hoist sling

A mobile hoist is mechanically a "block and tackle" which suspends the person's mass inside its own base to maintain stability during movement. Sometimes people complain about discomfort of a hoist sling, which is due to the position of their centre of gravity, just over the thighs, creating high pressure on the seams of the sling beneath them.

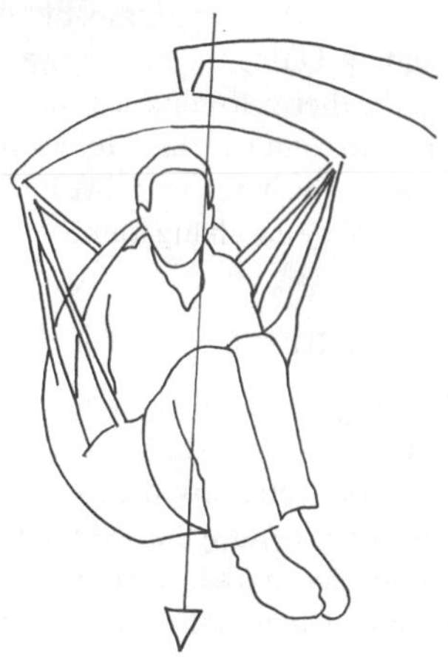

Humans performing advanced moves

Some humans now progress to extremes of movement, taking their body capability to either the strength or mobility ends of the continuum:

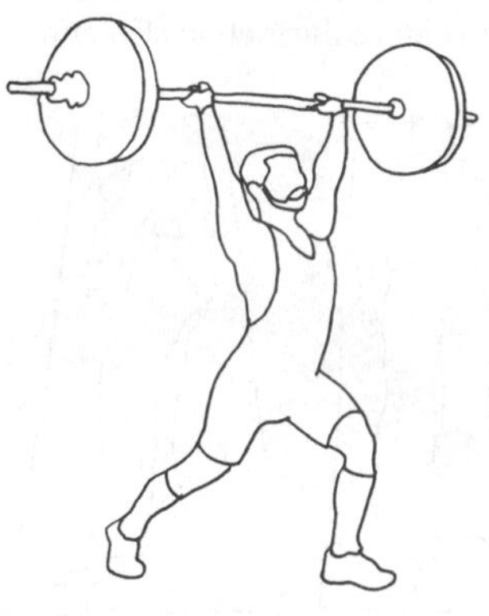

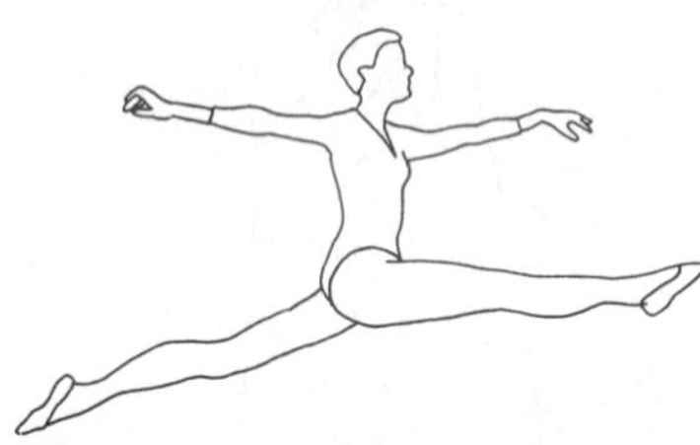

Humans who participate in sport make particular use of mechanical advantages:

- Divers and sprinters lean forwards to make themselves unstable in order to move faster, and speed skaters remain in this unstable position while moving over a low friction surface to increase their velocity even further.

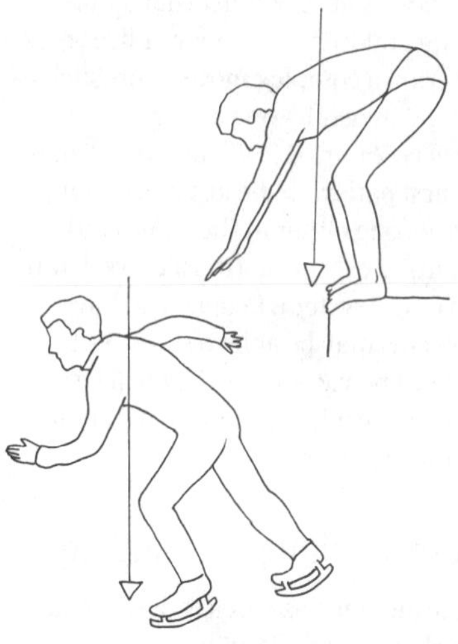

- Female ballet dancers and gymnasts suspend their entire body weight through a very small area of their toes. This creates huge pressures and again makes them very unstable.

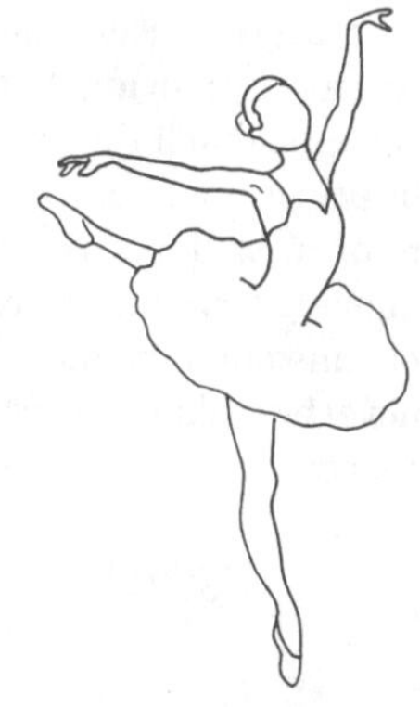

- Racing wheelchair athletes do not grip the tyres, they use contact with the heel of the palm only while they perform head extension to make use of the powerful scapular and chest muscles.
- Male ballet dancers suspending their partner's full body weight will have their hands around their partner's trunk to do so... and both feet on the floor.

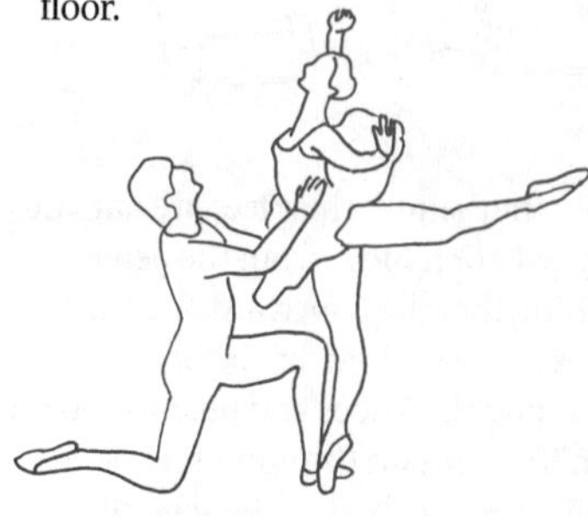

- Adults automatically lift babies and small children with contact points on the trunk, especially at the shoulder girdle and pelvis.

5 Calculating forces

Limitations of using biomechanical calculations

Forces can be calculated to give an approximation of how people face hazards not just from manual handling and the effort involved in moving loads and people, but also from static postures. However, it should be borne in mind that there are limitations to the use of biomechanical calculations as the sole criterion for measurement of a handling task:

- Many biomechanical measurements are gained from cadaver specimens (*Nachemson 1975*) and therefore bear little relationship to the body. They are consequently only an approximation of the forces that apply in living tissue
- Measurements gained may vary from study to study of the same task e.g. lifting tasks (*Gallagher et al 2002*) as humans differ in their performance. Many studies are done using a single task action, which avoids the possibility of the subjects either learning and improving or fatiguing and worsening.
- Biomechanical measurement is usually very precise, for instance, using a force plate for gait measurement, or wearing a spinal movement monitor. This necessitates human adaptation to fit into the measuring devices and produces what may be considered an "unnatural" movement, and a possible "Hawthorne" effect.
- Human movement is very complicated; each body segment possesses its own centre of gravity moving through three planes of movement around changing axes. There must therefore be an inevitable "simplification" factor, for instance, where only one joint is considered, where body mass is arbitrarily halved or where other forces and accelerations are ignored.
- Human performance is not reliant purely upon mechanical factors. Psychosocial, physiological and chemical factors all have a part to play and may provide enhancement or limitation to mechanical efficiency. Low back pain experience is multifactorial (*McGill et al. 2003*).

However, the mathematics are useful to gain some insight into the magnitude of forces within the body, and to use these figures as a guideline towards deciding at what point human tissue would be experiencing "excessive" forces which might create problems.

Example 1

This person is bending forwards but no movement is taking place, that is, they are in equilibrium.
So

$$\Sigma \mathbf{M} = \mathbf{0}$$

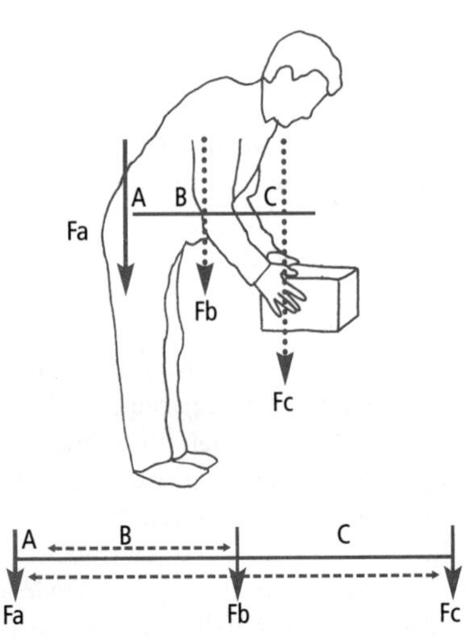

The moments occurring about the axis of the lumbar spine must be equal, which means that

force a (distance A)
= force b (distance B)

If the mass of this person is 60kg, then simplistically force b =30(9.81)N = **294.3N**

If distance B = 10(distance A) then force a = 10(294.3)N = **2943N**

If this person were then to lift an extra 10kg at the end of their outstretched arms, there would now be two summated forces to be counterbalanced by the internal forces produced by the muscles and ligaments:

ΣM = 0, therefore **Aa = (Bb + Cc)**

If distance C =20 times that of A, then a =10(b + 20(c)
where B = 294.3N and c = 10(9.81)N

so the muscle force (a) must equal 10(294.3) + 20(98.1) = **4905N**

Forces may be calculated in this way to give an indication of what limits should be considered for loads being repetitively handled, e.g. the equation developed by NIOSH (National Institute of Occupational Safety and Health (*NIOSH 1991, Waters et al. 1993*).

Static postures may all be analysed in this way, and the mathematics may be formulated into assessment systems, e.g. REBA (Rapid Entire Body Assessment – see appendix 1), (*Hignett and McAtamney 2000*) which can be immensely useful in comparing postures, especially in industry, without a complex mathematical sum.

Example 2

A care provider kneels and bends forward to perform leg dressings:

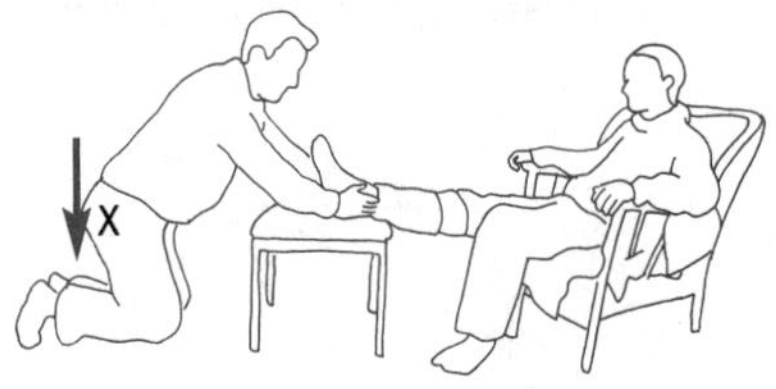

Again, there is no movement overall, so the moments created about the lumbar spine are in equilibrium.

Body weight of carer = 70kg
therefore
upper torso = 35kg

Gravitational force created =
35(9.81)N = **343.35N**

This force is acting approximately one metre from the lumbar axis, so the moment produced will be

343.35 (1) = **343.35Nm**

This is being counter-balanced by the force from the ligaments and musculature acting over a distance of only 0.01m from the lumbar axis, so

Force θ (0.01m) = 343.35Nm
therefore
force θ = 343.35
0.01m = **34335N**

This means that a force has to be created internally by ligament tension and active muscle contraction. In the spine, this muscle contraction produces a compressive force on the spinal discs, and it is the magnitude, speed and repetition of this compression that may lead to disc damage (*McGill et al. 1996*).

However, most forces, especially those in the body, do not act at 90°. Forces that act at an angle of incidence may still be calculated if the angle is known, using the *parallelogram of forces*. This gives equations for calculating the horizontal and vertical *force vectors* that combine trigonometrically to provide the *resultant force*. These equations are:

V = R (sine of angle)
and
H = R (cosine of angle)

This means that if a force of (say) 2000N is applied at an angle of 40°, a component of that force will move the object *horizontally* and a component will move the object *vertically* depending upon the angle. These two components can be calculated:

V = R(sine 40 °)
so the vertical effort will be 2000(0.64)
= **1285.575N**

H = R(cosine 40 °)
so the horizontal effort will be 2000 (0.767) = **1532.1N**

Therefore,the greater effort is being expended on moving this object horizontally.

These equations may also be used to calculate which angle is more efficient:

Example 3

A porter is pulling on a sheet to transfer a patient using a Pat slide at an angle of 60°. The patient weighs 70kg, so the porter must exert at least 70(9.81)N to begin moving the patient = 686.7N. The patient needs to move *horizontally* across the Pat slide, so the porter requires a horizontal vector of at least 700N or the patient will not move.

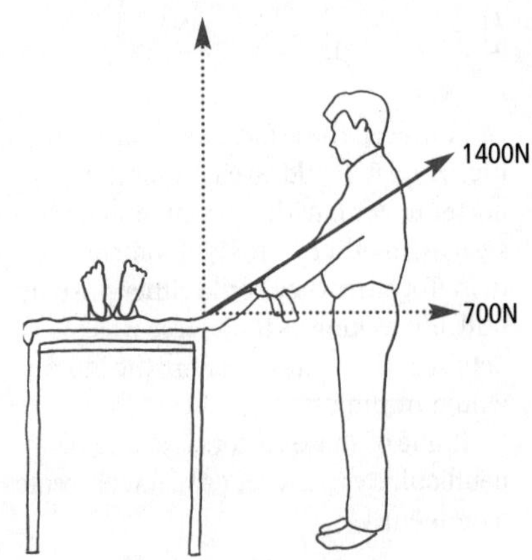

The cosine of 600 is 0.5, so if H = R (0.5) that is, 700 = R(0.5) then

$$R = \frac{700}{0.866} = \mathbf{1400N}$$

If the porter raised the bed so the angle was only 30° then the values would also change:

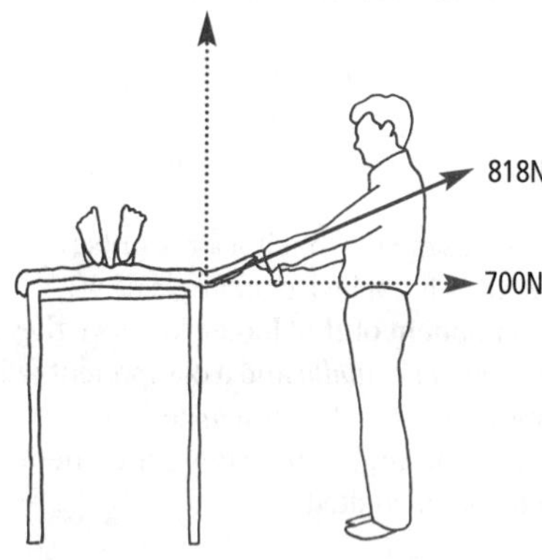

Cosine of 300 = 0.866, so now H = R (0.866), that is 700 = R (0.866) therefore

$$R = \frac{700}{0.866} = \mathbf{818.314N}$$

If the porter raised the bed still further so he was pulling at an angle even less than 30° then the force required would drop further, and obviously at 0° he would only need to produce the 700N.

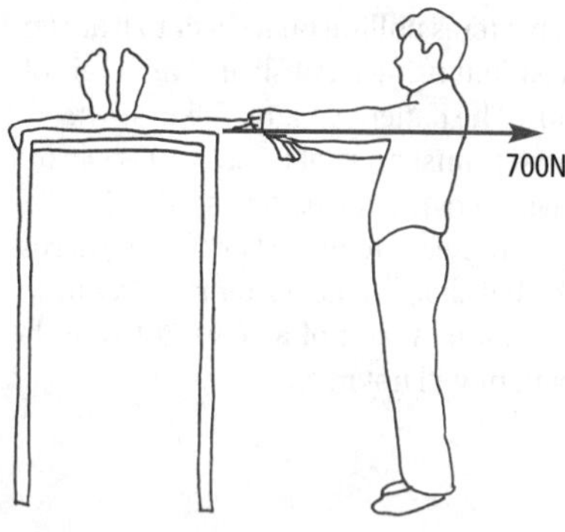

However, these force levels are still high, and it would be easier for the porter to work with a concurrent force system, in other words, get someone to help. Together they could either push or pull, but as long as their force was acting in the same direction, the forces would summate.

If one of these vectors is acting perpendicularly to a lever arm, it will create a moment.

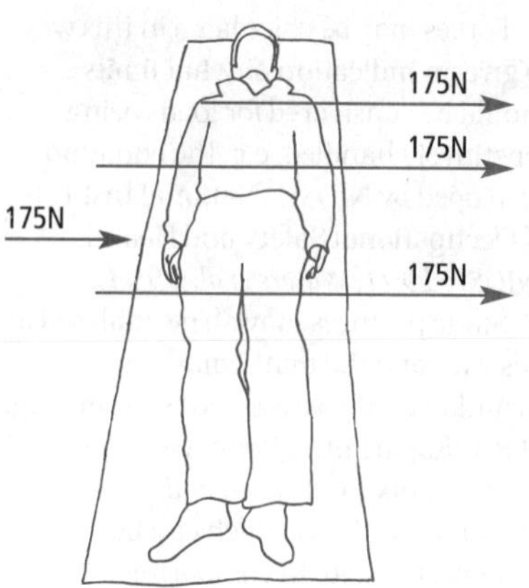

Example 4

If this is a porter pushing a cage trolley with their force applied at an angle, there may be a tendency for the trolley to tip forwards due to the effect of the moment created by the vertical vector:

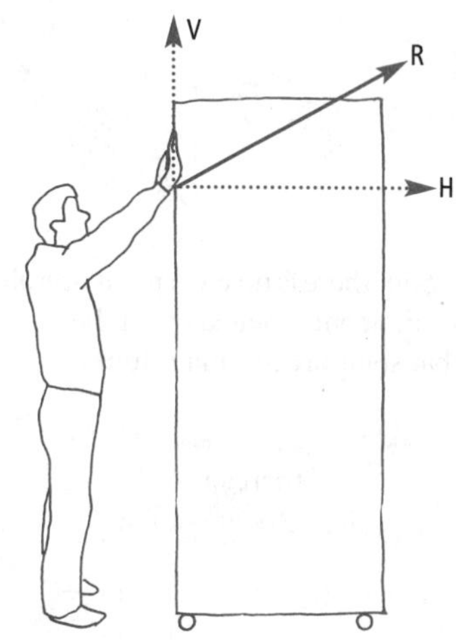

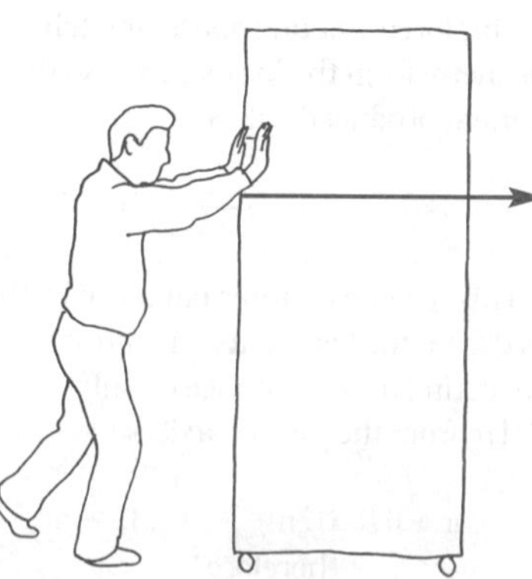

Structures within the body work very closely with vectors, as a force (for example at heel strike) will have a different point of application in two planes of movement. The vectors from these forces will in turn create moments which are resisted by muscular synergy. Many muscles in the body have more than one attachment and more than one action for this reason, many of these attachments work through angles that add up to 90° to make them effective in different planes of movement.

Example 5

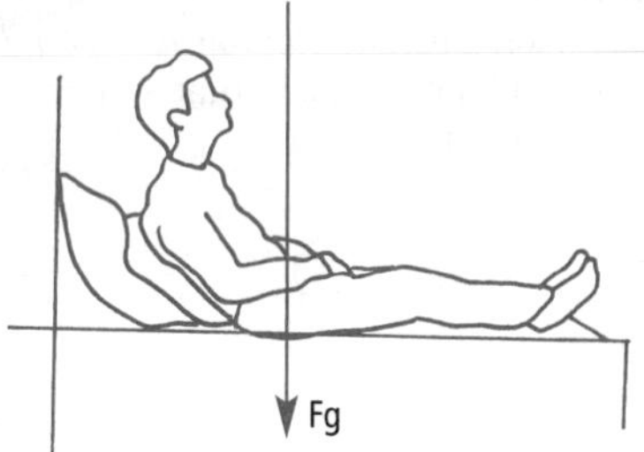

If this person weighs 60kg, then their inertial force will be:

$$60\,(9.81)\text{N} = 588.6\text{ N}$$

In order to move, this person must move their centre of gravity, which at present is beyond their parameters, so they must "fold themselves up" initially. They must then exert more than 588.6 N in order to achieve movement; in other words, break the equilibrium. If they do not have the strength to produce sufficient force (from their musculature and ligaments) then someone else will need to provide an assistive force for them.

When sitting there is also the problem of pressure; if this person's ischial tuberosities are approximately 0.2 square metres, then

$$\frac{588.6\text{N}}{0.2\text{ m}^2} = 2943 \text{ Pascals of pressure}$$

If this external pressure exceeds the internal pressure of the circulation (capillary hydrostatic pressure) over a period of time, then obviously this area will become ischaemic and begin to break down.

6 Conclusion

People assisting other people to move can use mechanical principles, wherever possible, to make their assistance mechanically efficient by:

- Putting effort into moving the centre of gravity which, in a person, is the *pelvic area.*
- Making points of contact on the trunk, preferably over the shoulder girdle and pelvis.
- Making use of friction-lowering to

reducing effort in horizontal movement, increasing it to reduce horizontal movement.

- Making use of stability-reducing it to get ready for movement, but ensuring both handlers' feet are in contact with the floor during effort.
- Making use of head movement to initiate body movement and assisting the arms in pushing.
- Avoiding too much muscular tension and using smooth movement.
- Keeping levers short by getting as close as possible to the weight.
- Keeping vertical effort to a minimum.
- Using the major muscle groups for effort.

These mechanical principles are easily used to determine the efficient movement of inanimate loads, which possess no other features apart from their mass, shape and surface properties, allowing straightforward calculations to be made regarding the magnitude of force required to effect movement. They may also be used to determine whether "techniques" or "manouevres" are efficient; (see chapter 18)

But the human body is much more than a mechanical structure; movement is determined not just by forces, but also by psychological, physiological and chemical stimuli. Mathematical measurement of this kind does not take into account the "human factors", for example, inevitable psychosocial elements such as the presence or absence of a relationship between the people involved and their level of motivation. Handling around the pelvis and holding the load close are mechanically efficient ideas, but socially the pelvis is a "taboo" area, especially with children, and being close involves intrusion into personal space, which may be unacceptable to handler, client, or both.

Therefore, biomechanics can be a useful tool in assessing, measuring and analysing manual handling procedures, but because humans are not merely a collection of levers, decisions based solely upon mathematical parameters may not always produce appropriate answers to people-handling problems.

References

Armfield DR, Stickle RL, Robertson DD, Towers JD, Debski RE (2003). Biomechanical basis of common shoulder problems. Semin. Musculoskelet Radiol. 2003 Mar;7(1):5-18.

Bonde-Petersen F, Henriksson J, Lundin B (1975). Blood flow in thigh muscle during bicycling exercise at varying work rates. Eur J Appl Physiol Occup Physiol. 1975 Aug 15; 34(3):191-7.

Brénière Y and Ribreau C (1998) A double-inverted pendulum approach of the human gait. Journal of Biomechanics Volume 31, Supplement 1 , July 1998, Page 86 Proceedings of the 11th Conference of the European Society of Biomechanics

Buckwalter JA and Cooper RR (1987). Bone structure and function. Instr Course Lect. 1987; 36:27-48.

Gallagher S, Marras WS, Davis KG, Kovacs K (2002). Effects of posture on dynamic back loading during a cable lifting task. Ergonomics. 2002 Apr 15;45(5):380-98.

Green EM, Mulcahy CM, Pountney TE (1995). An investigation into the development of early postural control. Dev. Med. Child Neurol. 1995 37(5) 437-438

Hignett S and McAtamney L (2000). Rapid Entire Body Assessment (REBA). Applied Ergonomics Volume 31, Issue 2 , 3 April 2000, Pages 201-205

Hollands MA, Sorensen KL, and Patla AE (2001). Effects of head immobilization on the coordination and control of head and body reorientation and translation during steering. Exp Brain Res. 2001 Sep; 140(2):223-33.

Kapandji IA (1974). The physiology of the joints vol. 3-the trunk and vertebral column. 2nd edition. Churchill Livingstone UK

McGill SM, van Wijk MJ, Axler CT and Gletsu M (1996). Studies of spinal shrinkage to evaluate low-back loading in the workplace. Ergonomics. 1996 Jan; 39(1):92-102.

McGill SM, Grenier S, Kavcic N and Cholewicki J (2003). Coordination of muscle activity to assure stability of the lumbar spine. Jnl. of Electromyography and Kinesiology 13(4), August 2003 353-359

Nachemson A (1975). Towards a better understanding of low-back pain: a review of the mechanics of the lumbar disc. Rheumatol Rehabil. 1975 Aug;14(3):129-43.

National Institute for Occupational Safety and Health (1991). A work practices guide for manual lifting Cincinnati: DHSS (NIOSH) publication no 81-122

Pisano F, Miscio G, Colombo R, Pinelli P (1996). Quantitative evaluation of normal muscle tone. J Neurol Sci. 1996 Feb; 135(2):168-72.

Smit TH Odgaard A and Schneider E (1997). Structure and function of vertebral trabecular bone. Spine. 1997 Dec 15; 22(24):2823-33.

van der Helm FC (1994). Analysis of the kinematic and dynamic behavior of the shoulder mechanism. J Biomech. 1994 May;27(5):527-50.

Waters TR, Putz-Anderson V, Garg A and Fine IJ (1993). Revised NIOSH equation for the design and evaluation of manual lifting tasks. Ergonomics July 1993 36:7 749-776

Recommended further reading

Latash ML (1998). Neurophysiological basis of movement Human Kinetics (US) 1998

Pheasant S (1991). Ergonomics work and health. Macmillan 1991

Scheck DJ and Bronzino JD (eds.) (2002). Biomechanical principles and applications CRC Press New York 2002

Tracy MF (1995). Biomechanical methods in postural analysis in Corlett EN and Wilson JR (eds.) Evaluation of Human Work (1990) ch. 23 571-605

Vasey JR and Crozier L (1982). A neuromuscular approach 1-6 Nursing Mirror April 28-June 2 1982

Wirhed R (1991). Athletic ability and the anatomy of motion. Wolfe Medical 1991

7 Occupational health in the NHS

Christine Pennington BA(Hons) MSc
Management Consultant

1 Introduction

The NHS employs over a million people and, under the *Health and Safety at Work Act, 1974*, is responsible for ensuring, as far as possible, their health, safety and welfare. But staff absence and sickness is a potential constraint on the NHS' ability to deliver the challenges of the *NHS Plan (Department of Health, 2004)*. The most common work related illnesses in the NHS are musculoskeletal disorders and stress *(Department of Health, 2002; Health Commission, 2004)*.

Within the NHS, Occupational Health Departments have a responsibility to:

"Contribute to the effectiveness of the organisation by enhancing staff performance and morale through reducing risks at work which lead to ill health, absence and accidents"

(The Management of Health Safety and Welfare Issues for NHS staff, NHS Executive HSC 1998/064 1998) and to provide rehabilitation, so minimising the period of absence and illness for the employee and reducing costs to the employer.

This chapter focuses on NHS Occupational Health Services for NHS employees. It describes how occupational health services are staffed and run, and the challenges facing occupational health services, setting out the case for a step change in the way NHS occupational health services are organised and delivered.

2 Setting the context

Work related ill health in the NHS

"The term work related ill health means physical and mental illness, disability or other health problems that are caused or made worse by work." *(paragraph 23 p8 HSE 2000)*.

The NHS staff survey *(The Commission for Healthcare Audit and Inspection (Healthcare Commission, 2004)* found that one in five staff reported some injury or illness as a result of work and that two in five reported suffering from work related stress in the previous year. Yet the prevention of ill health at work is not only beneficial to employees; it is cost effective for employers. For example, South West Water expects to save nearly £1 million over ten years though a programme to prevent one type of work related upper limb disorder *(HSE, 2000)*.

Sickness absence in the NHS averaged 4.9% in 2001 – higher than the average of 3.7% across the group of public administration, education and health employees *(NAO, 2003)*. The full costs of sickness absence in the NHS are estimated to be £1 billion each year *(NAO, 2003)*. In 1999 the Department of Health set a national improvement target for reducing sickness absence by 20% by 2001 and 30% by 2003 *(Department of Health, September 1999)*. These targets have not been achieved; in fact the numbers of incidents of violence and aggression, and of accidents, both increased *(NAO, 2003)*. It should be noted however, that in 1996 few trusts had systems for reporting accidents and injuries to NHS staff. This has improved, but procedures are still subject to under reporting, differences in systems, and inconsistencies in classifying, recording and reporting, both within and between trusts. This means that comparisons between trusts, or over time, are unlikely to be valid *(NAO, 2003)*.

Responsibilities for maintaining work related health

The NHS delivers its responsibility for the health and safety of its staff at work (arising under the *Health and Safety at Work Act, 1974*) through activity to assess and manage risks, prevent accidents and injury and provide occupational health advice and support. Although all NHS trusts provide an occupational health service for their staff, the quality, scale and accessibility of the service varies, and provision is largely reactive (*National Audit Office, 2003*). Not all NHS organisations have their own Occupational Health Department. All NHS employers are, however, required to provide occupational health services for their staff. Several NHS organisations therefore buy in their occupational health services from another local NHS trust. More recently, funding was made available to extend occupational health services to GPs and their staff (*Department of Health, 2001*).

In its 2003 report, the NAO identified the "statutory and management responsibilities for health and safety" of specific NHS employees, including the occupational health manager:

- Chief executive: overall statutory responsibility for managing health and safety risks and establishing clear lines of accountability throughout their organisation
- Human resources director: sickness absence
- Health and safety lead: all aspects of health and safety management: recording monitoring, reviewing and assessing root causes of incidents; facilitating health and safety training
- Occupational health manager: organises pre employment checks and access to support, including physiotherapy and counselling to help a speedy return to work
- Director of estates or facilities: ensures the maintenance and safe upkeep of the buildings and environment. *(paragraph 1.19, p11, NAO, 2003)*

The role of the occupational health service

The role of an occupational health service is set out in greater detail in government guidance to the NHS, "An occupational health service addresses the impact of work on health and of health on work. It seeks to reduce the incidence of illness and injury caused by work in the NHS" *(page 5 The Management of Health Safety and Welfare Issues for NHS staff, NHS Executive HSC 1998/064 1998)*.

Similarly, occupational health services exist to "promote and maintain the physical, mental and social well being of all staff" (*World Health Organisation OHS definition" (page13 The Management of Health Safety and Welfare Issues for NHS staff, NHS Executive HSC 1998/064 1998).*

In addition to the responsibilities to staff, there is also a wider organisational responsibility to, "Contribute to the effectiveness of the organisation, by enhancing staff performance and morale through reducing risks at work which lead to ill health, absence and accidents" *(page 13 The Management of Health Safety and Welfare Issues for NHS staff, NHS Executive HSC 1998/064 1998).*

The guidance emphasises that "Active co-operation and good communication between OHS, health and safety officers, line managers and personnel departments within the employing organisation is essential to ensure effective outcomes, both for individual staff members and for the organisation" *(emphasis as in the original p14 The Management of Health Safety and Welfare Issues for NHS staff, NHS Executive HSC 1998/064 1998).*

Included in the anticipated outcomes from such effective working are:

- Identifying where sickness absence is a concern and devising strategies for eliminating identified causes, consequently assisting in its management and reduction
- Awareness of the organisational and individual causes of work related stress and advice to management on the drawing up, implementation and monitoring of strategies for dealing with the causes and effects of these, *(page14 The Management of Health Safety and Welfare Issues for NHS staff, NHS Executive HSC 1998/064 1998).*

NHS Occupational Health Departments may or may not also encompass additional responsibilities, such as risk assessment, manual handling and health and safety. Although, conceptually, it makes good sense to group together the staff with responsibility for protecting and maintaining the health of the organisation's staff, the differing priorities and cultures of these groups has resulted in few, if any, examples of effective working together within a single department despite this being recognised many years ago in the *Health at Work in the NHS* initiative (September 1992) as a key ingredient to success. Despite the explicit guidance from the Department of Health a further, more recent, example of the lack of cohesion in staff support services is that over a third of trusts had a mismatch between the human resources department and the health and safety department in their information on accidents (*NAO, 2003*). The National Audit Office concluded "This highlighted a lack of communication and collaboration between the different parts of the trust that have a role to play in managing health and safety risks, including occupational health and estates" (*paragraph 12, page3 NAO 2003*).

NHS occupational health strategy

Although the Department of Health was one of the signatories to the long term strategy for occupational health (developed jointly by several government departments and published by the Health and Safety Executive in 2000) it developed its own strategy in 2004 (*Department of Health, 2004*) in response to the NAO report "*A Safer Place to Work" (NAO, 2003)*. The drivers for the strategy were stated to be:

- Direct and indirect costs of poor management of occupational health
- Changing attitudes to risk, redress, blame and compensation
- Requirement for the NHS to recruit and retain a healthy workforce to meet the challenges of the NHS Plan.

While stating that the advisory role of occupational health professionals is a key element of the strategy is to fully network occupational health into the management systems of the trust, the vision is that:

"The NHS should be recognised by other large employers as having embedded occupational health and safety into its organisational management systems and to be an exemplar in the field of human resource management." *(page 2, Department of Health, 2004).*

The first high level aim, derived from the NAO recommendations, is:

"To develop a more proactive, rather than a reactive approach to occupational health and safety" *(page 2, Department of Health, 2004).*

The draft strategy goes on to describe in detail the accountabilities and responsibilities of the Department of Health, NHS chief executives, NHS trust boards, all NHS senior managers, managers, occupational health professionals, health and safety professionals and employees *(Department of Health, 2004).*

3 Organisational role, staffing and structure

This section describes the role of occupational health in NHS organisations, the day to day work of an Occupational Health Department and its members . An important section on staffing levels and qualifications sets out indicative guidance and stresses that this must be used within the wider context of the responsibilities of the specific service. Evidence about the relationship between spend on occupational health services and sickness absence rates are presented and critiqued, and the ideal size for an occupational health department is discussed.

Organisational role

The role of an occupational health service in providing advice is independent from the organisation's hierarchy; it is independent from the member of staff, their line manager and the human resources department. Yet the service also has an organisational role.The balance between these perspectives has been made explicit:

"Wherever health issues arise in relation to employment and work in the NHS, the occupational health service should provide competent advice in support of the organisation's objectives. There is thus a clear requirement for an Occupational Health Department to work closely with others on a day to day basis. This includes particularly personnel, health and safety and health promotion departments. This working harmony does not compromise the professional independence of the OH service, the maintenance of the highest standards of medical confidentiality nor the requirement to safeguard and improve the health of the workforce. The best outcomes for staff, patients and others come from working together within an agreed robust framework." *(page 5 The Management of Health Safety and Welfare Issues for NHS staff, NHS Executive HSC 1998/064 1998).*

There is therefore a balance to be achieved by occupational health professionals between the potentially conflicting positions of staff, their line managers and the needs of the organisation. Clear and consistent communication between the different parts of the organisation (occupational health, human resources, line managers) is critical to the effective use of occupational health services *(Pennington, 2005 in press)*. Staff also need to be actively informed about the potential benefits offered by occupational health services. Indeed, under *Improving Working Lives (Department of Health 2000)* an increasing number of NHS organisations see occupational health services as an important staff benefit and are raising awareness of services.

Day to day work

The day to day contribution that the occupational health service should make to an NHS organisation is to:

- Assess the health of potential employees through a health screening (or pre employment) questionnaire, following up with a telephone call or consultation where necessary
- Ensure those starting work with the organisation have received the necessary immunisations and vaccinations (at no cost to the employee)
- Support managers in ensuring that adequate health surveillance is provided
- Provide advice on needlestick and other workplace injuries
- Undertake individual assessment of employees' fitness for work
- Assess the health requirements of particular jobs
- Rehabilitate staff into work following injury or illness
- Plan and deliver health improvement measures in the workplace
- Undertake health education
- Provide counselling
- Undertake workplace assessments *(NHS Executive, 1998, NAO, 2003)*.

Some departments provide further services to staff such as travel vaccinations.

Referrals

Occupational health professionals provide advice to other people in the organisation to enable them to make, and progress, decisions. For example, a professional may have a consultation with a member of staff who has been referred to them following a number of short periods on sickness absence. Following the consultation the occupational health professional's letter to the line manager may state that there is no underlying illness or condition giving rise to the absences. The manager then knows they are not required to establish workplace adaptations or changes to the work process to support the health of the member of staff. The manager may also then choose to address the number of absences with the member of staff in other ways using the processes set out in the organisation's human resources policies. It is, however, for the manager to decide what course of action should be taken, with the advice of the organisation's human resources department. Line managers who have not had previous contact with an occupational health department may not realise the advisory nature of the information they receive. Expectations of each party could be better managed through clearer communication about the role of the service. A member of staff can also refer themselves for a consultation or advice.

As with other NHS professionals in their day to day work, the consultation with the member of staff (or patient) is confidential: its contents should not be routinely shared with the member of staff's line manager, for example. The professional's opinion will usually be communicated by letter to the line manager. The contents of the letter may be agreed with the member of staff during the consultation, and be dictated in their presence. The member of staff may be encouraged to share information about their condition with their line manager, for example to enable suitable adaptations or other changes to be readily identified and put into place.

Specific advice on issues such as confidentiality, consent and disclosure for occupational health clinicians, NHS staff and line managers is available through their professional bodies or representatives.

4 Staffing levels and qualifications

The largest group of staff in an Occupational Health Department is nurses. This is followed by administrative support and doctors. Departments may also include *(HSE, 2001)*:

- Non-clinical manager
- Counsellor
- Occupational physiotherapist
- Ergonomist
- Safety officer
- Occupational hygienist.

This section describes staff levels and skill mix for occupational health services.

Staff numbers and departmental responsibilities

Staffing levels and skill mix in Occupational Health Departments should reflect the responsibilities of the service they provide to their own, and other, organisations *(NHS Executive, 1998; HSE 2004)*, however staffing levels vary widely *(NAO, 2003)*. The Department of Health has argued against providing indicative numbers of clinicians per thousand employees (for example): stating that staffing levels should not be determined on the number of employees alone, but on the number of sites, the type of work being undertaken and the responsibilities of the service(s); there must, however, be access to the advice of an occupational health physician *(NHS Executive 1998)*. Staffing levels and skill mix should be consistent with the levels of occupational health risks identified in the trust's risk assessment and the arrangements for health and safety *(Health and Safety Executive, 2004)*; and NHS trusts are required to appoint competent persons to assist them in complying with their statutory duties. Nevertheless some indication of staffing numbers is helpful to those establishing a service, and sets an independent baseline for those negotiating resources for an occupational health service.

Guidance on the numbers of occupational health physicians and nurses per 1,000 employees has been developed *(ANHOPS 2003)* and given credibility by being cited by the HSE in their advice to inspectors *(HSE 2004)*. This should not, however, be interpreted strictly: the guidance clearly states that staffing levels will be further influenced by the scale of the departmental responsibilities *(ANHOPS, July 2003)*:

- Management duties of the service
- Co-ordination of risk assessment, health and safety, fire, security, physiotherapy and psychology for staff
- Number and location of sites
- Income generation activities
- Provision of training and advisory services (such as first aid, induction, risk management, sickness absence, and so on), health promoting activities and counselling.

Box 7.2 Qualifications of NHS Occupational Health Staff *(HSE 2004)*

Doctors

- Professionally leading a department – the "responsible doctor": registered medical practitioner, eligible to be entered on the General Medical Councils' specialist register in occupational medicine. Appropriate qualifications are: Membership of the Faculty of Occupational Medicine (MFOM) or overseas equivalent; experience of health services
- All other doctors: current registration with the General Medical Council

Nurses

- All nurses hold current registration with the Nursing and Midwifery Council
- At least one nurse has experience of health services (advisable)
- At least one nurse should hold a post registration qualification in occupational health nursing at degree level or equivalent, recordable with the Nursing and Midwifery Council (for example, Occupational Health Nursing Certificate, Occupational Health Nursing Diploma, BSc Occupational Health/Public Health).

The HSE refers in a parallel way to 'clinical facility' time: staffing levels should be such as to allow adequate clinical facility time to undertake the range of activities required to meet the trust's own risk assessments and control measures, and will also be determined by the management arrangements for the service.

It is interesting to note that physiotherapy and psychology services are mentioned under the co-ordination activities of the department, but physiotherapists and psychologists (or counsellors) are not included as core staff in the table. Despite stress and back pain being the highest causes of work related ill health in the NHS there is, implicitly, little importance in the guidance attached to the potential role of other professional groups in the prevention and management of these conditions.

In following this guidance, the absolute minimum occupational health staffing a trust with 750 employees should have is 1.5 sessions a week of an occupational health physician, one full-time occupational health nurse adviser and 1.25 administrative staff; a trust with 2,750 employees should have an occupational health department with 4 sessions a week of an occupational health physician, 3.25 occupational health nurse advisers and 2.50 administrative staff.

Departments undertaking external work must ensure that this is not detrimental to the provision of their core service *(NHS Executive 1998: HSG 98(064); Department of Heath, 2001)*. Indeed, HSE inspectors are specifically alerted that "commitment to outside contracts can conflict with the ability to provide an effective service for the employing trust" and that "The level of staffing should be balanced against the volume of contracts and worker numbers using the service." *(Paragraph 18, HSE 2004)*.

The levels in the guidance are widely thought, within occupational health professions, to be too low. Nevertheless, the publication of such standards provides a useful benchmark.

Box 7.1 Summary of core staffing requirements *(ANHOPS, 2003)*

Post Title	Core staffing levels (for the first 750 employees)	Additional requirements (for every 1,000 additional employees)
Occupational Physicians (sessions per week)	Clinical activities: 1.00 Policy and strategy input: 0.50	A further: Clinical activities: 1.00 Policy and strategy: 0.25
Occupational Health Nurse Advisers (whole time equivalents)	1.00–1.25	A further: 0.75–1.00
Administrative staff (whole time equivalents)	1.25–1.50	0.25–0.50

Staff qualifications

The grades and qualifications of staff required will depend primarily on the responsibilities of the department and the extent to which work is effectively delegated and supervised. The Health and Safety Executive has developed guidance for its inspectors on the qualifications of NHS occupational health staff *(Health and Safety Executive, 2004)*.

Where a department has no member of clinical staff with specialist practitioner status as defined above, and does not have access to such advice, the HSE suggests an improvement notice should be considered where one of the following is found:

- No specialist physician input
- A physician, but no nurses with occupational health qualifications
- Clinical staffing appear competent (as defined above) but there are concerns regarding accommodation and facility time

Advice in the form of a letter should be considered. This would, however, be complemented by formal enforcement if an inspector encountered intransigence on the part of the trust concerning the advice. Occupational health staffing levels, skill mix and qualifications should reflect the risks identified in the organisation and the specific responsibilities of the service. As such, guidance on indicative staffing levels may be deemed unhelpful. Nevertheless, specific guidance provides a useful benchmark, and has been noted by the HSE. Professionals with specific skills relevant to addressing the two most common causes of work related ill health in the NHS (back pain and stress) that is, physiotherapists and counsellors, should, however, be included.

Departmental budget

Given the high costs to organisations of sickness absence and work related ill health it would appear sensible to invest heavily in occupational health services with a correspondingly wide remit. Although the *NAO (2003)* identified some correlation between higher occupational health spend and reduced sickness absence rates it is not clear from the report whether this figure relates to the actual departmental contribution from the trust or its budget, which may encompass a significant income generation target. The relationship between spend on occupational health services and sickness absence also appears dependent on a small number of high spending trusts. It would be helpful for all NHS organisations if this relationship were explored further. That is, to:

- Clarify the definition of occupational health spend
- Identify the trusts with low levels of sickness absence and low levels of occupational health spend to identify how they have achieved their outcome so efficiently.

5 Locality structure

An Occupational Health Department may have its base in one NHS trust and be commissioned to provide an occupational health service to several NHS organisations in the locality. The ideal size for an Occupational Health Department (as opposed to an occupational health service) has not yet been identified. Departmental size varies from a single, part time occupational health nurse to an in-house team of doctors, nurses, managers and support staff *(NAO, 2003)*. An important factor in changing departmental size was the re-organisation of trusts from April 2003. Several neighbouring departments (which may have previously been competitors for the same local non NHS work) became a single trust and, ostensibly at least, a single department.

Much larger Occupational Health Departments could become freestanding organisations, providing occupational health services to all NHS bodies in their area, echoing the shared services model. One department would provide services to all NHS organisations in up to three strategic health authority areas. As a consequence, the number of Occupational Health Departments would reduce from approximately 200 to around 10. This would have the critical mass necessary to provide a strategic overview and better address issues in quality of care, service developments and provide improved career opportunities for staff.

This section has described the main responsibilities and day to day work of NHS Occupational Health departments. Staffing levels and skill mix should follow from the risks identified within the trust, and the debate about the usefulness of developing staffing ratios per 1,000 employees has been discussed.

6 Service standards

There are currently four arenas in which standards for occupational health services have been generated:

- Guidance from professional bodies
- Evidence based clinical guidelines
- Management standards
- NHS Plus.

This section describes the different standards, and notes that clinically based strategic direction is a significant omission. This could be secured through the development of outcome targets; a tried and tested mechanism within the NHS to secure a user and stakeholder focus, and responsiveness to the needs of the wider NHS (see section 4).

Guidance from professional bodies

The most well known professional body in occupational health is the Faculty of Occupational Medicine. The Royal College of Nursing does, however, have members exclusively employed in taking forward the profession of occupational health nursing and has issued its own guidance. Physiotherapists employed in occupational health have their own occupational interest group, The Association of Chartered Physiotherapists in Occupational Health and Ergonomics (ACPOHE). In addition, there are the Association of NHS Occupational Health Physicians and the Association of Occupational Health Nurses. These organisations provide forums for the discussion of occupational health issues relevant to the individual professions and may provide training, validation, guidance and advice to their members. Most of these organisations have websites, which describe the guidance and services available to their members.

Evidence based clinical guidelines

The National Institute of Clinical Excellence (NICE) has established standards for the development of clinical guidelines for the NHS *(NICE, February 2004)*. These set out a specific methodology for identifying, reviewing and grading research evidence and thus developing evidence based clinical guidelines. To date, NICE has not commissioned any guidelines in occupational health topics.

The Department of Health has, however funded a number of clinical guideline projects that have used the NICE standards. These include:

- Pre employment health assessment
- Pregnant workers
- Chronic Fatigue Syndrome

The final reports will be published by NHS Plus.

Other guidelines using the NICE standards or those of the Scottish Intercollegiate Guideline Network (SIGN) have been commissioned by the British Occupational Health Research Forum (BOHRF). These are published by BOHRF. To date, those commissioned include:

- Occupational asthma
- Mild to moderate mental ill health at work
- Management of back pain at work
- Hand-arm vibration syndrome.

Other organisations may commission or undertake work to develop clinical guidelines in occupational health but do not state that they adhere to the NICE standards. These have therefore not been included here.

Management standards

In 2001 the Department of Health published management standards for the delivery of NHS occupational health services *(Department of Health 2001)*. The standards are:

1. Risk management: Comprehensive risk assessment is undertaken, a risk management policy and details of risk management activity are recorded

2 Risk assessment following accidents: All accidents are reported through the incident reporting system and followed up
3 Pre employment: Pre employment health questionnaires dealt with within two days of receipt (that is, the day of arrival or the day after) or an initial decision to be made on further action to be taken. Manager to be notified within two working days (that is, the day of arrival or the day after) of the need for potential new employee to attend for health assessment. First appointment for health assessment is within 7 working days
4 Immunisation of new starters: All new starters to be sent a letter prior to commencement requiring their attendance in the occupational health service within two weeks of their start date.
5 In-service referral (management or self): Appointment with occupational health nurse in five working days; appointment with occupational physician in ten working days
6 Immunisation: There is a written immunisation policy setting out requirements for different staff groups
7 Immunisation: All staff offered appropriate immunisation (appointment given at line manager's request; cost of immunisation is employer's responsibility). Minimum of one recall after failure to attend
8 Health surveillance: All staff requiring health surveillance to meet H&S legislation receive surveillance appropriate to their work or exposure
9 Ill health retirement: The protocol set out in *Managing Ill health retirement in the NHS* (Department of Health 2001) is followed
10 Counselling: Appointment within 48 hours; immediate access by telephone.

These were to be monitored annually by the Department of Health through the Improving Working Lives Standard and the Human Resources Performance Management Framework.

The Improving Working Lives assessments, however, have to cover a wide range of topics across the trust in a very short period of time. The extent to which evidence that the standards are being met is sought within Occupational Health Departments is likely to be variable.

A recent study to review achievement of the standards *(Pennington, 2004)* found that some departments neither used, nor had heard of the standards. And those that had heard of them did not audit their performance effectively. Nevertheless, the best performing departments shared six pointers towards good practice

- Responsiveness to stakeholders
- Ability to justify and secure resources
- Effective collection and use of management information
- Well designed forms and good written communication
- Good relationships with occupational health colleagues within the department and in other local departments
- Effective delivery of responsibilities and the use of influence.

These themes are expanded, with case studies and advice on undertaking an audit to assess performance, in three further articles *(Pennington 2005, in press)*.

The Department of Health standards should not be expected to remain at their current levels. An increase in the levels of performance expected from NHS Occupational Health Departments is therefore anticipated.

NHS Plus

Where NHS Occupational Health Departments have the capacity to do so, they provide services to local companies. Occupational Health Departments therefore hold important potential for the health of non-NHS employees across the country. This contribution to the wider economy was acknowledged in the NHS Plan, which described the launch of NHS Plus *(Department of Health, 2000)*. An NHS Plus Occupational Health Department has set standards for the delivery of their services *(Department of Health, July 2001)*. These include:

- Assurance that the service to NHS staff is adequate and that selling services to third party organisations will not compromise the service to the NHS
- Professional standards for accountability, ethics, security of information, confidentiality, clinical governance; appraisal, training and development
- Staff qualifications
- Facilities: Access, receptions, waiting, clinical, toilet, offices, clinical equipment; health and safety
- Business arrangements: written terms and conditions of business; finance, indemnity for staff, written list of services.

The standards have an entry level, that must be met to be accredited with the NHS Plus badge, and then higher levels of achievement. Departments' continued performance against the standards has not, however, been routinely monitored.

Clinically based strategic direction: Performance standards

This section has described four arenas in which standards for the work of Occupational Health Departments have been developed:

- Professional bodies or profession-based membership organisations
- Evidence based clinical guidelines
- Management standards from the Department of Health
- Standards to be met prior to delivering services to signing up to NHS Plus (to deliver services to non-NHS organisations).

Although professional bodies are responsible for maintaining the standards of their members there are not any systems in place to monitor the sustained achievement of the standards issued through other bodies that are delivered at the departmental level. There is therefore little incentive for departments to continue to invest resources in meeting these other standards.

The standards described in this section do not, however, relate to the outcomes of the service, for example, in terms of reduced sickness absence or improved management of sickness absence. Setting and monitoring such standards may help to improve the delivery of NHS occupational health services.

Much of the way NHS services are delivered has been modernised; that is, re-focused on the needs and preferences of patients. This has been achieved through the setting of high targets and active performance management of NHS organisations (for example, on waiting times for appointments and treatment). This has required the service to become much more responsive to patients' needs and to challenge the accepted ways of working. To date, NHS occupational health services (in the widest sense) have not been affected by these changes in ways of working. This has, perhaps, resulted in a concentration on day to day activities and a reactive rather than a pro-active stance in some departments. This is in contrast to Occupational Health Departments that take a more strategic role, focus on delivering the standards identified above, and anticipate and plan for changes in the levels of different work-related ill health (such as back pain and stress). An outline of the potential modernisation of occupational health services is in section 8 below.

7 Priority areas

Introduction

The two main causes of work related ill health in the NHS are back pain and stress *(Department of Health, 2002; Health Commission 2004)*. This section describes the scale of ill health currently being experienced by NHS staff with these conditions and the initiatives to address these, as set in place by the government, such as Back in Work *(Department of Health, 2002)*. Although there are some important examples of good practice in NHS trusts, not all trusts provide back care services or adequate levels of counselling (or other support services such as post traumatic event de-briefing) through their Occupational Health Departments to prevent and address the levels of ill health currently being experienced.

The NHS Staff Survey *(Commission for Healthcare Audit and Inspection (Healthcare Commission) 2004)* identified high levels of work-related injury and stress among NHS staff. One in five reported some injury or illness as a result of:

- Moving and handling (The epidemiology and biomechanics of musculoskeletal injury in nurses is described in greater detail in chapters 4, 5, 6 and 8).
- Needlestick and sharps injuries
- Slips, trips and falls
- Exposure to dangerous substances.

Fully twice the number experiencing ill health from these sources, two in every five NHS staff, reported suffering from work related stress in the previous year. Nurses, health visitors, midwives and Allied Health Professionals all reported high levels of work related stress.

In 1995 the cost to society of work-related illness was estimated to be £10 billion, with musculoskeletal conditions being responsible for about £5.5 billion of this *(HSE, 2000)*.

This section describes the current position of the NHS on the two largest causes of work related sickness absence: back pain and stress.

Back pain

Background information

The Department of Health has reported that 24 per cent of NHS staff regularly experience back pain *(Department of Health, 2002)*. This is a particular risk for nurses, 80,000 of whom hurt their backs each year *(Institute of Employment Studies 1996 in NAO, 2003)*. One in four nurses has taken time off work with a back injury sustained at work and for some this has meant the end of their career *(Department of Health, 2002)*. Back injuries are also associated with longer periods of sickness absence: one in twenty NHS staff have taken more than 20 days off work in a year due to back pain *(Department of Health, 2002)*.

Moving and handling is considered to be an important contributing factor to back pain. Moving and handling related incidents remain approximately 17%–18% of reported incidents/ accidents in the NHS *(NAO, 2003)* and they account for 40% of NHS sickness absence costs, estimated to be £400 million a year *(Department of Health, 2002)*. This therefore has important implications for NHS organisations. Since 1996 nearly half of NHS trusts (47%) have employed manual handling specialists, but increased workloads, staff shortages and heavier and more dependent patients are all perceived to have contributed to these statistics *(NAO, 2003)*.

Nevertheless, accidents resulting in more than three days absence from work have reduced year on year since 1996 and the proportion of these caused by moving and handling incidents has reduced. The NAO suggests this reduction may be attributed to:

- The HSE's focus on this issue during inspections
- Work by the Royal College of Nursing and the National Back Exchange
- NHS trusts introducing:
  - Patient handling policies
  - Mechanical handling equipment
  - Staff training programmes
  - Staff rehabilitation programmes.

Nurses, back pain and work instability

Nurses and nursing assistants have the highest rates of musculoskeletal disorders among NHS staff *(HSE 1995)*. The management of nurses with musculoskeletal disorders focuses on those who are off sick from work rather than those who are continuing in work despite their symptoms. Some individuals who are working may experience increasing difficulties with some or all of their work tasks because of their health problems; they could be said to be experiencing Work Instability.

The concept of Work Instability (WI) arose from the recognition that the vocational impact of any incapacity must relate to the individual's work demands, and has previously been explored in Rheumatoid Arthritis (RA) *(Gilworth et al 2003)*. The term WI was coined to describe the extent of any mismatch between functional (in)capacity and work demands at a point in time, and its potential impact on job retention and security. The following definition of WI has been proposed *(Gilworth et al 2003)*:

"Work Instability is a state in which the consequences of a mismatch between an individual's functional abilities and the demands of his or her job can threaten continuing employment if not resolved".

It is during this period of WI that the individual is vulnerable to sickness absence and possibly job loss or early retirement. This is, arguably, the time at which interventions and support in the workplace are of greatest preventive importance in relation to promoting work attendance and job retention.

A valid and reliable Work Instability Scale could provide an effective health surveillance and screening tool to facilitate early, appropriate referral for job retention measures to be implemented. A research project to validate a self-administered scale for nurses against a gold standard of full vocational assessment by occupational health physiotherapists and ergonomists is being undertaken at the University of Leeds. It is anticipated that the WI scale developed will reflect both the physical and psychosocial impact of coping with a musculoskeletal disorder at work.

Rehabilitation and return to work

In 2000 the HSE stated "interested parties recognise the importance of early interventions to provide rehabilitation" *(paragraph 29, p8 HSE 2000)*. Rehabilitation is multidisciplinary, with roles for managers, occupational health, doctors and/or nurses with a number of shared elements: return to work assessment, physiotherapy, counselling and retraining. Nevertheless, those with a mild illness of short duration may not require rehabilitation and employees unlikely to return to work may find the offer of rehabilitation distressing *(HSE, 2000)*. Nevertheless, there is great potential benefit to offering early rehabilitation to employees absent from work with work related ill health for both the employee and the employer.

Rehabilitation for musculoskeletal disorders is also addressed in chapter 8.

Back in work initiative

The Department of Health developed a Back in Work pack *(Department of Health 2002)* with the Royal College of Nursing, the British Medical Association, Chartered Society of Physiotherapy, UNISON and the National Back Exchange to raise awareness of back care and promote effective prevention and treatment for NHS staff. The wider Back in Work initiative has included workshops and recognition of good practice. Nevertheless, two years on, not all NHS trusts have back care services for their staff.

NHS employees would benefit from individual workplace assessments to identify those likely to suffer back pain and prevent this taking place, access to early treatment through occupational health services and rehabilitation.

Reasons for the lack of provision of back care services in NHS trusts include the following:

- Reasons for sickness absence may not be identified, so a pattern indicating a need for services is not detected
- There is a shortage of physiotherapists; treatment of NHS staff is given second place to meeting targets for the treatment of the public
- It is not necessarily clear within an NHS trust where the responsibility for preventing and addressing staff back pain lies: health and safety, occupational health, human resources, risk assessment
- Addressing sickness absence caused by back pain requires effective working together between human resources, physiotherapy, line managers and occupational health; there may be inadequate leadership or leverage to ensure this takes place
- Issues of line management and professional management of back care advisors may be perceived to be insurmountable.

While sickness absence from back pain and other musculoskeletal disorders remains high it will continue to be a priority for the Department of Health. Further work under the Back in Work initiative may be targeted to address these perceived barriers to providing services for NHS staff.

Physiotherapy in occupational health

Chartered physiotherapists work in some NHS Occupational Health Departments as part of the multidisciplinary team. Their primary responsibility is usually to provide an acute treatment and advice service to NHS employees who are suffering from musculoskeletal complaints and are able to remain at work, in addition to those staff who are absent from work as a result of musculoskeletal ill health. For the latter group, the overall goal is to enable a safe and timely return to work while reducing the risk of re-injury and/or chronicity. Physiotherapists provide health education and are well placed to support health promotion initiatives.

As mentioned above, physiotherapists provide the treatment and rehabilitation for staff on sickness absence who have the potential to return to work. They are able to design and implement functional restoration programs tailored to the needs of the individual and the demands of the job the staff member is to return to. The physiotherapist is also able to assist in the assessment of work suitability for staff in cases where redeployment or consideration of retirement on grounds of ill health are being considered. Physiotherapists have a specialist advisory role in the assessment and management of staff with musculoskeletal problems and as such play a key role in the multidisciplinary Occupational Health Team.

Physiotherapists are able to perform functional capability assessments to guide the rehabilitation program in the creation of return to work or alternative work programs. Physiotherapists also play a role in helping to determine and manage any psychosocial barriers to return to work through the use of a biopsychosocial model approach to case management.

The grades and qualifications of the occupational physiotherapists will depend on the responsibilities of the department and the extent that the work is effectively delegated and supervised. Physiotherapists working in the field of Occupational Health should have some post qualifying training in occupational health and ergonomics (see ACPOHE guidelines).

In certain circumstances, physiotherapists within Occupational Health Departments have additional qualifications and skills in ergonomics, risk assessment, risk management, health promotion and training programs such as manual handling and person handling.

Stress

Definition of stress and background information

The HSE defines work related stress as "the adverse reaction people have to excessive pressures or other types of demands placed on them." *(Paragraph 2.16 p26 NAO, 2003)*.

Several important reviews identifying the dramatic increase in work-related stress in the NHS are reported by the NAO *(NAO, 2003)*:

- One review identified over 20 reports that consistently showed that between a quarter and a half of NHS staff were reporting significant levels of stress, and that many stressors were unique to healthcare *(Weinberg and Creed 2000 and Anderson, Cooper and Willmott 1996 in NAO 2003)*

- Particular issues for senior nurses were staffing busy wards, competency of agency nurses, long hours, recruitment and retention problems and ward cleanliness. They blamed their increasing stress levels on organisational factors that were beyond their control *(Allen 2001 in NAO 2003)*
- Finally, an RCN survey assessed the psychological health of members. Just over one in ten had a profile associated with being in receipt of NHS therapies. This group had twice the sickness absence of other nurses surveyed but only half were receiving counselling or other treatment *(RCN 2002 in NAO, 2003)*.

While two thirds of occupational health managers reported that work related stress had increased over the last three years, they did not have data to verify this *(NAO, 2003)*. Nevertheless, only 8% of trusts' occupational health leads and 7% of health and safety leads identified stress as one of their top three priorities *(NAO, 2003)*.

Department of Health guidance

Identifying and addressing workplace stress is not, however, a new responsibility for Occupational Health Departments. Good practice in managing stress at work was described in guidance to all Occupational Health Departments and trusts *(NHS Executive 1998)*:

"Stress at work is now widely recognised as a significant problem in the health service." *(p77 The Management of Health Safety and Welfare Issues for NHS staff, NHS Executive HSC 1998/064 1998)*

This guidance also stated that the responsibilities of Occupational Health Departments include: "analysing data on sickness absences to identify possible problems at an early stage, such as stress related illness." *(NHS Executive 1998)*.

In 2000 The Department of Health published guidance on the provision of counselling services in NHS trusts, requiring trusts to provide access to counselling services to all staff *(Department of Health, August 2000)*. Counselling services may be commissioned by the human resources department or the occupational health service. There is, however, an occupational health responsibility to audit accessibility of the service. This does not imply that the occupational health service should provide the counselling service directly, nor that records of contact with the counselling service are kept in occupational health patient records *(Department of Health 2001)*. The National Audit Office reported in 2003 that, although all trusts provide counselling services, only one in seven provide a fast track referral system that enables staff to receive assistance at the earliest possible moment. It recommended that all NHS trusts should review their strategies for managing work-related stress and for providing counselling and other support to staff *(NAO, 2003)*.

Although counselling services for NHS staff are now widespread, emphasis should also be placed on the prevention of stress through safer and improved systems of work.

8 The future

Constraints on occupational health

NHS occupational health services have an important role in supporting the delivery of the NHS Plan. Constraints on the service can, consequently, limit the extent to which the NHS Plan is delivered. In this section the constraints on occupational health services are reviewed and potential mechanisms for overcoming these constraints are considered.

There are two main constraints on occupational health services:

- Resources: difficulties recruiting and retaining staff, financial pressures
- Lack of strategic direction within local departments.

Resources

There are two areas in which resource constraints are experienced: recruitment and retention of staff and financial pressures.

Just under half of occupational health managers reported problems with recruitment and those who contract services from other trusts identify resources as a key constraint *(NAO, 2003)*. Departments who deliver services to non-NHS organisations may also find themselves under pressure from raised income generation targets that are not related to changing local economic conditions.

Lack of strategic direction

It has been emphasised to Occupational Health Departments that their role encompasses working closely with other support departments, yet the HSE has identified only a small number of trusts that collect comprehensive data on occupational ill health and link accident and ill health data to sickness absence records *(NAO, 2003)*. This observation is not new. Nearly ten years earlier the NAO reported that few NHS trusts routinely analysed data to identify potential problems and none could provide information on trends in occupationally-related ill health among their staff *(NAO 1996 in NAO 2003)*. Although guidance was developed for Occupational Health Departments (such as HSG 94 (51) and HSG 98(064)) this position does not appear to have changed substantially. Only half of occupational health leads reported they had an annual plan or programme for improving the health and safety of staff and a quarter has a long-term strategy *(NAO, 2003)*.

It is clear from the evidence of the NHS staff survey *(Commission for Healthcare Audit and Inspection (Healthcare Commission) 2004)* that rehabilitation of musculoskeletal disorders and addressing issues of workplace stress are a priority of staff support services such as occupational health. The priorities of NHS employers and employees are not, however, necessarily reflected in the workload and direction of the Occupational Health department.

Modernisation

One potential means to address these constraints is to modernise the service. The aim of modernising NHS services is to make them more responsive to the needs of patients. This has been achieved through setting targets that are regularly monitored, and are achieved through reviewing existing processes and practices and making changes to increase the efficiency and effectiveness of services. This has, in some cases, also resulted in enhanced roles for staff.

NHS occupational health services could use these techniques to improve the delivery of services. These would include:

- Setting and reviewing performance against outcome targets relevant to the NHS such as: sickness absence, provision of back care advice and treatment and improved access to counselling
- Improving the quality of services to make them more responsive to users (NHS staff) and stakeholders (human resources managers, line managers)
- Developing and applying a diagnostic tool to identify departments' strengths and areas for development
- Process mapping: describing the individual steps in a single process to identify blockages and where delays arise (particularly from a user's perspective)
- Developing effective collection and interpretation of management information, and so improve decision-making
- Increase customer focus, such as genuine responsiveness to users and stakeholders
- Effective communication with users and stakeholders
- Developing capacity planning tools
- Mutually supportive relationships with staff in other local Occupational Health Departments
- Critically reviewing skills and competencies against the strategic aims and needs of the service: identifying the need to recruit other professional groups and enhanced roles for staff
- Developing a virtuous circle of good clinical practice (implementing clinical guidelines) and good management practice (meeting the current performance standards).

This modernisation is not, however, likely to come about unless there is greater importance on the role of occupational health in addressing the constraints on the delivery of the NHS Plan. Recommendations requiring radical change in the way departments work have been made in past years with a lack of success in achieving widespread coverage across the NHS. In addition, many departments' budgets include a significant element of external income generation. Occupational Health departments need to secure adequate resources for themselves, and to obtain the necessary efficiencies through service redesign, to deliver their organisational objectives. As an alternative, step change in the organisation of services may be required to deliver the outcomes of reductions in work related ill health in the NHS.

9 Summary and conclusion

Summary

This chapter describes NHS occupational health services. The chapter began with statistics indicating the scale of work related ill health in the country and in the NHS, and the cost benefits of addressing sickness absence issues. This was followed by a description the role, structure and function of NHS occupational health services including guidance on both staffing levels and qualifications, setting out the reasons why this guidance must be considered carefully against the specific responsibilities of the Occupational Health Department. Section 6 describes the standards to which NHS Occupational Health Departments deliver their services: guidance and advice from professional and membership bodies, evidence based clinical guidelines, management standards from the Department of Health and the NHS Plus standards (required for accreditation to NHS Plus).

It is of note that there are no outcome or performance standards for NHS Occupational Health Departments – unlike those for waiting times and clinical outcomes in other clinical areas.

The two most common reasons for work-related ill health in the NHS are back pain and stress. The prevalence of back pain in nurses is higher than any other NHS occupational group. Section 7 describes the levels of ill health currently being experienced and initiatives to address these. Section 8 describes the constraints on NHS Occupational Health Departments and outlines potential modernisation issues which would echo the changes to working practices experienced in other areas in the NHS and help to increase customer focus and responsiveness, and improve clinical outcomes through placing greater emphasis on the role of professionals, other than doctors and nurses, in addressing the high levels of back pain and stress.

Conclusion

Successive government guidance has emphasised the need for Occupational Health Departments to work effectively with stakeholders and to develop a strategic vision *(see HSG 94(51), HSG 98(064), Department of Health 2001)*. The lack of subsequent monitoring or follow up may have contributed to the lack of change in the past. A step change in delivering NHS occupational health services may be required to adequately address the clinical priorities of back pain and stress. This will have important positive consequences on the ability of the NHS to address difficulties in staff recruitment and retention and so contribute to meeting the targets for improving the health of patients described in the NHS Plan.

References

Where statements are unreferenced in this chapter they are made on the basis of the author's experience of undertaking consultancy projects; referencing these reports would compromise the confidentiality under which they were commissioned.

ANHOPS (2003). Assessing the Occupational Health Manpower levels for NHS Trusts (2) (P Verow and J Harrison) ANHOPS

Department of Health (1995). Health at Work in the NHS Department of Health

Department of Health (July 2000). The NHS Plan: A plan for investment, a plan for reform CM 4818-I Department of Health

Department of Health (August 2000). The Provision of Counselling Services for Staff in the NHS Department of Health

Department of Health October (2000). The Improving Working Lives Standard Department of Health

Department of Health (2001). The Effective Management of Occupational Health and Safety Services in the NHS Reference number 25770 Department of Health

Department of Health (2001). Managing Ill-health Retirement in the NHS Department of Health

Department of Health (25 July 2001).

NHS Plus (letter inviting Occupational Health Departments to join NHS Plus)

Department of Health (July 2002). Back in Work: Everything you need to know about the national Back in Work campaign Department of Health

Department of Health (2001). The Provision of Occupational Health and Safety Services for General Medical Practitioners and their staff Department of HealthDepartment of Health 2004 NHS Occupational Health and Safety Strategy for England (Draft) Department of Health

Gilworth G, Chamberlain MA, Harvey A, Woodhouse A, Smith J, Smyth MG and Tennant A (2003). Development of a Work Instability Scale for rheumatoid arthritis Arthritis and Rheumatism, 2003; 49: 3 349-354.

Health and Safety Executive (2004). Assessment of Clinical Staffing in Occupational Health Departments of NHS Trusts Sector Information Minute SIM 07/2004/04 HSE

Health and Safety Executive (2000). Securing Health Together: An Occupational Health Strategy for Great Britain HSE Books

Commission for Healthcare Audit and Inspection (The Healthcare Commission) (July 2004 Summary Report Analysis of the (2003). Staff Survey Commission for Healthcare Audit and Inspection London

National Audit Office (30 April 2003). A Safer Place to Work: improving the management of health and safety risks to staff in NHS Trusts National Audit Office

National Health Service Executive (1998). The Management of Health, Safety and Welfare Issues for NHS Staff HSC 1998/064 Leeds

National Health Service Executive (1999). The Working Together: Securing a Quality Workforce for the NHS: Managing Violence, Accidents and Sickness Absence in the NHS HSC 199/229 Leeds NHS E 1999

National Institute for Clinical Excellence (February 2004). Guideline Development Methods: Information for National Collaborating Centres and Guideline Developers London: National Institute for Clinical Excellence

Occupational Health Advisory Committee (2000). Report and Recommendations of the Occupational Health Advisory Committee on Improving Access to Occupational Health Support Health and Safety Commission

Pennington CM (2004). Pointers towards good practice Rowanmast Ltd, Bristol

Pennington CM (2004). The Effective Management of Occupational Health and Safety Services (1) in the NHS in Occupational Health Physiotherapy', Association of Chartered Physiotherapists in 'Occupational Health and Ergonomics (in press)

Pennington CM (2004). The Effective Management of Occupational Health and Safety Services in the NHS (2) in Occupational Health Physiotherapy Association of Chartered Physiotherapists in Occupational Health and Ergonomics (in press)

Pennington CM (2004). The Effective Management of Occupational Health and Safety Services in the NHS (3) in Occupational Health Physiotherapy Association of Chartered Physiotherapists in Occupational Health and Ergonomics (in press)

Royal College of Nursing Guidance on Occupational Health Practice Royal College of Nursing, London

Seccombe I and Smith G (1996). In the Balance: registered nursing Supply and Demand Institute of Employment Studies Report 315 reported in National Audit Office 30 April 2003 A Safer Place to Work: improving the management of health and safety risks to staff in NHS Trusts National Audit Office

8

The prevention and management of simple low back pain

Stephen May MA MCSP Dip MDT MSc
Senior lecturer in physiotherapy

1 Introduction

The aim of this chapter is to provide advice about how to try and prevent back pain from occurring and what to do about it should back pain occur. It is based on self-management principles, with the aim of equipping the reader with a knowledge of the most appropriate actions to help themselves.

An understanding of the context of back pain is important, including issues such as prevalence, natural history, risk and prognostic factors, some of these issues will be discussed first. All of these topics, the epidemiology and the management guidelines, will be described with recourse to recent available evidence.

At the present time nothing has been conclusively shown to prevent the onset of back pain, nonetheless, measures to limit the impact of back pain have become much clearer in the last few decades. Although the abolition of back pain appears at present to be something of a pipedream, the optimum self-management principles have become apparent.

2 Epidemiology

Modern epidemiological studies give us a clear idea about certain aspects of the back pain experience (see Box 8.1 on page 82 for terms used). Back pain is extremely common; most adults will experience an episode. In the UK there is a lifetime prevalence of at least 60%, about 40% of all adults have back pain in a single year, and about 20% have back pain at any one point in time (*Hillman et al. 1996, Papageorgiou et al. 1995, McKinnon et al. 1997, Walsh et al. 1992, Waxman et al. 2000*). Recurrences, relapses and episodes are very common – these occur in over 60% of those who have back pain (*Klenerman et al. 1995, van den Hoogen et al. 1998, Linton et al. 1998*). Traditionally it was thought that most people experienced brief and transient back pain and only a minority (7%) had chronic symptoms. Research now shows that 40% of those who experience back pain will have symptoms that persist for several months (*Linton et al. 1998, Hillman et al. 1996, Croft et al. 1998, Waxman et al. 2000*).

Research also shows that the majority of people with back pain do not seek any treatment, but cope by themselves (*Walsh et al. 1992, Hillman et al. 1996, McKinnon et al. 1997, Waddell 1994*). Evidence indicates that the back pain of individuals who seek care is no different from the back pain of those who do not in terms of severity, accompanying leg symptoms or disability (*Hillman et al. 1996, Croft et al. 1997*).

Thus, these studies provide an interesting insight into the back pain experience that could be summed up as follows:

- back pain is a normal experience common to the majority of adults
- episodes or recurrences are normal
- symptoms that persist for months are normal
- most individuals cope with back pain without seeking treatment.

3 Types of back pain and investigation

Back pain is a symptom not a diagnosis. It is not possible in most cases to identify the structure that is causing the pain by clinical examination. Terms like facet joint syndrome, discogenic pain, or sacro-iliac joint pain exist, and all these structures can certainly be a source of symptoms, but their recognition by clinical examination has not been demonstrated (*Schwarzer et al. 1994a, 1994b, 1995a, 1995b*).

Imaging studies have failed to demonstrate usefulness in identifying specific pathology. X-rays do not improve outcomes nor in general do they effect management (*Miller et al. 2002, Kendrick et al. 2001, Halpin et a 1991*). Radiographs, magnetic resonance imaging and computer-assisted tomography studies may be effective at identifying changes and abnormalities from 'normal' anatomy, however a great number of conditions that were thought to be pathological have been identified in asymptomatic individuals. No direct causal relationship has been found between spondylolysis, spondylolisthesis, spina bifida, transitional vertebrae, spondylosis (osteoarthritis of the spine), Scheuermann's disease, and back pain (*van Tulder et al. 1997, Roland & van Tulder 1998*). Disc herniations and spinal stenosis has been commonly identified in individuals with no back pain (*Boden et al. 1990, Jensen et al. 1994, Boos et al. 1995*). Thus, in general, further investigations for simple back pain are unnecessary, unhelpful regarding management, and a waste of resources. X-rays and more sophisticated imaging studies will simply identify normal changes that happen as we age, these changes were there before the onset of back pain and they will be there when the back pain goes – mostly they are irrelevant. X-rays also involve exposure to substantial quantities of radiation that is potentially harmful (*Waddell 2004*).

The following triage for back pain has been generally accepted (*CSAG 1994, RCGP 1999, Carter et al. 2000*). The majority of people with back pain have simple back pain, 5-10% may have nerve root pain and 1% or less have back pain due to serious spinal pathology (see Table 8.1). 'Red flag' features are aspects of the clinical presentation that might indicate serious spinal pathology. They are not diagnostic of serious pathology, but the existence of any of these features is an indicator to seek medical help urgently. If back and leg pain is accompanied by pins and needles, numbness or weakness in some of the muscles in the leg or foot, then nerve root pain or sciatica may be present. This is generally considered to be a more severe type of back pain, but in every other way should be managed in much the same way as described for simple back pain.

The majority of people will have 'simple' or mechanical back pain which can include pain in the buttocks and thighs. The term 'mechanical' simply means that symptoms will vary depending on activities or movements and over the course of time. This variability is helpful in identifying movements or positions to avoid and movements or positions to do more of; this will be discussed in more detail later. Despite the lack of structural diagnosis of this non-specific term it does not mean we do not know how to manage simple back pain.

Table 8.1. Diagnostic triage for back pain, including 'red flag' features possibly indicating serious pathology

Simple back pain (> 90%)
- age 20-55
- pain in back, buttocks, thighs
- pain varies with activities, movements and time
- generally well

Nerve root pain / sciatica (5-10%)
- leg pain worse than back pain
- leg pain radiates to foot or toes
- pins and needles or numbness in foot or toes
- limited straight leg raise test
- weakness in big toe extension, dorsiflexion or calf muscles

Red flag features for possible serious spinal pathology (1%)
- age > 55 for onset of back pain
- violent trauma
- constant, progressive pain that does not vary with activity or time
- thoracic pain
- history of cancer, systemic steroid, drug abuse, HIV
- systemically unwell / fever
- widespread weakness or pins and needles / numbness
- numbness around anus, perineum or genitals
- serious bladder dysfunction – urinary retention / overflow incontinence

Source: Carter et al. 2000

4 Risk factors and prognosis

Risk factors refer to characteristics that make individuals more susceptible to a condition, whilst prognostic factors affect the outcome after the onset of a condition. It is helpful to know about and understand these factors as this may help inform behaviour to avoid the onset of back pain, or to diminish its persistence. The four major types of risk and prognostic factors are:

- individual / lifestyle
- physical / biomechanical
- psychosocial
- clinical.

Individual and lifestyle factors include age, gender, weight, flexibility, smoking status, and marital status. The evidence for all such factors is contradictory or scant, and thus there is no clear link between any of these and back pain onset or prognosis (*Frank et al. 1996, Ferguson & Marras 1997, Burdorf & Sorock 1997, Nachemson & Vingard 2000*).

Certain *biomechanical* risk factors have been identified consistently across many studies (*Frank et al. 1996, Bombardier et al. 1994, Burdorf & Sorock 1997, Ferguson & Marras 1997, Hoogendoorn et al. 1999, Vingaard & Nachemson 2000*). These are occupational physical stresses occurring during work:

- heavy or frequent lifting
- whole body vibration (as when driving)
- prolonged or frequent bending or twisting
- postural stresses (high spinal load or awkward postures).

An individual is three to five times more at risk of back pain if their work involves frequent heavy lifting or other postural stresses (*Frank et al. 1996*). This has postural implications for the way manual handling and other activities are performed.

Biomechanical forces as prognostic factors have been less thoroughly evaluated, but are generally believed to perpetuate an episode of back pain as well as initiate it (*Adams & Dolan 1995, Dolan 1998*). The majority of spinal pain is seen as varying in intensity with the patient's activity, and is *almost always aggravated by mechanical factors* (Spitzer et al. 1987). This important report referred to *activity-related spinal disorders*, with the clear assumption of the importance of day-to-day activities and postures in affecting symptoms. Several studies have identified positions found by patients to aggravate existing symptoms (*McKenzie 1979, Biering-Sorensen 1983, Boissonault & Di Fabio 1996, Stankovic & Johnell 1990, van Deursen et al. 1999*). Most commonly these are activities that involve forward flexion, such as sitting and bending, whereas these virtually never have a relieving effect. Walking, changing position frequently and lying down commonly help relieve symptoms, but in some aggravate them. The posture adopted when sitting has been found to have a relieving or aggravating effect on leg and back symptoms (*Williams et al. 1990*), and avoiding bending activity in the morning has helped reduce chronic back pain (*Snook et al. 1998*). All these studies demonstrate the importance of postural concepts both to try to prevent the onset of back pain and to affect the outcome once back pain has occurred.

Psychosocial factors include depression, anxiety, beliefs and attitudes about back pain and activity, job satisfaction, relationships at work, and control at work. Although some studies highlight these issues, in general, the evidence for any of them as risk factors for back pain is contradictory or scant (*Burdorf & Sorock 1997, Ferguson & Marras 1997, Vingard & Nachemson 2000, Hoogendoorn et al. 2000*). Two prospective studies indicate that low levels of perception of general health are predictors of new episodes of back pain (*Croft et al. 1996, 1999*). The evidence would suggest that these factors might be weakly associated with back pain, but strongly associated with the *reporting* of back pain and seeking healthcare (*Linton 2000*).

However as prognostic factors psychosocial issues play a significant role in the transition from acute to chronic pain and disability (*Vlaeyen & Linton 2000, Linton 2000*). Issues, termed 'yellow flags', can act as barriers to recovery – meaning that if these issues are not addressed symptoms may become persistent and long lasting. Most studies that have looked at both psychosocial and clinical factors have found that chronic symptoms are predicted more by psychosocial than clinical factors, or a combination of both (*Burton et al. 1995, Klenerman et al. 1995, Gatchel et al. 1995, Deyo & Diehl 1988, Hasenbring et al. 1994, Thomas et al. 1999*).

Table 8.2. 'Yellow flag' features that are associated with chronic back pain and disability

- fear motivated avoidance of activity
- anxiety about back pain
- depression
- belief in passive coping strategies
- belief that back pain will have catastrophic repercussions
- belief that personal health is controlled by others rather than by self
- low level of belief in one's ability to achieve a particular outcome.

Source: Linton 2000

As will be noted from the list of 'yellow flags', individuals who are overly anxious about the pain, who avoid movement and activity because they fear it will hurt, those who think rest will make their back pain better, and those who expect others to make their back pain better all fare worse in the long run. Such beliefs are more likely to lead to chronic symptoms and disability. Conversely, individuals who use active coping strategies, believe in their ability to make themselves better, and maintain activity, even if it is painful, will get better more quickly. The bottom line is 'don't take back pain lying down'.

Finally there are *clinical* risk and prognostic factors; these include items such as history of back pain, features of back pain, and findings from physical examination. The most consistently identified risk factor for an episode of back pain is a previous history of back pain (*Frank et al. 1996, Ferguson & Marras 1997*). An individual with previous back pain is three to four times more likely to develop back pain again than someone without that history (*Frank et al. 1996*). This means that once you have had an episode of back pain it is particularly important to perform the preventative measures mentioned later.

Those who report leg pain may be more at risk of persistent symptoms (*Goertz 1990, Lanier & Stockton 1988, Chavannes et al. 1986, Cherkin et al. 1996, Carey et al. 2000, Thomas et al. 1999*). The single most important prognostic clinical factor is a phenomenon termed centralisation (*McKenzie 1981, McKenzie & May 2003*). Centralisation describes a symptom response to repeated movements or sustained positions, which is:

- lasting abolition of peripheral symptoms
- decrease and abolition of remaining back pain.

This improvement in symptoms has consistently been shown to be a reliable indicator of a good prognosis (*Donelson et al. 1990, Sufka et al. 1998, Long 1995, Werneke et al. 1999, Karas et al. 1997, Werneke & Hart 2001, Aina et al. 2004*). It has been found to be an even stronger predictor of outcomes than some 'yellow flags' (*Werneke & Hart 2001*). This means that if a position or movement can be found that first decreases and then abolishes your most distal symptoms or back pain, if only back pain is present, you have found a powerful and reliable tool to make yourself better.

In summary, in respect of risk factors it is apparent that there are no simple causal explanations for back pain. Onset of back pain in most instances is spontaneous and not related to any specific event (*Kramer 1990, Waddell 2004, Hall et al. 1998*). Although biomechanical risks appear of some importance, at most, all risk factors, individually or combined, can only explain a small proportion of back pain (*Mannion et al. 1996, Adams et al. 1999*). A past history of back pain is the factor most consistently associated with future back pain.

In summary, in respect of prognostic factors, multiple issues may be important. Attitudes and beliefs about back pain, activity, and the individual's belief in their ability to deal with it are clearly important. The more active you are the better the outcome. If you can identify specific movements or positions that abolish symptoms, even better.

5 Attitudes about work

It used to be considered that back pain is a justification for rest and sick leave from work. Such a notion is *no longer tenable*, and it is in the best long-term interest of the worker for both employer and employee to facilitate and promote an early return to work (*Carter et al. 2000*). It is clear that being off work for a long time is counter productive and unhelpful. The day someone goes off work with back pain they have a 1-10% chance of still being off work a year later (*Waddell 2004*). Once they have been on sick for 4-6 weeks they have a 20% risk of long-term disability, and if sick for 6 months a 50% risk. Once a worker has been on sick leave for a year or more they are unlikely to work again, regardless of the features of their back pain or the health care they receive (*Waddell 2004*). In other words long term sick leave is a slippery slope, easy to slide down but extremely difficult to claw back up to full-time employment.

Not surprisingly given the importance of psychosocial factors reviewed earlier there is increasing evidence that workers beliefs and attitudes to work affect their likelihood of return (*Waddell 2004, Main et al. 2000*). Just as the term 'yellow flags' has been introduced for the concept of psychosocial barriers to recovery, so have the terms 'blue flags' and 'black flags' been used to respectively describe *perceptions* of work and work *characteristics* that may act as barriers to recovery (*Main et al. 2000*).

Table 8.3. Perceptions of work ('blue flags') that may act as barriers to recovery

- high job demands / time pressure
- low control
- unhelpful management style
- poor social support
- low job satisfaction
- belief that work is harmful and will damage the back.

Source: Main et al. 2000

'Blue flags' are a matter of perception by the worker that may require careful attention from management and Occupational Health Departments aimed at the worker's beliefs. 'Black flags' are conditions of employment, both national and local, that may affect the worker's ability to return to work.

Table 8.4. Occupational factors ('black flags') that may act as barriers to return to work

- sickness policy
- entitlement to sick leave
- requirements of occupational health department for 'full fitness'
- organisational size and structure
- management style
- ergonomic demands of job
- number of working hours

Source: Main et al. 2000

The recent evidence based recommendations for the worker with back pain (*Carter et al. 2000*) are as follows:

- Encourage the worker to remain at work, or return as early as possible, within a few days or weeks at most.
- Consider temporary adaptations to the demands and pattern of work to facilitate this.
- Address the common misconception among workers of the need to be - pain free before returning to work. Some pain is to be expected and the early resumption of work activity improves the prognosis.

6 Self-management guidelines for simple low back pain

The following guidelines are for the management of simple low back pain both in its acute stage, during the first few weeks, and when symptoms have persisted for many weeks.

Medication

Non-steroidal anti-inflammatory drugs (NSAID), such as ibuprofen, and simple analgesics are both available over the counter as non-prescription medication. There is some evidence to support the value of NSAID medication in acute back pain to provide short-term benefit only, but they are not clearly better than simple analgesics. No NSAID has demonstrated superiority. There is less evidence to support the use of medication for sciatica or chronic back pain. (*Bogduk 2004, Smith et al. 2002, van Tulder et al. 2000b, NHS Centre for Reviews and Dissemination 2000, Koes et al. 1997*).

If the pain is very bad you might take paracetamol or ibuprofen, whichever suits you best, for a few days or a few weeks at most. Take them regularly so that the pain does not 'break through'. Painkillers can be used to help as you get active (*Roland et al. 2002*). No drug should be taken long term – the side effects of NSAID can be serious, especially if taken regularly or by the elderly (*NHS Centre for Reviews and Dissemination 2000*). Do not take ibuprofen or aspirin if pregnant, or if you have asthma, indigestion or an ulcer. Always read the instructions and warnings carefully, and if in doubt consult your GP. Do not rely on painkillers only; they may relieve the pain short-term, but they will not, by themselves, get you back to full function and normal activity.

Bed rest

Bed rest is not an effective treatment for back pain. If you are forced to rest this should be for a maximum of 2 days. Staying active generally produces faster recovery and fewer long term problems, and bed rest may lead to worse outcomes (*Hagen et al. 2000, 2002, Waddell et al. 1997*). Bed rest is not an effective treatment for sciatica either (*Vroomen et al. 1999*). Bed rest should never be considered for chronic back pain.

Activity modification

With an acute onset of back pain it may be necessary to modify some of your normal activities *temporarily*. The emphasis here is on the temporary nature of any activity modification. Staying active makes no difference to the level of pain, but leads to faster recovery, faster return to work, and fewer long term problems (*Carter et al. 2000, Waddell et al. 1997, Hagen et al. 2002*).

General advice about activity is as follows: keep on the move, do not stay in one position for too long, and try and do a bit more activity each day. Do not sit for too long, try a support in the small of the back, but get up and move about regularly (*Roland et al. 2002*).

As discussed earlier it is common for people with back pain to find that certain positions aggravate symptoms, most commonly sitting or bending, whilst certain positions or activities relieve them, most commonly walking or being on the move (*McKenzie 1979, Biering-Sorensen 1983, Boissonault & Di Fabio 1996, Stankovic & Johnell 1990, Williams et al. 1990, Snook et al. 1998, van Deursen et al. 1999*). This will be different for different individuals. Listen to your symptoms and *temporarily* avoid or decrease the amount you do the former and do more of the latter.

Work

If you can, stay at work, even if you have to adapt the way you do certain jobs or ask for some help. Usually your back will not get any worse at work than at home. If you have to take some time off work try to get back to work after a few days or a couple of weeks at the most. The longer you are inactive and off work the more likely you are to get long term pain and disability. It is

Box 8.1 Commonly used terms used in the description of back pain

Epidemiology	Study of the occurrence, distribution and course of a condition
Acute	A new episode of back pain
Chronic	Back pain that has persisted for more than 2 –3 months
Prevalence	The proportion of the population who have the condition in a lifetime, year or at one point in time
Incidence	The number of new cases of a condition
Natural history	The normal course of a condition
Recurrence	Relapse
Risk factor	Feature that makes a condition more likely to occur
Prognostic factor	Feature that affects the natural history one condition has occurred
Red flag	Features that might indicate serious spinal pathology
Yellow flag	Attitudes, belief and behaviours that are barriers to recovery

not necessary to be pain free before returning to work (*Carter et al. 2000*). Those with chronic back pain should not be off work.

Attitudes and beliefs

Recognition of 'yellow flags', psychosocial barriers to recovery, has demonstrated how attitudes and beliefs of people with back pain can affect the outcome (*Vlaeyen & Linton 2000, Linton 2000, Burton et al. 1995, Klenerman et al. 1995, Gatchel et al. 1995, Deyo & Diehl 1988, Hasenbring et al. 1994, Thomas et al. 1999*). In table 8.2 some of these 'yellow flags' are listed. In contrast it is therefore possible to list the attitudes to adopt that will help you recover more quickly and avoid long-term problems:

- do not avoid activity because you think it might hurt – a certain level of pain occurs during recovery
- do not be over anxious about your back pain – check there are no 'red flags' and you can be certain it is not a symptom of serious pathology
- use active coping strategies – keep on the move, walk regularly; rather than passive strategies, such as bed rest
- have belief in your ability to cope with back pain – most people do
- set yourself progressive goals in terms of activity to demonstrate to yourself that you can affect change.

Exercise

In general, systematic reviews have concluded that, whereas exercise is ineffective for acute back pain, it is effective for chronic back pain (*Smith et al. 2002, van Tulder et al. 2000a, NHS Centre for Reviews and Dissemination 2000, Maher et al. 1999, Hubley-Kozey et al 2003, Kool et al. 2004, Liddle et al. 2004*). However exercise should have a role in activation in acute back pain, and walking, swimming or any other form of exercise that you normally do should be continued as much as possible, or resumed as early as possible. For chronic back pain, no particular form of exercise appears best, but strengthening or general exercise regimes have been shown to be effective.

Monitoring symptoms

Monitoring symptoms during everyday activities may provide you with a reliable and valuable tool for self-management. Movements or positions that produce centralisation, abolition or reduction of symptoms should be done regularly. Centralisation describes the lasting abolition of leg symptoms or back pain in response to repeated movements or sustained positions (*McKenzie 1981*). Centralisation of symptoms has consistently been shown to be a reliable indicator of a good prognosis (*Donelson et al. 1990, Sufka et al. 1998, Long 1995, Werneke et al. 1999, Karas et al. 1997, Werneke & Hart 2001, Aina et al. 2004*). If a position or movement can be found that first decreases and then abolishes your most distal symptoms or back pain you have found a powerful and reliable tool to make yourself better. Sometimes when the leg pain goes the back pain can get temporarily more intense. The phenomenon of centralisation is explained more fully in a patient self-management book (*McKenzie 1980*).

Conversely if movements or positions cause the spread of pain into your leg or make activities more difficult these movements or positions should be temporarily avoided.

Patient booklets

There are a number of self-management booklets written for people with low back pain, just two will be recommended here. *Treat Your Own Back* (*McKenzie 1980*) gives advice about correct sitting posture and lifting, but also describes in detail a series of specific exercises that can be used and a system of monitoring symptoms to ensure you are doing the appropriate exercise. Following the advice in this book has been shown to be effective in decreasing the level of pain and the number of painful episodes in a cohort of individuals with chronic back pain,

Box 8.2 Key aspects of self-management of mechanical back pain

- keep work and activity limitation to a minimum
- avoid sick leave if you can, and if you have to have a few days off work keep it brief for a quicker return to normal function
- do not get over-anxious about your back pain or fearful about moving, some pain as you start to mobilise is normal
- active, rather than passive, coping strategies will help you more now and in the future
- to help you mobilise, if you need, take simple analgesics or ibuprofen regularly for a brief period only
- start light activity early (such as walking or swimming, or whatever you are comfortable with) and increase the amount you do each day
- keep on the move, do not sit for long periods, **don't take back pain lying down**
- sit with support in your low back, but get up regularly
- 'listen' to your symptoms and act on their 'voices'
- if you find a movement or position that decreases or abolishes some or all of your pain repeat that movement or position as frequently as you can, as long as it is helping
- if you find a movement or position that increases, or brings on your pain or causes it to spread, *temporarily* avoid this
- in the future keep fit, flexible and active
- in the future exercise regularly

both short and long-term, the majority of whom found the advice very valuable in managing their back pain (*Udermann et al. 2004*).

The Back Book (Roland et al. 2002) has advice for patients based on the latest research, much of which is summarised above. It advises about the value of general activity, keeping active rather than resting, and about how to use active coping strategies. The book has been shown to reduce high levels of fear of movement in patients with back pain (*Burton et al. 1996*). A useful website, which provides brief guidelines for the management of acute back pain, is: www.workingbacksscotland.com

Prevention of back pain

From an epidemiological perspective, as discussed above, it is known that back pain is rarely a one-off event. The strongest known risk factor for future back pain is a history of back pain in the past (*Croft et al. 1997, Shekelle 1997, Smedley et al. 1997*). At least fifty percent of those who have a first episode of back pain will have further episodes, many recurrences are common and at least a quarter of the back pain population have a long-term problem (*Klenerman et al. 1995, van den Hoogen et al. 1998, Linton et al. 1998, Hillman et al. 1996, Croft et al. 1997, 1998, Waxman et al. 2000*). Certain behaviours regarding exercise and posture may be important in helping to prevent future episodes or reduce their impact should they occur.

Exercise has been shown to have a protective effect against back pain and its effects. Exercise programmes have decreased the prevalence, severity and duration of back pain episodes, and decreased time off work due to back pain. There is consistent evidence that exercise may be effective in preventing back pain. (*van Poppel et al. 1997, Gebhardt 1994, Lahad et al. 1994, Karas & Conrad 1994, Zimmerman 1998, Minor 1996, Maher et al. 1999, Maher 2000, Linton & van Tulder 2001, Jellema et al. 2001*).

More general physical activity, for at least 3 hours per week, reduced the prevalence of back pain by at least 10% (*Harreby et al. 1997*). Those who maintained regular exercises after a rehabilitation programme had fewer recurrences of pain and less absence from work compared to those who were physically inactive (*Taimela et al. 2000*). Performing a series of extensions in lying exercises, like a modified push-up with the lower half of the body remaining on the floor, only once or twice a day has been shown to significantly reduce back pain episodes and health care seeking for back pain (*Larsen et al. 2003*). In those with a history of back pain, recurrence rate in the year was nearly halved compared to a control group not performing these exercises.

The optimal sitting posture for back care is one of lordosis, when the hollow in the small of the back is maintained, coupled with regular interruption of sustained sitting (*Harrison et al. 1999, Pynt et al. 2001*). This position is facilitated by sitting with the hips at an angle of 90 degrees or more, and the use of a support in the small of the back (*Pheasant 1998*). Likewise activities involving prolonged bending require interruption of that position, and regular restoration of the lordosis by a few repetitions of backwards bending. The structures of the spine like movement, any position that you are forced to maintain for long periods is best interrupted on a regular basis.

7 Summary

Back pain is a normal experience that happens to the majority of adults. Frequently it is recurrent and persistent. Mostly the structural basis for back pain cannot be clinically proven. Very rarely (1%) is back pain due to serious spinal pathology, this is recognised by 'red flag' features which, if present, are a reason for seeking urgent medical help. The majority (more than 90%) is simple or mechanical low back pain. Sometimes (5-10%), this is accompanied by nerve root symptoms – pain into the foot with pins and needles, numbness or weakness in the foot. Even though it is not possible to readily identify the cause of most back pain the appropriate actions to limit the impact of back pain are now well known, and have been summarised in this chapter (see box 8.2).

References

Adams MA, Dolan P (1995). Recent advances in lumbar spinal mechanics and their clinical significance. Clinical Biomechanics 10.3-19.

Adams MA, Mannion AF, Dolan P (1999). Personal risk factors for first-time low back pain. Spine 24.2497-2505.

Aina A, May S, Clare H (2004). The centralization phenomenon of spinal symptoms – a systematic review. Manual Therapy 9.134-143.

Biering-Sorensen F (1983). A prospective study of low back pain in a general population. 2. Location, character, aggravating and relieving factors. Scand J Rehab Med 15.81-88.

Boden SD, Davis DO, Dina TS, Patronas NJ, Wiesel SW (1990). Abnormal magnetic-resonance scans of the lumbar spine in asymptomatic subjects. JBJS 72A.403-408.

Bogduk N (2004). Management of chronic low back pain. Med J Aus 180.79-83.

Boissonnault W, Di Fabio RP (1996). Pain profile of patients with low back pain referred to physical therapy. J Orth Sports Physical Ther 24.180-191.

Bombardier C, Kerr MS, Shannon HS, Frank JW (1994). A guide to interpreting epidemiologic studies on the aetiology of back pain. Spine 19.2047S-2056S.

Boos N, Rieder R, Schade V, Spratt KF, Semmer N, Aebi M (1995). The diagnostic accuracy of magnetic resonance imaging, work perception, and psychosocial factors in identifying symptomatic disc herniations. Spine 20.2613-2625.

Burdorf A, Sorock G (1997). Positive and negative evidence of risk factors for back disorders. Scand J Work Environ Health 23.243-256.

Burton AK, Tillotson KM, Main CJ, Hollis S (1995). Psychosocial predictors of outcome in acute and subchronic low back trouble. Spine 20.722-728.

Carey TS, Garrett JM, Jackman AM (2000). Beyond the good prognosis. Examination of an inception cohort of patients with chronic low back pain. Spine 25.115-120.

Carter JT, Waddell, Burton K et al. (2000). Occupational Health Guidelines for the Management of Low Back Pain at Work. Faculty of Occupational Medicine, London.

Chavannes AW, Gubbels J, Post D, Rutten G, Thomas S (1986). Acute low back pain: patients' perceptions of pain four weeks after initial diag-

nosis and treatment in general practice. J Royal Coll GP 36.271-273.
Cherkin DC, Deyo RA, Street JH, Barlow W (1996). Predicting poor outcomes for back pain seen in primary care using patients' own criteria. Spine 21.2900-2907.
Croft P, Papageorgiou A, Ferry S, Thomas E, Jayson MIV, Silman AJ (1996). Psychologic distress and low back pain. Evidence from a prospective study in the general population. Spine 20.2731-2737.
Croft P, Papageorgiou A, McNally R (1997). Low Back Pain - Health Care Needs Assessment Radcliffe Medical Press, Oxford.
Croft PR, Macfarlane GJ, Papageoorgiou AC, Thomas E, Silman AJ (1998). Outcome of low back pain in general practice: a prospective study. BMJ 316.1356-1359.
Croft P, Papageorgiou A, Thomas E, Macfarlane GJ, Silman AJ (1999). Short-term physical risk factors for new episodes of low back pain. Prospective evidence from the south Manchester back pain study. Spine 24.1556-1561.
CSAG (1994). Clinical Standards Advisory Group: Back Pain. HMSO, London.
Deyo RA, Diehl AK (1988). Psychosocial predictors of disability in patients with low back pain. J Rheum 15.1557-1564.
Dolan P (1998). Associations between mechanical loading, spinal function and low back pain. In: Proceedings Third Interdisciplinary World Congress on Low Back & Pelvic Pain, November, Vienna. Eds Vleeming A, Mooney V, Tilscher H, Dorman T, Snijders C.
Donelson R, Silva G, Murphy K (1990). Centralisation phenomenon. Its usefulness in evaluating and treating referred pain. Spine 15.211-213.
Ferguson SA, Marras WS (1997). A literature review of low back disorder surveillance measures and risk factors. Clin Biomech 12.211-226.
Frank JW, Kerr MS, Brooker AS et al (1996). Disability resulting from occupational low back pain. Part 1: What do we know about primary prevention? A review of the scientific evidence on prevention before disability begins. Spine 21.2908-2917.
Gatchel RJ, Polatin PB, Mayer TG (1995). The dominant role of psychosocial risk factors in the development of chronic low back pain disability. Spine 20.2702-2709.
Gebhardt WA (1994). Effectiveness of training to prevent job-related back pain: a meta-analysis. Br J Clin Psychology 33.571-574.
Goertz MN (1990). Prognostic indicators for acute low-back pain. Spine15.1307-1310.
Hagen KB, Hilde G, Jamtvedt G, Winnem MF (2000). The Cochrane review of bed rest for acute low back pain and sciatica. Spine 25.2932-2939.
Hagen KB, Hilde G, Jamtvedt G, Winnem MF (2002). The Cochrane review of advice to stay active as a single treatment for low back pain and sciatica. Spine 27.1736-1741.
Hall H, McIntosh G, Wilson L, Melles T (1998). Spontaneous onset of back pain. Clin J Pain 14.129-133.
Halpin SFS, Yeoman L, Dundas DD (1991). Radiographic examination of the lumbar spine in a community hospital: an audit of current practice. BMJ 303.813-815.
Harreby M, Hesselsoe G, Kjer J, Neergaard K (1997). Low back pain and physical exercise in leisure time in 38-year-old men and women: a 25-year prospective cohort study of 640 school children. Eur Spine J 6.181-186.
Harrison DD, Harrison SO, Croft AC, Harrison DE, Troyanovich SJ (1999). Sitting biomechanics part 1: review of the literature. J Manip Physiological Therapeutics 22.594-609.
Hasenbring M, Marienfeld G, Kuhlendahl D, Soyka D (1994). Risk factors of chronicity in lumbar disc patients. A prospective investigation of biologic, psychologic, and social predictors of therapy outcome. Spine 19.2759-2765.
Hillman M, Wright A, Rajaratnam G, Tennant A, Chamberlain MA (1996). Prevalence of low back pain in the community: implications for service provision in Bradford, UK. J Epidem Comm Health 50.347-352.
Hoogendoorn WE, van Poppel MNM, Bongers PM, Koes BW, Bouter LM (1999). Physical load during work and leisure time as risk factors for back pain. Scand J Work Environ Health 25.387-403.
Hoogendoorn WE, van Poppel MNM, Bongers PM, Koes BW, Bouter LM (2000). Systematic review of psychosocial factors at work and private life as risk factors for back pain. Spine 25.2114-2125.
Hubley-Kozey CL, McCulloch TA, McFarland DH (2003). Chronic low back pain: a critical review of specific therapeutic exercise protocols on musculoskeletal and parameters. J Manual Manip Thera 11.78-87.
Jensen MC, Brant_Zawadzki MN, Obuchowski N, Modic MT, Malkasian D, Ross JS (1994). Magnetic resonance imaging of the lumbar spine in people without back pain. NEJM 331.69-73.
Karas BE, Conrad KM (1996). Back injury prevention interventions in the workplace. An integrative review. AAOHN 44.189-196.
Karas R, McIntosh G, Hall H, Wilson L, Melles T (1997). The relationship between non organic signs and centralization of symptoms in the prediction of return to work for patients with low back pain. Physical Therapy 77.354-360.
Kendrick D, Fielding K, Bentley E, Kerslake R, Miller P, Pringle M (2001). Radiography of the lumbar spine in primary acre patients with low back pain: randomised controlled trial. BMJ 322.400-405.
Klenerman L, Slade PD, Stanley IM et al. (1995). The predication of chronicity in patients with an acute attack of low back pain in a general practice setting. Spine 20.478-484.
Koes BW, Scholten RJPM, Mens JMA, Bouter LM (1997). Efficacy of NSAIDs for low back pain: a systematic review of randomised clinical trials. Ann Rheum Dis 56.214-223.
Kool J, de Bie R, Oesch P, Knusel O, van den Brandt P, Bachmann S (2004). Exercise reduces sick leave in patients with non-acute non-specific low back pain: a meta-analysis. J Rehabil Med 36.49-62.
Kramer J (1990). Intervertebral Disk Diseases. Causes, Diagnosis, Treatment and Prophylaxis. (2nd Ed.) Thieme Medical Publishers, New York.
Lahad A, Malter AD, Berg AO, Deyo RA (1994). The effectiveness of four interventions for the prevention of low back pain. JAMA 272.1286-1291.
Lanier DC, Stockton P (1988). Clinical

predictors of outcomes of acute episodes of low back pain. J Family Pract 27.483-489.

Larsen K, Weidick F, Leboeuf-Yde C (2002). Can passive prone extensions of the back prevent back problems? A randomised, controlled intervention trial of 314 military conscripts. Spine 27.2747-2752

Liddle SD, Baxter GD, Gracey JH (2004). Exercise and chronic low back pain: what works? Pain 107.176-190.

Linton SJ, Hellsing AL, Hallden K (1998). A population-based study of spinal pain among 35-45-year-old individuals. Spine 23.1457-1463.

Linton SJ (2000). A review of psychological risk factors in back and neck pain. Spine 25.1148-1156.

Linton SJ, van Tulder MW (2001). Preventive interventions for back and neck pain. What is the evidence? Spine 26.778-787.

Long AL (1995). The centralisation phenomenon. Its usefulness as a predictor of outcome in conservative treatment of chronic low back pain (a pilot study). Spine 20.2513-2521.

Maher C, Latimer J, Refshauge K (1999). Prescription of activity for low back pain: What works? Aus J Physio 45.121-132.

Maher CG (2000). A systematic review of workplace interventions to prevent low back pain. Aus J Physio 46.259-269.

Main CJ, Spanswick CC (2000). Pain Management. An Interdisciplinary Approach. Churchill Livingstone, Edinburgh.

Mannion AF, Dolan P, Adams MA (1996). Psychological questionnaires: Do "abnormal" scores precede or follow first-time low back pain? Spine 21.2603-2611.

McKenzie RA (1979). Prophylaxis in recurrent low back pain. NZ Med J 89.22-23.

McKenzie R (1980). Treat Your Own Back. Spinal Publications New Zealand Ltd, Waikanae.

McKenzie RA (1981). The Lumbar Spine. Mechanical Diagnosis and Therapy. Spinal Publications, New Zealand.

McKenzie RA, May S (2003). The Lumbar Spine. Mechanical Diagnosis and Therapy (2nd Ed). Spinal Publications New Zealand Ltd.

McKinnon ME, Vickers MR, Ruddock VM, Townsend J, Meade TW (1997). Community studies of the health service implications of low back pain. Spine 22.2161-2166.

Miller P, Kendrick D, Bentley E, Fielding K (2002). Cost-effectiveness of lumbar spine radiography in primary acre patients with low back pain. Spine 27.2291-2297.

Nachemson A, Vingaard E (2000). Influences of individual factors and smoking on neck and low back pain. In: Eds: Nachemson AL, Jonsson E. Neck and Back Pain. The Scientific Evidence of Causes, Diagnosis, and Treatment. Lippincott Williams & Wilkins, Philadelphia.

NHS Centre for Reviews and Dissemination (2000). Effective Healthcare: Acute and chronic low back pain. NHS Centre for Reviews and Dissemination 6.1-8.

Papageorgiou AC, Croft PR, Ferry S, Jayson MIV, Silman AJ (1995). Estimating the prevalence of low back pain in the general population. Spine 20.1889-1894.

Pheasant S (1998). Bodyspace. Anthropometry, Ergonomics and the Design of Work. Taylor & Francis, London.

Pynt J, Higgs J, Mackey M (2001). Seeking the optimal posture of the seated lumbar spine. Physio Theory & Practice 17.5-21.

RCGP (1999). Clinical Guidelines for the Management of Acute Low Back Pain. Royal College of General Practitioners, London.

Roland M, van Tulder M (1998). Should radiologists change the way they report plain radiography of the spine? Lancet 352.229-230.

Roland M, Waddell G, Klaber Moffett J, Burton K, Main C (2002). The Back Book. The Stationery Office.

Schwarzer AC, Aprill CN, Derby R, Fortin J, Kine G, Bogduk N (1994a). Clinical features of patients with pain stemming from the lumbar zygapophyseal joints. Is the lumbar facet syndrome a clinical entity? Spine 19.1132-1137.

Schwarzer AC, Derby R, Aprill CN, Fortin J, Kine G, Bogduk N (1994b). Pain from the lumbar zygapophyseal joints: a test of two models. J Spinal Dis 7.331-336.

Schwarzer AC, Aprill CN, Bogduk N (1995a). The sacroiliac joint in chronic low back pain. Spine 20.1.31-37.

Schwarzer AC, Aprill CN, Derby R, Fortin J, Kine G, Bogduk N (1995b). The prevalence and clinical features of internal disc disruption in patients with chronic low back pain. Spine 20.1878-1883.

Shekelle P (1997). The epidemiology of low back pain. IN: Low Back Pain, Eds Giles LGF, Singer KP, Butterworth Heineman, Oxford.

Smedley J, Egger P, Cooper C, Coggon D (1997). Prospective cohort study of predictors of incident low back pain in nurses. BMJ 314.1225-1228.

Smith D, McMurray N, Disler P (2002). Early intervention for acute back injury: can we finally develop an evidence-based approach? Clin Rehabil 16.1-11.

Snook SH, Webster BS, McGorry RW, Fogleman MT, McCann KB (1998). The reduction of chronic non-specific low back pain through the control of early morning lumbar flexion. A randomised controlled trial. Spine 23.2601-2607.

Spitzer WO, LeBlanc FE, Dupuis M et al. (1987). Scientific approach to the activity assessment and management of activity-related spinal disorders. Spine 12.7.S1-S55.

Stankovic R, Johnell O (1990). Conservative treatment of acute low-back pain. A prospective randomised trial: McKenzie method of treatment versus patient education in "mini back school". Spine 15.120-123.

Sufka A, Hauger B, Trenary M et al (1998). Centralisation of low back pain and perceived functional outcome. JOSPT 27.205-212.

Taimela S, Diederich C, Hubsch M, Heinricy M (2000). The role of physical exercise and inactivity in pain recurrence and absenteeism from work after active outpatient rehabilitation for recurrent or chronic low back pain. A follow up study. Spine 25.1809-1816.

Thomas E, Silman AJ, Croft PR, Papageorgiou AC, Jayson MIV, Macfarlane GJ (1999). Predicting who develops chronic low back pain in primary care: A prospective study. BMJ 318.1662-1667.

Udermann BE, Spratt KF, Donelson RG, Mayer J, Graves JE, Tillotson J (2004). Can a patient educational book change behavior and reduce pain in chronic low back pain patients? Spine J 4.425-435.

Van den Hoogen HJM, Koes BW, van Eijk JTM, Bouter LM, Deville W (1998). On the course of low back pain in general practice: A one year follow up study. Ann Rheum Dis 57.13-19.

Van Deursen LL, Patijn J, Durinck JR, Brouwer R, van Erven-Sommers JR, Vortman BJ (1999). Sitting and low back pain: the positive effect of rotatory dynamic stimuli during prolonged sitting. Eur Spine J 8.187-193.

Van Poppel MNM, Koes BW, Smid T, Bouter LM (1997). A systematic review of controlled clinical trials on the prevention of back pain in industry. Occupational & Environmental Med 54.841-847.

Van Tulder MW, Assendelft Wjj, Koes BW, Bouter LM (1997). Spinal radiographic findings and non-specific back pain. A systematic review of observational studies. Spine 22.427-434.

Van Tulder MW, Malmivaara A, Esmail R, Koes BW (2000a). Exercise therapy for low back pain. A systematic review within the framework of the Cochrane collaboration back review group. Spine 25.2784-2796.

Van Tulder MW, Scholten RJPM, Koes BW, Deyo RA (2000b). Nonsteroidal anti-inflammatory drugs for low back pain. A systematic review within the framework of the Cochrane Collaboration Back Review Group. Spine 25.2501-2513.

Vingard E, Nachemson A (2000). Work-related influences on neck and back pain. In: Eds: Nachemson AL, Jonsson E. Neck and Back Pain. The Scientific Evidence of Causes, Diagnosis, and Treatment. Lippincott Williams & Wilkins, Philadelphia.

Vlaeyen JWS, Linton SJ (2000). Fear-avoidance and its consequences in chronic musculoskeletal pain: a state of the art. Pain 85.317-332.

Vroomen PCAJ, de Krom MCTFM, Wilmink JT, Kester ADM, Knottnerus JA (1999). Lack of effectiveness of bed rest for sciatica. N Eng J Med 340.418-423.

Waddell G (1994). Epidemiology Review. Annex to CSAG Report on Back Pain. London: HMSO.

Waddell G, Feder G, Lewis M (1997). Systematic reviews of bed rest and advice to stay active for acute low back pain. Br J Gen Pract 47.647-652.

Waddell G (2004). The Back Pain Revolution (2nd Ed). Churchill Livingstone, Edinburgh.

Walsh K, Cruddas M, Coggon D (1992). Low back pain in eight areas of Britain. J Epidem Comm Health 46.227-230.

Waxman R, Tennant A, Helliwell P (2000). A prospective follow-up study of low back pain in the community. Spine 25.2085-2090.

Werneke M, Hart DL, Cook D (1999). A descriptive study of the centralization phenomenon. Spine 24.676-683.

Werneke M, Hart DL (2001). Centralization phenomenon as a prognostic factor for chronic low back pain and disability. Spine 26.758-765.

Williams MM, Hawley JA, McKenzie RA, van Wijmen PM (1991). A comparison of the effects of two sitting postures on back and referred pain. Spine 16.1185-1191.

Zimmerman T (1998). The effectiveness of different intervention strategies in preventing back pain in members of the nursing population and the general population. Work 11.221-231.

9

Manual handling risk assessment – theory and practice

Carole Johnson MCSP SRP Cert Ed
Manual Handling Consultant

1 Is a manual handling risk assessor born or made?

The range of what we think and do
is limited by what we fail to notice.
And because we fail to notice
that we fail to notice
there is little we can do
to change until we notice
how failing to notice
shapes our thoughts and deeds

R.D. Laing
(cited by Daniel Goleman in *Vital Lies, Simple Truths*)

Some people seem to be able to identify risks, factor in the surrounding issues, devise an acceptable action plan, communicate well with the other parties and save money with an awesome skill. Others struggle to find the particular difficulties, cannot separate out the risks, fail to communicate with the appropriate parties and over simplify the solutions. These people are constantly seeking affirmation from others that their decisions are right, prefer blanket polices and tight protocols and in the process are unable to manage the manual handling risks around them. Some know the answers but are constrained by other parties or factors.

This chapter focuses on the concept of manual handling risk assessment and begins to tackle the less discussed aspects of risk assessment alongside those that are well known. The aim is to assist the reader in improving their ability to assess risk whether they are 'born' or 'made'. This chapter will interlink with all the other chapters in this book and the reader will be directed to specific chapters for further detail as appropriate.

Manual handling risk assessment and management is sometimes oversimplified to just the completion of a form. This is an incomplete perspective and the hope that this will comply with regulation and local policy is naïve and dangerous. Manual handling risk assessment must be viewed as a holistic process, which has several inter-relating aspects and where the risk assessment record is just one part. It is the author's hope that by the time the reader has finished this chapter he/she will have a clearer understanding of the concept of risk assessment.

Noticing

The relevance of the above quote to risk assessment is apparent. The process of risk assessment in simple terms begins by 'noticing' the risk factors. The 'noticing' must then be followed by analysis, relevant risk reduction and review. The *ability* to 'notice' is based on the knowledge and experience of the assessor and the capacity of that assessor to recognise their personal limitations. A good assessor is already collecting information, watching and listening before they are even asked. Not 'noticing' may result in the difference between a successful outcome and a dismal failure. Some of the reasons why these difficulties occur will be explored as part of the risk assessment framework. Change management is also discussed in chapter 3.

A simple template for assessment is provided within *HSE (2004) Manual Handling Guidance on Regulations* (L 23) and Schedule 1, and with the appendices of that guidance, should form the foundation of the questioning process.

It is often *technically* possible to resolve a moving and handling issue where there is a risk of injury, but it may be more difficult to understand why the people involved are reluctant to adopt a change, find funding or follow safety measures over the long term.

Additional factors need to be considered when assessing the handling of people; this is one example:

Example

A young adult has multiple disabilities. She cannot see, hear or easily communicate with the people around her. She weighs 11 stones. She is in pain although various professionals have been unable to improve this significantly having tried many options. She has to be supported at all times in specially fitted equipment and cannot support her own head. She cries loudly all day. Staff try very hard to cope with this but have to be moved to work with different people every hour in order to achieve the best during the working day.

Staff have discovered that when the young lady is in the hydrotherapy pool she stops crying and visibly relaxes and therefore she is taken swimming twice a day. The employer was forward thinking and realising that there was a high risk of injury ensured that there were suitable hoisting facilities and equipment so that staff did not have to lift the young lady at any time. The facilities were checked and deemed to be suitable and safe. All staff had been trained and assessed as competent at using the equipment.

6 months after the installation of the equipment and the setting up of the safe systems of work at least 3 members of staff were injured. A re-assessment was requested and it was discovered none of the new equipment was being used.

The staff stated that they did not wish to use the equipment (although the technical reasons for not using the equipment given had all been resolved) and stated that they would only use a manual lift using two people, into and out of the water. The staff continued with this view even after retraining and the threat of disciplinary action. The situation seemed irresolvable until a psychologist offered an explanation for their behaviour:

The staff could not cure or remove the basic cause of pain, but only relieve it for a short period. The rest of the time they subconsciously felt guilty that they could not help and therefore felt that they carried a responsibility for that pain and should therefore 'suffer' with her.

This idea was not well received by some of the professionals involved, but when presented to the staff struck a chord. After discussion the handling plan was re-instated, with staff receiving support and counselling. No further injuries were reported.

In the scenario given above, it is evident that the staff themselves had not 'noticed' their own guilt feelings and were therefore prepared to take significant risks despite the outcome of the risk assessment. The professionals initially involved had also not 'noticed' (understood) the reason for non-compliance.

To some, the above example may seem fanciful and people may consider that there must have been other short-comings within the process such as inadequate training, poor management or other factors. Nevertheless, prior to the psychologist's intervention, injuries had occurred when all care had been taken to devise a safe system of work and provide appropriate equipment. After the psychologist's intervention the safe system of work could be truly implemented. Whether or not the 'diagnosis' of the problem was correct, it gave the staff a rationale that they could identify with and consider – a way out.

2 Setting the scene

Manual Handling Risk Assessment has grown as a subject and must be placed within the legal framework. Further information on the Legal Aspects and Balancing Risk can be obtained from chapters 1 and 2.

This chapter confirms that the manual handling assessment fits into a structure that includes health and safety legislation and other laws, including the *Human Rights Act 1998* and the *Disability Discrimination Act 1995*. There has been a tendency in the past to place the health and safety legislation 'above' other legislation, but it has become clear that the process is one of balancing rather than hierarchy.

Hutter (2001) explains that the purpose of health and safety legislation is to give structure, procedures and routines, which can be included in the everyday life of the individual. The risk assessment should be part of the employee's life and not a piece of paper locked away in a file.

She also emphasises that in order to make the risk assessment process work, the employer has a responsibility to find ways of communicating the structure, procedures and routines. She suggests walkabouts, i.e. face-to-face contact as the best method of imparting the importance of compliance.

'Health and safety regulation – a short guide' provides a summary on regulations as well as an explanation of the difference between the law, codes of practice and guidance, *HSE (2003)*.

A comprehensive list of relevant legislation is also provided in *Mandelstam (2002)*.

Manual Handling Operations Regulations 1992

The Manual Handling Operations Regulations (as amended) 1992 (MHOR), updated in 2004, provides the framework for the risk assessment process within manual handling. It allows a systematic assessment process of all the relevant subject areas with the aim of identifying the main areas of risk and then developing a plan (safe system of work) for those involved.

There is often criticism of these Regulations in that they are felt to be very load orientated and do not use terms that easily relate to people handling. However, in the guidance, it clearly states that a load is a 'discreet moveable object', which 'includes for example a human patient...' and it is therefore the role of the professional to use words that 'humanise' the load in order to make terminology more acceptable.

As the MHOR have been in place a number of years, there have been other documents and articles that discuss and analyse the Regulations and their impact, among these are *The Principles of Good Manual Handling (HSE 2003)* and the *Evaluation of the Six Pack Regulations (1998)* (both published by the HSE).

The requirements of the Regulations can be summarised as:

It is the duty of the employer as far as reasonably practicable to

- **Avoid** the need for his employers to undertake manual handling tasks where he may be injured
- **Assess** the risk where it is not possible to avoid the task
- **Reduce** the risk to the lowest reasonably practicable level
- **Review** if the circumstances change.

The acronym **AARR** is often given to aid the memory.

Standards

Alongside the legal framework, standards are available to assist in the process of the assessment of manual handling risk. Four important documents to consider are:

- *Risk Management Standard* DoH *(2003)*
- *Health and Safety Management Standard* DoH *(2003)*
- *Risk Management* SAI 4360 *(2004) (supersedes 4360:1999)*
- *Manual Handling Standard NBE (2004)*

Please note that the first two documents are health service based and the third is industry based, but the principles can be taken from all the documents and applied to social care in so far as all of the standards provide a general framework where risk can be analysed.

Further broader documents *Healthcare Standards*, DoH (2004) and *Health and Safety Commission – Strategic Plan 2001–2004* (Health and Safety Commission) have also been published and, although manual handling is not specifically mentioned, would be embraced by the core and developmental standards.

Criterion 6 from the *Risk Management Standard (2003)* states:
'A risk management process, based on the requirements of AS/NZS 4360: 1999 SAI (1999) and covering all risk, is embedded throughout the organisation at all levels, including the board, with key indicators to demonstrate performance. The whole system of risk management is continuously monitored and reviewed by management and the Board in order to learn and make improvements to the system'.

Criterion 13 from the *Health and Safety Standard* states:
'Manual handling operations that involve a risk of injury are, where possible, avoided. Risk of injury related to any remaining manual handling operations is reduced to the lowest level reasonably practicable'.

According to the Australian Risk Management Standard AS/NZS 4360: 1999, risk management is an 'iterative process consisting of well defined steps which, taken in sequence, support better decision-making by contributing a greater insight into risk and their impacts'. The term iterative is useful here as it suggests a process that is repeated and refined in order to gain a better idea of the problem. It details how this process should be conducted and the reasoning.

As well as the national and international standards available, it is likely that there are local standards and policies. It is important for the reader to access this information and apply it to the local process.

3 Identifying risks and the 'human' aspects

It is possible to produce a list of risk factors when assisting people and this section will give the reader some key questions to ask. It is also necessary to identify how that information will be collected and from which sources.

Sources of information

Information on risk factors listed in the next section can be obtained from:

- Interview with the person being assisted
- Interviews with carers/relatives
- Interview with staff
- Team meetings
- Medical notes
- Care Plans
- Personal profiles/plans
- Pen pictures
- Policies
- Written protocols/procedures
- Articles/books and research studies
- Expert opinion/experience
- Risk Registers
- Incident information including near misses
- Insurance claims
- Peer review

The level of manual handling risk assessment will determine the number of sources that need to be accessed.

TILE

The HSE guidance notes on the MHOR 1992 (L23) list many of the risk factors related to manual handling and this information provides a sound basis for identifying risk. The guidance gives information on principles, risk assessment filters, example checklists and an assessment tool to aid the assessor. A basic assessment should consider:

- Task
- Individual Capability
- Load
- Environment (other factors and the interaction between these components)

The above list is often summarised as TILE or sometimes LITE.

The following tables look at each component of TILE in more detail and gives examples to help the assessor understand that component. The tables are based on Schedule 1 from the HSE guidance on the MHOR. The load (as a person) is based on the Chartered Society of Physiotherapy publication list, *Guidance in Manual Handling for Chartered Physiotherapists (2002)*:

The task

Factor	Example (load)	Example (person)
What is the task?	Can a diagram or description be given to help explain?	Personal care, standing transfer, off the floor, transfer onto a trolley, specialist procedure, transfer to equipment
Does it involve…		
Holding or manipulating loads at a distance from trunk?	Lifting a sack of rubbish from a bin	Supporting a person's leg during a surgical procedure or treatment
Twisting?	Picking an object from a table without moving the feet	Performing a medical intervention while sitting on the side of a bed
Stooping?	Lifting an large object from the floor	Supporting a small child walking
Reaching upwards?	Reaching for files on a high shelf	Lifting a child who has climbed onto a table
Excessive lifting or lowering distances?	Lifting items from the floor to place on a high shelf	Attempting to lift a person from the floor
Excessive carrying distances?	Carrying equipment where no trolley is available	Carrying a child from a classroom to the toilet
Excessive pushing or pulling of loads?	Pushing a hospital bed along a corridor	Pushing the cassette on overhead tracking in a swimming pool
Risk of sudden movement of loads?	Insecure handles	Person being assisted slipping or falling
Frequent or prolonged physical effort?	Moving a delivery of incontinence pads	Supporting a person while walking

The task (cont.)

Factor	Example (load)	Example (person)
Insufficient rest or recovery periods?	Moving a delivery consignment	Assisting a number of residents to get up in the morning
A rate of work imposed by a process?	Lifting to/ from a conveyor belt	Busy domiciliary care or institutional care settings – getting a number of people up in a certain time frame/regular toileting regimes/ put-to-bed routines, especially where there is a shortage of staff
Are there exceptional circumstances to consider?	Equipment failure	Hoist or other equipment failure, evacuation of premises

The load (as an object)

Factor	Example
Is the object…	
Heavy?	Wheelchair or divan bed
Bulky?	Computer monitor
Difficult to grasp?	Large piece of medical equipment
Unstable or with contents likely to shift?	Bags of shopping, laundry or boxes with unsecured items
Sharp hot or otherwise potentially damaging?	Cooking pans, needles

The load (as a person)

Factor	Example
How much help does the person need?	Is the person able to perform all the tasks even without supervision? If they need help, how much help. Do they need equipment? Do you know what equipment is available? Do you know the benefits and dangers of the equipment or process you are using or recommending?
Client expectations/wishes	Does the client have requests or wishes that will affect the moving and handling? Have this been discussed and considered?
Does the method chosen encourage independence?	In the longer term, will the method of assistance encourage the person to be as independent as possible? Is it important to this person to be as independent as possible? Are the Physiotherapist and Occupational Therapist or other professionals involved? Does this handling plan need to be integrated with the therapy plan?
Able to weight bear?	Can the person stand and do so without the need for support or assistance? Does the person rely on standing to be able to transfer and move within their environment? Does the state of the person's feet affect weight-bearing ability?
Pain/ medication	Is the person in pain? Has the pain been diagnosed and a suitable system of pain relief established? Does the person need referral to their GP or a pain specialist? Does the person take any medication that affects their mobility? Does timing of drug administration need to be changed to ensure best effects occur during moving and handling tasks?
Tissue viability/ infection	Does the person need any special considerations related to their skin or need disposable equipment such as slings because of infection.
Ability to communicate with others	Can the person explain their situation to you and follow requests?
Predictability	Is the person always the same or are there times when they are better than others. Do they easily tire or have difficulty providing sustained effort? Does the variance mean that more than one action plan is needed?

Factor	Example
Is the person a child or vulnerable adult?	For example, do there need to be considerations because the person has been or may have been abused in the past?
Behaviour	Is the person likely to be anxious, passive, show inappropriate responses or be violent or aggressive? Are there any triggers to the behaviour?
Cultural issues	Possible differing expectations regarding gender of carers, authority & acceptance, methods of managing personal hygiene
Physical abilities/ operations or interventions	Has the person a disability or health problem that affects how much they can help? Are there any special considerations that need to be included? Is there a health problem that may intermittently affect their ability (e.g. epileptic seizures)? Does the person have any problems with muscle tone, spasm, tremor, contractures, and/ or stiffness? Has the person undergone surgery or had a recent heart attack? Can the person balance themselves in lying, sitting and standing? Do they have any muscle weakness?
Comfort	Is the method used comfortable and not causing any difficulties, for example skin damage, pain, undue stress on a part of the body?
Body shape	Does the person need specialist equipment because of their body shape, such as individually made hoist slings or postural equipment?
Height and weight of the person	How tall and heavy is the person? Will special equipment be needed to support them, such as beds, seats, hoists, commodes? Can that equipment support the combined weight of the person being assisted and the staff?
Falls	Does the person have a history of falls – is there a falls assessment tool that should be completed?

Individual capability (the handler)

Factor	Example
Does the job… Require unusual strength. Or height?	Is there an expectation for the tallest and/or strongest members of staff to perform particular tasks? E.g. lifting people up from the floor, working around beds, matching of staff to particular patients/clients
Create a hazard to those who might reasonably be considered to be pregnant or to have a health problem?	Are there aspects of the task that can be seen to constitute a risk to a pregnant woman, or, for example, to someone who already has a back problem or other health problem?
Ever need to be undertaken by a person who does not usually take part in moving and handling or who is an occasional visitor	E.g. Speech or music therapist, care manager, other professional. The assessment should consider these specialists and ensure that they understand the risks and are included in the policy and action plan.
Require special information or training	Does the person undertaking the task have sufficient knowledge and skill to continue safely? Has there been a consideration of the skill level required to do the task?
Additional Requirements	Does the handler/ employer need to consider a child protection policy for example the Criminal Records Bureau (CRB) check?

The environment

Factor	Example
Is there…	
Space constraints on posture?	This could be due to extra equipment needed in a small space, storage difficulties or due to design of the equipment, layout of furniture in a person's home.
Uneven, slippery or unstable floors?	Is there a leak or fluid/ ice on the floor, are there steps, thresholds or edges that make the moving and handling more difficult. Doers the surface make pushing equipment over it difficult? Are you working outside?
Variations in levels of floors or work surfaces?	Is the person or member of staff required to work on different levels or negotiate steps?
Extremes of temperature or humidity?	Does the temperature or humidity need to be recorded and investigated? What temperatures are needed for the comfort of dependent individuals, compared with those carers undertaking work tasks.
Ventilation problems?	Is there too little or too much ventilation?
Poor lighting?	Can the person and staff see sufficiently to get the job done?
Indoors/outdoors	Is the task being undertaken indoors or outdoors? Are there variable gradients, distances involved, weather conditions to consider, or assisting the person in public places?
Equipment?	Can the equipment assigned such as hoists, wheelchairs, standing frames be used easily in the space provided? Has the equipment been checked as part of a maintenance programme and does it comply with equipment regulations? Are there systems in place to obtain specialist equipment that may only be needed on an occasional basis?

Other factors

Factor	Example
Does clothing affect the task	Are the person being assisted and the handler(s) wearing suitable clothing? Has jewellery been removed, suitable shoes and clothing worn? Does protective equipment affect the task (e.g. gloves, plastic overshoes at a swimming pool)?
Have the views of the person being assisted been considered?	Does the person have any views or concerns about the task and the way it is being planned? Have they had negative experiences in the past that may mean they are reluctant to use equipment?
Are there other legal factors that need to be considered?	Does the moving and handling task infringe the person's human rights or could be considered discriminatory? Is the duty of care affected?
Are there other personal factors that need to be considered?	Has the handler or the person being handled expressed concerns or views about any aspect of the task? Have that person's values been taken into consideration?
Could a generic assessment save time and still meet the needs?	Some tasks may be same for a ward or department e.g. using a bath hoist to get into and out of the bath and anyone using that bath would follow the same procedure. Generic assessments can save time, but any variance must be documented and any form should have a question that leads the assessor to further assessment when required.
Does the handler undertake regular manual handling?	See Ergonomics section below

Ergonomics

It is important when looking at the assessment of manual handling risks to consider ergonomics and the effect of any ergonomics interventions. It is necessary not only to look at an individual task, but also frequency, duration and other influencing factors. It may also be necessary to look at the whole working day of a member of staff for example. An individual task may not constitute a great risk of injury, but an accumulation of exposure to risks over a working shift may be unacceptably high.

According to Silverstein, as cited by *Wilson (2002)*, 'we have evidence that the more risk factors combined in the same job, affecting the same tissues, the greater the risk of WMSD, and the longer the exposure the greater the risk of WMSD (**NB** *WMSD correlates to WRMSD or work related musculoskeletal disorders*). There is evidence that reducing the physical and psychosocial risk factors decreases the severity, and may also decrease the incidence of WMSD'. However, at times it can be difficult to identify the greatest risk, or where to begin in the risk reduction process – particularly where complicated ergonomic and psychosocial factors are perceived as affecting that risk.

The recognised risk factors for low back pain as listed by *Wilson (2002)* are:

- Heavy physical work
- Prolonged sitting
- Prolonged driving
- Lack of exercise
- Prolonged whole body vibration

With lesser factors listed as:

- Smoking
- Obesity
- Psychosocial factors

Ergonomic factors are listed as:

- Posture
- Forces
- Distance from the load being lifted
- Joint position
- Cumulative effects
- Duration of the work
- Rest breaks
- Static loading
- Generalised fatigue
- Environmental factors such as lighting, noise, temperature and possibly electromagnetic radiation.

There has been a great deal of research undertaken on particular risk factors and a number of useful documents, studies and books are available from such authors as *Kroemer/Grandjean (1997)*, *Troup (1985)*, *Adams (2002)* and *Wilson (2002)*.

This section gives an overview of Ergonomics (see also chapter 4).

Biomechanics

Although posture is often recognised as a significant factor by Back Care professionals, individuals performing the tasks themselves are not necessarily aware of the effects of poor posture, especially in the long term. *Wilson (2002)* explains that 'good posture should involve:

- minimum joint strain or biomechanical loading
- economy of energy – minimal muscular loading
- avoidance of prolonged, repetitive or awkward movements.'

He suggests that 'to minimise muscle tension, a person must:

- Keep their joints in the middle one third of range of movement as much as possible
- Keep their limbs close to the centre of gravity as much as possible
- Try and support body parts that move away from the mid range or centre of gravity.'

The bulleted lists above are useful adjuncts when assessing risk and are considered in a number of assessment tools (see also chapter 6).

Psychosocial factors

Psychological factors and options to decrease the risks are broadly considered in the guidance to the *MHOR (2004)*. The HSE list some of the factors on their website (http://www.hse.gov.uk /msd/ mac/psychosocial.htm) :

- Workers who have little control over their work and work methods (including shift patterns);
- workers who are unable to make full use of their skills;
- workers who, as a rule, are not involved in making decisions that affect them;
- workers who are expected to only carry out repetitive, monotonous tasks;
- work which is machine or system paced (and may be monitored inappropriately);
- work demands which are perceived as excessive;
- payment systems that encourage working too quickly or without breaks;
- work systems which limit opportunities for social interaction;
- high levels of effort that are not balanced by sufficient reward (resources, remuneration, self-esteem, status).

The HSE advises that in order to improve the risk of injury related to the psychosocial factors listed above, the following should be considered:

- reducing the monotony of tasks where appropriate;
- ensuring there are reasonable work load (neither too much or too little) deadlines and demands;
- ensuring good communication and reporting of problems;
- encouraging teamwork;
- monitoring and control shiftwork or overtime working;
- reducing or monitoring payment systems which work on piece rate;
- providing appropriate training;

Perception of risk

'...individuals respond to the risks which concern them, not to those which trouble the experts...'
Heyman (1998)

It is possible that the risk assessor, who has seen similar situations in the past, may have a perception of higher risk than the person doing the task. Risk assessment relies heavily on the experience and understanding of the person undertaking the assessment and the person performing the task.

This was evident in a study of occupational health and safety on the railways. *Hutter (2001)* states that 'those at most risk were sometimes the least likely to perceive the risks in their working environment'.

One reason for this she explains is that 'those further up the corporate hierarchy had more information available to them and thus had a broader view of the risks associated with the workplace'.

However manual handling may not be seen by those outside the field as a hazardous activity requiring skilled risk assessment. Lifting may be viewed as the 'thing' that has to happen to get from A to B in order to perform the 'real' task. There are many occasions, for example, lifting people of the floor, where staff can feel damned if they do manually lift the person from the floor (as they face the risk of musculoskeletal injury) and damned if they don't (a feeling of distress by the person on the floor or disbelief by others).

While the perception is 'just do it', the general expectation will continue to be that lifting people is not a high-risk activity. There is often anecdotal evidence from the staff themselves that they frequently request strategies to decrease manual handling risk, but that the employer does not acknowledge the workers' appeals. There must be an explanation as to why perception of risk is so variable. One theory presented by *M. Kip Viscusi (1998)* is that people will always over-estimate the small risks and under-estimate the greater risks, because people are not perfectly informed. 'They simply do not take the information presented to them at face value, and if they do, the full information model emerges as a special case'.

Case Study

Jim has been manually lifting another family member for some considerable time. He is offered a portable hoist that can be dismantled when not needed. He has back pain, which he says he has acquired from heavy lifting for a number of years at work. He insists that lifting the family member does not give him back pain. The professional is adamant on supplying the hoist and that it must be used. Jim very reluctantly agrees to the equipment. The first time he dismantles the hoist he sustains an injury that requires time off work and he now refuses to use the equipment.

How would you have dealt with this situation and what should happen now?

In the example above it would be important to ascertain the events leading up to the incident, such as:

- Had Jim been working all day adopting poor postures?
- Had the hoist been a co-incidental last straw?
- Had Jim been shown how to use the hoist?
- Did Jim follow those instructions?
- Were there other factors to consider?
- Was the type/model of hoist provided appropriate to the circumstances?
- Was in fact Jim right and his method of lifting lower risk than using and dismantling the hoist?

Hutter (2001) also explores the fact that workers will choose to break the rules in order to get the job done. If the rules and regulations restrict the work required, the worker may decide to, or feel pressured into, taking a short cut or using a less safe alternative. She uses the example of high visibility clothing and the reluctance of railway staff to wear these items. Examples in the health and social care arena of short cuts may include not using a second person in order to save time, avoiding using equipment or not preparing the area.

The quote by *Heyman (1998)* at the beginning of this section explains why there is at times a mismatch between what the person and the professional want and why resolution can be difficult. He goes on to say, 'For this reason health professionals need to inform themselves about clients' risk perspectives, even if they dismiss them as erroneous or unscientific'.

Example

A person is dependent on 2 handlers to assist them to the toilet; on a particular occasion only one handler attends. The handler realises that they and the person are at increased risk of injury if they attempt the transfer on their own, but the person says they are desperate for the toilet and can't wait for a second handler. What are the driving concerns for the person and the handler? What should the handler do at that moment? How could this particular situation be avoided?

A Back Care Adviser discussing a situation with another Back Care Adviser is likely to have a similar basis for evaluating risk. They will find it easy to communicate with each other. The professional may look at events and conduct the risk assessment on the basis of 'adverse events', the person requiring moving and handling, however, may have different values and priorities .

Heyman (1998) states'... when service users and professionals differ in their value priorities, and professionals uncritically externalise their own values on to events, service users will immediately reject professional expertise as oppressive.' This has already been expressed by *Cunningham (2000)*.

As well as consideration of the value systems of the people involved, it is also worth considering the effect of general perceptions relating to moving and handling. It is possible that by and large everyone expects a nurse or care assistant to get a bad back, because information on nurses and musculoskeletal injury has been disseminated over a long period of time. Therefore, the handler and the person being handled do not factor in the risk of musculoskeletal injury because it has become the expectation.

Combined with the idea mentioned earlier that lifting is not considered an activity requiring specialist knowledge in its own right; it is easy to see how the value placed on injury prevention can diminish.

Sometimes the response to staff or carers not following a safe system of work has been dealt with by disciplinary action. It is however possible that sanctions may not receive the desired effect. *Hutter (2001)* refers to one interviewee who had been reprimanded for not following the rules asking whether sanctions had made a difference and for how long. The interviewee replied by saying that the reprimand did make a difference 'for as long as it takes to forget it'. When asked whether it worried the person that they could be subject to disciplinary action, the interviewee said 'Well yes and no. Yes, it is always there at the back of your mind that if you do something wrong and you break one of the rules... you could get raked over the coals.... But on the other hand sometimes... it makes life just that little bit easier.'

Client/Carer relationship

The aim of this section is to alert the reader to the importance of the development of a positive relationship with the person being assessed/assisted. It does skim over some of the psychological aspects and is not meant to be an all-encompassing analysis of human nature. It may seem far easier to look at biomechanical factors in the risk assessment process rather than other, less clear factors such as the effect of human relationships. No member of staff wants to believe that the reason an assessment is incomplete or not adhered to is because of the effects of personality and inter-personal skills. However, the assessor needs to be aware of such factors as:

- The person being assessed may respond differently to a figure in authority than a carer or family member.
- The assessor may use language and terms the person being assessed does not understand.
- The assessor may have a different value system or priorities to the person being assessed.

Even...

- The assessor may remind the person being assessed of someone they do or don't like and vice versa.

The relationship between the person assisting or assessing and the person being assisted can be complex. Add to this relationship other professionals, family members, friends and statutory bodies, it is little wonder that sometimes the process of developing a suitable moving and handling strategy can be difficult. The perspective of all of those people mentioned above will be different and yet must somehow be pulled together for the benefit of all.

Example

When someone is dedicated to another person, there may be no limits to what they will do. Goleman (1996) gives an example:

'Ponder the last moments of Gary and Mary Jane Chauncey, a couple completely devoted to their eleven-year-old daughter Andrea, who was confined to a wheelchair by cerebral palsy. The Chauncey family were passengers on an Amtrak train that crashed into a river after a barge hit and weakened a railroad bridge in Louisiana's Bayou Country. Thinking first of their daughter, the couple tried their best to save Andrea as water rushed into the sinking train; somehow they managed to push Andrea through a window to rescuers. Then as the car sank beneath the water, they perished.'

He goes on to say, '...from the perspective of a parent making a desperate decision in a moment of crisis, it is about nothing other than love.'

Professionals should acknowledge that a family carer assisting a person may take risks that the professional considers dangerous and unwise. That professional may not understand why the practice continues when there is a weight of 'evidence' to the contrary. It must be understood that as well as the biomechanical factors, the person may feel there is no choice, may be driven by love, may not recognise the risks or have a different evaluation of those risks.

Another consideration that even with the best intentions, the client, carer and assessor involved may all have a 'blind spot'. This 'blind spot' may effect their ability to design an action plan that is acceptable to all, it may not even be the same one and anyone in this scenario can be affected as suggested by *Goleman (1996)*:

- 'The mind can protect itself against anxiety by dimming awareness.
- This mechanism creates a blind spot: a zone of blocked attention and self-deception.
- Such blind spots occur at each major level of behaviour from the psychological to the social.'

The skilled assessor will be able to identify these blind spots and support all the parties in recognising these areas (in a non-threatening manner) and to lead to a successful action plan.

Dignity and sensory needs

Touch and sensory input is vital for our well being and development. Babies not handled will sink into 'an irreversible decline' and adults who are deprived of sensory input may suffer a 'transient psychosis' as *Berne (1968)* explains. It is thought that emotional and sensory deprivation leads to physical changes in the brain and can then be part of a general physical deterioration.

Our risk assessment process and plan of action should include the consideration of all the senses and the corresponding needs of the person being assisted. Touch for example can be a very important factor to consider in a handling task and lack of touch and distancing from a person has been often stated by staff as a reason for not using equipment.

Touch may also have to be carefully considered in the assessment where the person being assisted has had negative experiences, had trust betrayed or has been sexually abused. Certainly when working with children or vulnerable adults, there must be systems in place to protect them. It is important that staff are aware of and comply with legal requirements, national and local policy. Staff may feel unsure of their responsibilities when working with some individuals such as children and vulnerable adults. Difficulties do at times occur when a policy states that there must be two staff with a child from a child protection perspective, but where for example, there is insufficient space to fit equipment or a second person. Solutions such as leaving the toilet door open because a second person cannot fit into the toilet area do little for the dignity of the child or young adult. If there is truly no alternative then every effort should be made to ensure that dignity is preserved by use of screens etc.

Employers now generally insist that Criminal Records Bureau (CRB) checks are completed before a member of staff works with these vulnerable individuals. Those who are self employed are strongly advised to initiate the process themselves.

Protecting dignity must not be forgotten and assessors should be reminded that in the face of many pressures, staff may forget how that person feels. From a risk assessment perspective it is vital that the assessor considers how a person's dignity is being affected by the handling task.

Example

Staff were manually lifting a very light but dying lady (one on either side of the bed) and holding her in the space directly above the bed while a third assistant changed the sheets. The staff were supporting the full body weight of this lady for up to 1.5 minutes leading to pain and discomfort and a feeling of insecurity for the client. The reason given for doing this task in this way was because the hoist sling was painful for the client. The lady was deaf and blind and too ill to speak and would only cry or smile to indicate comfort levels. Following specialist assessment and intervention an alternative sling with additional padding was found and combined with a member of staff cradling her arms around the lady, resulted in no pain or discomfort for the staff or client. Because of this intervention the client's and staff's last memories were deeply moving and positive.

Communication

Communication of the legal requirements, the handling risks, the individual's needs and wishes is vital to decrease the risk of injury to those involved in the moving and handling process. Communication includes the spoken and written word as well as the policy of the organisation. Skill is required to communicate appropriately with the client, staff or management in order to achieve a positive outcome. Sometimes the failure in communication can be difficult to spot.

Example

A client was well known to community staff and had been diagnosed with Alzheimer's disease some years before. At the time of initial assessment the client had requested that staff use his first name. Some years later an assessment was requested as the staff reported that the client was violent and that moving and handling had become unsafe. They requested further handling strategies to deal with the 'violent' behaviour. The assessor determined that no change was required in the manual handling strategy, but as the client no longer recognised the carers they should use his family name rather than first name. The strategy worked and was passed on to all staff.

Cultural perspectives and personal circumstances may affect the communication process and the professional would do well to have an understanding of those needs and incorporate them into the safe system of work/action plan.

It would be wonderful if mistakes or miscommunication never occurred but, if it does, the person being assisted may request that the professional or organisation apologises. Admitting a mistake is sometimes perceived as opening the way to litigation and the admission of negligence. No hard and fast rule can be given, but the capacity to say 'sorry' can have many benefits.

Game theory

Game theory has been considered by many different disciplines from psychology to engineering and can also be applied in the context of manual handling risk assessments.

The theory suggests that all humans need interaction and to do this, structure their time accordingly. The interaction options are defined as rituals, pastimes, games, intimacy and activity and the two most gratifying options are intimacy and games according to *Berne (1968)*. This section focuses on the 'games'.

The term 'game' does not necessarily mean it is fun – it can be very serious. The game has to be played with at least two players and will have clearly defined rules and less clearly defined, unspoken rules. The interaction with other human beings will have particular characteristics that can be recognised. The rules of the particular game will be influenced by the programming of parents (or significant carers), society and the individual themselves.

Berne (1968) defines games as 'a recurring set of transactions, often repetitious, superficially plausible, with a concealed motivation'. There are a number of different game styles both positive and negative and these can be investigated at the reader's leisure.

The potential importance of the 'game theory' in manual handling risk assessments is to recognise that there must be a social interaction between the assessor and the person being assessed and therefore the potential for a 'game'. How that interaction proceeds (the game) will include past experiences of both parties, their perceived role in that situation and the words they use to interact.

One example of a negative game led by the professional is the 'I'm only trying to help you' game. This is not the same as legitimate offers of help but occurs when:

'The worker or therapist, of whatever profession, gives some advice to a client or patient. The patient returns and reports that the suggestion did not have the desired effect. The worker shrugs off this failure with a feeling of resignation, and tries again. If he is more watchful, he may detect in himself at this point a twinge of frustration, but will try again anyway. Usually he feels little need to question his own motives, because he knows that many of his similarly trained colleagues do the same thing, and that he is following the 'correct' procedure and will receive full support from his supervisors.' *Berne (1968)* indicates that this 'game' will not lead to a successful resolution of the difficulty but rather to the worker shrugging his shoulders and giving up. 'I was only trying to help' being the final words.

By contrast, 'good games', which *Berne (1968)* describes as '...one which contributes both to the well-being of the other players and to the unfolding of the one who is 'it'', should be used to maximise outcomes for all concerned.

The good games include:

- 'Busman's holiday' (e.g. the doctor who goes out to Africa to help in a rural hospital),
- 'Cavalier' (e.g. knight in shining armour; bringing out the best in someone within the boundaries of good taste and social situation and not for sexual advantage),
- The altruistic 'happy to help',
- 'Homely sage' (e.g. a person who becomes known as someone to go to whatever the problem) and
- 'They'll be glad they knew me' (e.g. it was worth developing the relationship, a positive outcome was achieved)

In all of the above the benefits are positive and therefore to be encouraged, but it must be understood that any game can become negative, even after a positive start. It may be disconcerting to admit that playing games is an integral part of our lives, and it may be difficult to change the game, but recognition that game playing exists may encourage all players to work towards improving the situation to a positive end.

Attitude and personal outlook

The effect of an individual's personal outlook must also be considered. *Goleman (1996)* discusses the beneficial effects of a positive perspective on health outcomes for patients who have had a heart attack as well as the benefits of positive subliminal suggestion to patients while still sedated. It is obviously not possible or ethical to routinely pass subliminal messages to clients or staff, but recognition that outlook plays an important part can help the assessor in the search for an acceptable plan.

The professional must always be aware of his or her own prejudices and perspectives and those of others when undertaking an assessment. Again, perception and skill are required to be able to ascertain important factors that staff or family may be reticent to divulge. Only one example is given here, but there are many more examples of the effect of attitude that could be used.

Example

Staff requested a moving and handling assessment for a student with learning and physical difficulties. The student was hoisted for all moving and handling transfers. Staff reported that they were experiencing bruising and other injuries when attempting to hoist the student. The assessor sensed a reluctance of the staff to give further details, but eventually discovered that the difficulties occurred when the student was taken to the toilet prior to a long journey home on school transport. The transport left at 15.15 hrs and therefore he was taken to the toilet at 14.45 hrs to allow time for hoisting and for using the toilet. The student was regularly found masturbating and became violent when the staff tried to stop this activity. Staff were embarrassed and rightly did not feel they could explain the reason to the bus driver for the student always being late for the bus. The solution was to start the going home process earlier and allow the student time to masturbate if he so wished. There was little point in telling this student that his behaviour was considered inappropriate by some. A far better solution is to manage the situation by acknowledging that the student had a different perspective to the staff at that time.

Skill

The ability of the person undertaking the risk assessment and performing the moving and handling task will have a profound effect on the handling experience for all involved. As part of the evidence gathering for the practical chapters of this book, the team were asked to assign a skill level to the task being considered. As well as the descriptions, a ten-point scale was used, and the skill levels as described by *Benner (1984)*, which are often used in nurse education. The description of the headings can be found in chapter 11. The headings proved to be most useful in deciding skill level and are listed below:

- Novice
- Advanced Beginner
- Competent
- Proficient
- Expert

It is important to consider the skill level of the person required to undertake the task.

The *RCN* document *Safer Staff, better care (2003)* reproduced at appendix 3, places manual handling training into the context of 'a fully integrated risk management system that meets all the legal requirements'. The document also lists the broad competencies required by all levels of staff. *The Manual Handling Standard, NBE (2004)* also considers the broad standards that should be considered.

Evidence Based Patient Handling Hignett et al. (2003) provides summaries on studies that looked at the use of lifting teams to undertake the manual handling within a hospital setting. The conclusion was that there was 'moderate evidence that using the lifting team approach can be effective'. The inference here is that a well-trained team, experienced and used to the equipment available can respond quickly and efficiently to a moving and handling need with a much-reduced risk of injury. Perhaps as part of the assessment process the skills of those undertaking the task needs to be further considered.

Part of the development of skill may be to investigate different perspectives on handling that have grown from a human movement/biomechanical viewpoint.

Among the options to consider are:

- Neuromuscular Approach *Vasey, Crozier (1982)* which considers efficient movement patterns and movement re-education which has application in moving and handling tasks *National Back Pain Association (1997)*
- Manutension *(http://www.manutention.org.au)*
- Haptonomics (*Corpus 2003*) – 'a holistic approach to safer handling through tailored assessments, interventions and support programmes'
- Alexander Principle, *Barlow (1990)* who summarizes the principle as 'use affects functioning' and discusses how to improve 'use' and 'function' of an individual's own body.

This list is not meant to be exclusive but to offer the reader an opportunity to extend their knowledge and skills beyond the standard texts and ideas. It is important for the reader to investigate different approaches and weigh up the benefits and considerations.

Interestingly the first three are concerned with the interaction between the handler and the person being handled, within a human movement framework, and provide the handler with the time to get to know how the human body responds to handling and the skill to interact positively with the person being handled.

Empowerment

Perhaps working out the solution to a problem would be much easier if risks could be listed and then simply added together to indicate the risk level prior to suggesting the action plan. Unfortunately, not only are there differing views on the interaction of risks, there are also different views on the possible plan.

There is a growing framework of information that helps in that decision making process and through the change in presentation and perspective of this book, it is hoped that more information and options are available. However, there are always likely to be differences of opinions and those differences do not have to be simply right or wrong. Just as different roads can lead to the same destination, so different techniques or approaches can lead to successful handling outcomes.

Further along the line, dissent by members of a team performing a task can be viewed negatively or positively with perhaps hindsight over used as justification. Staff may recognise that there is a high risk of injury and pass that information on, only for it to be ignored. Even after an event such as a shuttle explosion as reported by *Goleman (1996)* on a NASA shuttle, where engineers had given strong warnings regarding the launch, those engineers were demoted following an enquiry, even though had they been listened to, the disaster could have been averted. The engineers were only re-instated after public pressure.

It must be understood that whatever the numerically calculated risk, the personal impact of a negative manual handling event is likely to affect the opinion of the individuals involved more than the documented risk analysis. If a person has been injured, for example using the shoulder lift, they are likely to have a negative view of that technique, a person who used the technique a great deal and never experienced a problem is likely to view that technique in a better light. Where there is disagreement, the most senior person will have to make an informed decision, weighing up all of the information. That decision may be tested in court and become part of the decision making process for the future. The worst outcome for all when disagreements do occur, is simply to ignore the problem and hope that it goes away.

When the MHOR first came into force, many staff felt great relief that there would be a better system that allowed them to undertake manual handling within their own ability. They and their employers at least felt that they could say 'no' to practice that put staff at risk, hence 'no lifting' or 'minimal lifting' policies emerged. Since then, various court cases and judicial reviews have challenged that perspective and sought to redress the balance for the person being assisted. It is important that the risk assessment empowers all parties to feel able to say what can and can't be managed and to bring that information together into a plan that can work for all.

Training and competency

Although the HSE Guidance on the MHOR states that all manual handling risk assessments should be completed by a competent person and that the assessments should be based on common sense, it is largely believed that people handling assessments require a greater skill, because people are more complicated than loads. There is a strong move towards competency and therefore the risk assessor for manual handling of people would be wise to complete courses that give them the assessment skills they require and evidences their qualification to assess moving and handling situations.

There is an increasing need to for the handler to demonstrate competency in moving and handling skills and the desire for a manual handling 'driving test', at least at a basic level is often requested by employees and employers alike. There are, however, still great differences of opinion on what constitutes correct handling and with the multitude of variables present in any handling situation, there will always be the scope for discussion on what is best (see also appendix 3).

4 Risk analysis

Definition of risk

To understand the term 'risk', it may be helpful to be reminded of some definitions:

- Hazard (risk factor) – a potential source of danger
  Risk – the possibility that something unpleasant or unwelcome will happen *Oxford Dictionary of English (2003)*

Other definitions of risk include:

- 'the projection of a degree of uncertainty about the future on the external world' *Heyman (1998)*
- 'the chance of something happening that will have an impact on objectives. It is measured in terms of consequences and likelihood' *Risk Management AS/NZ 4360:1999*
- 'the probability that a particular adverse event occurs during a stated period of time, or results from a particular challenge' *Risk, Analysis, Perception and Management, Royal Society (1992)*
- 'Risk = likelihood of the event x severity of the outcome' *Note on Risk Assessment at Work, Royal Society of Chemistry (2002)*

The definitions aim to quantify risk in order to assist in its measurement and analysis. One of the greatest difficulties when attempting to analyse risk is that the overall risk of a negative event may be very low, but the impact on that individual who has been injured may be very high.

The tendency has been to 'ban' or eliminate a method if there has EVER been a reported injury. Personal injury claims also influence this thinking. This could be likened to a road traffic accident leading to the permanent closure of a road or the banning of driving! The accident may have a very significant effect on the individual and the personal trauma cannot at times be under-estimated, but closing the road can lead to a catalogue of further incidents with even more individuals being affected.

Sudden, poorly thought out, reactions may only lead to the introduction of further risk, rumours and potentially a poorer service. Removal of slide sheets from service in the example would likely lead to tissue viability issues and increased manual handling risks. Processes should be set up to avoid a repeat of the incident rather than the removal of an otherwise very helpful piece of equipment.

Example

A member of staff slips and breaks a leg on a slide sheet that was placed on the floor by another member of staff who did not consider the consequences. The employer has now banned slide sheets because they are 'dangerous'.

Is this a wise decision?

What alternative strategies could be considered?

Tools

Qualitative tools

These tools will assist the assessor in producing a subjective assessment of the risk.

The following list can be used to assist the assessor in that process of choosing the written framework but will not provide an exhaustive inventory of all possible options:

- HSE schedule/checklists and appendices in the Guidance on the MHOR *(2004)*
- Risk Management charts from the Australian/New Zealand Standard SAI 4360 (2004) – these as part of a risk management framework allow the assessor to grade the likelihood of injury against the severity to produce a qualitative risk analysis matrix. This can be used to prioritise risk.
- All Wales NHS Manual Handling Training Passport and Information Scheme (2003) (also available on the internet). This package details the training requirements for staff involved in moving and handling but also includes a manual handling assessment form for objects and people.
- Care Handling of Adults in Hospitals and Community Settings – Derbyshire Inter-Agency Group *DIAG (2003)*. This code of practice includes the background to risk assessment, example forms and a practical guide to procedures.
- Royal College of Nursing *RCN* documentation such as Changing Practice – Improving Health (RCN (2001) can assist in providing the risk assessment framework.
- The RCN Manual Handling Assessments in Hospitals and the Community *RCN (1996)* gives example forms for risk assessment, including a management checklist.
- Chartered Society of Physiotherapy guidance on manual handling *CSP (2002)*

- Chartered Society of Physiotherapy *CSP (2002)* falls audit pack
- Protocol for the therapeutic handling of neurologically impaired adults (for therapy staff) *Gwent Healthcare NHS Trust (2003)*
- Guidance on Manual Handling in Treatment, Association of Chartered Physiotherapists in Neurology *ACPIN (2001)*
- Paediatric Manual Handling – Guidance for Physiotherapists *Association of Paediatric Physiotherapists (2002).*

Quantitative tools

The following specific tools may require training prior to use and can be used to either give a more detailed assessment of a particular aspect or to give a numerical measure of risk. They are not all considered pure quantitative measures and are not always necessary to ascertain the level and type of risk. They are, however, being increasingly used to support and shape handling decisions that have previously been taken on personal experience or current opinion.

- Rapid Entire Body Assessment (REBA) *Hignett, McAtamney (2000)* is a tool that can be used to assess posture and has been used within the practical chapters of this book to evaluate the posture of the handlers undertaking the moving and handling tasks (see appendix 1)
- Rapid Upper Limb Assessment (RULA) *McAtamney, Corlett (1993)*, is available on the Internet. This works on a similar basis as REBA and looks more specifically at the upper body.
- Borg scale of perceived exertion *Borg (1998)*. This may be helpful for staff to attempt to quantify the amount of effort required to undertake a task.
- Ovako Working posture Analysis System. OWAS *Engels (1977)* computerised version is also available. This is a method for evaluating postural load while performing a task.
- Manual Handling Assessment Charts. *HSE (2003)* MAC tool can be used to determine the level of risk related to handling objects by a person on their own, team handling or carrying an object. It is *not* suitable for assessment of people handling.
- Ergonomic Workplace Analysis *Finnish Institute of Occupational Health (1989)* allows a broad assessment of the work task and includes a worker's assessment as well as the assessor rating. This assessment tool is more useful for object handling, although the worker assessment could be easily incorporated into people handling assessments.
- Evaluating change in exposure to risk for musculoskeletal disorders – a practical tool *HSE (1999)*. This tool devised by the Robens Centre for Health Ergonomics for the HSE and is specifically designed to assist the assessor in evaluating the changes made through an intervention.
- Plibel *Kemmlert (1995)* – a method assigned for the identification of ergonomic hazards. This study includes a chart that may help to identify 'musculoskeletal stress factors'.
- Interview protocols and ergonomics checklist for analysing overexertion back accidents among nursing personnel *Engkvist (1995)*. The study gives an interview method to assist with the assessment process.
- The Work Ability Index *Finnish Institute of Occupational Health (1998)*. This index can be used with the worker to ascertain the ability of that worker to perform his/her work. It is an occupational health tool that can be used to assist in the individual capability assessment. It can also be used to 'predict the threat of disability in the near future'.
- National Institute for Occupational Safety and Health (NIOSH) Equation (also available on the Internet) *(Waters 1994)*.
- Likert 10 point scales for comfort and activity of the person being handled.
- Functional Independence Measure *Granger, Hamilton (1987)*.
- Event trees *(SAI 2004)*.

The Introduction to the Practical Chapters also explains the use of such tools as a 10-point Likert scale and independence measures that will not be further referenced here.

Analysis

The tools listed above will help the assessor collect information and use the data to compare different options. At some point in this process a decision has to be made on what will happen next. These decisions will be made at a number of different levels from the Board room to the handler assisting the person out of bed.

The analysis may be presented in the form of reports, graphs, tables, matrices and will give an indication of the level of risk, the potential consequences and the associated cost. The analysis should also focus on the positive benefits of a suggested change.

As part of the analysis the assessor should ask themselves some important questions:

- Is there a clear picture of the risks involved?
- Is further assessment and measurement necessary?
- Can the risk be eliminated?
- How confident are you of your ability to evaluate the information collected?
- Are the methods you have used to analyse reliable?
- Is it possible that the risk could increase or decrease?
- What are the limitations of your analysis?

The quality of the analysis will be directly related to the tools used and the ability of the assessor to interpret the information collected in the light of their own experience and current knowledge. The assessor must be able to gauge the effect on the analysis of their own personal perspectives.

Example

An assessor recognised that a hoist failure while transferring a particular person could have serious consequences for the person being assisted and the staff. The assessor believed that staff would attempt to lift the person out of the sling should the hoist fail to lower. She therefore ordered a hoist with a manual lowering system. She felt confident that she assessed the risk and devised a suitable plan that would mean the staff were never compromised into performing a manual lift.

She received a call one day from the staff who had hoisted the person successfully onto the floor, but when they came to use the hoist to lift from the floor, discovered that the hoist was not working. There was no other hoist available.

Should the assessor have foreseen this difficulty?

What strategy would you devise for this unusual situation?

Documentation

The qualitative tools listed will mostly give the assessor a written format that they can use to document the risk, the quantitative tools used, the analysis of risk and the suggested plan. I t must be noted, however, that many forms do not easily document individual capability and it is important that the ability of all the individuals assisting are considered. The documentation needs to allow the person reading it to be able to not only see the suggested plans, but also the 'working out' that took place to reach that conclusion.

It is important to remember that the HSE Guidance on MHOR states that 'Assessment may best be carried out by members of staff who are familiar with the operations in question, as long as they have the competencies to do so'. The guidance does also recognise that expert help may be required. Those responsible for the assessment should be familiar with the Regulations and should be able to:

- **a** 'identify hazards (including less obvious ones) and assess risks from the type of manual handling being done;
- **b** use additional sources of information on risks as appropriate;
- **c** draw valid and reliable conclusions from assessments and identify steps to reduce risks;
- **d** make a clear record of the assessment and communicate the findings to those who need to take appropriate action, and to the workers concerned;
- **e** recognise their own limitations as to assessment so that further expertise can be called on if necessary.'

It is difficult to give exact advice on the form that should be used and there is no perfect 'form' available. Examples of documentation systems are available from the *Derbyshire InterAgency Group (2003), the all WalesManual Handling Passport and Information Scheme (2003).* The reader may also find it helpful to share information with Trusts, Social Service Departments, members of National Back Exchange and Manual Handling Advisers.

The tables earlier in the chapter under 'TILE' give a good basis for the relevant questions that need to be asked as part of the assessment, but the exact format will depend on the particular needs of the organisation.

Some assessors have found it helpful to produce a task list for the initial interview. The example included is one the author has developed for initial interview with children and their carers:

Moving and handling assessment – Part 1

Child Details			**Assessor Details**	
Name	Height		Name	Designation
	Weight			
	Age		Signature	
Address/Location seen			Assessment date	
			Review date	

Checklist of handling tasks				
Task	**Is the child fully independent?**			
	Yes	**No**	**Variable**	**Comments**
Turning in bed				
Rolling in bed				
Lying to sitting in bed				
Repositioning up the bed				
Getting into bed				
Getting out of bed				
Getting onto a change table				
Getting off a change table				

Checklist of handling tasks – continued				
Task	**Is the child fully independent?**			
	Yes	**No**	**Variable**	**Comments**
On toilet/commode				
Off toilet/commode				
In bath/shower				
Out bath/shower				
Sitting to standing				
Standing to sitting				
Standing				
Walking				
In/out standing frame				
In/out walker				
Into wheelchair				
Out of wheelchair				
In armchair				
Out armchair				
To floor				
Up from floor				
In/out car				
On/off transport				
In/out swimming pool				
On/ off horse				
In/out ball pool				
In/out sensory room				
On/off wedge				
On/off waterbed				
Other				

Is the child fully independent for all tasks? If YES – end of assessment If NO – complete part 2
Fully independent means that the child needs no manual assistance

The task list can be adapted to suit the needs of those involved. The purpose of the initial form is for the assessor to determine the tasks that occur and whether further assessment is required and forms part of the data collection. This form was developed from the forms used within Lincolnshire. No sections should be left empty on such a table, if the task is not to be assessed or not relevant, it should be marked in order to show that it has not simply been forgotten.

The next stage will be to collect information on the environment, the individual being assisted, any additional factors and the staff needs. If the environment remains the same for multiple assessments (e.g. a hospital ward) this may be completed as a generic assessment, providing regular checks are

Table 9.1

Task	Risks	Action
Personal Care Mrs Bloggs is transferred to her wheelchair using a hoist with a universal sling from a fixed height divan bed that is supported in one corner by bricks.	• Staff are stooping and over reaching to apply the sling. • Staff often catch the hoist on the bricks and have to realign the bricks before continuing with the transfer. • There is a high risk of the bed collapsing which could injure Mrs Bloggs and staff. • The safe working load of the bed is not known. • Staff have to lift Mrs Bloggs forward in bed to place the sling in position	• Discuss with Mrs Bloggs and relatives whether an alternative bed is available for the immediate short term. • Discuss with Mrs Bloggs the possibility of using a profiling bed, then if appropriate contact the Occupational Therapist to discuss the possibility of issuing a profiling bed • Check that the bed fits into the space required and can be brought into the house Check that the hoist can be used with the bed • Ensure Mrs Bloggs's wishes have been considered • Ensure that bed is delivered and correctly installed • Set up maintenance and training programmes

made to ensure that circumstances have not changed.

Recording the staff information may need to be completed in individual staff files, but it is important to remember that the action plan should be devised to suit the people involved (e.g. different skill levels, heights, experience). Evidence of training received should also be documented.

A more detailed assessment of the tasks can be completed based on the part 1 assessment and these should detail the particular risks and the action. For example:

The table above gives a great deal of detail. The actual amount of information required will depend on the other supporting documents and procedures in place.

There may be a number of tasks that need to be considered and the same process could be undertaken for all of tasks required. It may be necessary to divide the action in to short and longer term plans (as in the example, find another bed for the next few days, while a profiling bed is ordered).

It is sometimes helpful to produce a summary sheet to avoid the need for all staff to read through all the data of the complete assessment.

For example:

Table 9.2 Andrew Brown summary sheet/action plan – Task – Sit to Stand (armchair and dining chair)

Risks
1 High risk of injury to Mr Brown's shoulders through using the drag lift when assisting to stand
2 High risk of injury to people assisting Mr Brown to stand because of the low seat
3 Danger of collapse of the armchair (joints unsafe)
4 High risk of injury to anyone assisting Mr Brown into his dining chair due to lack of space and Mr Brown's difficulty in judging distances.
5 High risk of injury to untrained staff attempting to assist Mr Brown
6 High risk of injury to Mr Brown and to staff if he loses balance when standing.

Action	Action by?	Outcome	Date
A Trial of alternative armchairs, preferably chairs that will help Mr Brown stand (Risks 1, 2,3 & 6)	Sophie Brown (Occupational Therapist)		
B Alteration of the dining chair to improve usability (addition of braked castors) (Risk 4)	Sophie Brown		
C Posture training for staff prior to skills training to achieve as safe handling procedures as possible. The training will not succeed in itself without a change in furniture. Family members should attend the training sessions wherever possible. (Risk 5)	Carole Johnson (Manual Handling Adviser)		
D Develop a strategy for assisting Mr Brown from the floor if he does not require medical intervention. Trial suitable hoist and possibility of using air-filled cushion to lift from the floor (Risk 6)	Sophie Brown with Carole Johnson and Mr Brown		
Signed: Carole Johnson		Date	

The examples are fictitious and do not show the complete assessment. The information on the person being assisted, the environment and staff would also have been completed. A summary sheet, with named people responsible and an outcomes box can help the assessor of the person responsible for the action to monitor progress.

Further development of section D may be required to give the specific detail on how the transfers will take place. These may include notes and pictures to remind the handler of the requirements.

It is important that the document is signed and dated and it may be helpful to indicate the number of pages. The assessment should then be kept where all staff can access it and whenever possible should be given to the person being assisted for his/her information. The document must be reviewed if there are any changes. This may be possible by adding an additional sheet.

5 Reducing the risk

Strategies

One aim that is often portrayed when discussing risk related to musculoskeletal injury, is that all risk must be eliminated, particularly when moving and handling people. While this is a laudable aim, as with any other area of life, zero risk is unlikely to be possible. The Health and Safety Executive website (www.hse.gov.uk/msd) gives a useful summary:

'HSE's key messages about musculoskeletal disorders (MSDs) are:

- you can do things to prevent or minimise MSDs;
- the prevention measures are cost effective;
- you cannot prevent all MSDs, so early reporting of symptoms, proper treatment and suitable rehabilitation is essential.'

Prevention, however, will include the need to obtain a complete picture of the risks and therefore it is important to consider the legal influences, known risk factors, values, perspectives and trade-offs for the people involved.

Protocols, generic assessments and the use of standard procedures can help the assessor choose the strategy for a particular situation but in many cases an individual plan is required. This plan must be updated if circumstances change.

Devising an Action Plan

In simple terms, once the risks have been identified, the next stage will be to decide on the safe system of work and prioritise the actions required. This can range from something as simple as a non weight bearing person being admitted to hospital and therefore a hoist is used for all transfers to a very specific plan with short, medium and long term aims.

One perspective that has been considered by a number of groups (National Back Exchange Oxford Group and Hertfordshire Partnership NHS Trust for example) is the setting up of standard procedures or generic protocols that can be used for handling tasks. The assessor must consider whether the person needs assistance with handling in the first place and whether the generic protocol is suitable or needs further assessment and a specific procedure. The argument for this type of system is that most situations do follow standard predictable patterns and a great deal of time and effort can be saved by the assessor at the time by categorising the moving and handling. Conversely, some would say that everyone is different and therefore you will always have to adapt generic protocol.

The assessor should be aware of the range of resources available to them locally as well as the broader information and support. These would include:

- Handling Homecare *(HSE, 2001)*
- Disabled Living Foundation Equipment files
- Safer Handling in the Community *(National Back Pain Association 1999)*
- Joining specialist forums such as National Back Exchange
- Back Care/Manual Handling Adviser
- Books such as *Evidence Based Patient Handling (2003)*

However, it is also important to understand that while the aim should always be for all involved to be unharmed, the risk is unlikely to ever be zero.

The assessment and action plan must be part of a whole strategy dealing with the issues at micro and macro levels. There will always be more than one perspective to consider if an injury does occur or there is a near miss. The assessor must consider what level of residual risk is acceptable. For many people this is difficult, because a judgement has to made and the individual may be afraid that should an adverse incident occur, all involved will point the finger to blame that person for 'missing' that important piece of evidence. It must be remembered that hindsight gives us all a dimension that is not available to the person at the time and providing the assessor has considered the known factors, followed accepted procedure, is able to undertake the analysis, he or she is unlikely to be able to do much more.

The action plan can also be considered at two levels:

1 As a part of the overall strategy and risk management structure of the organisation

2 What the handler and the person being handled actually do

The overall strategy will consider such topics as a managed bed service, community equipment provision criteria, supervision practices, training needs analysis, other equipment design and occupational health perspectives.

The action plan for the handler on site has to adapt at that moment to the particular situation and will always require some flexibility.

Having 100 beds replaced may be the strategy, but actually 10 beds may be replaced at a time to control cost and minimise disruption. The actual strategy must include what is going to happen to the handlers working with the other 90 beds, now.

The person performing the handling task may not be 'interested' in the fact that 100 beds are being replaced, if their beds are not included in that wave, they will be concerned regarding how they manage their current non adjustable beds and must be given an action plan for this situation.

Person-handling action plans

The action plan must be relevant to the circumstances and must reduce the risk to the lowest level reasonably practicable. Whenever possible the risk should be addressed immediately, but it is recognised that this may not always be possible. Reasons such as no access to equipment are less of an issue these days as often equipment can be supplied very quickly for the short term. The more difficult situation will occur when specialist equipment must be acquired (e.g. special hoist slings), or where the person being handled needs to build up familiarity with the action plan. Nevertheless, the action plan must cover both situations.

The manual handling risk management plan will be available as a policy to all staff.

The person-handling action plan may be available in the care plan or person specific file, it may also be feasible to put it in specific places e.g. behind a wardrobe door. The person-handling action plan should include a summary of the main risks, the associated action and where a method is required, details of that method.

One of the common ways of passing specific information regarding the person being handled is the 'procedure sheet'. This can be a combination of pictures e.g. to show the placement of a sling with bullet points of advice to remind the handler of the key safety points. Pictures can be very useful and reduce the amount of explanation but need to be clear and accurate. It must also be noted that a picture will only show a point in time, rather than the flow of a process.

The action plan should be directly related to the risks identified and consideration must also be given to the effect of changing one element and any knock on effect or change to other risk factors.

The following list may be helpful when devising the plan:

- Know the options available to eliminate or reduce the risk (e.g. equipment options), methods available and suitability.
- Recognise that there is a difference between eliminating the risk through a clear logical process and risk avoidance due to a risk-averse strategy. It is worth remembering that the avoidance of a particular risk may also result in a lost opportunity. See sections on equipment and therapy handling.
- If the options are not clear, seek further advice
- Break down the risks into smaller units where possible; this will help stage the action plan in more complex situations
- Can the risk be shared?
- Is there an expectation of the individual, the staff, the organisation or even society that needs to be considered (e.g. not lifting a person from the floor without equipment)
- If necessary use additional tools to assess whether the risk has actually been reduced by the action plan, simply changed or in fact increased
- Communicate the action plan with the relevant parties to ensure that the plan is workable (e.g. does the plan fit in with the rehabilitation or the behaviour management of the person being handled)
- If residual risk remains ensure this is documented
- Produce specific guidelines if required (e.g. which loop to use on a hoist sling) to help the handler
- Decide on the review system and date that the action should be taken by and by whom. Decide on a default review time if no review request has been made.
- Show the 'working out', it may be obvious now what the reasoning was for a decision, but will it be obvious in the future?
- Ensure that the information is signed and dated for future reference. It would be wise to have this information on every page. It may also be helpful to indicate how many pages there are supposed to be for the document e.g. Page 1 of 8
- If an action plan is failing or there is a near miss/accident ensure that this information is reported in writing to the line manager and the review process initiated.
- Is skills training required? Does the training need to show competency?
- Could a different approach be used such as a specialist team within the workforce to do the handling tasks? ('lifting teams' i.e. teams of people trained in moving and handling and who are confident with equipment and handling methods. See *Evidence Based Patient Handling 2003*). There is evidence to suggest that such a strategy reduces the risk of injury.
- Have any unusual circumstances been considered?

Exceptional circumstances

Many moving and handling situations are predictable and foreseeable; however, there is a group of scenarios that may be unusual but foreseeable. These may, for example, include hoist failure during a transfer or between separate tasks of a whole procedure, fire evacuation, lift or equipment failure. Prevention is always better than cure, but reality indicates that sometimes the 'cure' may be all that staff have available.

The philosophy in exceptional circumstances should be principle-based i.e. should follow the basic safety rules, but cannot be completely prescriptive as it is unlikely the assessor would be able to predict the exact scenario. Where of course the action is being planned on the basis of a near miss, it will be easier to be prescriptive.

Some examples of exceptional circumstances may include:

- A person sitting down in the middle of a road
- Hoist failure part way through a transfer
- Sudden loss of strength part way through a transfer
- Equipment failure (damage to a wheelchair or bed)
- Fire evacuation
- A person having a seizure part way through being hoisted
- A fall in a confined space
- A person fainting while a blood sample is being taken
- Retreiving a person who has attempted self-strangulation by hanging
- Evacuation from a car/aeroplane seat
- Evacuation from a swimming pool
- Breakdown of a specialist vehicle
- Unexpected violence

Some of these scenarios are covered in chapter 17 of this publication

Example

A 12 stone person who is unable to weight bear or support himself in sitting is being pushed across a busy road in his wheelchair by one member of staff.

Part way across the road one of the front wheels shears off. This is a completely unexpected event for the staff involved.

What should he do?

It could be argued that wheels are unlikely to shear off and therefore there must have been some indication that there was a potential problem. One could also ask if the wheelchair had been regularly maintained and for future reference these points would be very important.

In this particular scenario the handler will have to decide:

1 Are they in immediate danger, in which case that must be the first priority?
2 Can he safely move the person in the wheelchair to the footpath or side of the road?
3 Can he affect a repair sufficient to get to the destination?
4 Can he call for assistance where the additional people are not going to placed at risk of injury?

In this particular scenario the handler tipped the wheelchair onto the back wheels to take the chair to the side of the road and then used his mobile telephone to call for a tail-lift vehicle to come and collect them. A spare wheelchair was found to replace the broken one. The maintenance contract on the chair was checked and safety checks were set up.

Equipment

It is often assumed that the introduction of equipment will resolve the issues related to manual handling. Any equipment will introduce positive and negative aspects in its use and the risk assessor needs to be aware of both perspectives before advocating any handling aid. This requires an intimate knowledge of the equipment, alongside an analysis of its capability. For example, a standard toileting sling may allow a person to transfer from a wheelchair directly to the toilet, but for that aid to be suitable the person may require upper body strength and head control. A good risk assessor should be able to list the uses and dangers of the equipment and modify that list when further information becomes available.

Example

Sliding Board
Standard wooden board with tapered ends on the lower surface.

Uses

- Allows a non weight-bearing person to transfer from one seated position to another

Benefits

- Allows the person to transfer independently or with minimal help
- Transfer is an active rather than passive process
- Surface of the transfer board allows easy movement

Precautions

- Person must have upper body strength and be able to move their body weight off centre without losing his/her balance
- Person must be able to coordinate his/her movement to achieve a transfer
- The person may slide off the board if they experience difficulties part way through the transfer
- The person may need time to learn and practice the skill
- The heights of the two surfaces must be similar in order for a transfer to be effective
- The board must be checked for damage
- The safe working load of the board and the weight of the person using it should be known
- A standard board cannot be used with chairs that have armrests
- The transfer is sometimes undertaken with a handler and transfer belt which introduces further precautions to consider.

The above example illustrates the benefits and precautions to consider when using a sliding board and similar lists can be devised for other equipment. The risk assessor and staff using equipment should also be able to locate easily the manufacturer's handbook and be able to have a good working knowledge of its content.

Sometimes handlers are not keen to use equipment because of the extra time involved. In some settings the use of equipment may result in a more than acceptable increase in the amount of time required.

Example

Teaching and support staff at a special needs school teach a class of 7 children with profound and multiple disabilities. None of the children are able to weightbear and each require 2 people to assist with personal care. The heaviest child weighs 28 kg. If the children were hoisted for every task, (such as personal care, therapy, activities, meals) the teacher has calculated this would take the two staff present 5½ hours each day. The school day is 6½ hours. Therefore teaching time would be ½ hour. If the staff manually lift the children, this takes only 1½ hours. There have been no staff injuries/days off sick in the last 7 years. The area has difficulty recruiting staff. The school has medium term plans to rebuild the facilities, which would allow overhead tracking and sufficient change beds and other equipment. Ofsted on the last visit said that insufficient time was being spent teaching and developing the children.

- How would the assessor determine the level of risk?
- How can the staff reconcile the teaching needs and the manual handling needs?
- What opportunities are lost if hoisting is undertaken?
- What would you suggest for the immediate short term?

In this example a balance needs to be made on the needs of the staff and the needs of the students. Manual handling is not the only consideration in this situation. The child may lose the opportunity to develop communication, learn a new skill, and spend time with their peers. This is not to undervalue the need to protect the staff but, as mentioned at the beginning of the chapter, zero risk is not possible. Balancing that risk will always produce discussion and in each set of circumstances a justifiable decision is the aim.

Therapy handling

This area of handling is often cited as an area of tension between therapists and carers. The therapist may have an aim for the person being handled such as relearning to walk, while others wish to ensure that this person and they are safe. It is still necessary for the therapist to perform an assessment that identifies the risk, analyses those risks and develop a strategy. The emotive aspects should be identified and addressed. Therapy staff must recognise that there may be instances where they feel confident in their abilities to support a person in their rehabilitation process, but others may not have this skill and this must be addressed in the action plan.

Example

An assessment was completed for a 12-year-old student who had been manually lifted into a standing frame. It was decided to use a walking harness with the overhead tracking. This worked well for 3 years. The student had a tracheostomy, but the walking harness did not interfere with the workings of this piece of vital equipment.

Over a summer holiday the student now aged 15 lost flexibility at the hips and knees to such an extent that she was chair shaped. The physiotherapy staff insisted that the staff hoist her into the standing frame to attempt to reverse the deformities. The staff struggled for 3 weeks to use the frame but felt that because of her shape the student was at risk of blocking her airway while in the frame. The physiotherapist and the staff felt that they must continue to try. The manual handling risk assessment was updated and the external manual handling risk assessor felt that using the standing frame should stop as the student could no longer achieve a sufficiently upright position to use the prone standing frame without obstructing the student's airway. The staff were experiencing a variety of musculoskeletal injuries trying to support the student while attaching security straps. This was because of the increased flexion deformities at the hips and knees

- Should the student stop using this standing frame?
- Could the conflict be resolved by using a different type of standing frame?
- Who would fund the additional equipment and what is the interim plan?

Example

A person suffers a stroke and is unable to weight bear on one side. The therapist has recognised the importance of retraining the standing and walking patterns in order for the person to be able to go home. They have identified that at the moment they have to offer considerable support to that person, but believe that he will improve and be discharged home. Other members of the team indicate that this person is likely to suddenly collapse at the knees and the risk of injury to the staff is too high to consider a standing transfer and that he will have to be sling hoisted until he shows signs that he is unlikely to collapse.

- If the person uses the hoist will he ever get stronger?
- By not retraining the standing would the staff be committing this man to being hoisted in the longer term and taking away his independence?
- Are there any other options?

The *Chartered Society of Physiotherapy (2002), ACPIN (2001), APCP (2002)* for example, have issued guidance on manual handling in therapy situations which may assist the risk assessor. As already listed, the *Gwent (2002)* protocol may also assist in making an informed decision.

The therapy staff must be aware of his/her responsibility to protect the staff and not devise therapy that places the staff at risk of injury. They must consider the capabilities of the staff combined with their experience and his/her professional duty of care to the staff they are delegating responsibility to or advising.

6 Monitoring the risk

It is necessary to review an assessment both from an overall risk management perspective and the individual action plan. This review can be conducted in different ways:

- **Regular review** – the specific risks and action plan review can be undertaken by a number of people including the person being assisted, the handler and/or his/her manager. The review will use the relevant tools already listed and must occur if the risks have changed and may need frequent reviewing where the ability of the person being assisted changes quickly and to ensure that best practice is being followed, alerting staff to new equipment and techniques as an integral part of update training content. Departments where this occurs (e.g. Intensive Care) may use written procedures/protocols to assist and the handler will need to have the ability to apply the principles and change plans with little notice. The risk management strategy must also be subject to review. The use of adverse incident reporting, generic assessments and equipment reviews alongside interviews and walkabouts will help modify the overall strategy when this is needed

- **Inclusion of new advances** – new ideas and equipment are being developed all the time. A formal system of keeping up to date with a method for testing and disseminating the findings will help keep moving and handling on the agenda for the handler and assist in making sure that current best practice is being followed. National Back Exchange local and special interest groups and the product review panel can provide some of this information.

- **Outcome analysis and review** – if an action plan has been implemented, perhaps reviewing the outcomes with the person being assisted would help the handler develop their expertise. The person being assisted may be positive or negative about the handling they receive, but avoiding the discussion can lead to a build up of resentment and therefore a breakdown in trust and ability to improve the service of the service. If the handler is afraid to ask for the person's honest opinion on the assistance they receive, they must not be surprised if that person takes action against the plan.

- **Adverse incident/near miss analysis** – the purpose of investigating these situations is to determine cause and influencing factors at the time of the incident to establish whether the incident could have been avoided or could be repeated. A decision would then need to be made on the basis of the findings. There has been a tendency to just stop an activity if there has been an adverse incident, but as already discussed the knock-on effect must also be considered of removing that piece of equipment or method.

- **3rd party audit** – this may be undertaken by a body such as the Health and Safety Executive, but could also be undertaken by external reviewers and may raise concerns or provide ideas on areas that may have been overlooked.

7 Summary

There are many facets to assessing manual handling risks and designing safer systems of work. The ability to design strategies that will work is a skill that needs to be based on the evidence available. However, there needs to be recognition that sometimes the risk is not the mechanical factor that can be easily spotted and measured, but comes out of the value systems of the people involved. No amount of technical solutions will work without that value system at least being acknowledged, if not in fact understood.

Noticing is everything

Acknowledgements

With thanks to:
Mark Johnson
Jennie Johnson
National Back Exchange
Mary Muir
Nicola Hunter
David Couzens-Howard

References

A number of web sites are quoted in this chapter and it is important for the reader to note that these details were correct at the time of writing. The reader's ability to reach these sites and the associated potential difficulties of using the World Wide Web are not the responsibility of the author.

ACPIN (2001). Guidance on Manual Handling in Treatment, UK, Association of Chartered Physiotherapist Interested in Neurology.

Adams A, Bogduk N, Burton K, Dolan P (2002) The Biomechanics of Back Pain, Edinburgh, Churchill, Livingstone.

All Wales, (2003). All Wales NHS Manual Handling Training, Passport and Information Scheme, Wales. All Wales Trust Manual Handling Advisers Group

APCP (2002). Paediatric Manual Handling – Guidelines for Paediatric Physiotherapists, UK, Association of Paediatric Chartered Physiotherapists.

Barlow W (1990). The Alexander Principle – The definitive Explanation of the World Famous Alexander Technique by its Foremost Practitioner, London, Victor Gollancz.

Benner P (1984). From novice to expert: Excellence and power in clinical nursing practice. Menlo Park: Addison-Wesley.

Berne E (1968). Games People Play – The Psychology of Human Realationships, London, Penguin.

Borg G (1998). Perceived exertion and painscales, USA, Human Kinetics

Corpus (2003). Foundation Haptonomics, UK, Corpus

CSP (2002). Guidance in Manual Handling for Chartered Physiotherapists, London, Chartered Society of Physiotherapy

CSP CoT, (2002). Falls Audit Pack – guideline for the collaborative, rehabilitative management of elderly people who have fallen, London Chartered Society of Physiotherapy and College of Occupational Therapists

Cunningham (2000). Disability, Oppression and Public Policy, Keighley, Sue Cunningham

DIAG, (2003). Care Handling of Adult in Hospitals and Community Settings – A code of practice, UK, Derbyshire Inter Agency Group

Disability Discrimination Act 1995 HMSO

DoH (2003). Risk Management Standard, London, Controls Assurance Unit, Department of Health

DoH (2003). Health and Safety Management, London, Controls Assurance Unit, Department of Health

DoH (2004). Healthcare Standards for Services under the NHS, London, Department of Health

Engels J (1994). An OWAS-based analysis of nurses working postures, Ergonomics Vol 37 No 5 pp 909 – 919

Engkvist (1995). Interview protocols and ergonomics checklist for analysing over exertion back accidents among nursing personnel, Applied Ergonomics 26, No 3 pp 213 – 220

Finnish Institute of Occupational Health (1998). Workability Index, Finland, Finnish Institute of Occupational Health

Finnish Institute of Occupational Health (1998). Ergonomic Workplace Analysis, Finland, Finnish Institute of Occupational Health

Goleman D (1996). Emotional intelligence – why it can matter more than IQ, London, Bloomsbury

Goleman, D (1998). Vital Lies, Simple Truths – the psychology of self-deception, London, Bloomsbury

Granger, Hamilton (1987) The Functional Independence Measure. In: McDowell I, Newell C, eds. Measuring Health: A Guide to Rating Scales and Questionnaires. 2nd edition. New York: Oxford University Press;115-121.

Gwent (2003). Protocol for the Therapeutic handling of Neurologically Impaired Adults, Gwent Healthcare NHS Trust

Heyman B Risk, Health and Healthcare – A Qualitative Approach, London, Arnold

Hignet S, McAtamney L (2000). Rapid Entire Body Assessment, Applied Ergonomics 31 201 – 205

Hignett et al, (2003). Evidence-Based Patient Handling – Tasks Equipment and Interventions, London, Routledge

HSC (2001). Health and Safety Commission – Strategic Plan 2001 – 2004, London Health and Safety Commission

HSE (1998). Evaluation of the Six-Pack Regulations 1992, London Health and Safety Executive

HSE (2001). Handling Homecare, London Health and Safety Executive

HSE (2003). Health and safety regulation – a short guide, London, Health and Safety Executive

HSE (2003). The Principles of Good Manual Handling: Achieving a consensus, London, Health and Safety Executive

HSE (2004). Manual Handling Operations Regulations 1992 (as amended) – Guidance on Regulations, 3rd Edition, London, Health and Safety Executive

HSE (1999). Evaluating Change in exposure to risk for musculoskeletal disorders – a practical tool, Surrey, HSE

HSE (2003). Manual Handling Assessment Charts, London, Health and Safety Executive

Human Rights Act 1998 HMSO

Hutter B (2001). Regulation and Risk – Occupational Health and Safety on the Railways, Oxford, Oxford University Press

Kemmlert (1995). Method assigned for the identification of ergonomic hazards – PLIBEL, Applied Ergonomics, Vol 35, No 3 , 199 – 211

Kroemer K, Granjean E (1997). Fitting The Task To The Human: A Textbook Of Occupational Ergonomics, 5th Edition, London, Taylor Francis

Mandalstam M (2002) Manual Handling in Health and Social Care – An A – Z of Law and Practice, London, Jessica Kingsley

McAtamney L, Corlett N (1993) RULA -: A survey method for investigation of work-related upper limb disorders. Applied Ergonomics 1993, 24(2), 91-99

National Back Pain Association(1997). The Handling of Patients – introducing a safer handling policy, 4th Edition, London RCN

National Back Pain Association (1999).

Safer Handling of People in the Community, London, BackCare
NBE (2004). Manual Handling Standard, Interoim Document for Healthcare Providers, Towcester, National Back Exchange
Oxford (2003). Oxford Dictionary of English, 2nd Edition, Oxford, Oxford University Press
RCN (2001). Changing Practice – Improving Health: an integrated back injury prevention programme for nursing and care homes, London, Royal College of Nursing
RCN (1996). Manual Handling Assessments in Hospitals and the Community – An RCN guide, London, Royal College of Nursing
RCN (2003). Safer Staff, Better Care – RCN Manual Handling Training Guidance and Competencies, London, RCN
Royal Society of Chemistry (2002). Note on Risk Assessment at Work, London, Royal Society of Chemistry
Royal Society (1992). Risk analysis, perception and management, London, The Royal Society
SAI (1999). Risk Management – Australian and New Zealand Standard 4360, Australia, Standards Australia International
SAI (2004). Risk Management – Australian and New Zealand Standard 4360, 2nd Edition, Australia, Standards Australia International
Troup J, Edwards (1985). Manual Handling – a review paper, London HMSO
Vasey, Crozier, (1982). A move in the right direction, Nursing Mirror, May12:28 – 31
Viscusi MKip (1998). Rational Risk Policy – The Arne Ryde Memorial Lectures Series, Oxford, Clarendon Press
Waters (1994). Applications Manual for the Revised NIOSH Lifting Equation, Ohio, U.S. Department of Health and Human Services
Wilson A (2002). Effective Management of Musculoskeletal Injury – A clinical Ergonomics Approach to Prevention, treatment and Rehabilitation, Edinburgh, Churchill Livingstone

Websites

http://turva.me.tut.fi/owas/
http://www.cdc.gov/niosh/94-110.html
http://www.dh.gov.uk/assetRoot/04/08/60/58/04086058.pdf
http://www.ergonomics.co.uk/Rula/Ergo/index.html
http://www.hcsu.org.uk/
http://www.hse.gov.uk
http://www.legislation.hmso.gov.uk
http://www.legislation.hmso.gov.uk/acts1995/Ukpga_1995_en_l.htm
http://www.wales.nhs.uk/documents/NHS_manual_handling_passpor.pdf
www.rscorg/lap/reccom/ehsc/ehscnotes.htm
www.manutention.org.au

10 Evidence based practice

Emma Crumpton MSc (Ergs) BSc MCSP
Sue Hignett PhD MSc MCSP MErgS Eur Erg

Summary

Increasingly in the world of healthcare there is an emphasis on evidence based practice. This chapter will explain what it is and why it is important for professional practice in manual handling. Specifically, it will consider the importance of, and need for, an evidence base for patient handling. The following questions will be considered.

- Why have an evidence base?
- What is evidence-based practice?
- How is evidence used?

1 Introduction

Evidence-based practice (EBP) falls within the portfolio of clinical governance together with risk management, health outcomes, lifelong learning, clinical guidelines and research and development *(Wright and Hill, 2003)*. Clinical governance was established in 1998 to provide 'a framework through which NHS organisations are accountable for continuously improving the quality of their services and safeguarding high standards of care by creating an environment in which excellence in clinical care will flourish' *(Department of Health, 1998)*. It brings together the factors required for organisational (top to bottom) cultural change within a simple concept, which is underpinned by complex components involving patients, health professionals, managers and policy makers.

Most health professionals are altruistic and keen to do their best for patients. One of the elements of being a professional is having a self-questioning attitude, with a desire to be self-correcting and self-regulating. As much of our professional satisfaction derives from being involved, identifying where improvements can be made and taking steps to effect these, EBP provides a framework for questioning our professional practice. The onus for patient handling information is often left within the remit of Back Care Advisers (BCAs), as they are the experts in their organisations. However, patient handling is a core skill for all health professionals, therefore the information should be of interest to all clinicians.

2 Why have an evidence base?

An evidence base is the accepted body of knowledge that underpins practice and from which guidelines and professional best practice are derived. The world of health care is an environment of increasing information and there is bombardment on a daily basis with guidelines, articles, peer-reviewed papers, word of mouth etc. and the quantity of information continues to increase. In 1948 there were about 4,700 scientific journals in publication by 1990 there were more than 100,000 scientific journals (http://www.hsl.unc.edu/lm/ebm/whatis.htm).

Gorman et al (1994) reported on the use of information from an observational study. Text books were claimed to be used by 39% and were actually used by 12%. Journals were claimed to be consulted by 18% and were observed being used by 7%. Human sources of information were claimed by 33 % but actually observed by 55%. This would seem to fit with the pattern seen in BCAs as there are no dedicated scientific peer-reviewed journals available. To review all the literature would therefore necessitate reading many journals. National Back Exchange (NBE) run an annual conference and local Back Exchange groups convene regular regional meetings. The topics discussed are very varied, based on the "local groups" reports in The Column, However, it does not appear that evidence or practice is systematically critiqued. Therefore, it is suggested that evidence-based patient handling is needed for the following reasons:

- There are many patient handling problems in a wide range of clinical specialities.
- There are too many journals to access all the information.
- BCAs feel as if they are in information overload.
- BCAs have limited time to read.
- BCAs read what they are familiar with e.g. The Column.
- BCAs tend to avoid difficult or complicated papers.

3 What is evidence based practice?

Firstly, evidence-based medicine will be considered, and then the way in which this model is being transformed for nursing practice, and finally an example of a specific patient handling activity will be given.

Evidence based medicine

The concept of evidence-based medicine (EBM) began in the medical profession in the 1970s with Archie Cochrane who argued that as healthcare resources would always be limited they should be used to provide services that had been shown to be effective *(Reynolds, 2000)*. He drew on his personal experience of applying research results to individual patients, suggesting that the application of scientific principles had been largely absent in the development and evaluation of new treatment methods. He went on to pioneer the use of systematic reviews and meta-analyses in medicine. The development of EBM aimed to help doctors to (1) interpret and use research findings and (2) use research to inform practice throughout their careers *(Reynolds, 2000)*. The most common definition of EBM is "*the conscientious, explicit and judicious use of current best evidence in making decisions about the care of the individual patient. It means integrating individual clinical expertise with the best available external clinical evidence from systematic research*" *(Sackett et al, 1997)*. EBM required that research should be classified into one of the following types of research: aetiology, therapeutics, diagnosis, prognosis, quality improvement, or economic evaluation, each with specific methodological criteria. This leads to a final hierarchy of evidence, whereby the randomised controlled trial (RCT) is considered to be the best method followed by controlled trials, cohort studies, case-control studies, surveys, qualitative studies and finally professional opinions *(Hamer and Collinson, 1999)*.

Reynolds (2000) summarised some concerns about EBM, one of which suggests that it presents a distorted and partial view, from a particular viewpoint (or ontology), of the use of science in medicine. This is reflected in the hierarchy of evidence with RCT gaining a higher ranking than an experimental case study. Another concern was that EBM rejected much that was central to the scientific method by focusing on quantitative research methods, resulting in the values, experiences and preferences of patients being mostly ignored. This trend is reversing with the inclusion of qualitative research *(Murphy et al, 1998; Green and Britten, 1998)* and a changing attitude within EBM whereby '*the principle which determines what kind of research is of value is dictated by the specific clinical question*' *(Reynolds, 2000)*.

Evidence based nursing

Evidence based nursing (EBN) is a developing area and so clinical decision-making tends to be based on a combination of clinical experience, observation, training, peer group teaching, published articles and personal research *(Blomfield and Hardy, 2000)*. *DiCenso et al (1998)* give a pragmatic definition of EBN as '*the process by which nurses make clinical decisions using the best available research evidence, their clinical expertise and patient preferences in the context of available resources*'. The evidence, by itself, does not allow the nurse to make a decision, but it does support the process. The integration of the three components into decision-making increases the likelihood of successful problem solving and so both patient care and staff health are improved.

The value of EBN is the emphasis it places on rational action through a structured appraisal of empirical evidence rather than the adherence to blind conjecture, dogmatic ritual or private intuition. However there are again real concerns about EBN related to the restricted view of nursing, and the nurse-patient relationship, which is derived from the concepts developed in EBM. So nursing is not unquestioningly adopting the medical model definition of EBP, instead nurses are setting a broader definition of evidence, which includes a wider range of methodologies as discussed earlier. This will be helpful when considering how EBP can be used for patient handling practice.

EBP in Patient Handling

BCAs have perhaps been more involved with some of the other areas of clinical governance, e.g. risk management, than EBP. It seems to be the case that some BCAs still work with a paradigm of practice that is based on the following assumptions:

- Clinical experience and peer group discussion are a valid way of building and maintaining one's knowledge about the efficacy of manual handling equipment, techniques or interventions.
- The study and understanding of basic mechanics, ergonomic principles and musculoskeletal disease is a sufficient guide for practice.
- A combination of manual handling training and common sense is sufficient to allow one to evaluate new equipment and techniques
- Expertise and experience form a sufficient base from which to generate valid guidelines for clinical practice.

According to this paradigm BCAs have a number of options for tackling the problems with which they are presented. They can reflect on their own clinical experience, talk to colleagues, reflect on the underlying principles, go to a guidance document, or ask a local expert or expert group such as National Back Exchange. This reflects how many BCAs work, using local NBE groups as a support network for peer group discussions and affirmation of practice. As the expert in their work place BCAs are usually sought out as a source of information and expertise by staff. According to the new paradigm outlined below the advice they give should be based on evidence.

The assumptions of a new evidence-based paradigm (www.cche.net/usersguides/ebm.asp) are as follows:

- Clinical experience and the development of clinical instincts are crucial and necessary parts of becoming competent in manual handling. Many aspects of clinical practice cannot, or will not, ever be adequately tested, therefore clinical experience and its lessons are particularly important in these situations. At the same time systematic attempts to record observations in a reproducible and unbiased way increase the confidence one can have in knowledge about equipment, techniques and interventions.
- In the absence of systematic observation one must be cautious in the interpretation of information derived from clinical experience and intuition for it may, at times, be misleading.
- The study and understanding of basic mechanisms of disease, injury, biomechanics and ergonomics are necessary but insufficient guides for practice.
- Understanding certain rules of evidence and its interpretation are necessary to correctly interpret literature.
- It follows that BCAs should regularly consult the original literature (and be able to critically appraise it) in solving problems and providing optimal care. It also follows that BCAs must be ready to accept and live with uncertainty and to acknowledge that management decisions are often made in the face of relative ignorance of their true impact.

The new paradigm puts a much lower value on authority as the underlying belief is that BCAs can gain the skills to make independent assessments of evidence and thus evaluate the credibility of opinions being offered by experts.

4 How is evidence used?

The practice and teaching of EBP requires skills that are not traditionally part of healthcare or manual handling training. These include:

- Defining a patient handling problem.
- Identifying what information is required to resolve the problem.
- Conducting a detailed search of the literature.
- Selecting the best of the relevant

studies and applying rules of evidence to determine their validity.
- Being able to present to colleagues in a succinct way the content of an article, its strengths and weaknesses (critical appraisal), the clinical message and its application to a person handling problem.

These steps will now be described in more detail using a person handling example.

Defining a person handling problem

The first step involves converting the need for information about prevention, diagnosis, prognosis, therapy, causation, etc. into answerable questions for example:

We need to do a risk assessment of a very heavy hemiplegic patient who can weight-bear and needs to be sat out in a chair (from their bed) due to a chest infection. It is desirable to promote independence but there is concern about the manual handling risks to staff, so our question is:

"What techniques and equipment can be used to achieve this transfer and promote safety for the person and handlers?"

Identifying what information is required to resolve the problem

In order to address this question we need to track down the best available evidence. Hignett et al produced a systematic review of patient handling activities in 2003 and this will be used as our starting point. The evidence was summarised into different sections so we would need to look at different sections to source the relevant information for our question. We should also consult professional guidelines and discuss the problem with experts and colleagues to ensure that we are accessing as much information as possible.

Conducting an efficient search of the literature and selecting the studies

Traditional reviews of the published evidence have usually relied on experts or researchers in the field to tell us the answer. However this method has two main weaknesses as the reviewer may have a particular prejudice or prior belief and/or the review can miss evidence that can contribute to the answer. So simply searching, for example Medline, could miss evidence that is published as conference abstracts or research theses (grey literature).

Hamer and Collinson (1999) and *Wright and Hall (2003)* describe the key components of a systematic review as being:

1. Definition of the research question with clear and precise objectives.
2. Methods for identifying the research studies with an explicit and rigorous search of published and grey (unpublished) literature.
3. Selection of studies for inclusion with explicit inclusion and exclusion criteria.
4. Quality appraisal of included studies using transparent appraisal processes and consistent data collection.
5. Extraction of the data.
6. Synthesis of the data with clear method of combining results (statistical or narrative).

Hignett et al (2003) described the search strategy for the patient handling systematic review as taking an unusual philosophical stance by appraising studies within a study type rather than comparatively, this means that the previously mentioned hierarchy (with RCTs as the gold standard) was not applied. A string search was run on eight databases (including Medline, CINAHL, EMBASE and Ergonomics Abstracts) and supplemented by searching the grey literature. They give a detailed description of the processes of inclusion, exclusion, appraisal, extraction and synthesis.

In order to select the studies which are relevant for our question it would be more useful to use *Hignett (2003)* which focuses on transfers starting from lying, sitting and standing positions. The number of studies for starting in the sitting position is reduced to 23 and this is further reduced to only 14 papers (listed below) for our specific question.

Critical appraisal of content of the article, and its strengths and weaknesses

Before looking at the evidence from *Hignett (2003)* we should carry out a critical appraisal of the review itself. The advantage of using *Hignett (2003)* rather than *Hignett et al (2003)* is that the former was published in a peer-reviewed academic journal, whereas the latter is a book that has not undergone a formal peer review process. Many books suggest critical appraisal questions for different study types. Figure 10.1 gives an example of the sort of questions that should be applied to in order to increase our confidence in the quality of the evidence.

Figure 10.1. Critical appraisal questions for a review (*Wright and Hill, 2003*)

Are the results of the study valid?
1. Did the review address a focused clinical question?
2. Were the criteria used to select articles for inclusion appropriate?
3. Is it unlikely that important, relevant studies were missed?
4. Was the validity of the included studies appraised?
5. Were assessments of the studies reproduced?
6. Were the results similar from study to study?

What are the results?
1. What are the overall results of the review?
2. How precise were the results?

Will the results help me in caring for my patients?
1. Can the results be applied to my patient care?
2. Were all clinically important outcomes considered?
3. Are the benefits worth the harms and costs?

Findings

The following evidence statements have been selected from *Hignett (2003)* to address the question.

- Moderate evidence from five studies *(Benevolo et al, 1993; Garg et al, 1991; Garg and Owen, 1994; Marras et al, 1999; Zhuang et al, 2000)* that a walking belt with two carers should be used for weight-bearing patients to transfer them from a sitting position to another sitting position.
- Moderate evidence from two studies *(Gagnon et al, 1986; Marras et al,*

1999) that a walking belt should not be used with one carer for weight-bearing patients. Additional evidence for this statement from two lower quality studies *(Gagnon and Lortie, 1987; Pan and Freivalos, 2000).*

- Moderate evidence from two studies *(Roth et al, 1993; Zhuang et al, 2000)* that using a belt lifter (standing hoist) is preferable to manual methods.
- Limited evidence from one study *(Owen and Fragala, 1999)* that sliding between a bed and stretcher chair may be easier than using either a gait belt or hoist.
- Limited evidence from one study *(Elford et al, 2000)* that using one or two handling slings with two carers is preferable to no slings.
- Limited evidence from one study *(Gingher et al, 1996)* that using a gantry hoist is preferable to mobile hoists for bed-chair transfers.

We would then want to integrate this information with our clinical expertise, our unique circumstances and the patient assessment, so the question may become more complex when we then consider whether:

- The recommended equipment is available.
- It has been maintained.
- The clinician has been trained to use it.
- The environment is suitable.
- It is suitable for the current condition of the person.

These questions may change the chosen technique and form the wider risk assessment/clinical judgement that needs to be considered with the research evidence. However by using the available evidence we can say that the preferred equipment and technique for this scenario would be a walking belt with two carers. If this option is not available then a standing hoist, sliding technique or gantry hoist could be used although the evidence to support these options is weaker than for the walking belt with two carers.

5 Conclusion

We can see that there are both internal and external drivers for using an evidence base for patient handling activities. The external drivers include the framework of clinical governance (and associated audit processes) the internal drivers are related to professional attitudes and behaviour. However we must bear in mind that evidence will go out of date and new treatment and technologies will be introduced so we should always be seeking new evidence to make sure that we are working with the most relevant information. The availability of evidence for patient handling is relatively new so we hope that practitioners and researchers will take the challenge forward to investigate those areas of patient handling about which there is currently limited or no evidence available. This presents an opportunity for us to embrace the new paradigm and learn methods for appraising and interpreting research literature.

References

Benevolo E, Sessarego P, Zelaschi G and Franchignoni F (1993). An ergonomic analysis of five techniques for moving patients [Italian]. Giornale Italiano di Medicina del Lavoro 15, 139-44.

Blomfield R and Hardy S (2000). Evidence-Based Nursing Practice. In Trinder, L. and Reynolds, S. (Eds.). Evidence-based practice. A critical appraisal. Oxford: Blackwell Publishing Ltd. 111-137

Department of Health (1998). A First Class Service: Quality in the New NHS. Health Service Circular: HSC (98)113. London: Department of Health.

DiCenso A, Cullum N and Ciliska D (1998). Implementing evidence-based nursing: some misconceptions. Evidence-based Nursing. 1, 38-40

Elford W, Straker L and Strauss G (2000). Patient handling with and without slings: an analysis of the risk of injury to the lumbar spine. Applied Ergonomics 31, 185-200.

Gagnon M, Sicard C and Sirois JP (1986). Evaluation of forces on the lumbo-sacral joint and assessment of work and energy transfers in nursing aides lifting patients. Ergonomics 29, 3, 407-421.

Gagnon M and Lortie MA (1987). Biomechanical approach to low-back problems in nursing aides. In Asfour, S. (Ed.). Trends in Ergonomics/Human Factors IV. Elsevier Science Publishers BV, North Holland 795-802

Garg A, Owen B, Beller D and Banaag J (1991). A biochemical and ergonomic evaluation of patient transferring tasks: wheelchair to shower chair and shower chair to wheelchair. Ergonomics 34, 4, 407-419.

Garg A and Owen B (1994). Prevention of back injuries in healthcare workers. International Journal of Industrial Ergonomics 14, 315-331.

Gingher MC, Karuza J, Skulski MD and Katz P (1996). Effectiveness of lift systems for long term care residents. Physical and Occupational Therapy in Geriatrics 14, 2, 1-11

Gorman PN, Wykoff L, Ash J (1994). Can primary care physicians questions be answered by using the medical journal literature? Bulletin of the Medical Library Association. 82, 2, 140-146.

Green J and Britten N (1998). Qualitative research and evidence based medicine. BMJ. 316, 18 April. 1230-1232

Hamer S and Collinson G (1999). Achieving Evidence-Based Practice. London: Harcourt Publishers Ltd.

Hignett S (2003). Systematic review of patient handling activities starting in lying, sitting and standing positions. Journal of Advanced Nursing. 41, 6, 545-552

Hignett S, Crumpton E, Ruszala S Alexander P, Fray M and Fletcher B (2003). Evidence-Based Patient Handling. Tasks, Equipment and Interventions. London: Routledge

Marras WS, Davis KG, Kirking BC and Bertsche PK (1999). A comprehensive analysis of low-back disorder risk and spinal loading during the transferring and repositioning of patients using different techniques. Ergonomics 42, 7, 904-926

Murphy E, Dingwall R, Greatbatch D, Parker S and Watson P (1998). Qualitative research methods in health technology assessment: a review of the literature. Health Technology Assessment. 2, 16. http://www.soton.ac.uk/~hts

Owen BD and Fragala G (1999). Reducing perceived physical stress while transferring residents: An ergonomic approach. American Association of Occupational Health Nursing Journal 47, 316-323.

Pan CC and Freivalos A (2000).

Ergonomic Evaluation of a new patient handling device. Proceedings of the IEA2000/HFES 2000 Congress. The Human Factors and Ergonomics Society, Santa Monica, California. 4, 274

Reynolds S (2000). The Anatomy of Evidence-Based Practice: Principles and Methods. In Trinder, L. and Reynolds, S. (Eds.). Evidence-based practice. A critical appraisal. Oxford: Blackwell Publishing Ltd. 17-34.

Roth PT, Ciecka J, Wood EC and Taylor R (1993). Evaluation of a unique mechanical client lift. Efficiency and perspectives of nursing staff. American Association of Occupational Health Nursing Journal. 41, 5, 229-234.

Sackett D, Richardson WS, Rosenberg W, Haynes RB (1997). Evidence Based Medicine: How to Teach and Practice EBM (1st Ed.). Edinburgh: Churchill Livingstone

Wright J and Hill P (2003). Clinical Governance. Edinburgh: Churchill Livingstone

Zhuang Z, Stobbe TJ, Collins JW, Hsiao H and Hobbs GR (2000). Psychophysical assessment of assistive devices for transferring patients/residents. Applied Ergonomics 31, 35-44.

11

Introduction to practical chapters

Emma Crumpton MSc (Ergs) BSc MCSP
Freelance Ergonomist
Carole Johnson MCSP SRP Cert Ed
Manual Handling Consultant

The practical chapters that follow are presented in a new way, with the intention of moving us forward from *The Handling of Patients 4th Edition (HOP4)*. This introduction explains why and how the information is laid out, and will give details of a very simple evidence gathering exercise that was carried out on each technique presented.

1 Practical chapters

Why?

In the 7 years since HOP4 was published there has been a lot of activity in the field of manual handling, including research, best practice guidance and legal considerations. This new edition gives a long overdue complete revision of structure and content, particularly for the practical chapters. A task based approach has been used, focusing on risk assessment and giving a summary of the available scientific evidence for each task. This has highlighted weaker areas in the evidence base for professional practice in manual handling, and shows where further work is needed.

How?

The authors for each chapter were selected for their accomplishment and experience in the field. They were instructed to use peer reviewed evidence to back up their content and where there is no available evidence, they were asked to use documented professional best practice, for instance the Derbyshire Interagency document *(Derbyshire Interagency Group Guidelines, 2001)*. All evidence was required to be in the public domain and available to readers.
Authors were instructed to first consider with an active (independent) person and progress through all relevant stages of dependency through to a person who is fully dependent.

Chapter structure

Each grade of each technique is detailed, and all potential applications noted so that the indexing system refers readers to the relevant section if beginning with a person's problem/ diagnosis rather than the task.

2 Evidence gathering process

Why?

Many techniques used and recommended by professional practice do not have a solid evidence base behind them. Therefore, the editorial team decided to attempt to evaluate the techniques listed in the chapters. The idea was to both give a start to readers wishing to judge the value of each manoeuvre, and also to demonstrate a first attempt at generating some research into the manoeuvres that are favoured by best practice guidelines. As stated in chapter 10 the evidence, by itself, does not make a decision for you, but it can help support the process. A detailed risk assessment is essential in all cases as the basis for decision making. The integration of the following three components into manual handling decision making increases the likelihood of successful problem solving, and so patient care and staff health are both improved

- Clinical expertise
- Patient values
- Best evidence.

Evidence-based practice is the integration of best research evidence with clinical expertise and patient values. This decreased emphasis on authority does not imply a rejection of what one can learn from colleagues and teachers whose years of experience have provided them with insight into techniques, equipment and intervention strategies which can never be gained from formal scientific investigation. It must be recognised that there is an "art" to patient handling and that a great deal of skill and judgement, and success in the field is gained by experience and professional insight. However practice must be evidence based as far as possible. Indeed, the professional judgement approach has already led us astray since the main approach to back pain in health care staff has been to provide techniques training and the only strong evidence that we have in the area states very clearly that techniques training in isolation is ineffective *(Hignett et al, 2002)*.

How?

Approximately 8 days of evidence gathering were organised and were attended by volunteer Back Care Advisers, who met strict criteria. Prior to undertaking the evidence gathering, all assessors completed a test to ensure inter-assessor reliability.

Method

The information and details on the techniques provided by the authors were assessed using the following tools.

- Functional Independence Measure
- Mobility Gallery
- Rapid Entire Body Assessment
- 10 point comfort scale
- 10 point activity scale
- Skill Level (Benner)

Full details of these tools are given in the summary table below.

The methodology is not ideal, but given the time and resource constraints it is a step in the right direction and begins an evidence base from which we can build. The main critical appraisal points are listed briefly below.

Results

Delegates were asked to complete an analysis of each manual handling technique by using the measurement tools. The results are presented at the end of each task in a table. It is hoped that all readers, particularly back care advisers, will take this as a starting point and conduct further small projects and/or audits of local practice, and in this way more evidence will be generated.

Evidence gathering method critique

- The photographs used for the REBA analysis of techniques were provided by the authors and are the ones from which the drawings included in the chapters were taken. They were not standardised, other than they were to be taken at the point of most risk during the manoeuvre. However, the photographs varied in their quality and angle as well as the accuracy of the timing of the snapshot.
- Analysis for each technique is based on a single still photograph.
- Many compromises and assumptions were made in order to complete the assessment. For instance, the position of a hidden wrist or obscure angle of the trunk. These were made by consensus of the experts attending the evidence gathering days.
- The results generated were based on a very small sample of self selected Back Care Advisers with prior knowledge of REBA.
- Models were used not real patients.
- The environment on the assessment days was spacious and time and work pressure did not affect handling.

Analysis

It was not possible to collect evidence for all the techniques supplied. Some analysis has been given where there is clear indication from the evidence that a certain technique has benefits over others within the section, however, the reader must always ensure that they have undertaken their own assessment in their particular circumstances. The reader may also have variations on particular methods discussed and it is hoped that the tools used in this book will aid evaluation of those differences.

New assessment tools are in process of development and it is always possible to complete more research and to extend and broaden the evidence collected, and the authors look forward to the expansion of possible evidence gathering in this important field.

Table 11.1 Summary of measurement tools

MEASUREMENT TOOL	PURPOSE	EVIDENCE FOR USE	SCORING
FIM	A slightly more complex assessment of dependence than the mobility gallery.	This is a widely used tool, particularly within the field of rehabilitation and involves the classification of a persons function according to 7 levels of function, from independence to total assistance. *Granger CV, Hamilton BB, Linacre JM, Heinemann AW, Wright BD. Performance profiles of the functional independence measure. Am J Phys Med Rehabil 1993;72:84-9.*	1–7

DESCRIPTION OF THE LEVELS OF FUNCTION AND THEIR SCORES	
INDEPENDENT	**Another person is not required for the activity (NO HELPER).**
7–Complete Independence	All of the tasks described as making up the activity are typically performed safely, without modification, assistive devices, or aids, and within a reasonable time.
6–Modified Independence	Activity requires any one or more than one of the following: an assistive device, more than reasonable time, or there are safety (risk) considerations.
DEPENDENT	**Another person is required for either supervision or physical assistance in order for the activity to be performed, or it is not performed. (REQUIRES HELPER)**
5–Supervision or Setup	Subject requires no more help than standby, cuing or coaxing, without physical contact. Or, helper sets up needed items or applies orthoses.
4–Minimal Contact Assistance	With physical contact the subject requires no more help than touching, and subject expends 75% or more of the effort.
3–Moderate Assistance	Subject requires more help than touching, or expends half (50%) or more (up to 75%) of the effort.
COMPLETE DEPENDENCE	**The subject expends less than half (less than 50%) of the effort. Maximal or total assistance is required, or the activity is not performed.**
2–Maximal Assistance	Subject expends less than 50% of the effort, but at least 25%.
1–Total Assistance	Subject expends less than 25% of the effort.

MEASUREMENT TOOL	PURPOSE	EVIDENCE FOR USE	SCORING
Mobility gallery	To grade the level of dependence of the person to be handled. This is a very simple scale and has potential for use by all skill levels of handler.	This tool has been developed by LOCOmotion (H. Knibbe and N. Knibbe, (19) The Mobility Gallery, Arjo Ltd) – see appendix 4. It has a strong evidence base in the Resident Assessment Instrument and the International Classification for Impairments, Disabilities and Handicaps by the World Health Organisation. The mobility gallery uses 5 levels of function, A–E, where A indicates total independence and E indicates total dependence.	A–E

SEE APPENDIX 4

MEASUREMENT TOOL	PURPOSE	EVIDENCE FOR USE	SCORING
REBA	A postural measurement technique	This widely used tool was designed to evaluate tasks where postures are dynamic, static or where gross changes in position occur. It is therefore suitable for patient handling (see appendix 1). *(Hignett and McAtamney 2000, Applied Ergonomics 31, 201–205)*	Risk levels 1–15 Action levels 0–4

RISK LEVELS			ACTION LEVELS		
1	=	Negligible risk	0	=	None necessary
2–3	=	Low risk	1	=	Maybe necessary
4–7	=	Medium risk	2	=	Necessary
8–10	=	High risk	3	=	Necessary soon
11–15	=	Very high risk	4	=	Necessary NOW

MEASUREMENT TOOL	PURPOSE	EVIDENCE FOR USE	SCORING
Patient comfort / dignity scales	10 point likert scale	Comfort and dignity were measured to get an idea of how the person being handled feels about the manoeuvre. When patients are handled inappropriately it causes pain and discomfort, the resultant associated defence reactions within their physical body (muscular contractions, respiratory blocking, reactions of start or withdrawal) can then be seen. People deserve to be respected, physically and emotionally. *Glaude D (2002)* Introduction to Haptonomy *Veldman F (2001)* Confirming affectivity; the dawn of human life The International Journal of Prenatal Psychology and Medicine Vol. 6 no 1, (1994), pages. 11–26.	0–10

0–10 LIKERT SCALE

0 -- **5** -- **10**

extreme discomfort ... extreme comfort

Introduction to practical chapters

MEASUREMENT TOOL	PURPOSE	EVIDENCE FOR USE	SCORING
Patient activity scales	10 point likert scale		

10n POINT LIKERT SCALE

0 -- 5 -- 10
no patient activity full patient activity

MEASUREMENT TOOL	PURPOSE	EVIDENCE FOR USE	SCORING
Benner scale	Benner's Application to Nursing of the Dreyfus Model of Skill Acquisition The Dreyfus model posits that in the acquisition and development of a skill, a student passes through five levels of proficiency: novice, advanced beginner, competent, proficient and expert.	Scale used to ascertain the skill level of handlers *Benner P (1984)*. From novice to expert: Excellence and power in clinical nursing practice. Menlo Park: Addison-Wesley, pp. 13-34. *Dreyfus H, Dreyfus S (1977)*. A Five-Stage Model of the Mental Activities Involved in Directed Skill Acquisition. University of California-Berkeley. *Dreyfus HL, Dreyfus SE (1986)*. Mind over Machine, New York: Free Press.	Novice – expert

BRIEF DESCRIPTION OF EACH LEVEL IN BENNER PAPER	
Novice	Beginners have had no experience of the situations in which they are expected to perform. Novices are taught rules to help them perform. The rules are context-free and independent of specific cases; hence the rules tend to be applied universally. The rule-governed behaviour typical of the novice is extremely limited and inflexible. As such, novices have no "life experience" in the application of rules. "Just tell me what I need to do and I'll do it".
Advanced beginner	Advanced beginners are those who can demonstrate marginally acceptable performance, those who have coped with enough real situations to note, or to have pointed out to them by a mentor, the recurring meaningful situational components. These components require prior experience in actual situations for recognition. Principles to guide actions begin to be formulated. The principles are based on experience.
Competent	Competence, typified by the nurse who has been on the job in the same or similar situations two or three years, develops when the nurse begins to see his or her acitons in terms of long-range goals or plans of which he or she is consciously aware. For the competent nurse, a plan establishes a perspective, and the plan is based on considerable conscious, abstract, analytic contemplation of the problem. The conscious, deliberate planning that is characteristic of this skill level helps achieve efficiency and organisation. The competent nurse lacks the speed and flexibility of the proficient nurse but does have a feeling of mastery and the ability ot cope with and manage the many contingencies of clinical nursing. The competent person does not yet have enough experience to recognise a situation in terms of an overall picture or in terms of which aspects are most salient, most important.
Proficient	The proficient performer perceives situations as wholes rather than in terms of chopped up parts or aspects, and performance is guided by maxims. Proficient nurses understand a situation as a whole because they perceive its meaning in terms of long-term goals. The proficient nurse learns from experience what typical events to expect in a given situation and how plans need to be modified in response to these events. The proficient nurse can now recognise when the expected normal picture does not materialise. This holistic understanding improves the proficient nurse's decision making; it becomes less laboured because the nurse now has a perspective on which of the existing attributes and aspects in the present situation are the important ones. The proficient nurse uses maxims as guides which reflect what would appear to the

BRIEF DESCRIPTION OF EACH LEVEL IN BENNER PAPER	
	competent or novice performer as unintelligible nuances of the situation; they can mean one thing at one time and quite another thing later. Once one has a deep understanding of the situation overall, however, the maxim provides direction as to what must be taken into account. Maxims reflect nuances of the situation.
Expert	The expert performer no longer relies on an analytic principle (rule, guideline, maxim) to connect her or his understanding of the situation to an appropriate action. The expert nurse, with an enormous background of experience, now has an intuitive grasp of each situation and zeroes in on the accurate region of the problem without wasteful consideration of a large range of unfruitful, alternative diagnoses and solutions. The expert operates form a deep understanding of the total situation. The chess master, for instance, when asked why he or she made a particularly masterful move, will just say: "Because it felt right; it looked good." The performer is no longer aware of features and rules; his/her performance becomes fluid and flexible and highly proficient. This is not to say that the expert never uses analytic tools. Highly skilled analytic abiltiy is necessary for those situations with which the nurse has had no previous experience. Analytic tools are also necessary for those times when the expert gets a wrong grasp of the situation and then finds that events and behaviours are not occurring as expected. When alternative perspectives are not available to the clinician, the only way out of a wrong grasp of the problem is by using analytic problem solving.

References

Benner P. (1984). From novice to expert: Excellence and power in clinical nursing practice. Menlo Park: Addison-Wesley pp.13-34

Dreyfus H, Dreyfus S (1977). A Five-Stage Model of the Mental Activities Involved in Directed Skill Acquisition. University of California-Berkeley.

Dreyfus HL, Dreyfus SE (1986). Mind over Machine, New York: Free Press.

Glaude D (2002). Introduction to Haptonomy

Granger CV, Hamilton BB, Linacre JM, Heinemann AW, Wright BD (1993). Performance profiles of the functional independence measure. Am J Phys Med Rehabil;72:84-9.

Hignett and McAtamney (2000). Applied Ergonomics 31, 201–205

Veldman F (2001). Confirming affectivity; the dawn of human life The International Journal of Prenatal Psychology and Medicine Vol. 6 no 1, (1994), pages. 11–26.

12 Sitting to standing

Sara Thomas DipCOT PGD SROT
Consultant Back Care Adviser

1 Introduction

Many personal and external factors influence the success of a person standing up from a seated position. This chapter will evaluate the determinants of the task of rising from a seated position into standing, giving consideration to the evidence available related to the achievement of this fundamental movement.

For the majority of individuals, rising from sitting is an automatic activity that requires no conscious thought or undue physical effort. However, for certain people, movement to a standing posture from sitting can be extremely difficult. *Eriksrund and Bohannon (2003)* suggest that sit to stand (STS) performance is reduced in many older individuals, particularly women and those who have various medical conditions, and conclude that difficulty in rising from a sitting position is a predictor of future disability, falls, nursing home use and mortality.

Many falls in the frail and elderly occur during activities in which they change position, e.g. standing up, sitting down or initiating walking (see chapter 17 for the management of such situations). *Vander Linden et al (1994)* suggest that it is the transitional phase involving the movement of the centre of mass against gravity during the STS transfer that causes such difficulties. *Cheng et al (1998)* sees a correlation between the task of STS and subsequent falls in stroke persons, finding more than a third of falls occur while they are rising or sitting down.

The World Health Organisation (1980) cited in *Eriksrund and Bohannon (2003)* has recognised the inability to rise from a sitting position as a disabling condition. Indeed, the ability to perform an independent STS movement is a skill that helps to determine the subsequent functional level of a person in relation to more complex mobility tasks such as walking and transfers, *Janssen et al (2002)*. This is supported by *Alexander et al (1991)* who found that there was a direct relationship between the ability to rise from a chair and performance in different functional activities.

The Medical Devices Agency (2002) suggest that "*Difficulty in standing from a seated position may be far more than a nuisance factor. It may erode a person's ability to mobilise safely, to participate in meaningful activity and to remain independent. It can cause distress, low self esteem, frustration and discourage people from making further attempts to stand*".

2 The hazards of assisted sit to stand (STS)

Sander (2003) suggests that the most common manual handling procedure performed by staff with people presenting with vascular dementia is assisting them to rise from sitting to standing. The frequency of undertaking this task will vary and depend upon the area of work and the functional level and requirements of the individuals.

Yip (2001) found "*biomechanical strain developed during repeated lifting and transferring of people between beds and chairs, onto trolleys, repositioning on beds and assisting them while walking.*" He concluded that these were the four most common activities putting nurses at high risk of low back pain.

A *Royal College of Nursing study (1996)*, entitled 'The Hazards of Nursing', asked the study group to describe people's mental and physical state at the time of the handling accident. The results showed that 92% of people were unable to stand up from sitting unaided. This would indicate that providing physical assistance to those individuals who cannot stand unaided poses an increased risk of injury to the handlers.

Hignett et al (2003) cites *Khalil et al (1987)* and indicates that when calculating the force acting on the erector spinae muscles of the handler, assisted standing from a chair resulted in most strain to nurses. *Marras et al (1999)* concluded in his study that in comparison with two person assisted stand techniques, the single person 'hug method' of assisting a person from sitting to standing required the greatest muscle force, and hence presented the highest risk of low back injury. However, caution should be used in interpreting 'laboratory' results. *Ruszala (2001)* warned how the results found in this study may be limited, as a person's ability to participate; normal patterns of movement and free arm movements were not considered.

3 Why stand?

The movement of standing from sitting enables an individual to engage in more complex movements and activities of daily living. Many people who use wheelchairs may, of course, undertake daily routines completely independently, but rising into a standing position, and maintaining that position, is both physiologically and psychologically beneficial to the person concerned. *Walter et al (1999)* in his study found that individuals with spinal cord injury who stood 30 minutes or more per day had significantly improved quality of life; fewer bed sores; fewer bladder infections; improved bowel regularity and decreased lower limb contractures than those who stood for less time – see table 12.1.

4 The task of sit to stand (STS)

The biomechanics of sitting to standing are also discussed in chapter 6. The following section provides information on the sequence of 'normal patterns of movement' which will enable a successful STS transfer.

Trew and Everett (2001) suggest that the movement from sitting to standing involves two distinct phases, a seated phase and a stance phase, the stance phase is further broken down into weight transfer and extension.

- In the seated phase the person prepares for standing by adjusting the position of their limbs and upper

the position of their limbs and upper body so that the centre of gravity moves forward until it is almost over their feet.
- A stance phase, where weight is taken through the lower limbs and the centre of gravity is transferred forwards and upwards.

On average, adults will complete the two phases of moving from sitting to standing in approximately 1-3 seconds. *Millington et al. (1992)* splits the overall task into three phases and uses different terms;
- weight shift
- transition
- lift

The results of the Millington study suggest that this characterisation of the sit to stand motion serves as a basis for identifying problems in elderly persons who demonstrate difficulty getting up from a chair.

Whilst it is recognised that this sit to stand sequence occurs in the general healthy population, individuals with conditions affecting mobility and, hence, function will adapt and find their own way of achieving and prolonging functional independence in STS tasks.

Galli et al. (2000) and *Sibella et al. (2003)* found that the STS task in very heavy persons was characterised by them leaning forward less than subjects with an average Body Mass Index (BMI). It was also noted that they required to move their feet further back and showed greater strain in the knee joints than the hip joints on moving from sitting to standing, the opposite being true in subjects with an average BMI.

Ramsey et al. (2004) found that people with mild to moderate Parkinson's disease exhibited asymmetrical movement when performing STS transfers. The inability to produce constant equilateral force when performing functional tasks such as STS could be an indicator for the increased propensity of falls or other instabilities in this group. This asymmetry in weight distribution was also noted by *Cheng et al. (1998)* when observing and measuring the movements of stroke persons. The stroke persons also required a significantly longer time to perform the rise and sit down (an average of 4.5 to 5.0 seconds).

Complexities such as these make it vital that practitioners are aware of the normal patterns of movement when providing verbal and/or manual assistance to people within their care. *Tarling (1997)* advises that staff should be aware of normal patterns of movement and the necessary preparations normally made for standing in order to be able to provide informed and effective assistance. *Sander (2003)* also advises the use of a number of key elements when assisting people with vascular dementia to rise from sitting. Primary among these is to facilitate and encourage *active* movement and to utilise *normal* patterns of movement and hence achieve a successful STS task.

The ability to sit down from standing is as essential as being to stand up, although there is little research in this area. Sitting from standing involves the function of the same muscles as are required for standing from sitting. *Tyldesley and Greive (2003)* state that sitting down moves the body from a less stable to a more stable position, and as the movement does not go against gravity it involves less physical effort. Whilst this movement may place less strain on knee and hip extensor muscles we should note that, people with weak muscles or limited joint movement may develop a technique of sitting, which involves 'falling' back into a chair rather than controlling the movement to its completion. This particularly happens as a result of the seat height being too low.

The *Neurodevelopmental Approach*, developed by Karel and Bertha Bobath in the 1940s, is commonly used by therapists and trained staff with individuals

Box 12.1

Benefits of standing/ weight bearing	Evidence
Improves/maintains bone density and joint range of movement	Eng *et al.* (2001)
Decreases occurrence of muscle contractures	O'Dwyer *et al.* (1996) Turner *et al.* (1998)
Decreases the incidence of 'functional' incontinence	Knibbe (2000), Staats (1998)
Improves/maintains digestion	Eng *et al.* (2001)
Maintains/improves cardiac function and circulation	Walter *et al.* (1999), Eng *et al.* (2001)
Prevention of skin breakdown	Walter *et al.* (1999), Eng *et al.* (2001)
Improvement/maintains quality of life	MDA (2002) Tyldesly and Greive (2003)
Maintains overall function in mobility	Monger *et al.* (2002). Gerdhem *et al.* (2003)

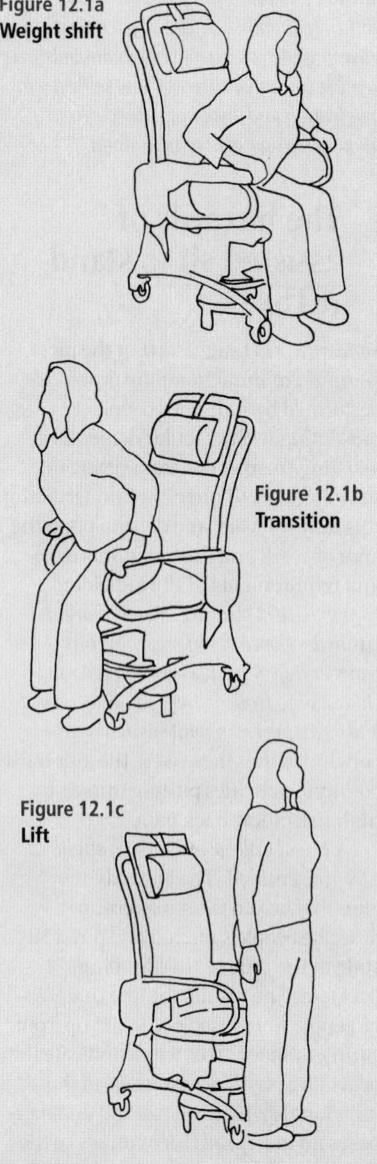

Figure 12.1a Weight shift

Figure 12.1b Transition

Figure 12.1c Lift

(adults and children) with neurological disorders. The approach makes use of positions that inhibit abnormal patterns of movement, facilitates normal equilibrium, balance and righting reactions and encourages normal movement patterns. Its basic principles are developed from neurological learning theory and from theories of normal human movement, (*Turner et al 2002*). This approach attempts to encourage the affected individuals to apply these principles in all aspects of activity throughout the day. *Ruszala (2001)* states that STS rehabilitation and the facilitation of normal patterns are essential elements of physiotherapy and vital to the promotion of independent movement. *Borgman et al (1991)* concluded that:

"the care of the stroke person is most rewarding when the nurse understands and practices, following appropriate training and under adequate supervision, rehabilitative nursing care. This care is based on neurophysiologic and neurodevelopmental principles of normal movement."

Clinicians are often required to assist with, and improve a person's STS ability, in addition to improving a person's ability to transfer to other surfaces. STS activities are an integral component of rehabilitation, which may be performed several times during one treatment session, *Ruszala (2001)*. A number of different handling techniques may be utilised with the aim of improving STS function. Such techniques allow the person to re-learn basic motor patterns through touch and positioning. One such method involves the clinician standing in front of the person to be assisted, positioning themselves in order to provide support and sensory stimulation of appropriate areas of the person's body, promoting symmetry and normal movement sequences. Success of this STS task relies on mutual and reciprocal activity of handler and person. *Tarling (1997)* however, provided sound advice by stating that staff should not undertake this type of handling without sufficient training. We should also consider *Gagnon et al (1986)* who concluded that handlers were subjected to unacceptably high vertical forces when involved in assisting a STS from the front of the person.

However, we should not disregard the clinical reasoning in skilled professionals and the importance of being able to make a suitable and sufficient risk assessment (see chapter 9) of the handling situation and goals of intervention. *The Chartered Society of Physiotherapy (2003)* states that:

'Whilst manual handling is an integral part of the role of a physiotherapist, the clinician must balance the potential benefits (utility) to persons arising from their intervention involving manual handling with the potential risks to themselves.'

It is also worth noting that the method described above is a very different one to the 'pivot transfer', as described in chapter 18 as a controversial technique, and by *Mutch (2004)*.

5 Factors involved in successful STS

The success of an independent STS and the time required to complete the movement are dependent upon a number of factors, which include the height of the chair (*Hughes et al, 1996*), muscle strength (*Riley, 1997*), use of the upper limbs (*Alexander et al, 2001*), balance (*Eriksrund and Bohannon, 2003*), foot placement and position (*Brunt et al, 2002*) and pain and stiffness (*Edlich, 2003*).

When considering what enables individuals to rise from a sitting position we should consider that there are many factors at play; *personal* factors and *external* factors.

6 Personal factors effecting STS

The personal factors effecting STS include a person's motivation to be active, emotion, cognitive skills (sequencing and depth perception), proprioception, medical condition and motor skills (i.e. balance, muscle tone, and strength). An individual is more than a physical being and issues such as motivation and intention (personal goal) will have a significant impact on a persons desired and presenting function.

Frail elderly people, those with neurological disorders and those who may be permanently or temporarily affected by orthopaedic conditions often have difficulty rising against gravity to standing without assistance, (*Cheng et al 1998, Sander, 2002*). The symptoms of such conditions include; reduced balance, reduced muscle tone and strength and reduced range of joint movement. *Trew and Everett (2001)* report that rising from a chair requires greater joint range of movement and muscle torque than walking and most stair climbing.

To be successful a person needs to have more than 90° flexion at the hip and knee joints and an almost full range of dorsiflexion (the ability to lift the feet upwards). It is the presence of pain, reduced joint range of movement, stiffness and muscle weakness that often limits the ability for elderly and arthritic people to achieve *STS, Edlich (2003)*.

Proprioception (the loss of postural or position sense) can also have a profound effect on the success of a STS movement. *Sander (2003)* describes a common difficulty when helping people with vascular dementia to stand up, which is their tendency to lean backwards when asked to lean forward due to poor position and postural sense. She recommends that staff develop effective communication skills and also suggests placing an object in front of the person to encourage the forward movement.

In addition *Bernardi et al (2004)* provide a number of personal criteria on which successful STS depends:

- trunk bending momentum
- centre of gravity
- position before the body rises
- lower limb extensor muscle strength

7 External factors effecting STS

There are many 'external' reasons why a person cannot manage a STS task, i.e. factors to do with the persons seating, their immediate environment, attitudes of family and/or handlers or resources available.

The STS activity may be carried out from a variety of surfaces such as an armchair, dining chair, toilet, bed, plinth etc. As a general rule the following guidelines on seat height, seat depth and armrest height and position can apply to many surfaces and do not relate only to an armchair.

8 Seating

According to *Janssen et al (2002)* the ability to do a STS movement is strongly influenced by the type of chair and its dimensions, i.e. height of seat and position and height of arm rests.

Rising from a chair when the design is inappropriate can be biomechanically demanding. For example, if the seat is soft, deep or low, there is posterior tilt (i.e. the seat is lower at the back than the front) or the backrest is reclined.

Seat height

Seat height has been found to be a determinant of a person rising successfully from a chair (*Eriskrund et al 2003, Edwards 1996, Edlich 2003, Alexander et al 2001*). However *Ruszala (2001)* cites *Kerr et al (1991)*, who suggests that while disabled people may benefit from a higher chair, (as well as using their arms to assist with the lift), the degree to which the height of the seat of the chair contributes to a successful stand varies according to the type and the degree of disability.

Hennington et al (2004) found that children with Cerebral Palsy (CP) took significantly longer to rise to standing than children without disabilities (1.71 seconds in comparison to 1.24 seconds), with the speed at which they extended against gravity being slower. However, he concluded that seat height did not affect the overall ability to stand for either children with CP or children without disabilities.

The Medical Devices Agency (2002) provides information and advice regarding the recommended heights of chairs, stating that the seat height is measured relative to the person's sitting knee height (popliteal region) taking account of the softness and thickness of a cushion or mattress. *Tarling (1997)* provides a guideline for seat height of between 350mm and 450mm from knee to floor, suggesting a seat height of 460mm high for elderly people with weakness in the legs. *Pheasant (2001)* suggests that the optimal seat height for many purposes is close to the popliteal height (back of the knee), and where this is not achieved a seat that is too low is preferable to one that is too high. He recommends for many purposes, a 400mm seat height is the best compromise. It is however preferable to have a seat height to suit the individual's body dimensions (anthropometrics). It is also necessary to find a balance between good rising height and sitting comfort as a seat which is too high can create problems with peripheral circulation (swollen feet and 'pins and needles') and postural instability, (*Weiner et al 1993, Pheasant 2001*).

Seat depth and angle

Very little published evidence was found regarding seat depth and success of standing from sitting. However the *Medical Devices Agency (1999)* suggest that seat depth should allow the user to make full use of the backrest and have a gap (to allow two fingers to pass) from the front edge of the seat to the back of the users knees (popliteal area). *Tarling (1997)* suggests a depth of between 432mm and 558mm, however the depth of the chair should correspond with the length from the back of the hips to the back of the knee in sitting. *Pheasant (2001)* suggests a seat depth of 435mm to enable the user to engage the backrest adequately.

It is suggested that people will have ease of STS if the seat is not too deep and they do not have to move too far forward to initiate the centre of gravity coming toward the edge of the seat and into the extension phase of standing. The deeper the seat the greater the problems of standing up and sitting down, *Pheasant (2001)*

If the seat is angled down towards the backrest, whilst this improves a person's contact with the backrest, achieving a standing position will require greater effort from the knee and hip extensors as well as greater effort from the upper limbs for pushing forwards and upwards, *MDA (2002)*.

Armrests

Ruszala (2001) suggests that when the upper limbs are used to assist with the rise phase of STS the forces in the knee joints are significantly reduced. *Eriksrund and Bohannon (2003)* state that upper extremity assistance at the time of standing will decrease the knee extension force for the task.

The MDA suggest that for comfort, the armrest height should allow the user to rest their arms whilst sitting without raising or dropping their shoulders, the length of the rest should also support the full length of the forearm. Increasing seat height and use of the arms decreases muscle and joint forces at the hips and the knees when rising from sitting, *Edwards (1996)*.

Finally, difficulties in standing up and sitting may also be reduced if the space beneath the front of the chair is unimpeded, allowing the user to place his feet beneath his centre of gravity, hence achieving a more effective upwards thrust into standing or a more controlled descent into sitting.

Assisted STS

People rise from a seated position approximately 90 times a day *MDA (2002)*. Altering and improving the person's immediate environment, i.e. providing them with the appropriate chair, handrails, shower seat with arms, raised toilet seat and/or toilet frame will assist to prolong independence in many other areas of daily living. This should be of primary consideration. However in many cases the provision of equipment to enable independence will not suffice and the person will require the use of more assistive devices and/or physical assistance from a handler. *Yassi et al (2001)* suggest that the use of handling equipment can reduce the risk of injury. *Keir et al (2004)* also advise the use of equipment to relieve some of the physical burden of manual handling, but due to the time involved in the use of such equipment suggest that there may be " increased cumulative loading in spite of a reduction in peak spinal loads".

The initial stage in the process of providing equipment to, or manually assisting a person in STS is to undertake a risk assessment (see chapter 9), this should identify the skills of the person and the areas in which they require help.

There are additional factors to consider, other than the ability to take weight through the feet, which will dictate whether a person can stand.

Dynamic sitting balance, the ability to sit unsupported by a chair and to lean forward and sideways without the loss of balance, move the centre of gravity over the feet, understanding and comprehension and motivation toward independence will all influence the ability to STS.

If the person is unable to lean forward in their seat, this may be a good indicator that they will have difficulty in STS or maintaining a standing posture without considerable support. In this instance equipment should be used rather than manual assistance. *Sander (2003)* suggests that the manoeuvre

(STS) is only possible where the person who is being facilitated to move can bear their own weight, perhaps with a little steadying once on their feet. Where reliable weight bearing is not possible then hoists become the only safe option.

Hignett (2003) et al found moderate evidence to suggest that mechanical hoists should be used for dependent, non weight bearing persons.

The following table illustrates the type of equipment, which may be used to assist people in the STS task. The different levels of activity (function) are described using the Mobility Gallery (see appendix 4) and the Functional Independence Measure (FIM) (see chapter 11).

Table 12.2

Mobility Gallery	Functional Independence Measure (FIM)	Suggested Equipment
A (Albert) **Independent**	1+2 Independent and Modified Independence	Raised toilet seat Chair raisers Arm rests on easy chair Shower seat with handrail
B (Barbara) **Minimal Assistance**	3 Supervision Minimal Assistance	Toilet frame with raised toilet seat Shower chair with arms Variable height bed Powered seat on chair Standing device Standing/turn device Handling belt with 1 handler
C (Carl) **Moderate Assistance**	4 Moderate Assistance	Variable height bed/plinth Powered rising chair Stand-aid (active) hoist Adjustable height shower chair with arms Standing bed/chair Handling belt with 2 handlers Walking harness with passive hoist Specialised walking hoist Tilt table Standing frame
D (Doris) **Maximum Assistance**	5 Maximal Assistance	Tilt table Standing frame
E (Emma) **Total Assistance**	6+7 Total Assistance	Not applicable

Practical Techniques

Task One

Sit to stand – help with one handler from the side of a chair without handling belt

DEPENDENCY LEVEL

Mobility Gallery B
FIM 4

- The person should be encouraged to move himself or herself through verbal guidance to move towards the edge of the chair and lean forwards to initiate the stand.
- The person should also have cognitive ability to understand and follow instructions from the handler.
- The person must be able to place full weight on their feet and move their own feet into position. The person should be able to maintain own balance when in full standing.

- The person should be able to place at least one hand onto the arm of the chair to help push into standing.

DESCRIPTION

- The person brings their bottom close to the edge of the seat and moves their feet into a position to allow them to push into standing and stand without losing balance. The handler's feet should be in a 'step' stance, i.e. one foot in front of the other facing the direction of movement.
- The person leans forward in the seat.
- The handler stands at the side of the person and encourages the person to place both hands onto the arms of the chair to push himself or herself into sitting on given commands.
- The handler faces direction of movement and places their nearest arm to the person across the person's back at around waist level, and leaves their hand open against the person's back. The handler should not grasp the person or the person's clothing. Ensure good contact with the person along the forearm against the person's back. The other hand can be placed onto the front of the person's nearest shoulder for added comfort and guidance.
- Using commands direct the person to lift their own head to initiate the stand, and at the same time place forward pressure on to the person's back to assist the normal movement in to standing.
- To complete the move the handler should move both feet to stand at the side of the person. The handler should remember to transfer his or her weight from their rear foot to their front foot and utilise their own weight to guide the person forwards and upwards.

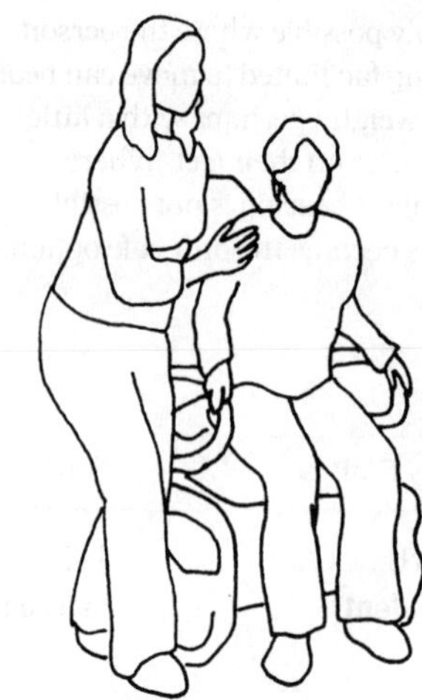

FIG 12.2a

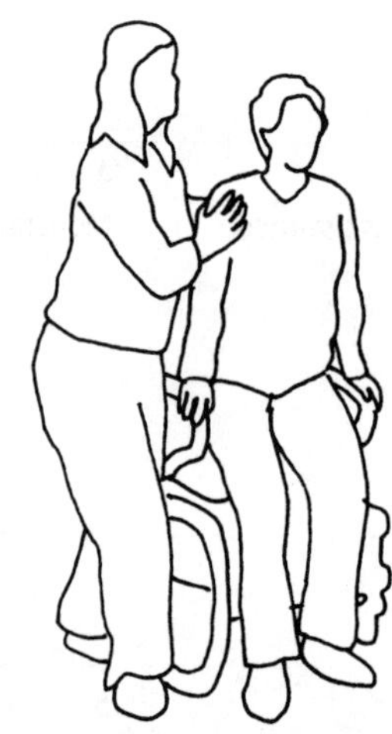

FIG 12.2b

OPTIONS AND VARIATIONS

1 This transfer may also be carried out with the use of a handling belt. The handler may stand at either side of the person and place their nearest arm across the person's back at around the level of the person's waist, ensuring good contact with the person and their forearm.

2 The handler may wish to stand facing the person and transfer his/her weight 'sideways' when the person stands. The weight transfer should be from the foot nearest to the back of the chair, towards the front of the chair.

PERCEIVED EXERTION FOR HANDLER

- The person should be encouraged to be active during the movement
- There should be little physical exertion for the handler.
- The handler should remember that they are to exert a forward and upward pressure for the person to bring himself or herself into standing.

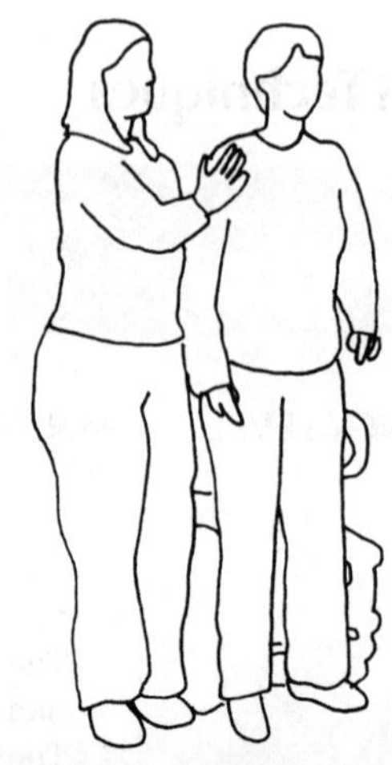

FIG 12.2c

	• It is important the handler works at the speed of the person as carrying out the procedure too quickly or too slowly will not allow the person to be active during the transfer. • The handler should work in collaboration with the person as a team and be aware not to hurry the person or lift them into standing.
COMFORT OF THE PERSON	• The method should be comfortable for the person and the handler should not grasp the person or their clothing. If handling belt is used: • Handlers should take care when placing a belt around the waist of people with abdominal problems as it may cause discomfort. • People who are underweight (according to the BMI chart) may find the belt 'digs' into their waist area. • Large people may find that the belt rises up towards their chest due to the shape of their waist area, in which case an alternative method and equipment should be sought.
SKILL LEVEL OF HANDLER	• The handler should have received basic manual handling training, be aware of assessment for people who require the use of a belt and also have understanding of patterns of normal movement for sit to stand. • If they are assisting a person with a hemiparesis (following a CVA) then they should be aware of management of the stroke patient.
EVIDENCE AVAILABLE	1 *Hignett (2002)* states that there is moderate evidence from 2 studies that a walking belt should not be used with one handler for weight bearing people. 2 *(BackCare 1999)* Safer Handling of People in the Community. 3 *Tarling C (1997/8)* in Fourth Edition of The Guide to the Handling of Patients.
DANGERS/ PRECAUTIONS	• If the person is unable to maintain weight on their feet or assist sufficiently to push into standing this will place too much strain onto the handler. The handler should be aware to allow the person to sit onto chair and not hold the weight of the person. Lowering the person slowly may cause strain on the handler. • If the person has weakness on one side, the handler should consider which side she is to stand so as not to take the full weight of the person leaning onto her. • The handling belt should be fitted firmly around the person's waist so as to prevent movement and sliding upward. • The handler should take care not to place their whole hand through the handle on the belt as this is likely to cause injury should the person move suddenly or fall back into the chair.
FURTHER OPTIONS	This method would be appropriate in a variety of situations such as from an armchair, dining chair, commode or toilet, if sufficient space is available.

Evidence review

Technique	REBA	Activity	Comfort	FIM	Mobility gallery	Skill level	Comment
HELP WITH ONE HANDLER FROM THE SIDE OF A CHAIR WITHOUT THE HANDLING BELT							
Fig 12.2a	4	9	9	4	B	Advanced beginner	One handler with one hand on the person's shoulder – this requires skill by the handler and is comfortable for the person. It is better to have person in a chair than to assist from a bed

Task Two

Sit to stand – help with two handlers from the side of a chair with handling belt

DEPENDENCY LEVEL

Mobility Gallery B
FIM 4

- The person should be encouraged under verbal guidance to move towards the edge of the chair and lean forwards to initiate the stand.
- If the person cannot move their bottom to the edge of the chair then one handler may assist them (see task three).
- The person should also have cognitive ability to understand and follow instructions from the handlers.
- The person must be able to place at least partial weight on their feet and move their own feet into position.
- The person should be able to maintain most of his or her own weight and balance when in full stand.

DESCRIPTION OF TRANSFER

- The person leans forward in the seat.
- If the person cannot move their own hips to the edge of the seat then one handler may assist by kneeling in front of the person and with the person leaning forward in the chair, ask the person to rock from one hip to another. The handler will exert a forward pressure on the side of the hip that the person has lifted. This movement will be repeated until the person is in the desired position near to the edge of the seat (explained fully in task three).
- The handler places handling belt around the person's waist and makes secure.
- The handlers stand at each side of the person and encourage the person to place his hands onto the arms of the chair to push himself or herself into sitting on given commands.
  If the person cannot place one hand onto the arm of the chair then one handler may support the person's hand by taking a palm to palm hold (avoiding holding the person's thumb, see chapter 13, figure 13.2a)
- The handler faces the direction of movement and places their nearest arm to person over the person's back and grasps the handle of belt near to the person's mid back. Ensure good contact with person along the forearm against the person's back.
- The other hand remains free or can be placed onto the front of the person's nearest shoulder for added support.
- Using commands, the person is directed to lift their own head to initiate the stand, and at the same time the handler places a

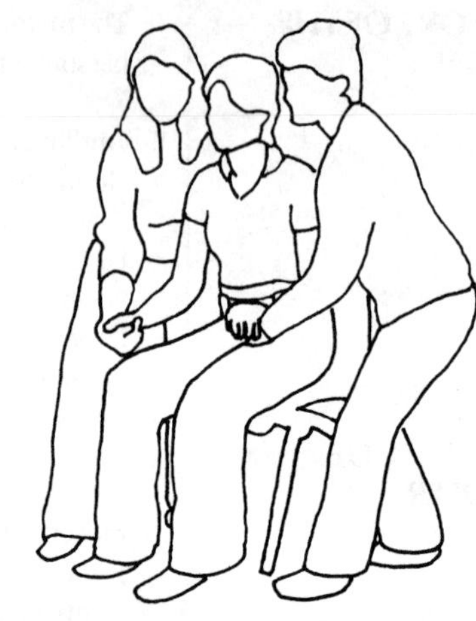
FIG12.3a

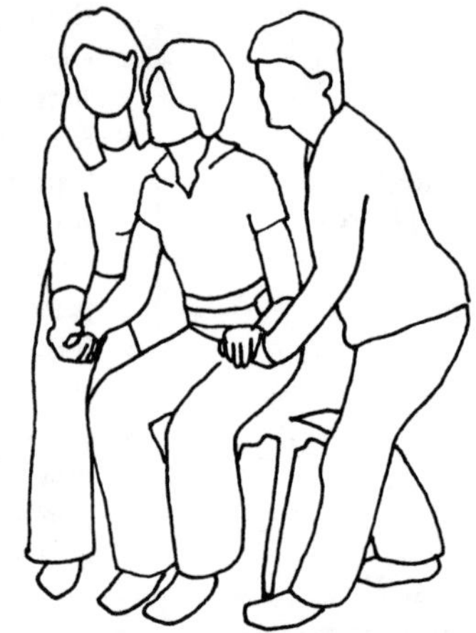
FIG12.3b

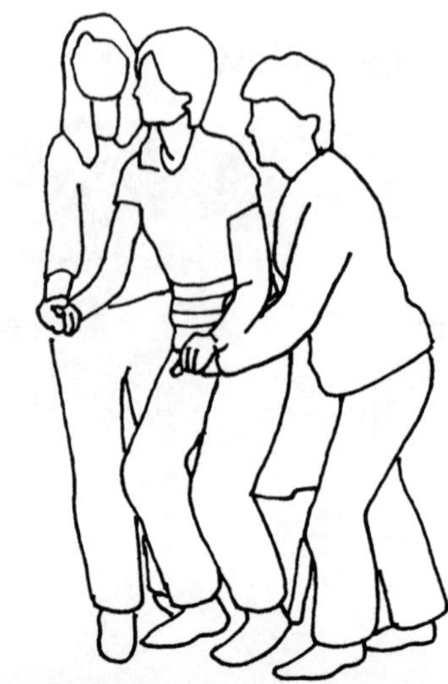
FIG12.3c

	forward pressure on the person's back and assists the normal movement into standing. • To complete the move the handlers should move their feet to stand at the side of the person. The handler should remember to transfer their weight from their rear foot to their front foot and utilise their own weight to guide the person forwards and upwards.	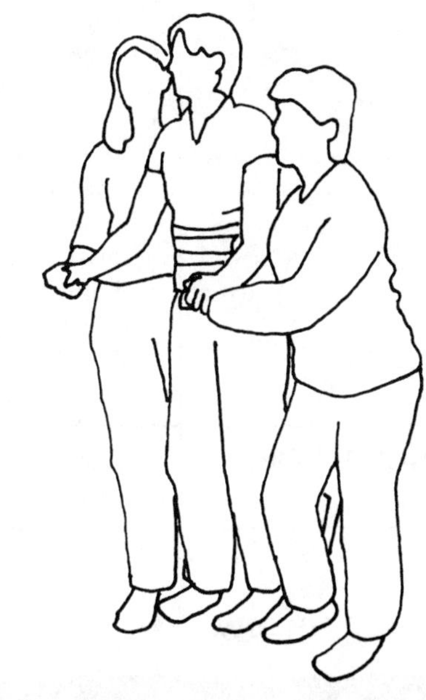 FIG12.3d
OPTIONS AND VARIATIONS	• This transfer may be carried out without the use of a handling belt. The handlers will stand at the side of the person and place their nearest arm across the person's back at around the level of the person's waist, ensuring good contact with the person and their forearm. The handlers should keep their hand open and not grasp the person or the person's clothing. • The handlers may wish to stand facing the person and transfer their weight 'sideways' when the person stands. The weight transfer should be from their foot nearest to the person's bottom towards the front of the chair.	
PERCEIVED EXERTION FOR HANDLER	• The person should be encouraged to be active during the movement. • There should be little to moderate physical exertion for the handlers. • Handlers should remember that they are to exert a forward and upward pressure for the person to bring himself or herself into standing, they are NOT TO LIFT with the belt. • It is important the handlers work at the speed of the person as carrying out the procedure too quickly or too slowly will not allow the person to be active during the transfer. • Clear commands should be given so the transfer is carried out in unison. • Achieving a kneeling position when assisting a person to the edge of the chair may be difficult for some handlers and therefore an alternative method should be found or equipment used. • The handler who is assisting the person to the edge of the chair should also be aware not to use upper body to pull the person forward, but lean back utilising their own body weight.	
COMFORT OF THE PERSON	• Handlers should take care when placing a belt around the waist of people with abdominal problems as it may cause discomfort. • People who are underweight (according to the BMI chart) who may find the belt 'digs' into their waist area. • Large people may find that the belt rises up towards their chest due to the shape of their waist area, in which case an alternative method, equipment should be sought.	
SKILL LEVEL OF HANDLER	• Handlers should have received basic manual handling training, be aware of assessment for persons who require the use of a belt and also have understanding of patterns of normal movement for sit to stand. • If they are assisting a person with a hemiparesis they should be aware of management of the stroke patient.	
EVIDENCE AVAILABLE	1 *Tarling C (1997)* in Fourth Edition to the Guide to the Handling of Patients. 2 *Hignett (2002)* states that there is moderate evidence from 5 studies that a walking belt should be used with two handlers for weight bearing persons to transfer them from a sitting position to another sitting position. 3 *(Back Care 1999)* Safer Handling of People in the Community. 4 *Garg et al (1991)* states that the walking (handling) belt would not work on those persons who cannot weight bear and those who are heavy, have contracture or confused. A two person technique with a walking (handling) belt was the preferred method out of the 5 different techniques evaluated.	

DANGERS/ PRECAUTIONS	• If person is unable to maintain weight on their feet or assist with the push into standing this will place too much strain onto the handlers. • Handlers should be aware to allow the person to sit back onto chair and not hold the weight of the person. • If the person has weakness on one side, the handlers should consider the method of assistance in order not to take the weight of the person leaning onto them. • The handling belt should be fitted firmly around the person's waist in order to prevent movement and sliding upward. It is advisable to use a handling belt with a choice of handles, which will accommodate different handler's reach. • Handlers should take care not to place their whole hand through the handle on the belt as this is likely to cause injury should the person move suddenly or fall back into the chair. • If this method is being used to assist the person to stand/sit in the toilet area, handlers should not try to support the person in standing whilst adjusting clothing. Either a third handler should be used or the choice should be to use a different technique utilising standing equipment.
FURTHER OPTIONS	This method would be appropriate for use to assist the person from a toilet seat, where there is sufficient space at the side of the toilet.

Evidence review

Technique	REBA	Activity	Comfort	FIM	Mobility gallery	Skill level	Comment
HELP WITH 2 HANDLERS FROM THE SIDE OF A CHAIR WITH HANDLING BELT							
Fig 12.3a	4	9	9	4	B	Advanced beginner	Analysis shows a twisted trunk, this can be reduced by altering foot position to be similar to Fig. 12.1a. Having 2 handlers does not appear to reduce the postural risk to the handlers in this scenario.

Task Three

Moving near to the edge of the seat (in preparation to stand from sitting)

DEPENDENCY LEVEL

Mobility Gallery C
FIM 4

- The person should be encouraged to move himself or herself through verbal guidance to move towards the edge of the chair and lean forwards to initiate the stand.
- If the person cannot move their bottom to the edge of the chair then one handler may assist them.
- The person should also have cognitive ability to understand and follow instructions from the handlers.
- The minimal physical requirements of the person are that he is able to lean his weight forwards and able to move his weight (with guidance and help) from side to side without falling over, the person requires trunk control and sitting balance.

DESCRIPTION

- The person leans forward in the seat and

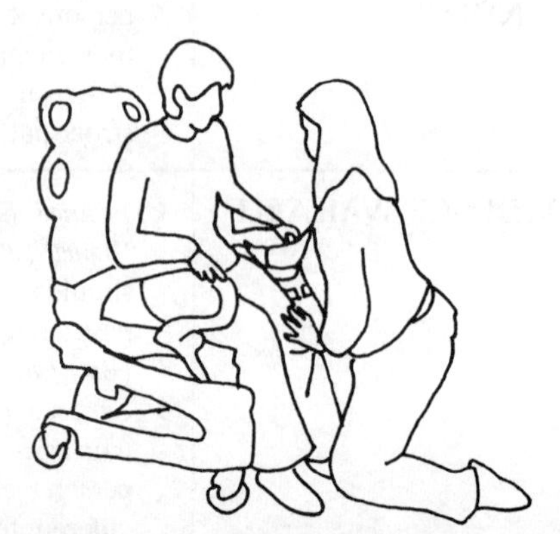

FIG 12.4a

takes hold of the arms of the chair (if possible with both hands or just one hand)
- The handler kneels in front of the person (on one knee). The person in the chair is asked to lean slightly forwards and to rock away from the side nearest the handler. The handler places one hand close to the person's hip and their other hand onto the front of the person's knee. As the person raises their weight off the seat the handler will exert a forward pressure against the person's hip, and a slight pressure to the person's knee, adducting the side raised off the seat to facilitate the forward movement of the thigh. This movement is repeated until the person is in the desired position closer to the edge of the seat.
- The handler places the handling belt around the person's waist and makes secure prior to the stand.

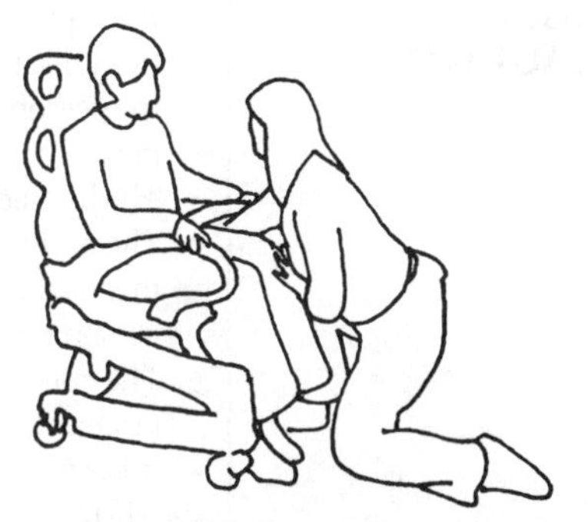

FIG 12.4b

OPTIONS AND VARIATIONS

- If the person requires excessive assistance then consideration must be given to a lifting chair or cushion to help push the person into standing without bringing them closer to the edge of the seat.

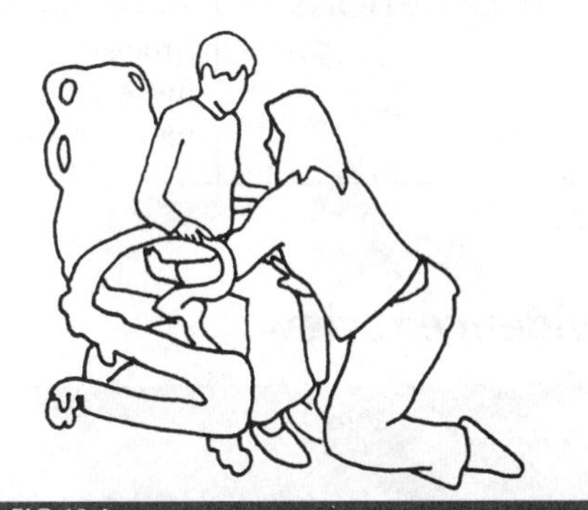

FIG 12.4c

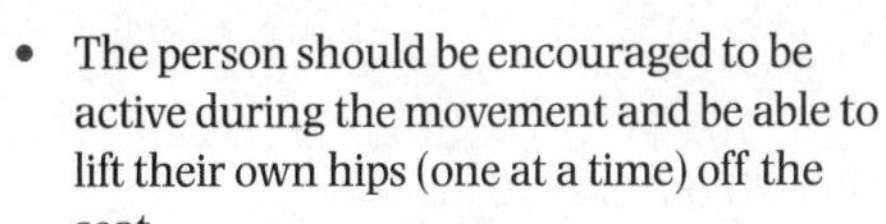

PERCEIVED EXERTION FOR HANDLER

- The person should be encouraged to be active during the movement and be able to lift their own hips (one at a time) off the seat.
- There should be little to moderate physical exertion for the handler.
- There should be a clear command so the transfer is carried out together.
- Achieving a kneeling position for some handlers may be difficult, hence a different method should be found or equipment used to assist the person into standing.
- The handler who is assisting the person to the edge of the chair should also be aware not to use their upper body to pull the person forward, but lean back utilising their own body weight.
- The handler should also not overstretch to reach around the person, as this stretching will place them at a biomechanical disadvantage.

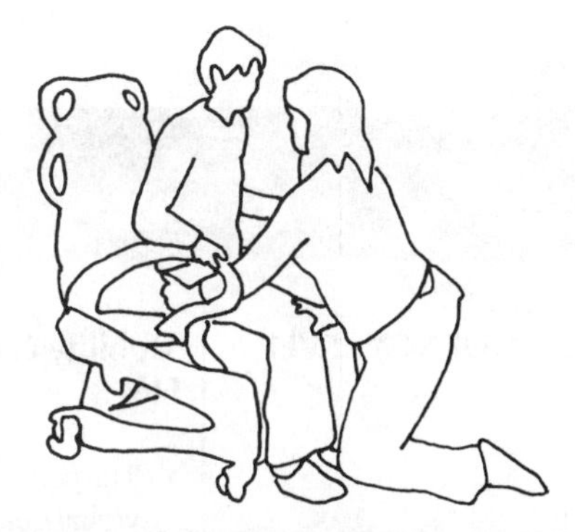

FIG 12.4d

COMFORT OF THE PERSON

- The movement should be carried out when the person indicates that they are ready to move, i.e. when they have lifted one hip off the seat of the chair.
- There should be no grasping of the person's hips or clothes. The handler should have their hands open but in good contact with the person's hips near to the back of the seat.

SKILL LEVEL OF HANDLER

- The handler should have received basic manual handling training, be aware of assessment for persons who require the use of a handling belt (if used), and also have understanding of patterns of normal movement for sit to stand and moving forward in the chair.
- If they are assisting a person with a hemiparesis they should be aware of management of the stroke patient.

EVIDENCE AVAILABLE

1 *Tarling C (1997/8)* in Fourth Edition of The Guide to the Handling of Patients.

DANGERS / PRECAUTIONS	• If the person is unable to maintain 'active' sitting balance and unable to move themselves from side to side without losing balance then equipment must be used for the STS transfer. If the person has no active sitting balance on a seat, the handler must question whether the person has the suitable skills to be assisted manually into standing. • The handler may be tempted to pull the person forward in one go – this must be avoided. • The handler may be tempted to use a handling sling to increase their reach, however this still means that the handler is working too far from themselves and may be tempted to pull the person forward. • The material of chair may prevent the movement forward in the seat – consider more appropriate seating. • If the person is sitting on a one way glide sheet to prevent slipping forward off the seat this will prevent this movement being performed within comfort levels for the handler and lead to excessive strain. • Some people have considered using a slide sheet to move the person forward, this is NOT advisable as the person may slide off the front of the seat. • The chair should also be suitable to accommodate the person leaning from side to side.
FURTHER OPTIONS	This method would normally be used to initiate the person to stand from an armchair. It is strongly advised that the type of seat being used is considered so the person can come forward in the seat themselves. This technique can be used in reverse to encourage a person to move back in the chair after sitting down or slipping forwards.

Evidence review

Technique	REBA	Activity	Comfort	FIM	Mobility gallery	Skill level	Comment
HELP WITH 2 HANDLERS FROM THE SIDE OF A CHAIR WITH HANDLING BELT							
Fig 12.4c	10	7	7	4	C	Advanced beginner	

Task Four

Sit to stand – help with one handler from the side of a bed without handling belt

DEPENDENCY LEVEL

Mobility Gallery B
FIM 3

- The person should be encouraged through verbal guidance to move towards the edge of the bed and lean forwards to initiate the stand.
- The person should also have cognitive ability to understand and follow instructions from the handler.
- The person must be able to place full weight on their feet and move their own feet into position (they should only require assistance to 'push' up into the standing position).
- The person must be able to maintain his or her own active sitting balance on the edge of the bed. Person should be able to maintain own balance when in full stand.

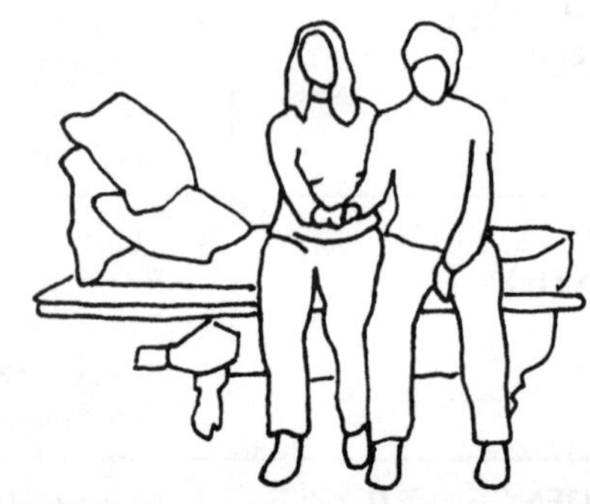

FIG 12.5a

DESCRIPTION OF TRANSFER

- The person supports himself or herself on the edge of the bed by placing his hands either side of him.
- The handler sits at one side of the person, so they are in contact with the person.
- The handler faces direction of movement and places their nearest arm to person around the person's back, ensuring good contact with person along their forearm.
- The other hand can be placed onto the front of the person's nearest shoulder for added support. If by doing this the handler feels they are twisting the handler can encourage the person to place their hand into the handler's free hand, using a palm to palm hold (avoiding holding each other's thumbs).
- The handler should sit with the farthest foot forward and near foot back slightly to provide the push into standing.
- Using commands, the person is directed to lift their own head and initiate the stand and at same time the handler places a forward pressure on the person's back and assists the normal movement into standing.
- To complete the move the handler should move both feet to stand at the side of the person. The handler should remember to transfer their weight from their rear foot to the front foot and utilise her own weight to facilitate the person forwards and upwards.

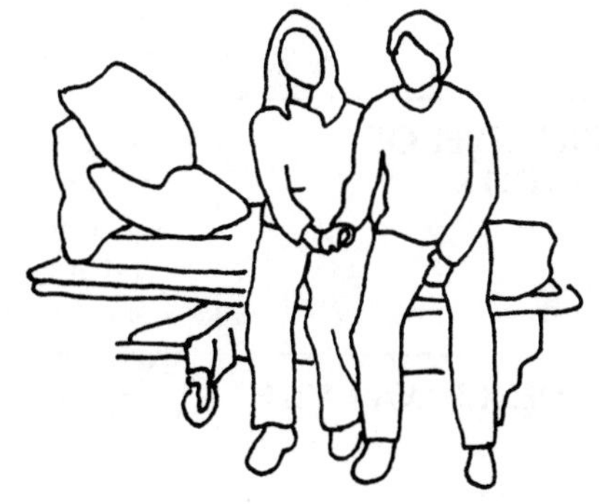

FIG 12.5b

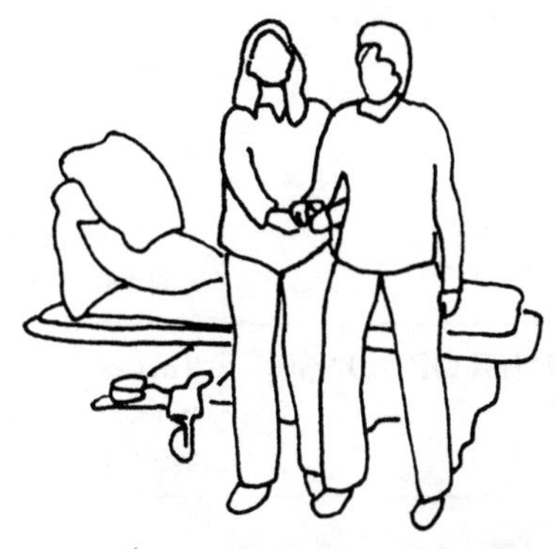

FIG 12.5c

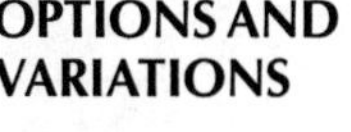

OPTIONS AND VARIATIONS

- This transfer may be carried out with the use of a handling belt. The handler will sit at the side of the person and place their nearest arm across the person's back at around the level of the person's waist, ensuring good contact with the person and their forearm and then grasp the handle of the belt in the middle of the person's back. The handlers should not place their whole hand through the handle/s on the belt, but only take a 'cylindrical' or 'power' hold of the handle.
- Additionally, a bed lever is a useful device which, when attached to the side of the bed, can assist a person in STS tasks both out of and on to the edge of the bed.

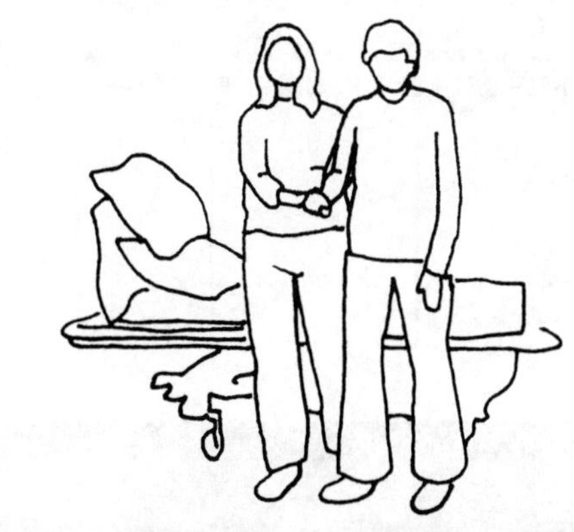

FIG 12.5d

PERCEIVED EXERTION FOR HANDLER

- The person should be encouraged to be active during the movement.
- There should be little physical exertion for the handler. The handler should remember that they are to exert a forward and upward pressure for the person to bring himself or herself into standing.
- It is important that the handlers work at the speed of the person carrying out the procedure, too quickly or too slowly will not allow the person to be active during the transfer. If the person is rushed this may lead to the handler taking undue physical strain.

COMFORT OF THE PERSON

- Handlers should take care when placing a belt around the waist of people with abdominal problems as it may cause discomfort.
- Also people who are underweight (according to the BMI chart) may find the belt 'digs' into their waist area. Large persons may find that the belt rises up towards their chest due to the

	shape of their waist area, in which case alternative methods and equipment should be considered.
SKILL LEVEL OF HANDLER	• Handlers should have received basic manual handling training, be aware of assessment for persons who require the use of a belt (if being used), and also have understanding of patterns of normal movement for sit to stand. • If they are assisting a person with hemiparesis (following a CVA) then they should be aware of management of the stroke patient.
EVIDENCE AVAILABLE	1 *Hignett (2002)* has limited evidence from one study that adjustable height beds should be used to assist a sitting to standing move from the side of the bed. 2 *Hignett (2002)* has moderate evidence from two studies that a walking belt should not be used with one handler for weight bearing persons.
DANGERS / PRECAUTIONS	• If the person is unable to maintain weight on their feet or assist with the push into standing this will place too much strain onto the handler, in addition this could be a sudden movement. The handler should be aware to guide the person back onto the bed and not hold the weight of the person. • If the person has weakness on one side, the handler should consider which side she is to stand so as not to take the full weight of the person leaning onto them. • The handling belt should be fitted firmly around the person's waist so as to prevent movement and sliding upward. • The handler should take care not to place their whole hand through the handle on the belt as this is likely to cause injury should the person move suddenly or fall back into the chair.
FURTHER OPTIONS	This method would be appropriate for use also on a variable height bed or treatment plinth where the height of the bed can be raised or lowered to 'grade' the activity in rehabilitation settings.

Evidence review

Technique	REBA	Activity	Comfort	FIM	Mobility gallery	Skill level	Comment
HELP WITH ONE HANDLER FROM THE SIDE OF A BED WITHOUT HANDLING BELT							
Fig 12.5a	7	9	9	4	B	Advanced beginner	From the side of the bed rather than chair appears to increase the postural risk without affecting the person

Task Five

Sit to stand – help with one handler from the side of a bed with a standing device

DEPENDENCY LEVEL

Mobility Gallery B
FIM 3

- The person should be encouraged to move himself or herself through verbal guidance to move towards the edge of the chair and lean forwards to initiate the stand.
- The person should also have sufficient cognitive ability to understand and follow instructions from the handler.
- The person must be able to place full weight on their feet and move their own

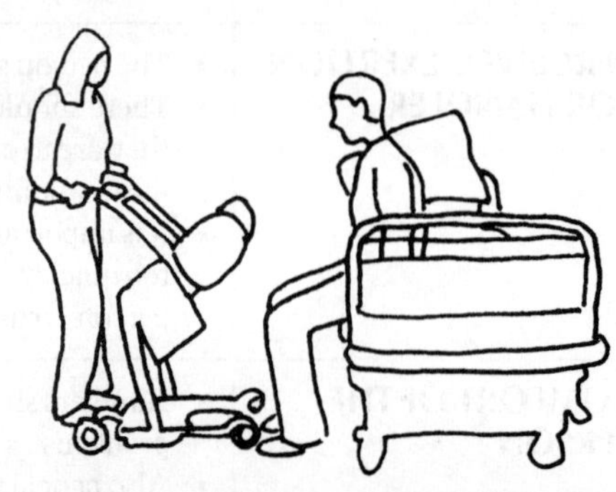

FIG 12.6a

	feet into position. The person should be able to maintain own balance when in full stand, but perhaps has difficulty in walking distances. • The person should be able to place both feet onto the foot platform, and hold onto the handle of the equipment. • The person should have good upper body strength and have adequate grasp to be able to hold onto and pull themselves up into standing.	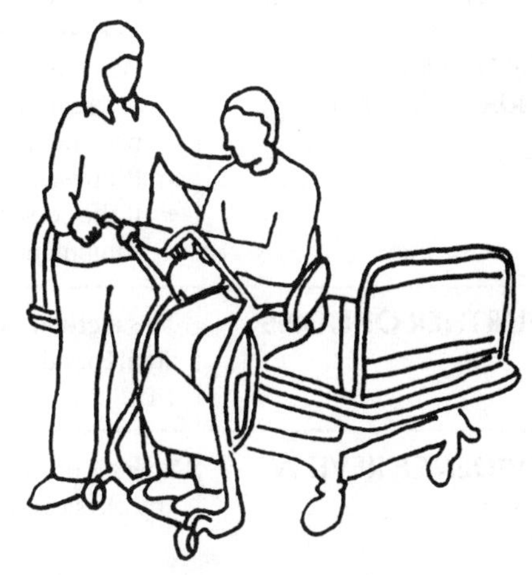 FIG 12.6b
DESCRIPTION OF TRANSFER	• The person brings their bottom close to the edge of the seat. • The person leans forward in the seat. • The handler brings in the equipment in front of the person and asks the person to lift their feet onto the platform. (If the person is unable to lift their feet onto the platform the handler should question this technique and whether a more assistive piece of equipment is required.) • The handler ensures the person's feet are fully on the platform and locks the brakes to stop the equipment from moving away from the person. • Using commands, the person is directed to hold onto the handle of the device and, whilst leaning forward, pull themselves into standing, lifting their own head to initiate the stand. • The handler, whilst standing at the side of the person, may wish to place a reassuring hand onto the person's back, only to communicate the need to move into standing. • When the person is in full standing the handler should drop down the seat flaps and instruct the person to perch themselves onto the seat. • The handler may wish to use a sheepskin sling to go around the person's back to provide additional support when transporting – however this is optional.	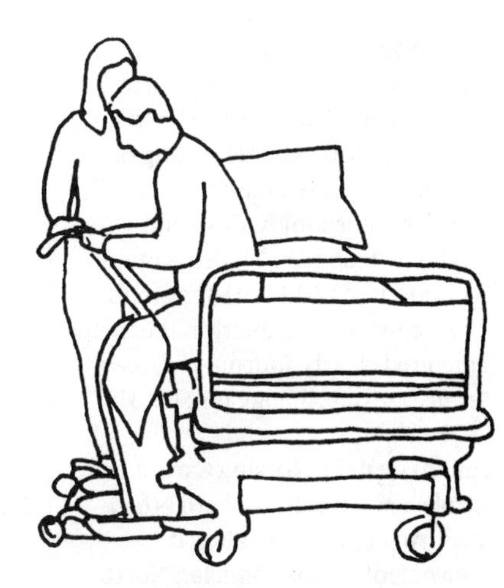 FIG 12.6c
OPTIONS AND VARIATIONS	• The device may be used in a variety of settings, such as the toilet area, shower, off the side of the bed or plinth, or any situation which involves the need for STS transfer.	
PERCEIVED EXERTION FOR HANDLER	• The person should be encouraged to be fully active during the movement. • There should be no physical exertion for the handler. • The handler should work with the person as a team and be aware not to hurry the person and assist or lift them into standing.	
COMFORT OF THE PERSON	• The method should be very comfortable to person, as the task is being carried out in the person's own time with no physical assistance. • Handlers should take care when placing a belt around the waist of people with abdominal problems as it may cause discomfort.	
SKILL LEVEL OF HANDLER	• The handler should have received basic manual handling training. The handler should also be aware of assessment for people who require the use of such a standing device and also have an understanding of patterns of normal movement for sit to stand. • If they are assisting persons with hemiparesis (following a CVA) then they should be aware of management of the stroke patient.	

EVIDENCE AVAILABLE	None found
DANGERS/ PRECAUTIONS	• When handling people with knee problems (arthritis, replacement etc) the handler should be aware that the use of the standing device requires the person's knees pressing against a knee pad and hence should be used with caution. • People with balance problems may find the movement of the device unnerving. • If the person requires assistance to stand (i.e. lift their bottom off the seat) then alternative equipment, i.e. a stand aid hoist should be used.
FURTHER OPTIONS	This method would be appropriate to assist the person from a toilet seat, bedside, plinth, shower area. For additional STS techniques using equipment please also see tasks 8, 9 and 10 in chapter 14.
EVIDENCE REVIEW	There is no evidence review for this task as the person's use of this equipment does not require any physical assistance from the handler.

References

Alexander NB, Scultz AB, Warwick DN (1991). Rising from a chair: effects of age and functional ability on performance biomechanics. Journal of Gerontology May;46(3):91–98

BackCare (1999). Safer Handling of People in the Community

Bernardi M, Rosponi A, Castellano V, Rodio A, Traballesi M, Delussu AS, Marchetti M (2004). Determinants of sit-to-stand capability in the motor impaired elderly. Journal of Electromyogr Kinesiology Jun;14(3): 401–10

Borgman (1991). Nursing Care of the stroke person using bobath principles. An approach to altered movement. Nurse Clinician North America Dec; 26(4):1019–35

Brunt D, Greenberg B, Wankadia S, Trimble MA, Shechtman O (2002). The effect of foot placement on sit to stand in healthy young subjects and persons with hemiplegia, Archive of Physical Medical Rehabilitation Jul;83(7):924–9

Busse M (2000). Access to appropriate hoisting equipment can be essential for effective rehabilitation: a case study, Nursing and Residential Care 2(4):168–73

Chartered Society of Physiotherapy (2002). Guidance in Manual Handling for Chartered Physiotherapists

Cheng PT, Liaw MY, Wong MK, Tang FT, Lee MY, Lin PS (1998). The sit-to-stand movement in stroke persons and its correlation with falling. Archive of Physical Medical Rehabilitation Sep;79(9):1043–6

Edlich RF, Heather CL, Galumbeck MH (2003). Revolutionary advances in adaptive seating systems for the elderly and persons with disabilities that assist sit-to-stand transfers. Journal of Long Term Effects of Medical Implants 13(1):31–9

Edwards (1996). Neurological Physiotherapy, A Problem Solving Approach. Churchill Livingstone. London

Eng JJ, Levins SM, Townson AF, Mah-Jones D, Bremner J, Huston G (2001). Use of prolonged standing for individuals with spinal cord injuries. Physical Therapy Aug;81(8):1392–9

Eriksrud O, Bohannon RW (2003). Relationship of knee extension force to independence in sit-to-stand performance in persons receiving acute rehabilitation. Physical Therapy Jun;83(6):544–51

Gagnon M, Sicard, Sirios J (1986). An evaluation of forces on the lumbo-sacral joint and assessment of work and energy transfers in nursing aides lifting persons. Ergonomics 29(3):407–21

Galli M, Crivellini M, Sibella F, Montesano A, Bertocco P, Parisio (2000). Sit-to-stand movement analysis in obese subjects. International Journal of Obesity and Related Metabolic Disorders Nov;24(11):1488–92

Gerdhem P, Ringsberg KA, Akesson K, Obrant KJ (2003). Influence of muscle strength, physical activity and weight on bone mass in a population-based sample of 1004 elderly women. Osteoporosis International Sep;14(9):768–72

Hennington G, Johnson J, Penrose J, Barr K, McMuklin ML, Vander Linden DW (2004). Effect of bench height on sit-to-stand in children without disabilities and children with cerebral palsy. Archive of Physical and Medical Rehabilitation. Jan;85(1);70–6

Hignett S (2003). Intervention strategies to reduce musculoskeletal injuries associated with handling persons: a systematic review. Occupational and Environmental Medicine. Sep;60(9)

Hignett S, Crumpton E, Ruszala S, Alexander P, Fray M, Fletcher B (2003). Evidence-Based Person Handling. Tasks, equipment and interventions. Routledge. London

Hughes MA, Myers BS, Schenkman ML (1996). The role of strength in rising from a chair in the functionally impaired elderly. Journal of Biomechanics Dec;29(12):1509–13

Janssen WG, Bussmann HB, Stam HJ (2002). Determinants of the sit-to-stand movement: a review. Physical Therapy Sep;82(9):866–79. Review

Keir PJ, MacDonell CW (2004). Muscle activity during person transfers: a preliminary study on the influence of lift assists and experience. Ergonomics Feb 26;47(3):296–306

Knibbe H (2000). Prevention of incontinence in nursing homes. A descriptive study into the possibilities for improving the continence policy in nursing homes

Marras WS, Davis KG, Kirking BC, Bertsche PK (1999). A comprehensive analysis of low-back disorder risk and spinal loading during he transferring and repositioning of persons using different techniques.

Ergonomics Jul;42(7):904–26
Medical Devices Agency (1999). Electric Riser Seats and Chairs. A comparative evaluation. EL2.
Medical Devices Agency (2002). Chair and Bed Raisers. An evaluation. MDA 02117. EL10
Millington PJ, Myklebust BM, Shambes GM (1992). Biomechanical analysis of the sit-to-stand motion in elderly persons. Archive of Physical Medical Rehabilitation Jul;73(7):609–17
Mutch K (2004). Changing manual-handling practice in a stroke rehabilitation unit. Professional Nurse Mar;19(7):374–8
Monger C, Carr JH, Fowler V (2002). Evaluation of a home-based exercise and training programme to improve sit-to-stand in persons with chronic stroke. Clinical Rehabilitation. Jun;16(4): 361–7
National Back Exchange, Essex Group (1996). Paediatric Moving and Handling. Report on Workshops
National Back Pain Association (1997). Fourth Edition to the Guide to the Handling of Persons. Royal College of Nursing
O'Dwyer N, Ada L, Neilson PD. Spasticity and muscle contracture following stroke. Brain
Pheasant S (2001). Bodyspace. Anthropometry, Ergonomics and the Design of Work (Second Edition). Taylor and Francis, London
Ramsey VK, Miszko TA, Horvat M (2004). Muscle activation and force production in Parkinson's persons during sit to stand transfers. Clinical Biomechanics (Bristol, Avon). May;19(4):377–84
Riley PO, Krebs DE, Popat RA (1997). Biomechanical analysis of failed sit-to-stand. IEEE Trans Rehabilitation Eng. Dec;5(4):353–9
Royal College of Nursing (1996). Hazards of Nursing, personal injuries at work (000692)
Ruszala S (2001). An evaluation of equipment to assist person sit-to-stand activities in physiotherapy'. Unpublished MSc dissertation, University of Wales: School of Health Care Studies
Sander R (2002). Standing and moving: helping people with vascular dementia. Nursing Older People. Vol 14 no1 2002
Sibella F, Galli M, Romei M, Montaseno A, Crivellini M (2003). Biomechanical analysis of sit-to-stand movement in normal and obese subjects. Clinical Biomechanics Oct;18(8):745–50
Staats PGM, Tak E, Hopman-rock M (1998). Nature, degree and treatment for involuntary loss of urine in care homes, an attempt towards a protocol, TNO-PG, Leiden
Tarling C. in National Back Pain Association (1997/8). Fourth Edition to the Guide to the Handling of Persons. Royal College of Nursing
Trew M, Everett T (2001). Human Movement (Fourth Edition). Churchill Livingstone. London
Turner A, Foster M, Johnson SE (2002). Occupational Therapy and Physical Dysfunction. Fifth Edition. Churchill Livingstone. London
Tyldsley B, Greive JI (2003). Muscles, Nerves and Movement in Human Occupation (Third Edition). Blackwell Publishing. Oxford
Vander Linden DW, Brunt D, McCulloch MU (1994). Variant and invariant characteristics of the sit-to-stand task in healthy elderly adults. Archive of Physical and Medical Rehabilitation Jun;75(6):653–60
Walter JS, Sola PG, Sacks J, Lucero Y, Langbein E, Weaver F (1999). Indications for a home standing program for individuals with spinal cord injury. Journal of Spinal Cord Medicine Fall;22(3):152–8
Weiner DK, Long R, Hughes MA, Chandeler J, Studenski S (1993). When older adults face the chair-rise challenge. Journal of American Geriatrics Society. Jan;41(12): 1429–34
Yassi A, Cooper JE, Tate RB, Gerlach S, Muir M, Trottier J, Massey K (2001). A randomized controlled trial to prevent person lift and transfer injuries of health care workers. Spine Aug 15;26(16):1739–46
Yip Y (2001). A study of work stress, person handling activities and the risk of low back pain among nurses in Hong Kong. Journal of Advanced Nursing Dec;36(6):794–804

13

Assisted walking

Sara Thomas DipCOT PGD SROT
Consultant Back Care Adviser

1 Introduction

Walking is an action, which enables individuals to achieve daily living activities. It is thought to contribute to the maintenance of bone density, joint function, muscular strength, cardiovascular fitness and also psychological well being. It is also a leisure activity enjoyed by a large percentage of the population, from a walk in the park to a coast to coast ramble. The ability to walk allows people to be engaged in many areas of daily living and social interaction. Many public areas, which have not been adapted for wheelchairs, remain inaccessible to those who are unable to rise from a seat and walk. (Hopefully, this will change as a result of the full implementation, in October 2004, of the Disability Discrimination Act 1995 and the requirement for public places to be accessible to those with a sensory or physical disability).

Walking can be described as the use of repetitive muscular actions to achieve a progressive forward upright movement of the whole body. It is a complex muscular and cognitive (usually unconscious) task. The typical walking cycle involves repetitive concentric and eccentric muscle actions of pelvis, trunk, shoulder girdle and the lower limbs with periods of single and double support, i.e. when one or both feet are on the ground. Such a walking cycle requires that the individual is able to balance during all movements as well as change direction to avoid obstacles and even walk backwards to negotiate the environment in which they live *(Tyldesley and Grieve, 2002)*.

2 Difficulties with walking

The factors impacting on the inability to walk are numerous, and are not always associated with perhaps the most obvious causes such as the lack of muscle strength or joint range. People with balance and/or proprioceptive problems (inability to feel the position of their body/limbs), brain injury or disease, fear of falling, lack of confidence etc. can all experience difficulty with aspects of walking. *Finnie (2000)* suggests that the new born baby makes 'splendid stepping actions', however, the reason he or she does not walk, and falls if unsupported, is due to an inability to balance. Independent walking can only begin when balance reactions (which emerge between 6 to 10 months) have started to develop (see also chapter 6).

Many disabling conditions, for example multiple sclerosis, Parkinson's disease, dementia, cerebral palsy, and arthritis in its various forms affect the ability to walk independently and in some severe cases effect the ability of the person to take weight on their feet at all. The normal ageing process also affects walking patterns and ability. *Koller et al (1985)* estimates that around 15% of elderly people experience problems with walking with no specific diagnostic cause.

Jones and Barker (2002) have identified a number of age related changes in walking, typically occurring between 60 and 70 years of age, with some of the changes occurring as a result of attempting to increase stability:

- shorter step and stride lengths than younger people.
- lower average walking speeds.
- greater variation in stride width.
- wider base of support.

Jones and Barker (2002) suggest that there are features of 'normal walking' in relation to children, which may also effect the way in which assistance is provided. In children, contact with the ground is made with a flat foot (until 2 years of age); the base is wider and there is no reciprocal arm swing (until approximately 4 years of age); stride length and speed is less than in adults; the number of steps per minute are less and there is reduced knee flexion in the stance phase.

The gait differences in adults and children must be considered when the person requires assistance in walking. For example, a fit and healthy handler may not fully appreciate the needs of the person requiring help and may attempt to assist the person to walk at the handler's individual manner and speed.

Each individual has their own pattern of walking due to personal factors such as height, leg length, joint range of movement, previous injuries, pain etc.

Even a person's intention and mood may influence the way in which they walk. Consider for example, that you may often recognise a person at a distance from their stature and the way in which they walk long before you have visual cues from their facial features. Walking in step with another person is a difficult task due to these personal differences, tall people for example will take long strides and shorter individuals will take smaller (and quicker) strides. These personal factors may be contributory to the reported physical difficulties and number of incidences of back and upper limb injuries occurring during assisted walking.

3 Assisted walking

Maintaining mobility and preventing the associated physiological and psychological effects of immobility is a desirable outcome within any health and social care setting. *Cheng et al (1998)* suggest that rising, sitting down and walking are among the most common activities in daily life. Hence, assisting people to walk is likely to be one of the most common tasks undertaken by care and rehabilitation staff in a wide variety of settings. A *Royal College of Nursing (RCN) (1996)* study reported that 91% of patients involved in accidents reported by nursing staff, were unable to walk without assistance (other than with a walking aid such as a stick or frame).

Love (1996) found that twice as many accidents occurred when assisting the patient to mobilise than when the patient was in bed. The *RCN (1996)* found that half of all lifting/handling accidents occurred whilst nurses were carrying out one of only three manoeuvres, the shoulder lift, the orthodox lift and providing support in walking. A more recent study by *Yip (2001)* lists assisted walking as one of the four most common activities putting nurses at risk of low back pain.

To date a number of legal cases have been brought forward as a result of a physical injury to a handler when assisting a person to walk *(Bayley v Bloomsbury Health Authority, Hadfield v Manchester Health Authority, Stainton v Chorley and South Ribble NHS Trust)* in *Mandalstam (2002)*. Such cases highlight the apparent danger to handlers when assisting people with walking, and specifically in respect of attempting to support the person if they fall (see chapter 17 for the management of such situations). Indeed, recent professional guidelines such as those produced by the *Derbyshire Interagency Group (DIAG, 2003)* advise that:

'a person who is at significant risk of falls should not be supported manually in walking'

Professional guidelines have provided handlers with advice regarding assisting people to walk for a number of years, *(NBPA 1992, NBPA 1997, BackCare 1999, DIAG 2003)*. There have been a number of generally accepted methods of providing such help by using handling/walking belts with one or two handlers, the use of specific handholds and the use of more assistive equipment such as walking harnesses and hoists. However, *Hignett (2003)* and *Hignett et al (2003)* state that the lack of research found relating to patient handling in standing is of particular concern, with no research literature being found to support the existing professional guidelines.

Evidence shows that providing manual assistance in walking is a hazardous activity for handlers, hence the person should be encouraged primarily to maintain 'modified independence,' that is, independence with equipment, according to the Functional Independence Measure (see chapter 11 for further information). If manual assistance is required then the handler should be aware of the 'normal patterns' of movement during walking *(Turner et al, 2002)*, and should also be aware of methods of providing appropriate assistance without lifting or carrying the weight of the person. It is also recommended that the handler be aware of strategies appropriate for the individual they are assisting and what to do if the person is unable to continue supporting their own weight *(NBPA 1997, BackCare 1999, DIAG 2003)* also see chapter 17.

4 Walking aids

In many cases the provision of an appropriate walking aid will enable a person to maintain their independence in walking. The use of a walking aid will assist the person by improving balance and stability, improving confidence in walking as well as assisting with general weakness of the lower limbs. A walking aid will transfer some of the weight off the legs onto the upper limbs, and may therefore also relieve some weight from a painful limb(s). Handrails are also extremely helpful for those with difficulties in walking, especially on slopes or ramps. In some instances, an appropriate height handrail on a wall will provide sufficient support for the person to continue with independent walking (in addition to or instead of a walking aid).

There are many types of walking aid including sticks, crutches, elbow crutches, quadrupods, walking frames, rollators and three-wheeled walkers. The type of walking aid chosen will depend on the age of the user, their disability and general physical condition, and the duration for which the walking aid is to be used. *Laufer (2003)* found that the use of a quad cane appeared to be more effective than a standard cane in reducing postural sway in people with moderate impairment following a stroke (CVA). In general it is recognised that walking sticks provide the least support, and are suitable for people who have good upper limb use and good grip. Walking frames are considered to provide the greatest support as they have the largest base, hence are commonly used for the elderly or younger individuals immediately following surgery or children with neurological or musculoskeletal dysfunction *(Jones and Barker, 2002)*. *Yohannes and Connolly (2003)* found that the use of a gutter frame reduced the functional disability in older people following hospital admission with acute chronic obstructive pulmonary disease.

Children who require support in walking may use wheeled walkers (David Hart type walkers) which support their body weight and enable the child to maintain a standing position, thus promoting function in standing and enhancing social integration with peers.

Prescription of any walking aid must be undertaken by a suitably qualified individual who is aware of the personal requirements and guidelines for measurement in addition to the benefits and attributes of the different types of walking devices.

Many authors propose that one of the most important factors in the prescription of a walking aid is the height of the equipment in relation to the user *(Turner et al 2002, Oddy 2003, Jones and Barker 2002, Tyldsey and Greive 2002)*.

The height of the walking aid will vary depending on the reason for use, e.g. a walking aid that is prescribed to reduce weight bearing on a painful limb will be shorter than one prescribed to improve balance. *Mulley (1988)* produced guidelines, which are now generally adopted by therapists and people who prescribe walking aids. Mulley suggested that the walking aid should measure to the ulnar styloid (the prominent bone in the side of the wrist) of the person who is standing erect with their shoulders relaxed and the elbow(s) flexed to 15°. A walking aid that is too short will result in the person leaning forwards in spinal flexion during walking, and an aid which is too long will result in the user elevating their shoulders, thus reducing stability and comfort.

People may have difficulty with walking as a result of a sensory impairment. Ensuring corridors and stairwells are well lit, flooring is secure and free of obstacles and using coloured strips on stair nosings (the edges of the steps), will assist the individual to negotiate their environment with or without a walking aid, independently and in safety.

5 Manual assistance during walking

Tappen et al (2000) found that when assisting people with Alzheimer's disease, the combined use of manual assisted walking and conversation can contribute to maintenance of functional mobility. However, there will be occasions when the person may require more than verbal guidance and the use of a walking aid to mobilise.

Manual assistance may be required from a handler in addition to (or instead of) the use of a walking aid within the care environment or during rehabilitation. Providing manual assistance requires careful assessment and, due to the extent of the known risk should only be undertaken by a suitably trained and experienced handler.

The Derbyshire Inter-agency Group (2003) suggest the assessment may include the following criteria prior to assisting a person to walk:

- trunk and upper limb control
- co-operation and comprehension
- appropriate balance and control
- asymmetrical posture or shape, or uneven effort
- appropriate footwear/orthotics
- walking aids
- stamina and distance capabilities and route
- attachments, i.e. catheter
- medical complications
- floor surface and slipping/tripping hazards

although additional factors may be relevant in specific situations.

When providing physical assistance handlers must be aware of providing the appropriate amount of assistance. Too little, and the person will not be supported adequately, too much, and the handlers are at risk of 'carrying' the person, posing a high risk of injury, both to the handler and the person being assisted.

Handlers should continuously use appropriate verbal instructions (wording and tone of voice), and guidance to encourage the person to be as independent as possible. Cues such as 'look ahead', 'head up', 'shoulders back' etc may provide enough guidance and stimulation to enable the person to stand and walk the required distance. *Oddy (2003)* suggests providing 'positive instructions', specifically when working with people with dementia. For example, rather than instructing a person 'not to sit down', instruct them to 'stand up' or 'stay standing'. She suggests that such positive commands are much more likely to produce the desired results.

Some handlers may choose to use equipment to assist them to gain a secure hold onto the person, such as a handling belt (see figure 13.1). Handles on the belt are positioned so that the handler does not have to hold onto the persons clothing or directly onto their body. Handlers are advised not to place their full hand through the handle of the belt as this will prevent the release of their hold of the person in the event of a sudden movement *(NBPA, 1997)*. Some professional guidelines do not advise the use of handling belts *(DIAG 2003)* possibly for such a reason.

Handling belt

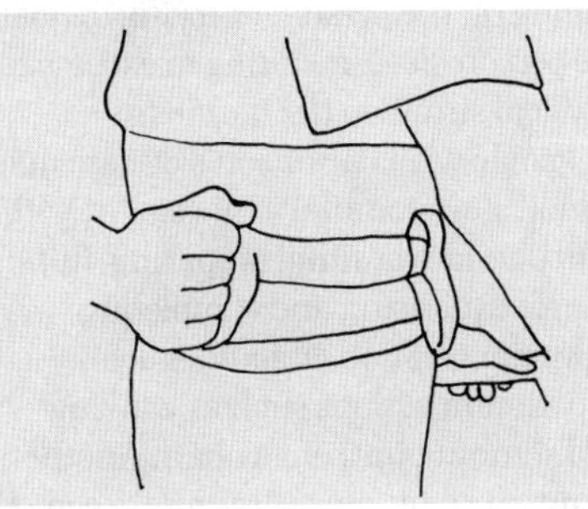

Figure 13.1 When using a handling belt, the handler must always take care not to exert a lifting force and must not attempt to hold the person off the floor should they be unable to continue holding their own weight. The handling belt should never be worn by the handler for the person requiring support to hold on to.

The *NBPA (1997), BackCare (1999)* and *HSE (2001)* have advocated the use of handling belts to provide support in walking. However, all manufacturers and suppliers provide warnings regarding inappropriate use and advise handlers to undertake a specific risk assessment in respect of the weight bearing ability of the person and other relevant factors. For instance, handlers should also be aware that using a walking belt with a confused individual may provide the person with the feeling of total support, hence they may lean heavily onto the handler or pull away suddenly, thus increasing the risk of injury to the handler.

The use of handling/walking belts has been advocated during chair to chair transfers, *(Garg et al 1991, Hignett et al 2003* – see also chapter 14*)*. Currently there does not appear to be any research evidence in respect of the use and efficacy of handling belts for mobilising people.

In conjunction with the use of a walking belt, handlers may also wish to hold onto the person's hand or nearside forearm providing good contact, and additional guidance and support for the person. No evidence was found relating to the use of specific handholds, however, professional texts have provided us with a number of different handholds (figures 13.2a, b and c) to consider, subject to an adequate risk assessment *(NBPA 1997, BackCare 1999, HSE 2001, Oddy 2003)*.

Palm to palm avoiding thumb hold

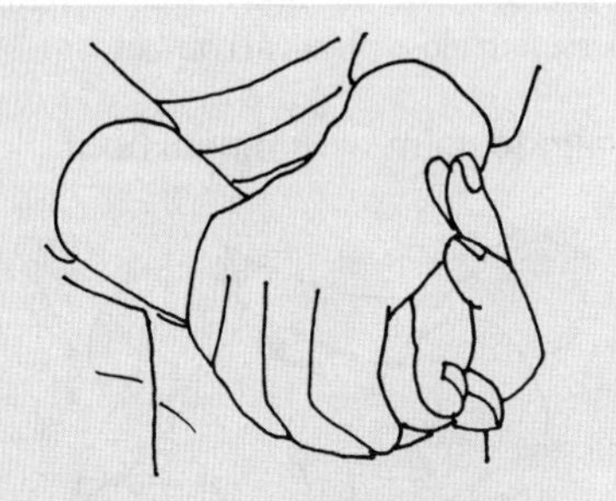

Figure 13.2a This handhold provides support for the person by allowing them to place their adjacent hand into the palm of the handler. Should the person try to grip the handler too tightly then this hold allows the handler to release their hand by bringing their hand towards their body in a downwards direction.

Palm and forearm support

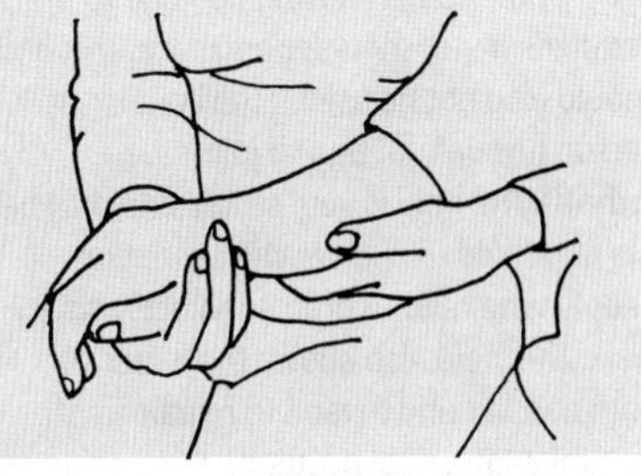

Figure 13.2b This handhold may be used for individuals who are a degree taller than the handler or who have poor grip or painful wrists or hands. The handler 'cupping' the forearm just below the elbow provides some of the support. Handlers should be aware not to grip the person's elbow as this may cause skin damage and bruising. Under no circumstances must the handler's forearm be allowed to rise above the elbow or into the person's axilla, even if the person falls. A variation of this method of holding is for the handler to 'cup' the person's nearest forearm in their furthest hand as described by *DIAG (2003)*.

Oddy (2003) describes a technique for assisting people to walk that involves the handler holding both hands of the person and walking backwards. Oddy calls this technique 'towing' and strongly advises against its use, particularly for people with dementia. Walking backwards can be extremely dangerous for the handler and for people with dementia, the use of this method may result in the person leaning backwards and resisting forward movement. In such circumstances *Oddy* recommends walking in unison with the person. This involves walking to one side and in step with the person in close physical contact.

Palm to palm with thumb hold

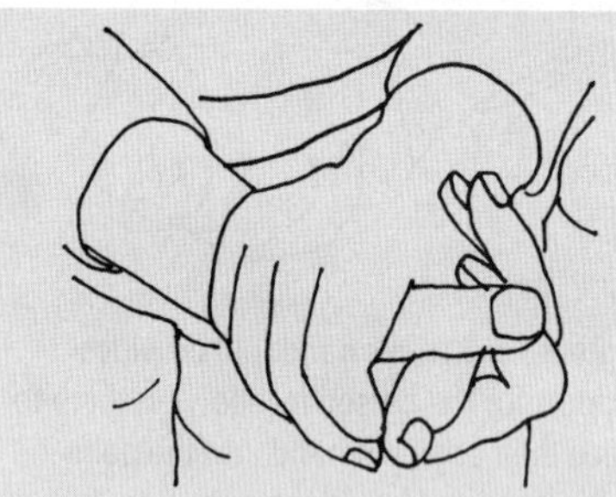

Figure 13.2c Caution must be exercised with the use of this handhold as it does not allow the handler to release her grip quickly in the event of the person losing balance or falling to the ground. In such an instance the person may try to grip the handler tightly, potentially causing damage to the handler's hand, shoulder and back. This hold should also not be used if the handler or person has painful thumb joints, i.e. arthritis. The hold is very secure and may be the handhold of choice when assisting people who tend to grab at objects as they walk. This hold also allows the hands of both handler and person to remain in a natural anatomical position.

Assisting people with specific needs

Rather than the generic prescription of standard methods of handling, every person should be treated as an individual and should receive assistance appropriate to their functional level. Knowledge of specific symptoms of common conditions may assist handlers provide more appropriate guidance and support when mobilising people.

Managing people who lean onto the handler

Some people may lean heavily (often backwards or onto the handler) when being assisted to walk. In such a case the handler should consider the benefit of assisting the person to walk with an additional handler, or consider whether more supportive equipment should be used, such as a hoist and walking jacket, see task three. Sometimes it is the method of assistance used by the handler that allows the person to lean towards or away from them. In such instances extreme care should be taken when considering the use of a walking belt as this may involve the handler pulling on the person, or trying to hold the person close, resulting in excessive physical strain on the handler.

People with Parkinson's disease may exhibit slow voluntary movement with difficulty in planning, preparing, initiating, sequencing and completing movements. Such difficulties are apparent in actions such as walking and standing up from a chair. Another common symptom is 'freezing', seen where a person stops and reports feeling as though their feet are stuck to the ground. People with Parkinson's often walk with small shuffling steps and their body leaning forward as if about to topple over. *Mutch (1986)* cited in *Turner et al (2003)* found that 78% of people with Parkinson's reported slowness in walking, 66% shuffling and stooping when walking and 65% had difficulty starting movements. Assisting a person with such symptoms can be physically challenging for the handler who will need to employ special techniques to assist with the person's mobility. Walking in unison with the person and pausing for a moment when the person stops (rather than pulling them forward) may assist the task. Walking can also be initiated by urging the person to lift one foot as if to climb a step or providing a visual cue such as the handler raising his or her foot as if to step.

People who have suffered a cerebrovascular accident (CVA or Stroke) may also require assistance in walking. *Moseley et al (2003)* suggest that approximately one third of people who survive an acute stroke are unable to walk three months after admission to a general hospital, and the inability or impaired ability to walk after a stroke is a significant contributor to long term disability. Commonly, people who have had a stroke have decreased walking speed, take smaller strides, have poor coordination, are not able to maintain weight bearing on the affected side for as long as the non affected side, and they may also tend to 'hitch' their affected hip. Handlers who are assisting people to walk with this condition should take these limitations into account. Methods of holding should consider the possible weakness of muscles and pain in limbs, for example around the shoulder. *Marras et al (1999)* found that the use of a handling/walking belt for a two handler transfer only reduced the spinal loading for the handler on the right side of the person, while the handler on the left side of the person had the same loading equivalent to a single person transfer. Such research indicates why perhaps the prescriptive advice regarding the side on which to stand (of a person who has had a stroke) is so inappropriate and instead it should be based on individual circumstances and person factors. Handlers should also position themselves sufficiently close to the person and on the side of the person assessed as appropriate in order to provide adequate assistance.

Assistance in walking may be given to both adults and children. When assisting adults, the adult handler can maintain an upright posture. Providing assistance to children or to individuals of a different stature to the handler presents additional problems, specifically the static load on the spine due to maintained, stooped posture, at the same time as providing some support. Using wheeled therapy stools may be one way of combating such postural strain. *Cromie et al (2000)* described equipment used by therapists to reduce strain on their body while working and reported that 45.3% of therapists used a wheelie stool and 16% used handling belts. Handlers should however be warned that assisted walking undertaken by a handler in sitting, places the handler at a biomechanical disadvantage. In such an instance the handler will only able to use their upper limbs and will have a tendency to work away from their body to accommodate the position of their knees in front. Conversely, if the handler is a great deal shorter than the person who is being assisted to walk then this may involve overstretching and taking excessive physical load. If this is the case, then the handler is advised not to undertake the task and to find the person alternative assistance.

The task of assisting people to walk is carried out in a variety of settings and with a number of different objectives. Assisting a person to mobilise to gain access to the toilet/bathroom/ sitting room is a commonly performed task by handlers within a care establishment. This type of assistance may be required on a frequent basis, and at a time when the person may not be concentrating on the task of walking but instead, on the reason why they are mobilising, i.e. they require to go to the toilet. If the person feels they need to go to the toilet urgently and requires manual assistance it may be wise to take them in a wheelchair and allow them to be assisted back when they are able to concentrate on the task in hand. Consideration should also be given to issues such as the time of day in which the person is being assisted.

Rehabilitation and assisted walking

Walking with assistance may be undertaken to enable the person to regain balance or improve active walking ability. *The Chartered Society of Physiotherapy (CSP) (2002)* defines the aim of rehabilitation handling as:

> *The encouraging of patients to move themselves or being allowed the opportunity to actively contribute to their own movement.*

Therapists and handlers undertaking physical handling as part of their treatment with an individual should heed accident statistics and trends and also research such as that carried out by *Cromie et al (2000)*. Results showed a 91% lifetime prevalence of musculoskeletal injuries in physiotherapists, with 1 in 6 therapists moving out of the profession as a direct result of work related musculoskeletal injuries. Physiotherapists, who were asked to state their job related risk factors, identified that 'assisting patients during gait activities' was a major contributor to their work related musculoskeletal disorder.

The *CSP (2002)* advises handlers to consider the 'utility of the act' and states that judicious use of equipment can significantly reduce the extent of the risk posed by frequent and hazardous manual handling.

In the same publication the CSP state:

> *'if the use of equipment can significantly reduce any risks as far as is reasonably practicable, then the physiotherapist must use the equipment or alternative methods may need to be devised. Alternatively the provision of more staff might be indicated. This does not mean that a hoist must be used for all transfers. Assessment and treatment should be part of a graded process, requiring less assistance to the patient as the treatment progresses'.*

For example, a walking harness may be required at the start of the rehabilitation programme, after which, assisted walking may progress to two members of staff assisting and a third pushing a wheelchair behind, to, eventually, walking independently with the walking harness being used only as a 'safety net' in case of unpredictable occurrences.'

A case study report by *Busse (2000)* concluded that '*the utilisation of hoists meant that therapists and carers were able to progress rehabilitation. Indeed the reduced burden of care for the nursing staff could not have been achieved safely without the use of hoists*'.

Ruszala (2001) undertook an evaluation of equipment to assist patient STS activities in physiotherapy. She concluded that an active hoist and the walking harness – see tasks three and four, were both identified as of potential benefit to physiotherapists during the acute phase of rehabilitation, with the additional options for standing balance and assisted walking seen as highly desirable'. The findings of the study also indicated that, whilst the walking harness was seen as least favourable by both physiotherapists and patients for assisted STS (as it did not promote the normal movement pattern), it was seen as the most beneficial when combined with other treatment activities, such as standing balance and walking re-education.

Assisting on steps/stairs

Extreme care should be taken when considering assisting a person to mobilise on stairs. Therapists should make a suitable and sufficient risk assessment when considering to undertake this task with a person. Hazards associated with assisting people with this task are many, such as handling in a confined space, difficulty handling the person close to the body and poor stability of the handler if the person topples forward (or backward), leading to a tendency of the handler to try to 'catch' or hold onto the person.

Oddy (2003) suggests guidance for people with dementia to negotiate steps and stairs with the handlers acting as 'gap fillers'. Partially blocking the sight of the descent of the stairs may assist people to have more confidence in negotiating the stairs independently. Handlers should however be aware that standing in front of the person descending stairs places them in an extremely vulnerable position. Wherever the handler positions themselves they should be able to guide the person to sit onto the stairs should they feel they are losing balance. Alternatively, allowing the person to walk down the stairs sideways, holding onto the handrail with both hands may also assist with the person's confidence.

The Derbyshire Inter-agency Group (DIAG 2003) states that it is not safe to give a person physical support in managing steps or stairs as the handler would have no control over the person's stability and hence be in a very vulnerable position. Therefore, ideally, with people who cannot independently negotiate the stairs, alternative methods for achieving access to additional floors of a building should be sought e.g. a stair lift, ramps, vertical lift etc. or a different route.

6 Summary

Assisting a person to walk may pose a high risk of injury to the handler(s). *Love (1996)* suggests that the problem in respect of reducing accidents that occur when a person is assisted to walk, unlike other manual transfers, is that it is not merely a matter of 'not lifting'. Both the role and the function of the handler, when assisting people to mobilise, needs to be reviewed. This should identify not only whether the person can bear weight on their feet and the handler has the required expertise to assist the person, but also what management strategies are in place to detect, and prevent the occurrence of possible causes of falling.

Manual handling risk assessment and resulting management strategies must be based on clinical knowledge, information appropriate to the person, the situation and the extent of the skills, knowledge and experience of the therapists and carers. Handlers assisting people to walk in therapeutic situations should assess specifically the 'utility of the act' *(CSP, 2002)*, and utilise appropriate handling equipment to assist them to continue with the person's rehabilitation, without placing themselves under undue risk.

Practical techniques

Task One

Assisted walking with 1 handler – with or without handling belt

DEPENDENCY LEVEL

Mobility Gallery B
FIM 4

- The person should also have cognitive ability to understand and follow instructions from the handler.
- The person must have head support, trunk support and be able to sit upright unsupported and be able to weight bear through both legs.
- The person should be able to place at least one hand onto the arm/s of the chair to help push into standing.
- The person must be able to place full weight on their feet and move their own feet into position. The person should be able to maintain own balance when in full standing.
- The person should be able to place one foot in front of the other and step forwards, and move the walking aid (if applicable) with only minimal assistance.

DESCRIPTION

- If the person is using a walking aid, they should be encouraged to stand using the arms of the chair and then hold onto the walking aid once in standing. Ensure the walking aid is close to the person to avoid stretching and overbalancing.
- The handler should stand at one side (dependent on use of walking aid and appropriate side for person), and face the direction in which the person and the handler is to walk.
- Care should be taken by the handler that they do not walk and impede the person's natural stepping or the walking aid which may be being used.
- The handler may place one hand on the centre of the person's back (or hold onto the centre of the walking belt if being used). The further hand of the handler may either be placed onto the front of the person's nearest shoulder or they may hold onto the person's nearest hand (using one of the handholds previously described).
- If the person is using a walking aid then the handler should walk on the opposite side.

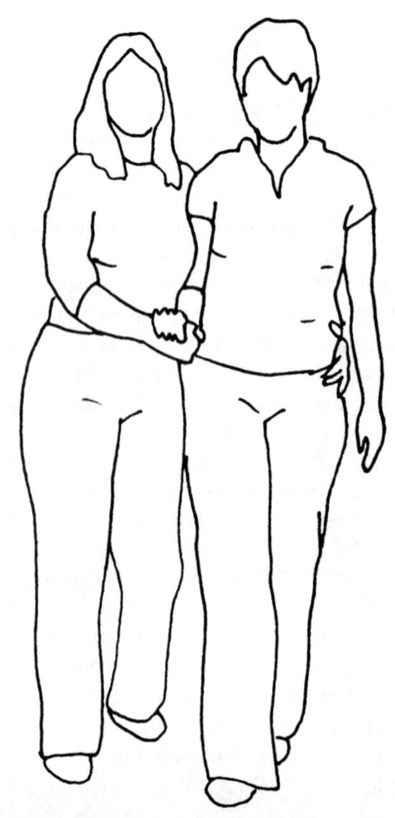

FIG 13.3

	• The handler should walk at one side and slightly behind the person.
OPTIONS AND VARIATIONS	1 You may wish to undertake this task with the use of a walking belt (figure 13.1). The handler will stand at one side of the person and place their nearest arm across the person's back at around the level of the person's waist, ensuring good contact with the person and their forearm and holding the handle nearest to the persons mid-waist. 2 If the person is using a walking frame to assist with balance then the handler may wish to walk behind the person (but slightly to one side so they are able to see where they are going). In this instance the handler may place both hands onto the person's waist/hips to provide guidance and assistance.
PERCEIVED EXERTION FOR HANDLER	• The person should be encouraged to be active during the movement. • There should be little physical exertion for the handler. • The handler should remember that they are to exert a slight forward pressure to the person to indicate a direction of movement,however, the person should be able to move forward under their own effort and at their own speed. • It is important the handler works at the speed of the person as carrying out the procedure too quickly or too slowly will not allow the person to be active during the task.
COMFORT OF THE PERSON	• Method should be comfortable to the person and the handler should not grasp the person or their clothing. If handling belt is used: • Handlers should take care when placing a belt around the waist of people with abdominal problems as it may cause discomfort. • People who are underweight (according to the BMI chart) may find the belt 'digs' into their waist area. • Large people may find that the belt rises up towards their chest due to the shape of their waist area, in which case an alternative method/equipment should be considered. • The speed of the walking pace should be governed by the person, not the handler as this will make the task comfortable for the person.
SKILL LEVEL OF HANDLER	• The handler should have received basic manual handling training and be aware of the assessment for people who require manual assistance in walking. • The handler should be aware of the use of a belt and also have understanding of patterns of normal movement for walking. • If they are assisting people with hemiparesis (following a CVA) they should be aware of the management of the stroke patient and be able to make the appropriate assessment as to which side to walk, and follow the manual handling plan. • The handler should have received instruction and specific guidelines as to the management of the falling/fallen person.
EVIDENCE AVAILABLE	1 *BackCare (1999)* Safer Handling of People in the Community. 2 *Tarling C (1997/8)* in Fourth Edition of The Guide to the Handling of Paitents . 3 *Derbyshire Inter-agency Group Guidelines (2003).*
DANGERS / PRECAUTIONS	• If the person is unable to maintain full weight on their feet this will place too much strain onto the handler. • If the person has weakness on one side, the handler must be aware of which side they are to walk to facilitate the task and minimise the risk. • If the walking belt is being used then it should be fitted comfortably but firmly around the person's waist in order to prevent movement and sliding upward. • Handlers should take care not to place their whole hand through the handle on the belt as this is likely to cause injury should the person move suddenly or fall or move away from the handler. • The handler should allow the person to move their own feet and they should not assist the person to walk by moving the person's feet. • The handler should be aware not to walk in front of the person as this may result in the person being pulled forward rather than being allowed to be active and 'lead' the movement.
FURTHER OPTIONS	This method would be appropriate to assist the person to walk short distances from one room to another.

Evidence review

Technique	REBA	Activity	Comfort	FIM	Mobility gallery	Skill level	Comment
ASSISTED WALKING WITH 1 HANDLER – WITH OR WITHOUT HANDLING BELT							
Fig 13.3	7	9	9	4	B	Novice	

Task Two

Assisted walking with 1 or 2 handlers, with or without belt, and with or without frame

DEPENDENCY LEVEL

Mobility Gallery B, C
FIM 4

- The person should have sufficient cognitive ability to understand and follow instructions from the handlers.
- The person must have head support, trunk support and be able to sit upright unsupported and be able to weight bear through both legs.
- The person should be able to place at least one hand onto the arm/s of the chair to help push into standing.
- The person must be able to place full weight on their feet and move their own feet into position. The person should be able to maintain own balance when in full stand.
- The person should be able to move their feet independently to step forwards and move their walking aid (if applicable) with only moderate assistance.

DESCRIPTION

- If the person is using a walking aid, they should be encouraged to stand using the arms of the chair and then hold onto the walking aid once in standing. Ensure the walking aid is close to the person to avoid stretching and overbalancing.
- The handlers stand either side of the person, and face the direction in which the person is to walk.
- Care should be taken by the handlers that they do not walk and impede the person's natural stepping or the movement and placing of any walking aid which may be being used.
- The handlers may place one hand on the centre of the person's back (or hold onto the centre of the walking belt if being used). The further hand of each handler may either be placed onto the front of the persons nearest shoulder or they may hold onto the person's nearest hand (using one of the handholds previously described) if a walking aid is not being used.
- The handlers should walk slightly behind the person.

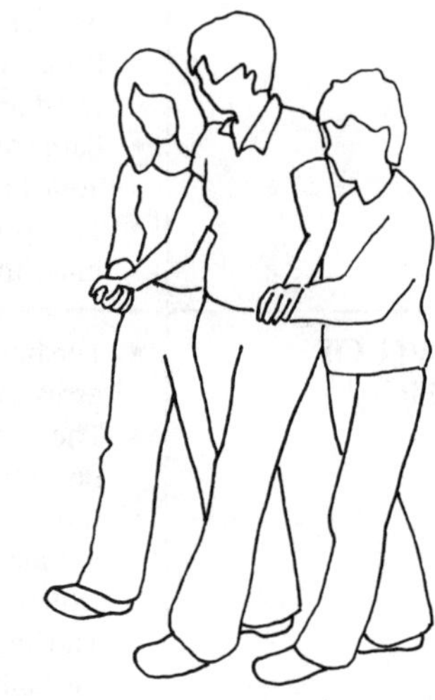

FIG 13.4

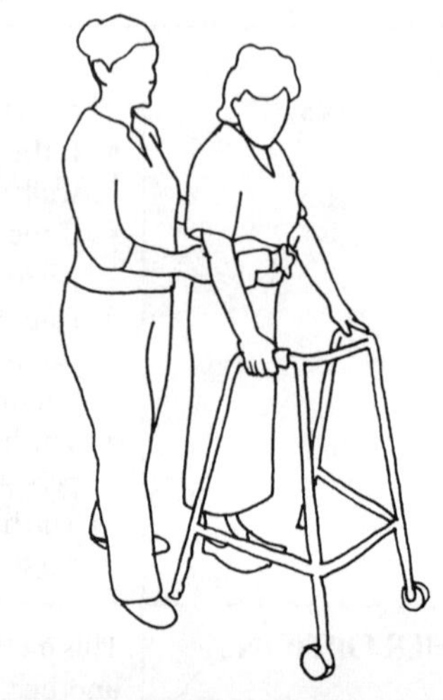

FIG 13.5

OPTIONS AND VARIATIONS	1 You may wish to undertake this task with the use of a walking belt. The handlers will stand at either side of the person and place their nearest arm across the person's back at around the level of the person's waist, ensuring good contact with the person and their forearm and holding the handle nearest to the person's mid-waist. 2 If the person is using a walking frame to assist with balance then the handlers may wish to walk slightly behind the person and to one side so they are able to see where they are going.
PERCEIVED EXERTION FOR HANDLER	• The person should be encouraged to be active during the movement. • There should be little physical exertion for the handlers. • The handlers should remember that they are to exert a slight forward pressure to the person to indicate a direction of movement, however the person should be able to move forward under their own effort and at their own pace. • It is important the handlers work at the pace of the person as carrying out the procedure too quickly or too slowly will not allow the person to be active during the task.
COMFORT OF THE PERSON	• The method should be comfortable to the person and the handlers should not grasp the person or their clothing. If handling belt is used: • Handlers should take care when placing a belt around the waist of people with abdominal problems as it may cause discomfort. • People who are underweight (according to the BMI chart) may find the belt 'digs' into their waist area. • Large people may find that the belt rises up towards their chest due to the shape of their waist area, in which case an alternative method/equipment should be sought. • The speed of the walking pace should be governed by the person, not the handlers as this will make the task comfortable for the person.
SKILL LEVEL OF HANDLER	• The handlers should have received basic manual handling training and aware of assessment for people who require manual assistance in walking. • The handlers should be aware of the use of a belt and also have understanding of patterns of normal movement for walking. • If they are assisting people with hemiparesis (following a CVA) they should be aware of management of the stroke patient and be able to make or follow the appropriate assessment as to the method used to assist the person. • The handlers should have received instruction and specific guidelines as to the management of the falling/fallen person.
EVIDENCE AVAILABLE	1 *BackCare (1999)* Safe Handling of People in the Community. 2 *Tarling C (1997/8)* in Fourth Edition to the Guide to The Handling of Patients. 3 *Derbyshire Inter-agency Group Guidelines (2003).*
DANGERS/ PRECAUTIONS	• If the person is unable to maintain full weight on their feet this will place too much strain onto the handlers. • The handlers should remember that the person is to be active during the task and should not take the weight of the person should they lean onto them. • If the walking belt is being used then it should be fitted firmly around the person's waist so as to prevent movement and sliding upward. • The handlers should take care not to place their whole hand through the handles on the belt as this is likely to cause injury should the person move suddenly or fall or move away from the handlers. • The handlers should allow the person to move their own feet, they should not assist the person to walk by moving the person's feet. • The handlers should be aware not to walk in front of the person as this may result in the person being pulled forward rather than being allowed to be active and 'lead' the movement. • The handlers should be aware of the route they are walking as assisted walking a person with two handlers (one either side) may be difficult where there are narrow doorways or environmental restrictions. In such an instance consideration should be given to the use of a wheelchair to negotiate restricted space. • The handlers should not hold onto each others hands/arms to support the person in walking or prevent the person from falling.
FURTHER OPTIONS	This method would be appropriate to assist the person to walk short distances from one room to another.

Evidence review

Technique	REBA	Activity	Comfort	FIM	Mobility gallery	Skill level	Comment
ASSISTED WALKING WITH 2 PEOPLE							
Fig 13.4	2	8	8	4	B	Advanced beginner	
ASSISTED WALKING WITH FRAME AND 1 HANDLER							
Fig 13.5	5	9	9	4	C	Novice	

Task Three

Assisted walking with hoist and walking harness, with 1 or more handlers

DEPENDENCY LEVEL

Mobility Gallery C
FIM 4

The person may be assisted to walk with the above equipment but requires some weight bearing ability.

DESCRIPTION

- The correct specified sling should be selected and applied in approved manner.
- This harness can often be applied in sitting, and as the person is raised to their feet the hoist is moved away to encourage them to lean forward as they rise.
- A handler will be required to move the hoist, if a mobile is used, and usually another handler is required to steady/assist with walking.

PERCEIVED EXERTION FOR HANDLER

If the person is heavy, use of gantry or tracking hoist must be considered. One or more handlers may be required, as may a walking aid to assist.

COMFORT FOR PERSON

- People with painful joints or delicate skin may find the walking harness uncomfortable.
- Padded leg supports are usually provided to ensure comfort.

SKILL LEVEL OF THE STAFF

- The handler requires communication skills.
- Use of this equipment requires special skill, and is usually confined to rehabilitation staff.

EVIDENCE AVAILABLE

1 *Ruszala (2001)* states that this equipment is suitable for early rehabilitation, although its use could constitute a high risk of injury for staff.

2 *Busse (2000)* suggests that the harness could be useful for people with unreliable

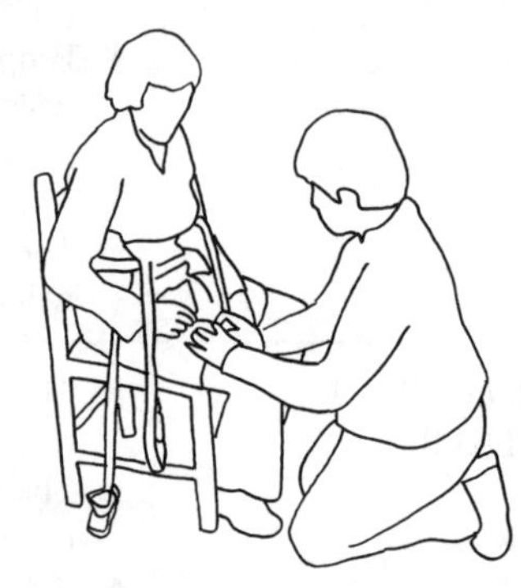

FIG 13.6a

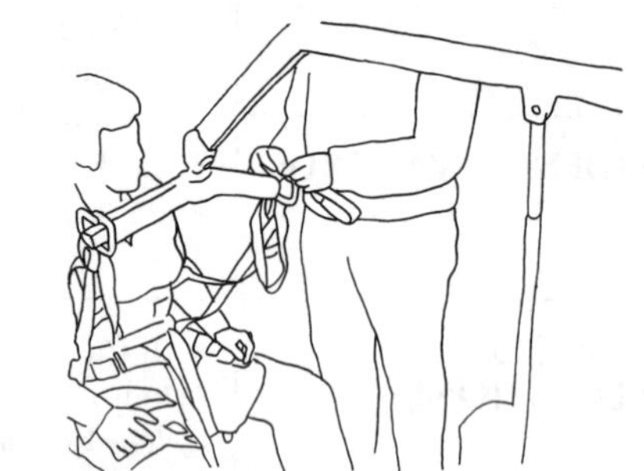

FIG 13.6b

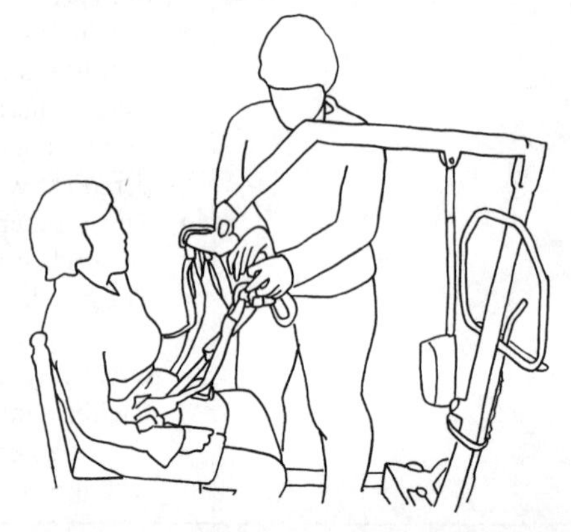

FIG 13.6c

balance or for positioning in a standing frame.

3 Standing harnesses were mentioned in *The Guide to the Handling of Patients (4th edition 1997/8)* and *Safer Handling of People in the Community (1999)* suggesting them as useful adjuncts for rehabilitation.

4 *National Back Exchange, Essex Group (1997)* advise that a walking harness could be used to access various types of paediatric equipment, including standing frames.

5 *Malouin et al (1992), Gardner et al (1998), Hesse et al (1999), Cherniak et al (1999), Kendrick et al (2001)* all discuss the use of a walking harness over a treadmill, with improvments in walking.

DANGERS/ PRECAUTIONS

- Mobile hoists should not be moved long distances with the person suspended. They may not raise a taller person to their feet sufficiently to be useful.
- Heavy/tall people may require ceiling tracking or gantries to enable handlers to assist them to walk safely.
- The sling must be correct size/type/ purpose for each person.
- Some people may benefit by careful selection of style of a compatible harness, as some harnesses bear weight on different parts of body (*DIAG 2001*).

FURTHER OPTIONS

Ceiling tracking or gantries remove the need to push mobile hoists any distance, but must be strategically positioned for optimum convenience.

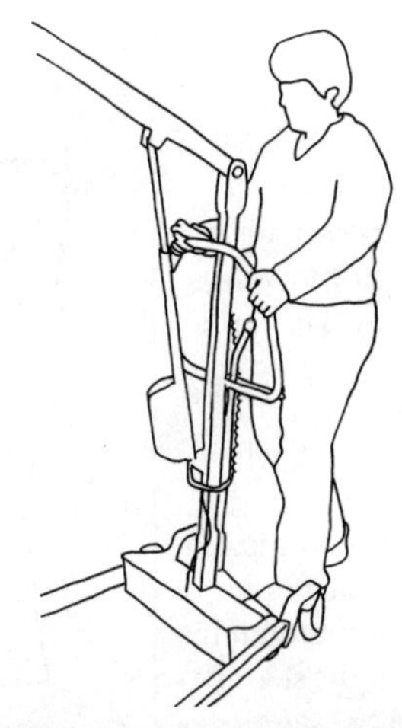

FIG 13.6d

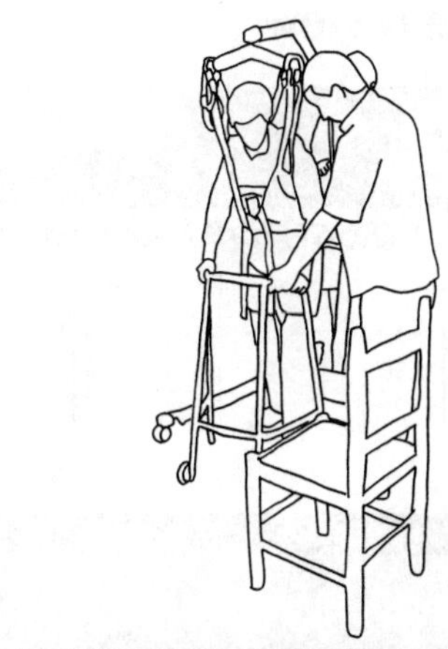

FIG 13.6e

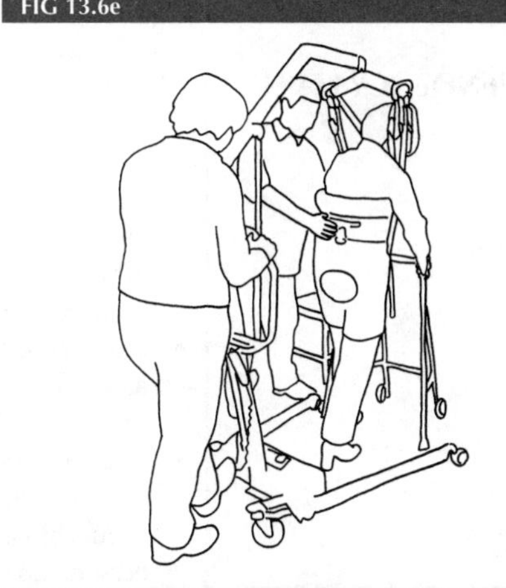

FIG 13.6f

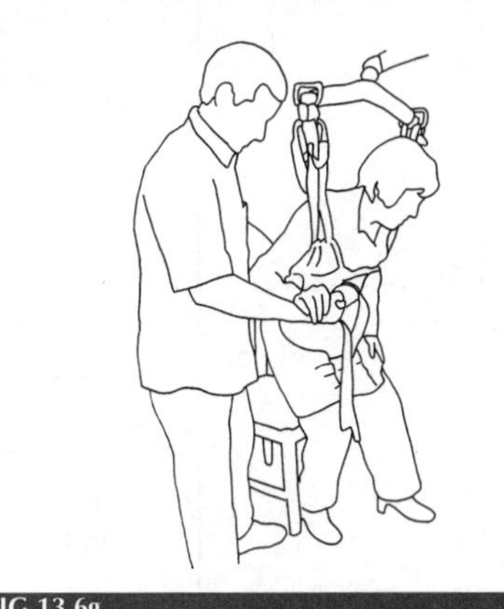

FIG 13.6g

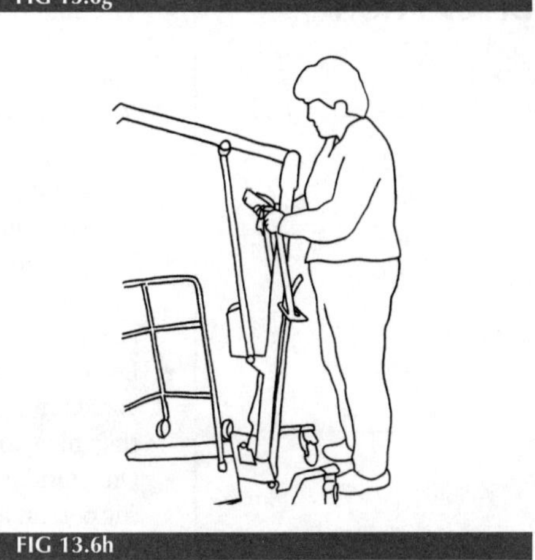

FIG 13.6h

Evidence review

Technique	REBA	Activity	Comfort	FIM	Mobility gallery	Skill level	Comment
TRANSFER WITH HOIST AND WALKING HARNESS WITH 1 OR 2 HANDLERS							
Figs 13.6 a–h	2	6	6	4	C	Competent	Use of a hoist gives a low postural risk for the handlers, but gives low activity and comfort for the person.

Task Four

Assisted walking with an active hoist

DEPENDENCY LEVEL

Mobility Gallery C
FIM 3

- The client should be encouraged to participate as much as possible with the whole task of rising from the chair and bearing weight onto his or her own feet.
- The person should have sufficient cognitive ability to understand and follow instructions from the handler(s).
- The person should have the 'desire' to stand and the goal of standing and walking should be clear and understood by both the person and the handler(s).
- The person should have head support and tone and use of their upper limbs, specifically their shoulders.
- The person should have the tone and strength in their upper body to be able to sit upright whilst in a chair with moderate support only. This equipment would not normally be used where the person required considerable support in sitting with the use of a brace or integral seating system.
- The person must be able to place both of their feet onto the ground and maintain contact with the floor.

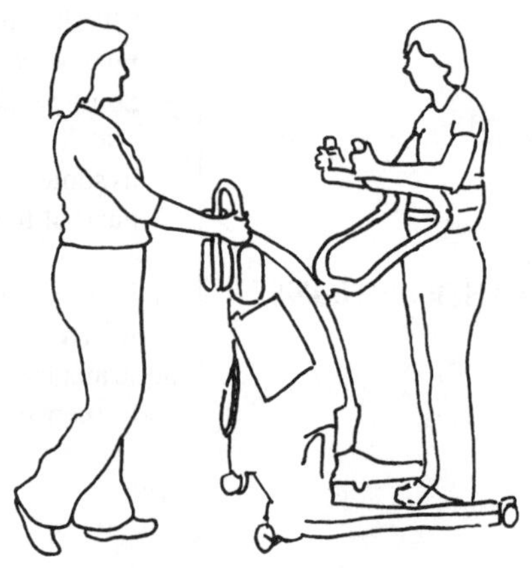

FIG 13.7a

DESCRIPTION

- The material support (back support) will normally be fitted onto the person whilst they are in a sitting position. In such an instance it is desirable for the person to be able to at least assist with leaning forward in the chair, to allow the handlers to fit the support comfortably.
- The person should be encouraged to utilise the patterns of 'normal' movement' when rising from the seat.
- Ensure that the person's feet are positioned correctly so they may utilise what power they have to assist the 'push' into standing.
- One handler may wish to sit at the side of the person and to stand up at the same time as the person. This may provide the

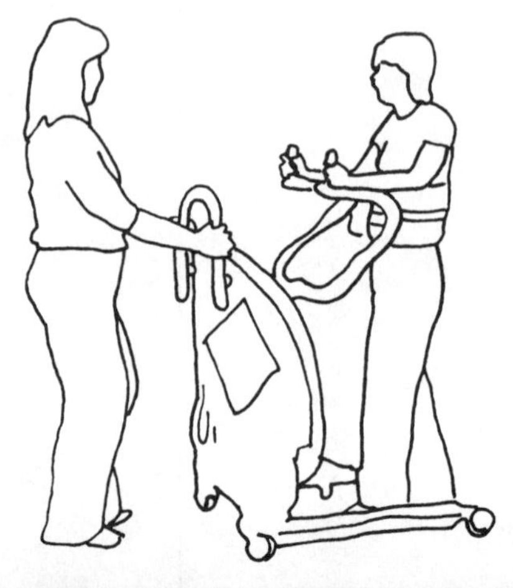

FIG 13.7b

person with visual demonstration of what is expected of them. This handler may place their closest hand onto the person's back for reassurance only.

- One handler attaches the back support to the hoist system and prepares the person for the standing action by raising the hoist to take the 'slack' out of the support. At this point the handler may wish to stop the lifting action and ensure that the person is ready for the stand.
- If the hoist has an 'arc rest' for the arms and hands then the handler(s) should ensure that the arms are fully supported, using the additional safety straps if appropriate to prevent the person's arms from falling off the arc rest.
- Once in standing the person may be encouraged to utilise 'normal gait' (or whatever is the intention of the person and handlers).
- The back support should now be adjusted for comfort to allow stepping/walking.
- It is important that the handlers adjust the height of the hoist to provide the correct amount of support for the person in standing. If the hoist is too high then the person's feet will be off the floor and there will be undue strain on the person's shoulders. If the hoist is too low then the person will not be supported or will step/walk in a stooped posture.
- The knee pad on the hoist may need to be removed where the person is to walk any distance. However, it is advised that the knee pad remain in position to undertake STS to provide extra support/stability.
- For reassurance, one handler may wish to walk behind the person with a wheelchair in case the person may wish to sit quickly.

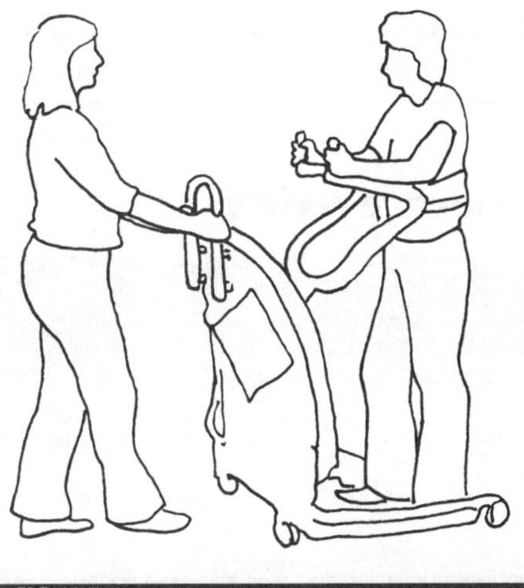

FIG 13.7c

OPTIONS AND VARIATIONS

1. This system may be used to assist therapists in the task of gait or weight bearing retraining.
2. Some walking hoists have an integral 'seat' which supports the person whilst they are able to move their legs to step/walk.

PERCEIVED EXERTION FOR CARER

- The system is designed to remove the hazards of assisting the person into standing and also to remove the effort of the handler(s) when assisting the person during walking, hence physical exertion of the handlers should be minimal.
- There may be some effort involved in the fitting of the back support on the person in the chair, especially if the person is unable to assist with leaning forward.
- There will however, be increased physical exertion by the handler who may be required to move the hoist. It is therefore advisable that a thorough risk assessment is undertaken as to the route and environment in which the task is taking place.
- It is important that the handler(s) work at the speed of the person as carrying out the procedure too quickly or too slowly will not allow the person to be active during the transfer.
- The handler(s) should work with the person as a team and be aware not to hurry and lift them into standing or move the hoist too quickly and not allow the person to fully experience walking.

COMFORT OF THE PERSON

- The task should be comfortable for the person. It is vital that the correct back support is used.
- As the person is required to place their knees against a knee pad, individuals with painful

	knees may find this system uncomfortable. • People with painful shoulder joints or reduced range of movement may also find the arc rest of the hoist uncomfortable.
SKILL LEVEL OF CARER HANDLER	• The handler should have received advanced manual handling training and be aware of the assessment for people who require the use of a walking hoist and also have an understanding of patterns of normal movement for STS and gait patterns. • The handler(s) should be aware of the treatment/handling plan and of the use and application of a walking jacket/harness. • If the handlers are assisting clients with hemiparesis (following a CVA) they should be aware of management of the stroke patient.
EVIDENCE AVAILABLE	*Ruszala (2001)* found that an active hoist (and the walking harness) provided a safer environment for physiotherapists and people whilst enabling them to facilitate movement during a range of activities including standing, balance and walking.
DANGERS/ PRECAUTIONS	• If the person is unable to maintain some of their weight on their feet and/or assist with the push into standing this may mean that a different sling is required (a passive sling), which will lift their full body weight. • If the person has weakness on one side, the handler should ensure that the person is able to place weight through their weak/painful shoulder. If they are unable to do so then an alternative system should be found to assist with walking practice.
FURTHER OPTIONS	This equipment allows the handler to assist the person to mobilise using the hoist to act as a 'safety net' should the person be unable to maintain weight-bearing.

Evidence review

Technique	REBA	Activity	Comfort	FIM	Mobility gallery	Skill level	Comment
STANDING AND WALKING WITH AN ACTIVE HOIST							
Fig 13.7a–c	4	6	7	3	C	Advanced beginner	

Task Five

Assisted walking a child (using a therapy stool)

DEPENDENCY LEVEL

Mobility Gallery C
FIM 3, 4

- The child should have sufficient cognitive ability to understand and follow instructions from the handler.
- The child must be able to place full weight on their feet and move their own feet into position. The child should be able to maintain majority of their own balance when in full stand.

DESCRIPTION

- The therapy stool may be used for the handler to sit on and assist/support the child whilst they are walking. As the child walks the handler will need to use their feet to move with the child and move the stool.

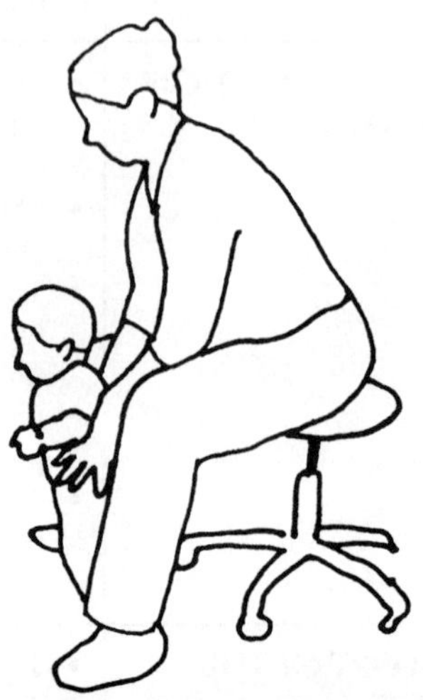

FIG 13.9

	• The child leans forward in the seat. • The handler stands at the side of the child and encourages the child to place both hands onto the arms of the chair to push himself into sitting on given commands. • The handler faces in the direction of movement and places their nearest arm to the child over the child's back at around waist level, leaving their hand open against the child's back and not grasping the child or the child's clothing. Ensure good contact with the child along the forearm against the child's back. The other hand can be placed onto the front of the child's nearest shoulder for added support. • Using verbal commands, the handler directs the child to lift their own head and initiate the stand, at the same time the handler places a forward pressure on the child's back and assists the normal movement into standing. • To complete the move the handler should move both feet to stand at the side of the child. The handler should remember to transfer their weight from their rear foot to their front foot and utilise their own weight to facilitate the child forwards and upwards. • The handler should remain close to the child whilst providing assistance in walking, providing support to the child at the shoulders and/or hips depending on the needs of the child.
OPTIONS AND VARIATIONS	You may wish to undertake this task with the use of a walking belt. The belt should be fitted comfortably on the child and reached comfortably by the handler.
PERCEIVED EXERTION FOR HANDLER	• The child should be encouraged to be active during the movement. • There should be little physical exertion for the handler. • The handler should remember that they are to exert a forward and upward pressure for the child to bring himself or herself into standing. • It is important the handler works at the speed of the child, as carrying out the procedure too quickly or too slowly will not allow the child to be active during the transfer. • The handler should work with the child as a team and be aware not to hurry the child and lift them into standing.
COMFORT OF THE PERSON	• The method should be comfortable to the child and the handler should not grasp the child or their clothing. If handling belt is used: • Handlers should take care when placing a belt around the waist of children with abdominal problems as it may cause discomfort. • Children who are underweight (according to the BMI chart) may find the belt 'digs' into their waist area. • Large children may find that the belt rises up towards their chest due to the shape of their waist area, in which case an alternative method/equipment should be sought.
SKILL LEVEL OF HANDLER	• The handler should have received basic manual handling training and be aware of assessment for children who require the use of a belt and also have an understanding of patterns of normal movement for sit to stand. • If they are assisting children with hemiparesis (following a CVA) they should be aware of management of the stroke patient.
EVIDENCE AVAILABLE	**1** The *Fourth Edition to The Guide to the Handling of Patients (1997/8).* **2** *Cromie et al (2000)* described equipment used by therapists to reduce strain on their body and stated that while working 45.3% of therapists used a wheelie stool.
DANGERS / PRECAUTIONS	• It is not advisable that the handler takes hold of the child's hands or supports them on walking whilst holding their hands above their head. • If the child feels as though they cannot continue to bear weight on their feet then the handler has the option to allow the child to lean/perch onto their lap for a short duration. • The handler should be aware not to overstretch and support the child away from their body as this will encourage considerable sustained flexion of the low back and hips and strain at the shoulders. • The handler should take regular rest breaks if handling a number of people (children) using this method, due to the cumulative static loading involved. • If a walking belt is used it should be fitted firmly around the child's waist/hips so as to prevent movement and sliding upward. • The handlers should take care not to place their whole hand through the handle on the belt

	as this is likely to cause injury should the child move suddenly away from the handler.
FURTHER OPTIONS	This method would be appropriate for use to assist a person of small stature (in relation to the handler).

Evidence review

Technique	REBA	Activity	Comfort	FIM	Mobility gallery	Skill level	Comment
WALKING WITH A CHILD							
Fig 13.10	8	7	8	3	C	Advanced beginner	
WALKING WITH A CHILD AT SHOULDERS							
	4	9	8	4	C	Proficient	Not covered in chapter
ASSISTED WALKING WITH A CHILD WITH BELT							
	7	8	7	4	C	Proficient	See Chapter 14
ASSISTED WALKING WITH A CHILD FROM THE FLOOR							
	10	5	7	3	C	Advanced beginner	See Chapter 14
KNEELING WITH A CHILD ON THE FLOOR							
	12	5	7	3	C	Advanced beginner	See Chapter 14

Acknowledgements

I would like to acknowledge Pat Alexander for the inclusion of task 5 in the practical section of this chapter.

I would also like to acknowledge Corpus UK, Mandy Clift, Trish Bartley and Corpus Holland for their kind and generous assistance in the development of these chapters and in the taking of the photographs used within chapters 12 and 13.

References

BackCare (1999). Safer Handling of People in the Community

Busse M (2000). Access to appropriate hoisting equipment can be essential for effective rehabilitation: a case study. Nursing and Residential Care 2(4):168–73

Chartered Society of Physiotherapy (2002). Guidance in Manual Handling for Chartered Physiotherapists

Cheng PT, Liaw MY, Wong MK, Tang FT, Lee MY, Lin PS (1998). The sit-to-stand movement in stroke persons and its correlation with falling. Archive of Physical Medical Rehabilitation Sep;79(9):1043–6.

Cherniak P, Caprio D, Fischer A, Tuckman J (1999). A novel device for walking training in elderly patients. Physiotherapy March. 85(3):144–148

Cromie JE, Robertson VJ, Best MO (2000). Work-Related Musculoskeletal Disorders in Physical Therapists: Prevalence, Severity, Risks and Responses. Physical Therapy April Vol 80(4): 336–351

Derbyshire Inter-agency Group (2003). Care Handling for People in Hospitals Community and Educational Settings. A Code of Practice

Finnie NR (2000). Handling the Young Child with Cerebral Palsy at Home. Third Edition. Butterworth Heinmann. Edinburgh

Gardener M, Holden, M Leikauskas RR (1998). Partial body weight support with treadmill location to improve gait after incomplete spinal cord injury, a single study experimental design. Physical Therapy 78(4): 36–1374

Garg A, Owen B, Beller D, Banaag J (1999). A biomechanical and ergonomic evaluation of patient transferring tasks: wheelchair to shower chair and shower chair to wheelchair. Ergonomics April;34(4):407–419

Hesse S, Konrad M, Uhlenbrock D (1999). Treadmill walking with partial body weight support versus floor walking in hemiparetic subjects. Archives of Physical MediceineRehabilitation. 80. April 1999: 421–427

Hignett S (2003). Intervention strategies to reduce musculoskeletal injuries associated with handling persons: a systematic review. Occupational and Environmental Medicine. Sep;60(9)

Hignett S, Crumpton E, Ruszala S, Alexander P, Fray M, Fletcher B (2003). Evidence-Based Person Handling. Tasks, equipment and interventions. Routledge. London.

HSE 2001 (2002). Handling Home Care. HMSO

Jones and Barker . Human Movement Explained. Butterworth Heinemann. Edinburgh

Love C (1996). Injury caused by lifting: a study of the nurse's viewpoint. Nursing Standard , August 7. Vol 10. (46)34–39

Kendrick C, Holt R, McGlashan K, Jenner JR, Kircher S (2001). Exercising on a treadmill to improve functional mobility in chronic stroke. Physiotherapy. 87(5):261–265

Koller WC, Glatt SL, Fox JH (1985). Senile Gait Clinical Geriatric Medicine :1: 661–669

Laufer Y (2003). The effect of walking aids on balance and weight bearing patterns of patients with hemiparesis in various stance positions. Physical Therapy . February. 83(2):112–22

Malouin F, Potvin M, Prevost J, Richards CL, Wood-Dauphines S (1992). Use of intensive task orientated gait training programme in a series of patients with acute cerbrovascular accidents. Physical Therapy. 72(11):781–789

Mandalstam (2002). Manual Handling in Health and Social Care. Jessica Kingsley Publishers. London

Marras WS, Davis KG, Kirkling BC, Bertsche PK (1999). A comprehensive analysis of low-back disorder risk and spinal loading during the transferring and repositioning of patients using different techniques. Ergonomics ; 42(7):904–926

Moseley AM, Stark A, Cameron ID, Pollock A (2004). Treadmill training and body weight support for walking after a stroke (Cochrane Review). In The Cocherane Library (2004), Issue 3. Chichister, UK: John Wiley and Sons Ltd

Mulley GP (1988). Everyday aids and appliances – walking sticks. British Medical Journal: 296;475–476

Mutch K (2004). Changing manual-handling practice in a stroke rehabilitation unit. Professional Nurse Mar;19(7):374–8.

National Back Pain Association (1997/8). Fourth Edition to the Guide to the Handling of Persons. Royal College of Nursing

Oddy R (2003). Promoting mobility for people with dementia. Second Edition Age Concern. England

Royal College of Nursing (1996). Hazards of Nursing, personal injuries at work (000692)

Ruszala S (2001). An evaluation of equipment to assist person sit-to-stand activities in physiotherapy'. Unpublished MSc dissertation, University of Wales: School of Health Care Studies

Turner A, Foster M, Johnson SE (2002). Occupational Therapy and Physical Dysfunction. Fifth Edition.
Churchill Livingstone. London

Tyldsley B, Greive JI (2003). Muscles, Nerves and Movement in Human Occupation (Third Edition). Blackwell Publishing. Oxford

Tappen RM, Roach KE, Applegate EB, Stowell P (2000). Effect of a combined walking and conversation intervention on functional mobility of nursing home residents with Alzheimer disease. Alzheimer Disease and Associated Disorders Oct-Dec;14(4):196–201

Yip Y (2001). A study of work stress, person handling activities and the risk of low back pain among nurses in Hong Kong. Journal of Advanced Nursing Dec;36(6):794–804.

Yohannes AM, Connolly MJ (2003). Early mobilisation with walking aids following hospital admission with acute exacerbation of chronic obstructive pulmonary disease. Clinical Rehabilitation Aug;17(5);465–471

14

Sitting to sitting transfers

Pat Alexander MSc LPD PGCE MCSP MIOSH
Consultant Back Care Adviser

1 Introduction

The normal method of achieving a transfer from one sitting position to another involves a mixture of physical, and psycho-social factors. These include motivation, balance, the ability to lean forward beyond the body's centre of gravity, to extend against the force of gravity and to regain balance in an upright position. This is followed by a move to another seat and the procedure is reversed. For those unable to achieve this change in position independently there are many ways of facilitating independence or providing assistance. Simple commands and standby supervision, alterations to the seating, and manual and mechanical methods may assist the person who is unable to transfer unaided. However, if handling aids are provided, *"they must also be easily accessible – an aspect which is remedied by good organisation" (Duffy 1999).*

Rising from a seated position is an essential requirement for everyday living for most people. It precedes functional mobility, and according to *Alexander (1991)* it is *"likely that increased dependency in transferring associates with institutionalisation and immobility-related diseases"*. According to *Laporte et al (1999)* the physiological and psychological benefits of mobilising can prevent a decline in well being, falls and a "critical decline in condition". Lack of confidence and difficulty in rising is accompanied by an increased risk of falling *(Alexander et al 1991, Tinetti et al 1990).*

About 2 seconds are required for healthy adults to achieve the action of rising from sitting to standing *(Kelley et al 1976)*. If this time is increased, due to pain or lack of stability, more strength is required, as less use is made of momentum *(Kotake et al 1993)*. The need for stability in rising is more important than that for momentum *(Schultz et al 1992)*, but the strength requirement can be lessened by various strategies.

There are a number of strategies for achieving seated transfers but the difficulty from a research point of view is comparing like with like. For example when investigating the use of a handling belt to assist in transferring, the extent to which a person may be able to weight bear is not always made clear. Some researchers *(Zhuang et al 1999)* consider six different methods, but concentrate mainly on measuring the force required to rotate and sit a person up from supine onto the edge of the bed prior to the actual transfer, as these activities by staff were believed to be the most strenuous part of the activity. However, person/handler perceptions as to comfort and effort required for the whole transfer were later identified by the researchers (ibid).

The method of choice for any particular manoeuvre will depend on the result of a risk assessment based on the TILE factors as suggested by the Health and Safety Executive (HSE). This will include factors such as the Task, the ability, knowledge and skill of the Individual (handler) and the availability of suitable assistive equipment, ability and choice of the person (Load) and the Environment *(Manual Handling Operations – Guidance on Regulations HSE 1992)*. All aspects of the intended movement must be considered before the move is attempted. The reason for the intended move may influence the method of transfer, for instance an urgent need to visit the toilet, may inform the risk assessment process and decision as to the nature and extent of the assistance required.

Training is essential before staff commence working with people with impaired mobility, and skills of observation should be encouraged, to ensure that staff are aware of and report any recent changes in the situation. Communication must be established in respect of the person's ability and wishes, before any assistance is offered and the manual handling plan included in the person's care plan (see chapter 9). All staff must be familiar with both the person and the use of any methods of assistance as recorded in the individual manual handling plan.

2 Location and type of seat

The successful performance of a seated transfer may depend on a number of factors all of which should be considered before the person sits down in the first place. The choice of the original chair and its location will present a variable environment. Its height, presence of arm rests and space around it will all affect the method of leaving it. The seat height should be sufficient for a person to get up with ease, and this may require the provision of a higher upright chair, or the use of blocks to raise the chair *(Chan et al 1999)*. The optimal height of a chair to facilitate rising may be higher than that considered the most comfortable position for sitting *(Chan et al 1999)*. Care must be taken that the pressure behind the knee does not impede the circulation *(Holden et al 1988)*. A decision should be made as to the possibly opposing needs for comfort and functional ability *(Rodosky et al 1989)*. The height of the destination chair relative to that of the original position may be critical to some methods of transfer.

Chair arms should project forwards far enough to allow a person to push up from them *(Munton et al 1981)*, and equipment may be supplied to provide an extended arm support where required. If people use their arms parallel to the body to push themselves up, then the muscular effort required by other parts of the body is lessened; however, when arms are abducted to push, stability is increased *(Schultz 1992)*. As with seat height, there is a trade off between the height of arm rests for sitting and that required to assist standing. These could slope up towards the front of the seat to effect a compromise *(Chan et al 1999)*. The provision of removable armrests will allow for a choice of methods of transfer for many people.

Riser seats could also assist in the sit to stand and stand to sit stages of the transfer, but care must be taken that the person is not left in an unstable position once standing. Although a forward rake to the seat could assist egress, it would not provide sufficient support in sitting for some people *(Holden et al 1988)*. An electric riser seat which alters the rake on assisting to rise could therefore be useful.

3 Facilitative measures for independent transfer

Various methods exist in which the person could be encouraged to be independent by increasing their mechanical advantage. These could include:

- The person moves closer to the edge of the chair to bring their centre of gravity closer to their base (requiring more space in front of the patella, as the knee moves forward during this movement). This involves the person extending the trunk and tilting the pelvis forward. This can also be achieved by rocking from side to side to move their buttocks forward, and may also be assisted by the person pressing down on the chair armrests to enable them to move their buttocks forward on the seat.
- The person places one or both feet under the trunk, increasing the degree of ankle dorsiflexion, thus reducing the horizontal movement necessary to produce stability in standing *(Schultz et al 1992)*.
- Encouraging the person to hold the head erect will also increase stability and shorten the time required *(Stevens et al 1989)*. During the lift-off stage of rising, the forward movement changes to an upward one, and looking down inhibits momentum and may increase the time and effort required (see also chapter 12).

If manual or mechanical assistance is needed, then space may be required around both sides of the chair. Should a standing and raising aid be used, there will need to be adequate space around or under the chair.

When assessing the assistance required to transfer a non weight bearing person of 50 kgs with strong arms, *Marras et al (1998)* concluded that the only safe way to assist was by using mechanical devices. All other methods, whether with 1 or 2 handlers entailed excessive compressive spinal loading on them. Similarly, *Ulin et al (1997)* investigated the transfer of a person weighing 56kgs and unable to weight bear or assist. These transfers from bed to wheelchair using a pivot transfer, a belt or a sliding board with 2 handlers, all involved spinal loads above the NIOSH Back Compression Design Limit (BCDL - 3400 N). Some transfers even exceeded the Back Compression Upper Limit (BCUL) of 6400 N *(NIOSH 1981)*. Jobs associated with compressive forces exceeding 6236 N show an eight-fold risk of workers developing low back pain when compared to those whose work only involved forces of 2673N or less *(NIOSH 1981)*.

Research by *Ulin (1997)* is specifically related to non weight bearing people unable to assist in their own transfer. Regardless of which of the six methods used, the forces involved were such that less than 53% of the female population, acting as the lead lifter would have sufficient strength to perform this, even if only taking 50% of the weight. During many 2 person lifts the lead handler can take up to 100% of the person's weight at different times. When measuring the forces involved in applying a sling and using both mechanical and electric hoists, none of these tasks exceeded the BCDL. Ulin concludes that *"regardless of patient weight, consideration should be given to completing the transfer with a mechanical lift to minimise back compression forces and subsequent risk of low back injury"* to the handler. Measurements were not taken of the forces required to move the person using the mobile hoist, only in applying the sling.

The use of equipment may reduce the physical demand on muscle strength from the person. This may assist mobility in people suffering pain or in a weakened state, but for others it may result in disuse atrophy. A balanced decision must be agreed by both assistant and person/family as to the use of adaptations and equipment. The effects of these strategies must be carefully monitored and modified if necessary.

4 Methods of transferring from a seated position to another seated position

The following offer facilitation for transfers not requiring physical intervention from another person

- Standby supervision with verbal prompts
- Chair raisers
- Extended chair arms
- Removable chair arms to enable independent sideways transfer
- Rotating discs
- Sliding/rolling boards
- Grab rails
- Mechanical seat raiser/riser chair.

Any of the above may also be used in conjunction with other equipment or direct physical intervention. The number of handlers required to assist may vary.

Practical techniques

Task One

Sitting to sitting through standing – no physical help from another person

DEPENDENCY LEVEL	Independent transfer if situation ideal, may require verbal supervision.
DESCRIPTION	• Person sitting in correct chair, destination chair appropriately placed, person sitting in optimal position, one foot back towards seat and feet apart, person sitting closer to front edge of seat (see task three, chapter 13), pushing up on armrests if necessary. • Person flexes at hip and knee, keeps head erect, achieves lift off, extends and stabilises. • Person steps around to stand in front of new chair, backs up to seat and reverses procedure to sit. See also task one, chapter 13.
PERCEIVED EXERTION FOR HANDLER	None
COMFORT FOR PERSON	Will depend on joint range and any associated pain in hips, knees and cervical spine, and possibly shoulder joint stability if arms are required to aid push off.
SKILL LEVEL OF STAFF	Clear verbal reminders.
EVIDENCE AVAILABLE	1 *Munroe and Steele (1998)* state that pushing on armrests reduces leg forces required. 2 *Weiner et al (1993)* identified that using a raised seat also reduces effort required. 3 The position of feet, pelvis, head and arms affects ease of rising *(Laporte et al 1999 pt 1).* 4 *Munroe and Steele (1998)* state that ejector devices in seating reduce muscle activity required, but that training in their use is recommended to ensure safety of users. 5 *DIAG (2001)* advice suggests use of handrails, frames etc and or one or two handlers for transfer.
DANGERS/ PRECAUTIONS	Person requires motivation and physical ability.
FURTHER OPTIONS	• This method could be used to access a bath seat or toilet. • Seat height can be improved by raising height of seat, lengthening arm rests to assist in push-off. • Person may require riser chair, with assisted lift-off.

5 Sideways transfers

Some people may be able to achieve independent transfers by using their arms. This is usually performed in a sideways direction, with any removable armrests detached for egress. Some prefer the chairs to be placed at right angles to each other so they can reach across to the other seat. This transfer can be facilitated by using a sliding board or patient roller across from one seat to another. The resulting reduction of friction can make this move easier. Care must be taken to ensure that the person has sufficient balance to effect this transfer safely. Amputees or people with no weight bearing ability can sometimes transfer themselves in this way.

To achieve an independent seated transfer the person may require help from a physiotherapist in order to improve their functional ability. An occupational therapist may offer advice in respect of improving the environment to facilitate the move. Should physical intervention from another person be necessary, the handler must be familiar with the use of any equipment required, and understand any contraindications in relation to its use.

Task Two

Sitting to sitting – no physical help from another person, independent sideways transfer

DEPENDENCY LEVEL	• Person requires balance, good upper body strength, ability to support weight on arms, ability to move hips across to another seat and motivation. • Ability to weight bear not required.
DESCRIPTION	• Transfer easier if chairs are side by side with armrests removed, but can be placed at right angles with fixed arms. • Person reaches across to other seat with outer arm, shuffles hips across and settles in new position.
PERCEIVED EXERTION FOR HANDLER	None
COMFORT FOR PERSON	This depends on upper limb joint range and arm strength/pain.
EVIDENCE AVAILABLE	*Safer Handling of People in the Community (1999)* states that the person must have good upper body strength.
DANGERS/ PRECAUTIONS	Chairs must be correctly placed and the person must have predictable balance and movement.
FURTHER OPTIONS	• This could be facilitated by using a slide or roll board under the buttocks to reduce friction (see task seven). • A turning disc under the feet, if the chairs are at right angles, may prevent the ankles twisting and the feet catching on each other. • Person could reach for grab rail, pull themselves to standing, step sideways and sit in adjacent chair. • These methods could be adapted to access a toilet or bath seat.

6 Seated transfers – some manual assistance or equipment required

- Repositioning person in chair
- Moving person up the bed when sitting
- Use of handling belt
- Use of sliding/roll board
- Turning disc
- Turning device with handle
- Turning device with fixed frame

Research on repositioning a slumped person in a wheelchair shows that performing this manually involves excessive spinal compression in the handler *(Varcin-Coad and Barrett 1998)*. Only manual techniques were involved in this research in which either1 or 2 people lifted the person back into the chair. The lift was carried out from behind the wheelchair, with the handler grasping the person's forearms to reposition their pelvis back in the chair, and was compared with other methods where another handler assisted *(Varcin-Coad 1998)*. The spinal loading when the second handler lifted at the person's knees was much higher than when the second handler pushed back horizontally at the knee. However, both methods resulted in an increased risk of injury to the first handler positioned behind. The one handler lift entailed less effort than the lift upwards at the knee with another handler. As the forces involved exceeded the BCDL, the use of mechanical equipment was recommended for this task. The use of the one way glide was not tested.

Some people will be able to assist in their own repositioning by edging their way back into the chair *(DIAG 2001)* or may require assistance to achieve this from 1 or 2 handlers. Alternatively, a handler can encourage the person to rock from side to side whilst assisting the person to edge back in the chair by applying pressure at the side of the ribs or hip *(DIAG 2001)*.

For some people, risk assessment will indicate that the safest and most comfortable option will be to use a hoist and sling for repositioning in their chair. If this is likely to be necessary it may be appropriate to leave the sling behind them in the chair, bearing in mind factors such as comfort, tissue viability, friction from frequent re-insertion, aesthetics and personal choice.

The use of the one way glide ("glide and lock") may help people with sitting balance and ability to push themselves, or be pushed back into the chair by another. It must be on the seat before they sit down and remain under them throughout their time in the seat, so it must not be creased.

Task Three

Reposition person in chair with one way glide

DEPENDENCY LEVEL	**Mobility Gallery C** **FIM 3** Person must have sitting balance, and be already sitting on the equipment prior to repositioning.
DESCRIPTION	Person either pushes themselves back into chair using one-way glide, or handler may assist by pushing gently on person's knees.
PERCEIVED EXERTION FOR HANDLER	Some people may require assistance from a handler in order to be repositioned. This effort should not be excessive, otherwise another method of repositioning should be selected.

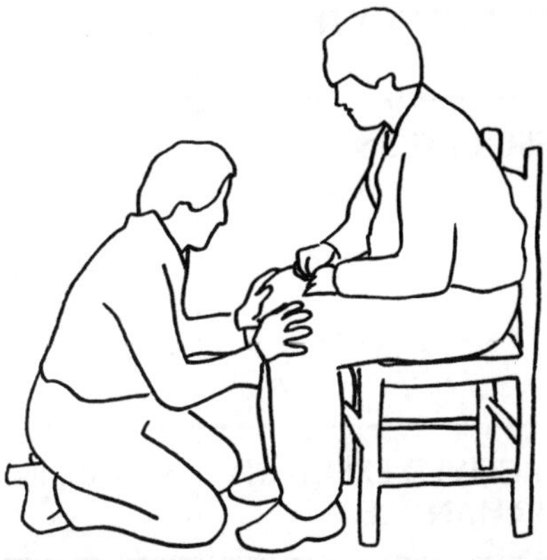

FIG 14.1

COMFORT FOR PERSON	If the person has painful knees this may prove uncomfortable when handler pushes on knees.
SKILL LEVEL OF STAFF	Staff must be familiar with equipment.
EVIDENCE AVAILABLE	No evidence found in use of one way glide, although *DIAG (2001)* recommends this equipment for prevention of slipping, as does *Safer Handling of People in the Community (1999)*. The latter publication cautions against this equipment for people with fragile skin or poor circulation.
DANGERS/ PRECAUTIONS	• If person has short legs, the handler may need to place person's feet on a box or similar to ensure their thighs are parallel with the floor, to allow for pushing directly back on knees. • Person must sit on one way glide, so tissue viability may be at risk with some. The use of the fleece covered cushion may help, although shearing forces on the tissues may still present problems.
FURTHER OPTIONS	• If person has ability to lift buttocks up alternately, the one way glide will not be needed, as they will be able to edge their own way back into the seat. Some people can sit on a non slip material such as Dycem to reduce slipping, but shearing forces may still present problems. • Should neither of these methods be applicable, a hoist could be used to effect this repositioning.

Evidence review

Technique	REBA	Activity	Comfort	FIM	Mobility gallery	Skill level	Comment
REPOSITION PERSON IN CHAIR WITH ONE-WAY GLIDE							
Fig 14.1	5	8	9	3	C	Advanced beginner	One way glide ensures the person is active and has a medium level of postural risk.

Task Four

Sitting to sitting through standing – with help from 1 or 2 handlers

DEPENDENCY LEVEL	Physically able, but requires some assistance to rise, can weight bear and move feet independently.
DESCRIPTION	• Person sits as above in task one of this chapter, handler(s) face same way as person, placing inner hand on person's upper back, outer hand at top of person's chest at front. • Handler(s) exerts some pressure from behind and may rock person back and forth, saying ready, steady, up (or similar agreed command) and restrain person from leaning too far forward with outer hand. Please also see task four, chapter 12. • Person moves to rise, as in task one, and is assisted to turn through 90 degrees and then to sit in another seat.
PERCEIVED EXERTION FOR HANDLER	Should only require minimal effort from handler.
COMFORT FOR PERSON	The handler's hand should not cause discomfort in this position.
SKILL LEVEL OF STAFF	Basic training required in communication and methods of assisting people.
EVIDENCE AVAILABLE	No research available, but recommended by *DIAG (2001)*.
DANGERS/ PRECAUTIONS	Handler's outer hand prevents person leaning too far forwards.

7 Sitting up in bed and moving

See chapter 15.

8 Use of equipment to assist transfers

Studies *(Moody and McGuire 1996)* suggest that nurses may be unable or reluctant to use equipment due to unavailability, lack of training and insufficient space. In another paper by *McGuire and Moody (1996 b)* it was shown that although nurses often believed that patients found aids frightening or uncomfortable, in fact most of the patients found them to be desirable and safe. They concluded that the design of some aids requires improvement, and that the needs of the people, the tasks the aid will be used for and the environment must all be considered. Despite training in safer methods of transfer *(Kane 1994)*, some nurses may also feel pressured into using poor techniques by other colleagues. The lack of resources for equipment in some settings may be due to a lack of full appreciation by management of the knock on costs following back injury to staff *(McGuire et al 1997)*.

Assisting a person to transfer using a handling belt

A wide belt with handles can be used to assist a weight bearing person to stand and transfer. If their weight bearing is unpredictable, this method would not be suitable. The selection of the correct size and shape of belt is important, as it must fit snugly around the person's waist and be fastened securely. A person with a spinal deformity may find a wide belt uncomfortable, and those belts without outside handles may prove painful if the handler's knuckles press against the person's body inside the belt. The belt handles should be held in such a way that the handler does not get her hands trapped if the person falls. Using a belt increases the reach of the handler, and gives a better grip and it also allows for a pain free grasp if a person has pain or tender skin. Use of the handling belt may entail some spinal twisting for the handler.

Some belts have a non slip lining to prevent them riding up the person's body. However, if this occurs, it may be due to an incorrect fit, asymmetry of the person's trunk or, more frequently because the person is sagging at the knees and not truly weight bearing. This would then involve an asymmetrical lift to the side of the handler's body and potentially a full body lift, should the person lose their ability to stand. *Dehlin (1975)* identified that lifting a patient manually from bed to chair and back exceeded the safe limits set by the International Labour Office and was often impossible to perform when attempting to lift 'correctly' with bent knees and a straight back.

Research on the use of a belt around the person's waist to assist in their movement is complicated by the research language. In most instances it is made clear that a 'gait belt' is a wide band of material affixed around the person and used by handlers inserting their fingers inside, against the person's body. A 'walking belt' is described as a wide band around a person's waist, with handles for handlers to use. *Garg et al (1991)* identified person discomfort and increased risk to handlers when the gait belt is used. *Owen and Fragala (1999)* researched bed to chair transfers using a gait belt, hoist or slide pad with profiling chair. Both handlers and people expressed perceptions that the slide pad method with the adaptable chair was easier, safer and more comfortable than the others.

Task Five

Sitting to sitting – 1 or 2 handlers assisting with handling belt

DEPENDENCY LEVEL	Person must be able to weight bear and move feet independently, but requires assistance to rise to feet.
DESCRIPTION	• Person sits as in task one, and handler affixes belt. Handler(s) assist from side by holding either person's hand in palmar grasp and outside of belt loop, or belt loops with both hands. • Handlers may rock person, saying ready, steady, up (or similar) and guide person to other seat and assist in sitting.
PERCEIVED EXERTION FOR HANDLER	Care must be taken to only assist person in standing. This method is unsuitable if a lift is required.
COMFORT FOR PERSON	• Person with painful chest, a stoma or pregnant person may find this uncomfortable. • Some people with asymmetry may find the belt does not fit well.
SKILL LEVEL OF STAFF	Basic training required in communication and methods of selecting appropriate equipment and assisting people to move.
EVIDENCE AVAILABLE	1 Originally recommended in *The Handling of Patients 4th edition (1997/8)* and *Safer Handling of People in the Community (1999)*. 2 The research available *(Zhuang et al 1999)* mostly measured the compressive force required to rotate a person from supine to sitting, prior to assisting them to a chair. Both handlers and subjects found them safe and comfortable to use, and using the belt was faster than other methods, except for manual lifting *(Zhuang 1999, Benevolo et al 1993)*. 3 Research by *Marras et al (1999)* shows there is very little difference between the under arm drag and the "gait belt" as to the handler's likelihood of falling into the high risk group membership, due to the high compression forces (both above the recommended NIOSH limits). However, the use of the belt reduces the shearing forces in both directions to handlers' spines . 4 *Garg et al (1991)* showed that belts without handles were uncomfortable for both the person and staff, but that use of the belt with handles and 2 handlers required less effort, increased comfort and security but it did take a little longer than manual methods alone. 5 Use of the handling belt by one handler from in front was determined to be unsafe by *Gagnon et al (1986), Gagnon and Lortie (1987)*.
DANGERS/ PRECAUTIONS	• If person ceases to weight bear, handler(s) may suddenly be taking all the weight of person. • If person sits down suddenly this may enforce stooping and twisting by handler(s).
FURTHER OPTIONS	This method can be utilised to access a bath seat or toilet.

Use of the turning disc on the floor

If a person has the ability to weight bear, but is not able to step from one chair to another, then a turning disc under their feet will facilitate this transfer. It can be assisted by one handler or two, but requires careful positioning to ensure that the person arrives safely at the destination seat. The person must have both good balance and reliable weight bearing and not have painful hips or knees on rotation of the trunk.

Task Six

Standing transfer with 1 or 2 handlers using turning disc

DEPENDENCY LEVEL	**Mobility Gallery** B **FIM** 3

Person must be able to weight bear and have good standing balance, but is unable to step around and requires assistance to rise to feet.

DESCRIPTION

- Transfer achieved by handler(s) assisting person to stand (with or without handling belt) with chairs carefully placed at right angles.
- Handler(s) stand at outside edge of chair facing forward (if 2 handlers required then there must be sufficient space between chairs).
- Handler(s) assist person to stand (see task one) then assist person to turn by standing in front or to the side of person). This may be achieved by firmly pushing at person's hip level, or a belt may assist if person's trunk is held rigid and does not rotate when pressure applied. If 2 handlers are available then one may be required to move the chairs to a suitable position.
- When person is correctly positioned the handler(s) may 'sidle' around to the side and assist to sit as per normal.

PERCEIVED EXERTION FOR HANDLER

If person is heavy, this may be hard work for handler(s).

COMFORT FOR PERSON

People with painful hips or knees may find this uncomfortable.

SKILL LEVEL OF STAFF

- Handler requires communications skills and ability to assist person with specific equipment.
- Handlers need to reposition furniture as required.

EVIDENCE AVAILABLE

The Guide to the Handling of Patients (4th edition) (1997/8) and Safer Handling of People in the Community (1999) recommend this method but there is no research based evidence as to its effects. Both publications caution against possible instability of person in its use.

DANGERS/ PRECAUTIONS

Handler must ensure that person will not collapse during transfer, by consulting risk assessment and enquiring as to balance and ability to cooperate, as well as weight bearing ability.

FURTHER OPTIONS

If 2 handlers are required to ensure safety whilst turning, then a third person may be required to move chairs around. Failing this another method of transfer should be considered. This method could be used to access a bath or toilet.

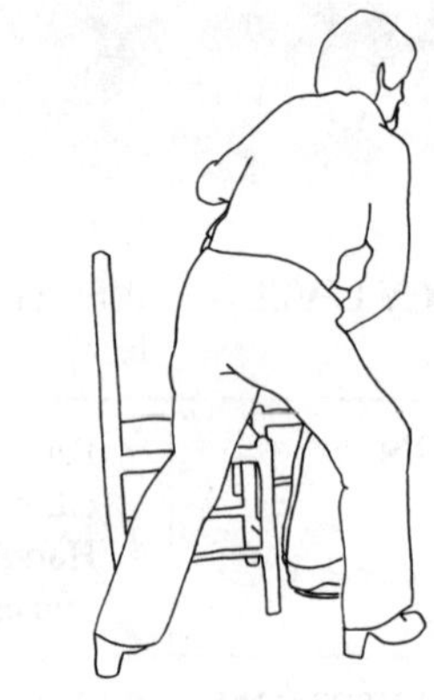

FIG 14.2a

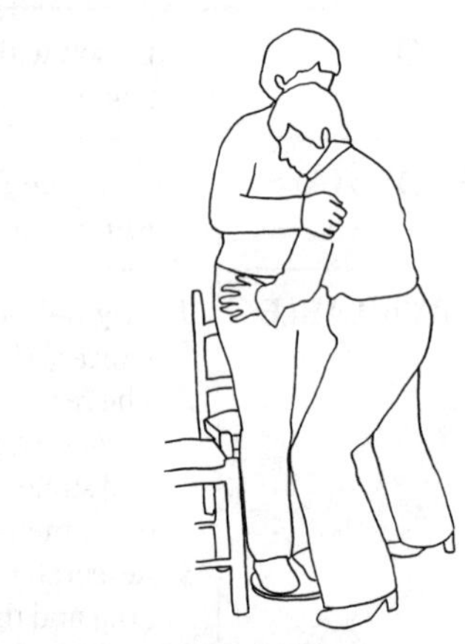

FIG 14.2b

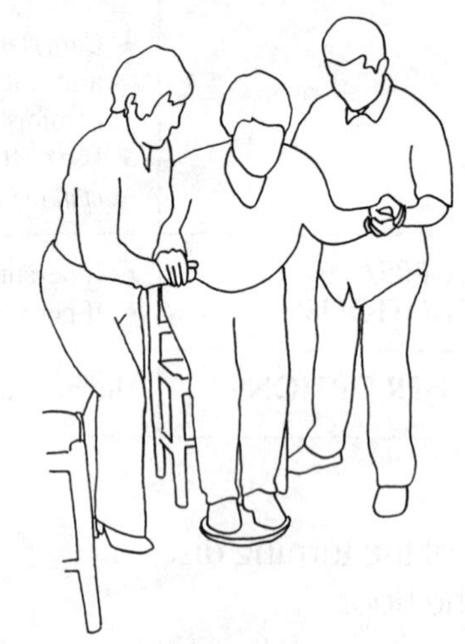

FIG 14.2c

Evidence review

Technique	REBA	Activity	Comfort	FIM	Mobility gallery	Skill level	Comment
USE OF TURNING DISC ON FLOOR – STANDING TRANSFER WITH 1 OR 2 HANDLERS							
Figures 14.2a – c	6	6	4	3	B	Competent	Turn table gives a medium level of postural risk, encourages some activity and gives a low level of comfort.

Use of a Sliding Board

Some people have the ability to perform independent non weight bearing transfers using a short slippery board to bridge the short gap between 2 seats, which must be close together (see earlier on relative seat heights). They require strong arms and good sitting balance as well as trunk control. *Safer Handling of People in the Community (1999)*, cautions against using a sliding sheet on top of the board as it may cause uncontrolled slipping.

Task Seven

Sideways transfer with slide/roll board and assistance of 1 handler

DEPENDENCY LEVEL

Mobility Gallery C
FIM 4

- Person requires balance, good upper body strength, ability to support weight on arms, ability to move hips across to another seat and motivation.
- Need not be weight bearing, but may initially require guidance across the board.

DESCRIPTION

- Transfer easier if chairs side by side with armrests removed, but can be placed at right angles with fixed arms if curved board is used.
- Person reaches across to other seat with outer arm, shuffles hips across and settles in new position.
- Handler ensures person remains on board by placing hand on person's hips, with verbal instruction and minimal manual guidance, kneeling/crouching in front of person.
- If person has good postural stability the handler's hands may be placed on or around the person's shoulders.

PERCEIVED EXERTION FOR HANDLER

Person requiring more than minimal assistance may require alternative method of transfer

COMFORT FOR PERSON

Care should be taken not to "pinch" person's skin when inserting the board.

SKILL LEVEL OF STAFF

Handler requires communications skills and ability to supervise person with specific equipment.

EVIDENCE AVAILABLE

1 Evidence *(Zhuang et al 1999)* shows that if assistance is required for this transfer by using a handling belt then the pushing forces are high. As this research described a supine lying to seated transfer to a chair with a person asked 'not to assist', it may not be applicable. The sliding board used had a seat that slid along a groove in the board. The handler was pushing 81 Newtons, measured by the pressure exerted by the feet on the force platform. People perceived the board as being unsafe and uncomfortable, and staff stated that it

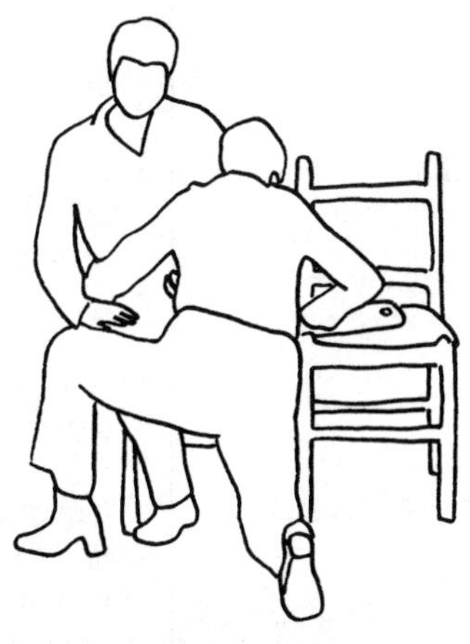

FIG 14.3a

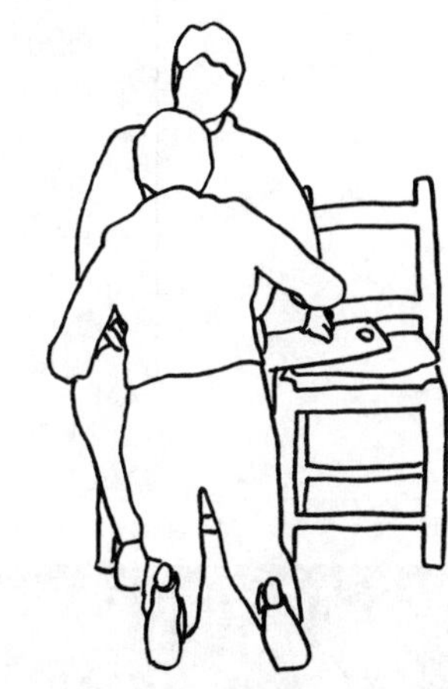

FIG 14.3b

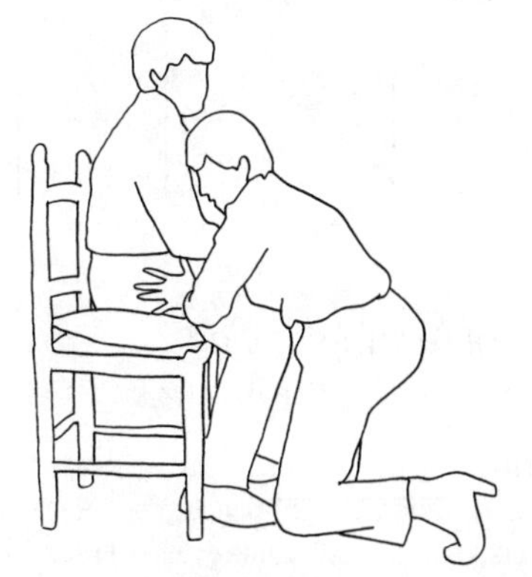

FIG 14.3c

was harder to use than the manual lift. It was, however, faster than hoisting.

2 Research by *Ulin et al (1997)* showed that with 2 handlers assisting, the force required exceeded NIOSH levels of back compression, however this was using a subject that was unable to assist at all on a wooden board.

3 *DIAG (2001)* advice suggests that only minimal assistance from one or more handlers should be required to achieve this transfer. *Safer Handling of People in the Community* cautions against using a roller slide sheet on top of a sliding board, as it may result in hazardous slipping.

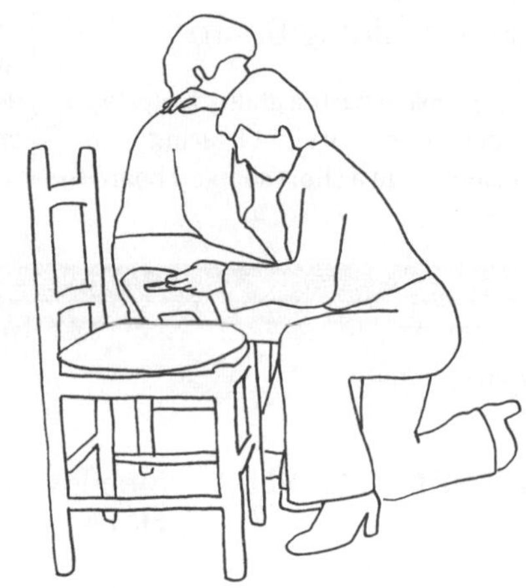

FIG 14.3d

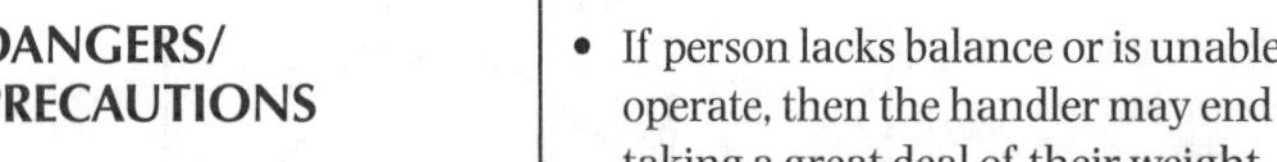

DANGERS/ PRECAUTIONS

- If person lacks balance or is unable to co-operate, then the handler may end up taking a great deal of their weight.
- The 2 surfaces must be adjacent to each other and similar in height.
- Not to be used in conjunction with a separate sliding sheet.

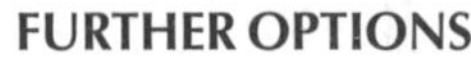

FURTHER OPTIONS

- It may help to have a turning disc under the feet, if the chairs are at right angles, to prevent the ankles twisting and feet catching on each other.
- If independent, the person may perform this transfer unaided. This method could be used to access a toilet, but bare buttocks do not always slide well on a board.
- Use of a board with a round aperture may allow for the person to use the toilet with the board in situ. When sliding onto a bath seat, care must be taken to see that the person has good sitting ability, and is able to lift, or have their legs lifted into the bath.

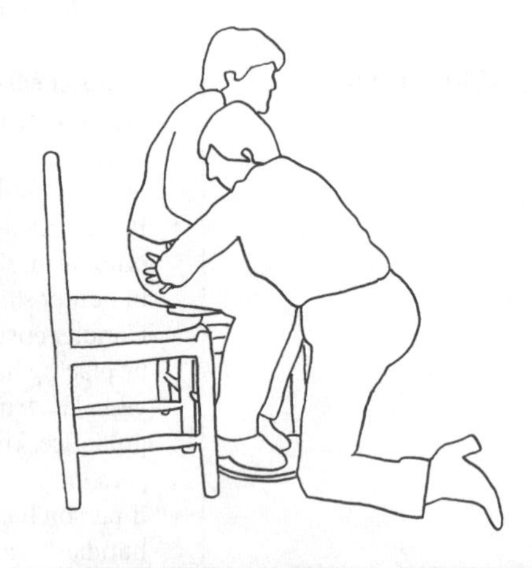

FIG 14.3e

Evidence review

Technique	REBA	Activity	Comfort	FIM	Mobility gallery	Skill level	Comment
SIDEWAYS TRANSFER WITH SLIDE/ROLL BOARD WITH THE ASSISTANCE OF 1 HANDLER							
Figs 14.3 a–e	11	8	7	4	C	Competent	The slide board has a very high REBA score. It requires a high level of activity and gives an acceptable level of comfort.

Use of turning device with central handle

The turning device with a tall central handle enables weight bearing people with a strong, predictable grasp to raise themselves with the help of a handler, before they are turned to lower themselves onto another seat. This equipment is only designed to turn, not to allow for the person being pushed around the room. However, there are now relatively new designs available which allow for transfer around the room by pushing, although this will require risk assessment as to the floor surface and pushing forces involved. It must also be clarified as to whether or not the person has sufficient standing balance for this, and that the equipment is designed for this purpose.

Task Eight

Transfer with turning device with handle and 1 handler

DEPENDENCY LEVEL

Mobility Gallery B
FIM 5

Person requires balance, good upper body strength, ability to weight bear, and have a strong, predictable grasp and be able to understand/cooperate with instructions.

DESCRIPTION

- With chairs carefully placed at right angles the turner is introduced from in front of the person, ensuring that it goes sufficiently under the person's feet and that the knee rest is against the upper end of the tibia.
- With the handler's foot on the 'brake' the person is asked to reach forward and grasp the handle, and pull themselves to their feet. A second handler could assist with clothing if required.
- Once the person is standing, the handler removes foot from brake, rotates person to position in front of destination chair, replaces foot on 'brake' and asks person to lower themselves onto seat.
- The turner is then carefully removed and wheeled away.

PERCEIVED EXERTION FOR HANDLER

Handler should not feel a strain, particularly if stride stand foot position is adopted.

COMFORT FOR PERSON

Should feel comfortable for the person, as they only expend the effort required.

SKILL LEVEL OF STAFF

Handler requires communications skills and ability to assist person with specific equipment.

EVIDENCE AVAILABLE

1. Advised in *Safer Handling of People in the Community (1999)* and recommended because it encourages the person to assist themselves.
2. *Ruszala (2001)* identified that this device could help functional activities. It was found easy to use and effective by staff.

DANGERS/ PRECAUTIONS

- Person must have reliable grasp to help themselves up and hold on whilst being turned.
- If person is much heavier than handler then handler will not be able to hold turner whilst person pulls against them.

FURTHER OPTIONS

This method could be used to access a toilet or bath seat.

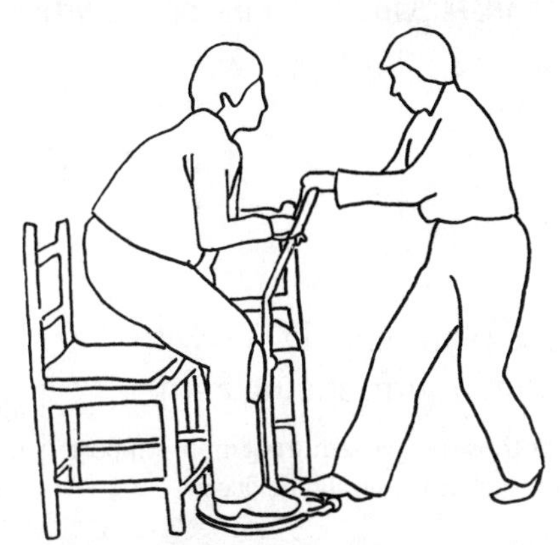

FIG 14.4a

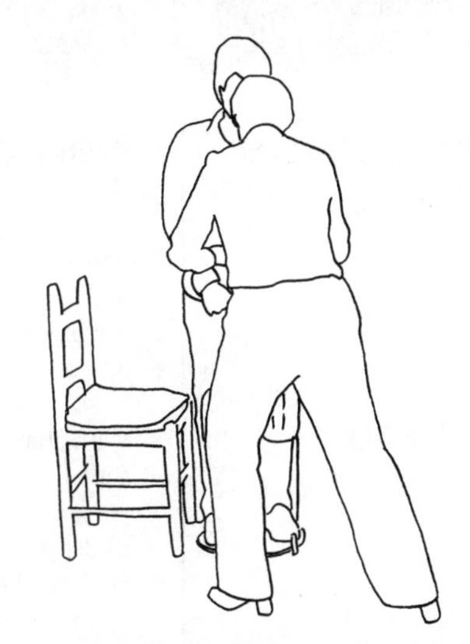

FIG 14.4b

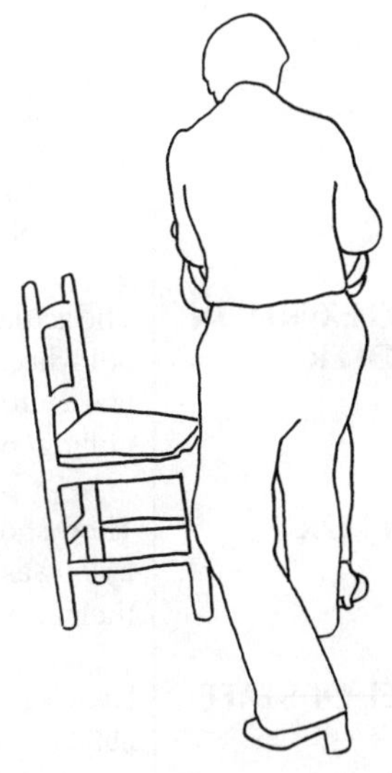

FIG 14.4c

Evidence review

Technique	REBA	Activity	Comfort	FIM	Mobility gallery	Skill level	Comment
TRANSFER WITH A TURNING DEVICE WITH A HANDLE AND 1 HANDLER							
Figs 14.4 a–c	5	9	9	5	B	Advanced beginner	The **stand** and **turn** disc gives a medium level of postural risk and maximises the input from the person

Use of turning device with built in surrounding frame

For those people requiring more support and stability a similar device with a frame around it can be used. Although much heavier to ensure stability, it can also be wheeled to the person before use, the person pulls themself up, then the handler releases the brake before rotating the frame to the desired position. After the person has lowered themselves to a seat, the frame can be wheeled away.

Task Nine

Transfer with turning device with frame and 1 handler

DEPENDENCY LEVEL

Mobility Gallery B
FIM 5

Person requires balance, good upper body strength, ability to weight bear, and have a strong predictable grasp and be able to understand/co-operate with instructions.

DESCRIPTION

- With chairs carefully placed at right angles the turner is introduced in front of the person, ensuring that it goes sufficiently under person's feet.
- With the handler ensuring the hand "brake" is applied, the person is asked to reach forward, grasp the frame and pull themselves to their feet.
- Once the person is standing the handler removes hand brake, rotates person to position in front of destination chair, re-applies hand brake and asks person to lower themselves onto seat
- The turner is then carefully removed and wheeled away.

PERCEIVED EXERTION FOR HANDLER

The actual turn should entail very little effort, but wheeling the device into and out of the place into the correct position may require pulling/ pushing.

COMFORT FOR PERSON

There should be no discomfort for the person, as long as they have sufficient strength in their arms to pull up.

SKILL LEVEL OF STAFF

Handler requires communications skills and ability to assist person with specific equipment.

EVIDENCE AVAILABLE

No research found, but *DIAG (2001)* suggests

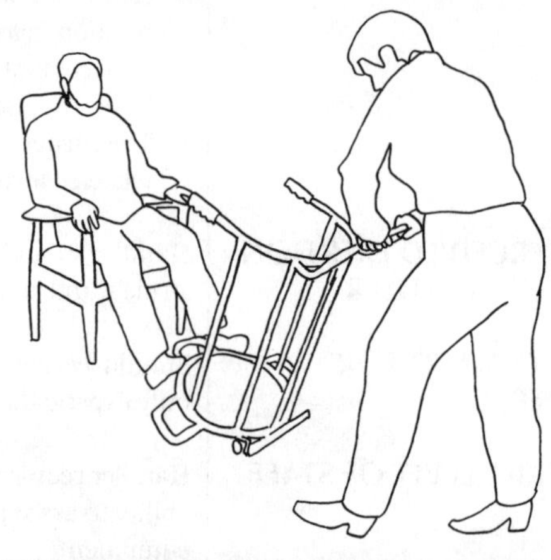

FIG 14.5a

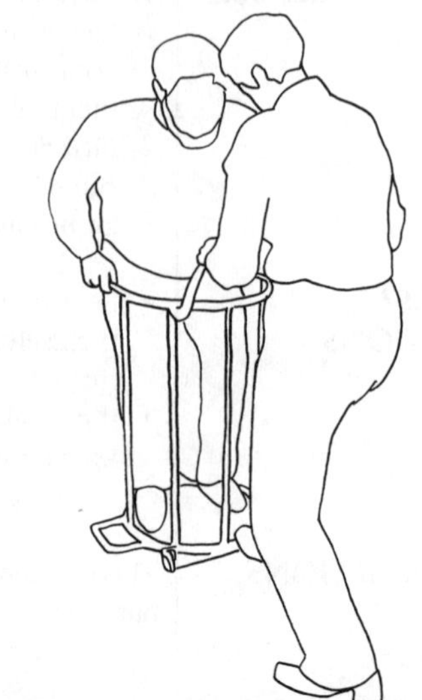

FIG 14.5b

DANGERS/ PRECAUTIONS

1 or 2 handlers, with one assisting the person to stand, and also states that this device should not be replaced by a flat turning disc. Person must have reliable grasp to help themselves up and hold on whilst being turned. The framed turner is heavy and must be manoeuvred with care when moving to/from person.

FURTHER OPTIONS

This equipment could be used to access the toilet or a bath seat, if space allows.

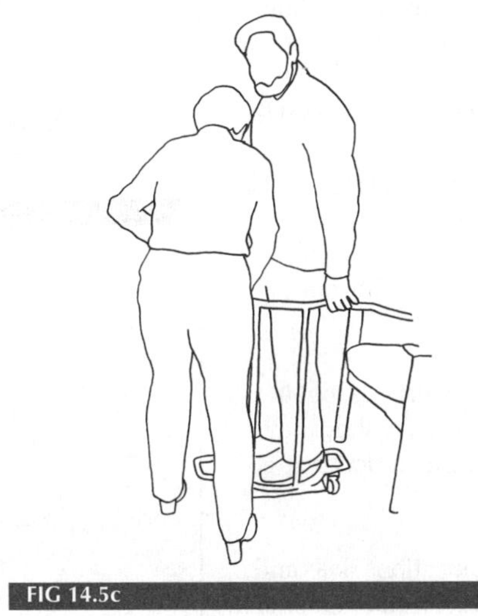

FIG 14.5c

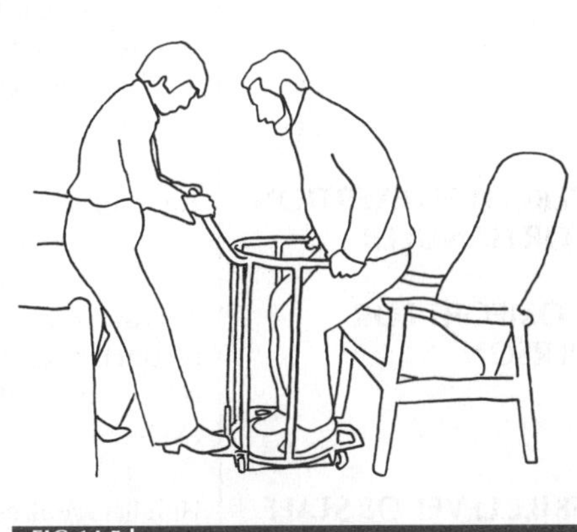

FIG 14.5d

Evidence review

Technique	REBA	Activity	Comfort	FIM	Mobility gallery	Skill level	Comment
TRANSFER WITH TURNING DEVICE WITH FRAME AND 1 HANDLER							
Figs 14.5 a–d	3	9	9	5	B	Advanced beginner	This turning device gives a low level of postural risk and maximises the input from the person.

Equipment available for more dependent people

- Standing and raising aid.
- Hoist and sling.
- Tracking/gantry/mobile hoist and walking harness.

In order to use a standing and raising aid, the person must have some weight bearing ability and, in most cases, the ability to hold onto the handles with both hands. They do not have to pull themselves up, as this is done either mechanically or electrically.

Task Ten

Transfer with standing and raising aid and handler(s)

DEPENDENCY LEVEL

Mobility Gallery C
FIM 3

- Person must have some weight bearing ability and be able to cooperate by reaching for handles and holding on whilst aid mechanically raises them to their feet.
- Both arms must remain outside the sling, unless otherwise specified by manufacturer.

- If person pulls themselves upright the sling may slide up, so they must usually remain leaning back against the sling.

DESCRIPTION

- Correct specified sling to be selected and applied in approved manner.
- The sling should then be connected to hoist and person asked to grasp handles and remain holding on whilst raised to an inclined standing position.
- The person is raised from supporting surface (clothes removed as appropriate if accessing toilet) and moved, then lowered to receiving surface.
- Sling should be detached and removed to ensure comfort.
- If person is to be returned to original seat this process is repeated.

PERCEIVED EXERTION FOR HANDLER

Applying sling may require twisting and reaching for handler.

COMFORT FOR PERSON

This transfer should be comfortable, but if person is not sufficiently able the sling may ride up on their back and pull under their axillae.

SKILL LEVEL OF STAFF

Handler requires communications skills and ability to assist person with specific equipment.

EVIDENCE AVAILABLE

1. This equipment was recommended by *Busse (2000)* for people able to support a limited part of their weight to reinforce a sit to stand movement.
2. *Ruszala (2001)* showed that this equipment was suitable for early rehabilitation.
3. *Fragala (1993)* showed that use of standing and raising aids (and sling lifters) reduced occupational injury.
4. *Roth et al (1993)* showed that use of the standing and raising aid for changing incontinence pads, toileting and bed/chair transfers was found easier by staff than manual lifting or use of the full hoist.
5. Use of the standing and raising aid saves time, and was seen as more comfortable than manual lifting by people (*Zhuang et al 2000*). However, as the forces measured were of a dependent person being rotated to sit at the bed edge, and this equipment is designed for a partially assisting person, *Zhuang* states that forces required may be less than in his work. He found no significant differences in moving a standaid or a hoist around with a person aboard.
6. *DIAG (2001)* states that the person must have some weight bearing ability, trunk and upper limb control and some ability to cooperate.

DANGERS/ PRECAUTIONS

- Mobile standing and raising aids should

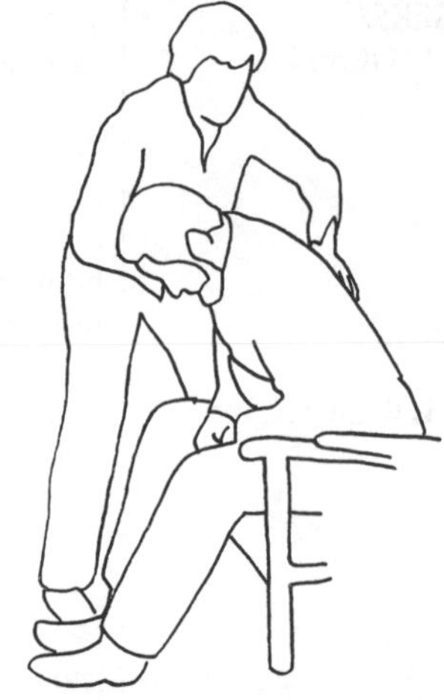

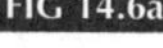

FIG 14.6a

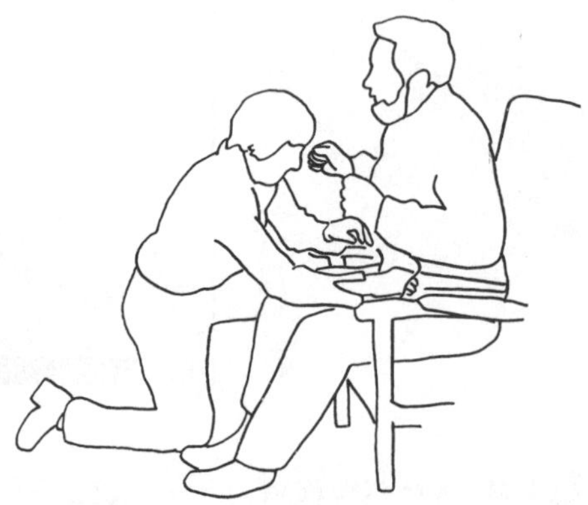

FIG 14.6b

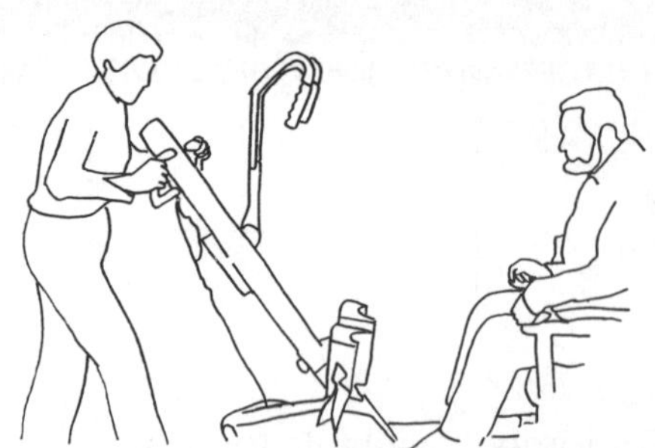

FIG 14.6c

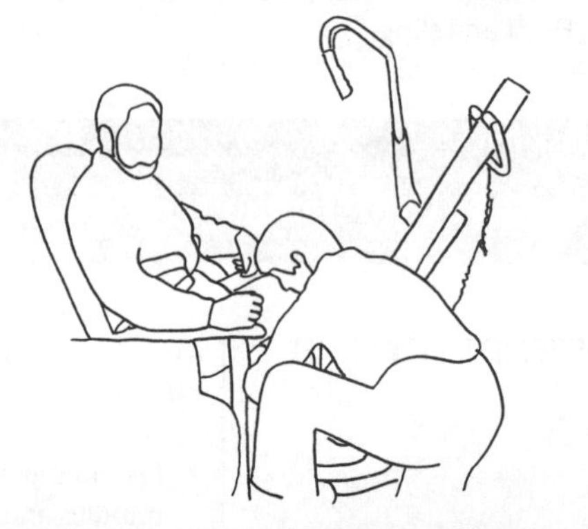

FIG 14.6d

not be moved long distances with person suspended.

- An en-suite bathroom may be considered close enough in some instances.
- Some have a removable seat that can allow the seated patient to be transferred to another location in a comfortable and dignified way.
- Heavy people may require more handlers to move them safely.
- Sling must be correct size/type/purpose for each person.

FURTHER OPTIONS

Equipment must be strategically positioned for optimum convenience.

- These "belt" slings may facilitate toileting/dressing if person has requisite ability.
- This method may be used to access the toilet or a bath seat.
- Some can be used to assist walking. The risk assessment must show that the person has requisite ability. The footplate must be removed beforehand and person raised sufficiently upright.

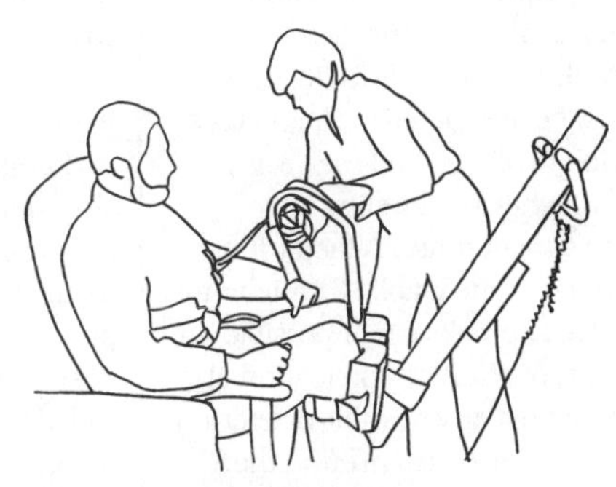

FIG 14.6e

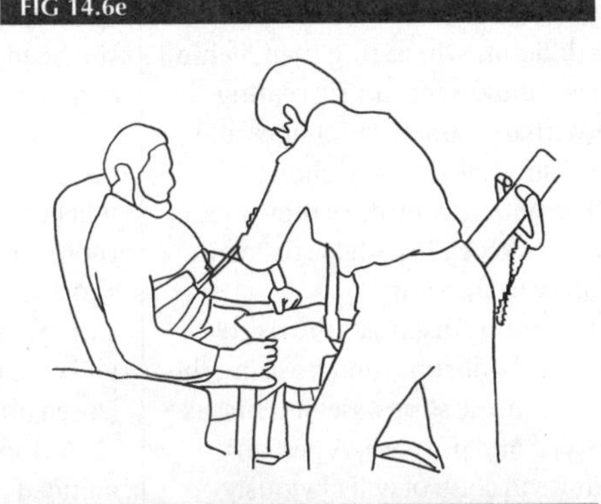

FIG 14.6f

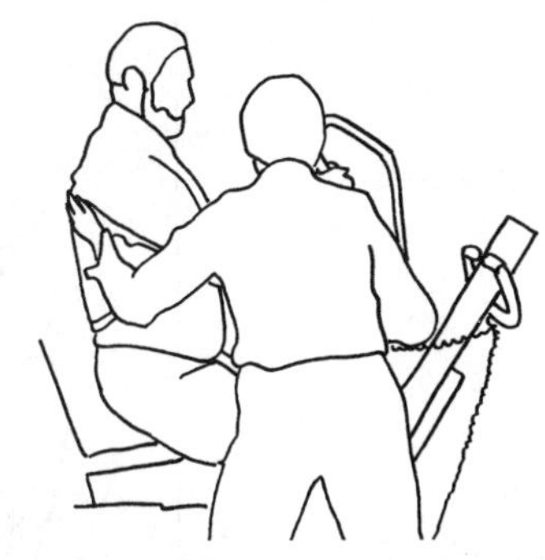

FIG 14.6g

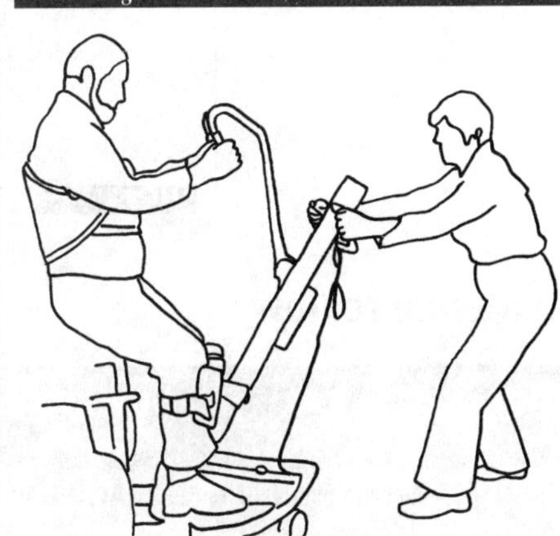

FIG 14.6h

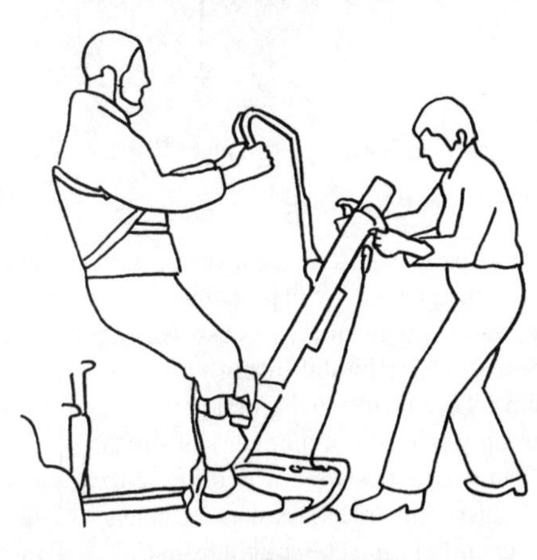

FIG 14.6i

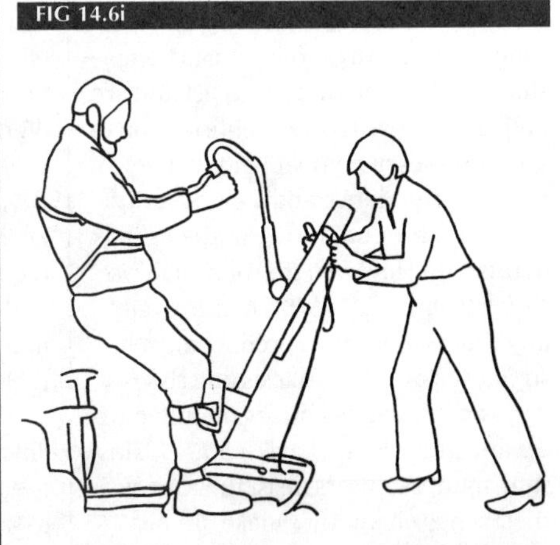

FIG 14.6j

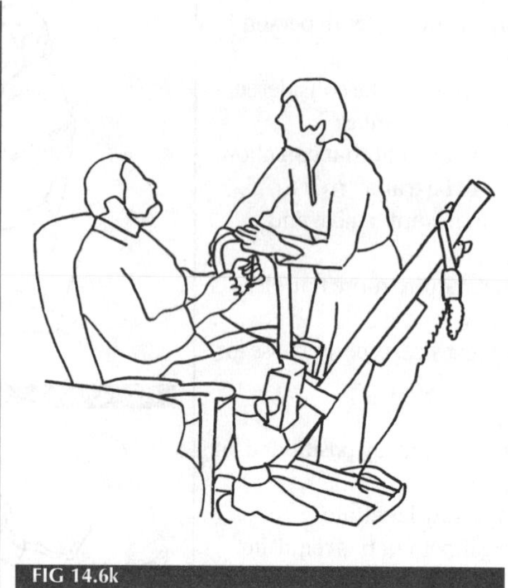

FIG 14.6k

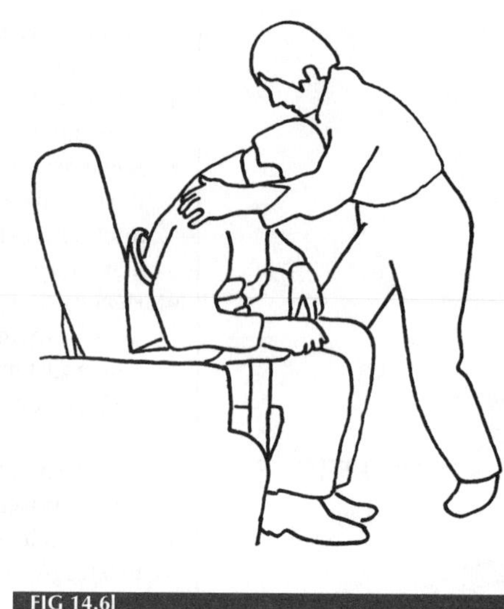

FIG 14.6l

Evidence review

Technique	REBA	Activity	Comfort	FIM	Mobility gallery	Skill level	Comment
TRANSFER WITH A STANDING AND RAISING AID AND HANDLER							
Figures 14.6 a – l	5	4	7	3	C	Competent	The stand aid had a medium postural risk level, and a low activity level.

Transfers involving use of hoist and sling

Those people with no ability to assist in their own transfer will probably, following an adequate risk assessment, be transferred by staff using a hoist and sling. There is much discussion and anxiety around compatibility of slings. If slings are to be used with other makes of hoists and are assessed as suitable, information must be sought from the supplier of slings (BS EN 10535). Some sling manufacturers have tested their slings with other makes of hoist and are prepared to give written confirmation of specific cases of compatibility. Others may issue guidance and an indemnity insurance around the use of their slings in this way. However, the *Medical Device Regulations (MDR 1993)* require that any claims made for a product must be supported by relevant tests and risk assessments carried out by manufacturers and importers *(Handley 2004)*. Most sling manufacturers insist that use of their slings on another make of hoist will also depend on an assessment by a competent person to ensure safety during use. This risk assessment is also a requirement of *LOLER 1998*. It is essential that the correct type and size of sling is used, and that the fabric is comfortable and suitable for its purpose. Staff must be instructed in the correct application of slings, and the decision made as to whether the sling is to remain in situ after use. A factor to be considered is tissue viability, which must also involve appreciation of possible skin damage by constant re-application of slings as against any possible deleterious effects of pressure if left around the person. Other factors include comfort, dignity, aesthetics and person choice, as well as difficulties inserting them behind people in moulded or matrix seating. People with asymmetrical shapes may require a specially tailored sling to fit, and those with involuntary movements may require specialist advice to ensure their safety in the sling.

DIAG (2001) discusses the use of different types of sling, emphasising the need for accurate sling assessments, as to size, type and purpose. A person without head control will obviously require a sling with head support. A toilet (access or dressing) type of sling may be unsafe if used on a person with low tone, trunk instability, an inability to keep their arms outside the sling, an amputee, or someone lying flat on the floor.

Slings can be applied in a variety of situations, in sitting or lying on a bed or the floor. Some staff may find it difficult to apply a sling on the floor due to problems with their own knees when kneeling. If a person cannot easily be rolled from side to side to apply a sling in lying, the sling could be inserted between 2 flat slide sheets that have been unrolled under the person from the head down or the feet up (see chapters 15 and 16).

A ceiling mounted hoist will remove the need to move the hoist around, but will limit the location of transfers unless room covering tracking is available. As a short term option the provision of a gantry, over the area vital for transfers will ease matters, and can often be leased and erected at short notice.

As long ago as *1984, Bell* recommended that not only should an equipment officer be appointed, and teaching packages should include instruction in the use of hoists, but that equipment selection must ensure compatibility with existing "fittings and furnishings". *Bell* also comments on other factors influencing hoist use, such as individual patient needs, environmental problems, staffing levels and attitude and knowledge in the use of equipment. *Duffy (1999)* also suggested that after classroom instruction in the use of equipment, this should be followed up by practice in simulated or real care settings.

Task Eleven

Transfer with hoist and sling, with 1 or 2 handlers

DEPENDENCY LEVEL

Mobility Gallery D
FIM 1

Person may be unable to assist with transfer.

DESCRIPTION

- Correct sling to be used in specified manner.
- The sling should then be connected to the hoist and the person raised from supporting surface and moved, then lowered to the receiving surface.
- Sling should be detached and either removed or tucked away to ensure comfort, dignity and safety.

PERCEIVED EXERTION FOR HANDLER

Most exertion is usually felt when moving a mobile hoist with a person suspended, especially on a floor surface such as carpet.

COMFORT FOR PERSON

Correctly sized and fitted slings should not be uncomfortable, although some people may require special fabrics to ensure comfort, e.g. silk, netting, fleece lined.

SKILL LEVEL OF STAFF

Handler requires communications skills and ability to assist person with specific equipment.

EVIDENCE AVAILABLE

1 *Garg (1991)* showed that although some hoists required less effort than others, very heavy and totally dependent people should be transferred by well designed hoists, despite the longer time factor required. Staff reported less effort was involved in using a gantry hoist *(Gingher et al 1996)* and this could often by used by one handler. People appeared less disturbed than by previous methods of transfer.
2 *Marras et al (1998)* concluded that a non-weight bearing person of 50 kgs should be transferred by mechanical devices, not manually, due to excessive spinal loading, whether with the assistance of 1 or 2 handlers.
3 *Zhuang et al (2000)* suggest that as slings/hoists varied in comfort and ease of use, care should be taken in selection/design.
4 *DIAG (2001)* recommends the use of electric hoists over manual, except in certain specified situations, for example, as

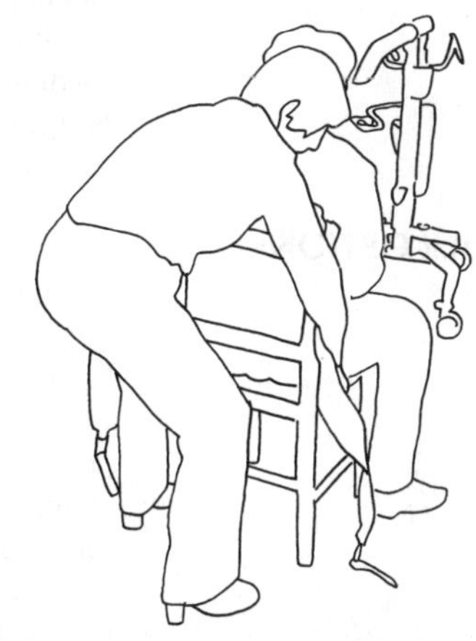

FIG 14.7a

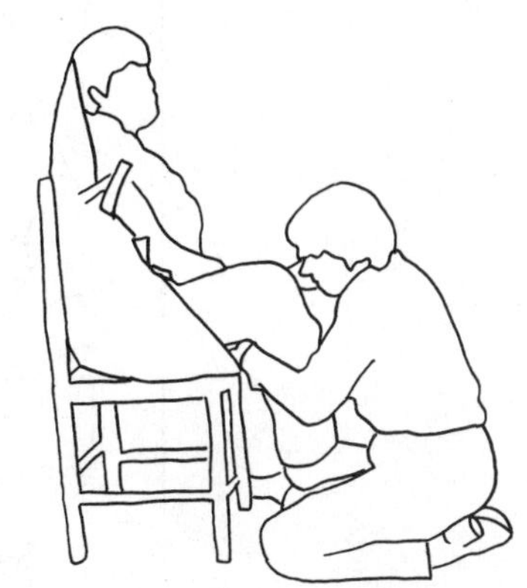

FIG 14.7b

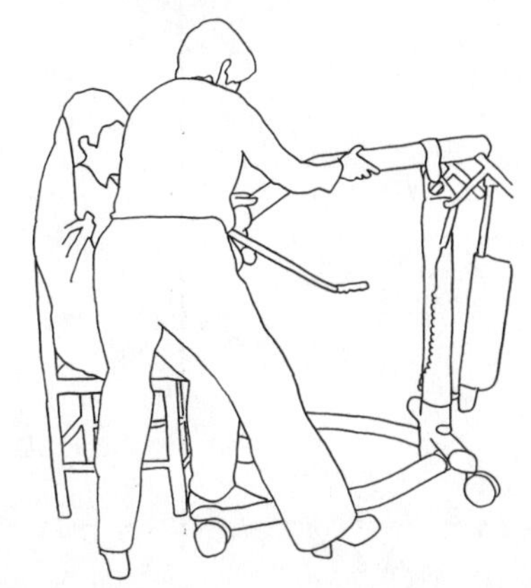

FIG 14.7c

an interim measure, infrequent use, no electric supply, where water may cause problems or difficulty in charging battery.

DANGERS/ PRECAUTIONS

- Mobile hoists should not be moved long distances with the person suspended.
- Risk assessment must inform the decision to transfer to a wheelchair and push to another room, although an en-suite bathroom may be considered close enough in some instances.
- Heavy people may require ceiling tracking or gantries to enable handlers to move them safely.
- Sling must be correct size/type/purpose for each person.

FURTHER OPTIONS

If person requires toileting, either an access sling can be used, or

- person can rock from side to side to allow for removal of clothing when placed on toilet.
- person can be hoisted onto a bed or changing table, undressed and the sling replaced prior to being hoisted onto a commode or toilet.
- this method can be used to access toilet or bath or bath seat.

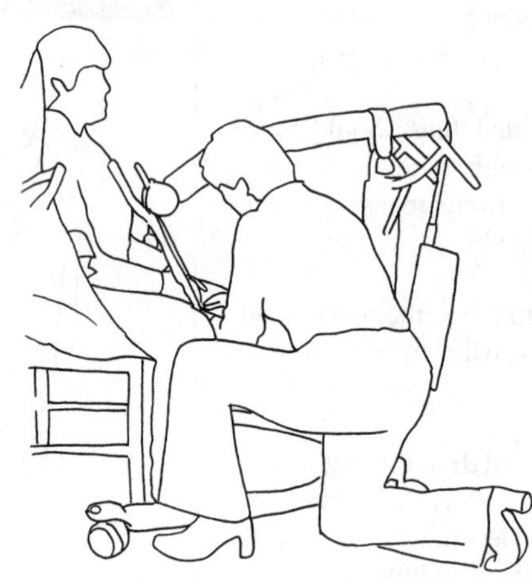

FIG 14.7d

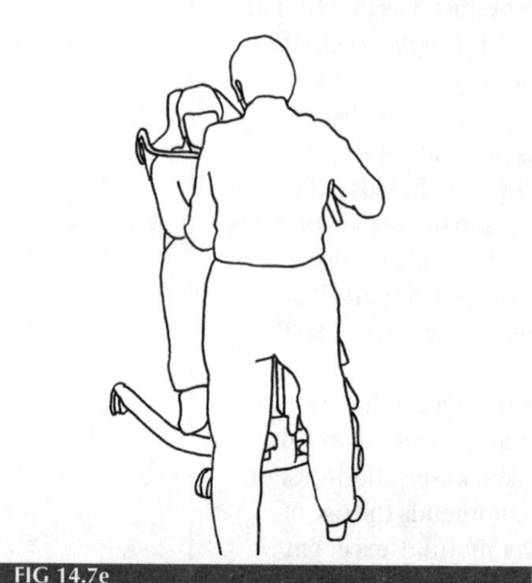

FIG 14.7e

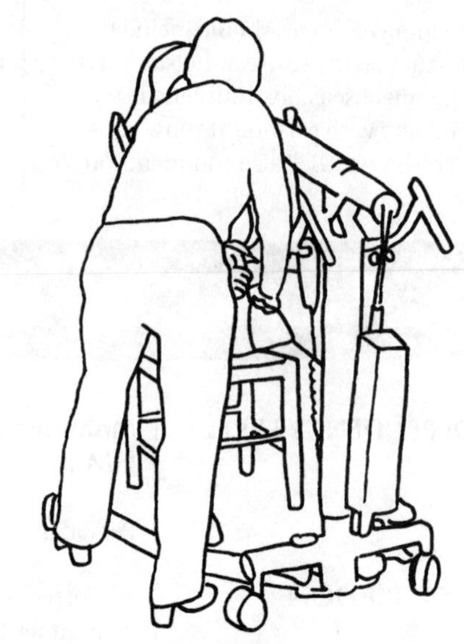

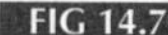

FIG 14.7f

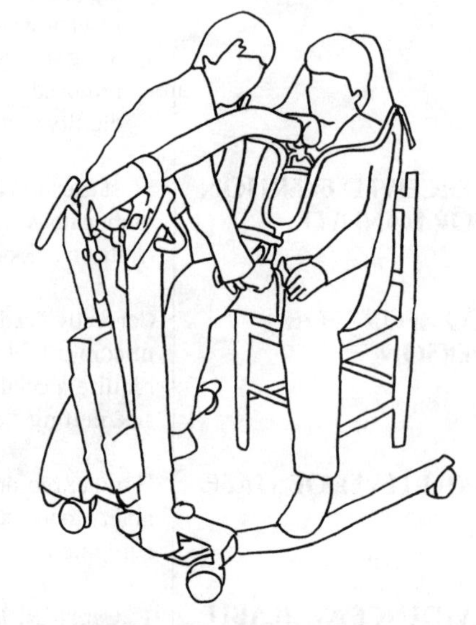

FIG 14.7g

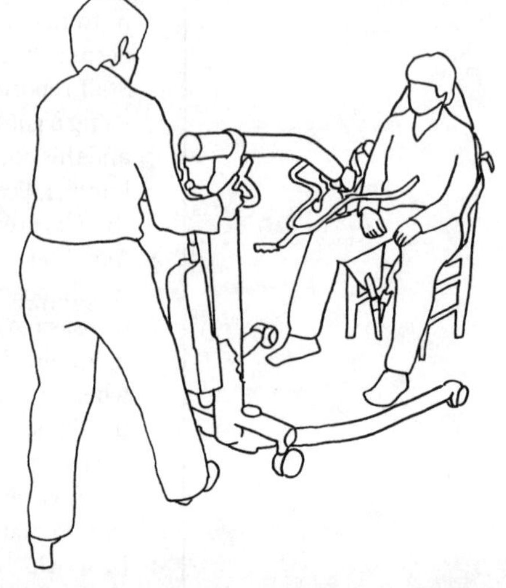

FIG 14.7h

Evidence review

Technique	REBA	Activity	Comfort	FIM	Mobility gallery	Skill level	Comment
TRANSFER WITH HOIST AND SLING WITH 1 OR 2 HANDLERS							
Figs 14.7 a–d	8	2	9	1	D	Advanced beginner	Hoist use is only appropriate for much less able people. The risk levels are high for both inserting the sling and moving the hoist.
PUSHING HOIST AND PERSON OVER A CARPET							
Figs 14.7 e–h	9	2	8	1	D	Advanced beginner	Hoist use is only appropriate for much less able people. The risk levels are high for both inserting the sling and moving the hoist.

Use of hoist and walking harness

Should a person require a transfer using a hoist but is able to assist in some weight bearing, even if unpredictably, then a therapist may advise the use of a hoist and standing harness. This must be prescribed, selected and monitored by a skilled person, and staff instructed carefully in the use of such apparatus. This method of transfer could also be used as part of a rehabilitation programme, or as a means of accessing specialised equipment such as a standing frame, walker, tricycle or equivalent (see also chapter 13).

Many physiotherapists use a walking harness and hoist as a rehabilitation tool. This support can be provided as tracking over a treadmill, allowing walking to be practised in safety *(Malouin et al 1992, Gardner et al 1998, Hesse et al 1999, Cherniak et al 1999, Kendrick et al 2001)*.

Of course there is overlap in the above methods, depending on the individual capability and professional judgement of the handler, the equipment available and staff skill.

Children may also require help with walking, and there are several ways to assist this. If possible, the child should be encouraged to rise to their feet with as little help as necessary, as lifting from the floor is a hazardous occupation. Some can be shown how to lean on strategically placed furniture to assist in rising.The above method of walking with a hoist and special harness, as detailed in task five, chapter 13, could be used, or a manually assisted lift with one or two handlers could be performed. Both handlers could crouch either side and assist a child with some weight bearing ability to their feet; use of a handling belt may assist with this task. Alternatively they could half kneel on one knee only, to each side and rise to their feet in a smoothly coordinated manner.

To assist a child to walk, the handler could use a wheeled stool and push themselves forward or backward by paddling with their feet (*Association of Paediatric Chartered Physiotherapists – APCP–1999*). Some schools of thought encourage the handler to grip the shoulder to enable keypoints of control to be utilised, or alternatively a handling belt could aid the grip.

Seated transfers in a community setting

Many of the above transfers would work equally in a care setting or in the community. It is often believed that hospitals are always spacious and the cubicles areas well planned, but modern nursing is often hampered by the amount of equipment around the bedside. It was even mentioned as a problem as long ago as 1984 by *Bell*, who noted that *"there was insufficient space between any of the beds in any of the wards to allow any of the mobile hoists to be used effectively if bed screens were drawn"*. However, the pressures in community work also involve negotiating with person and family as to the space required and the need for equipment *(Alexander 1998)*. According to *Bell (1987)* the need for smaller domestic hoists as opposed to those required for institutional use became apparent by the late 1960s.

There may be some local confusion concerning supply of equipment to peoples' own homes. In many areas the integrated Community Equipment Stores (ICES) are functioning well, but in some areas different types of equipment are supplied by various service providers. Residential homes and day care settings should have sufficient resources to acquire their own equipment as required, and will find it easier to supply aids that will meet the needs of several people, rather than a one off. Hopefully there will be more space in such purpose built care settings than in a person's own home. However, many of the en suite bathrooms provided in residential homes will not allow for a hoist, wheelchair and occupant and 2 handlers, although it is recognised that the dependency level of people in such homes will often require that assistance is given for personal care *(Care Standards Act 2000)*.

Many residential and domiciliary settings may have carpeted floors, which will clearly increase the effort of pushing around equipment such as hoists. Research by *Bell (1984)* showed that the design of the castors could also influence the pushing and pulling forces involved in moving patients around by hoist. One of the early references to the four aspects of assessment, "the patient, the attendant, the task and the environment" was from *Bell (1987)* when discussing a systems approach to patient handling.

The Health and Safety Executive in their publication *Handling Home Care (2001)* advises those staff working in a person's own home to ensure that they take into consideration the person's rights to autonomy, privacy and dignity. However, despite the need to respect the person's wishes wherever possible, the balanced approach is emphasised, and it states that care workers are not required to perform tasks that put them or other people at risk unreasonably.

The main exception to the use of tasks one to eleven, in a community setting, would be the availability of a walking harness and mobile or tracking hoist. Not only does this require special equipment, but the time and expertise required of staff is unlikely to be available in a domestic or residential setting. It is more commonly used in rehabilitation units to re-educate walking, either in a gym or set over a treadmill, and in schools, to access standing frames and walkers.

9 Seated transfers in bathrooms and toilets

Problems arising around seated transfers in bathrooms and toilets centre around 3 issues:

- the lack of space.
- the need for access to the person's body.
- differences in levels of seating and toilet/bath.

The use of a sanichair on wheels (commode frame with brakeable castors) reduces the number of transfers required and allows them to be performed in another room of sufficient size *(HSAC 1998, Garg et al 1991b)*. They can then be wheeled to the bathroom, instead of the commode being used with the pan in situ.

Bathing

Various adaptations to bathrooms are feasible, from fitting height adjustable baths to the use of a simple bath board to facilitate the person's entry. There are many types of bath seat which remove the need for a person to get right down to the bottom of the bath. Others rise from the bath floor to the rim, electrically or mechanically powered, to allow people to transfer at the bath edge and then be lowered to the bath bottom. Some actually have rotating seats to facilitate this entry. Should a very dependent person wish to be bathed this may be achieved by various means including the following:

- removing the cosmetic front bath panel to allow for mobile hoist access under the bath from the side.
- approaching a freestanding bath end-on by mobile hoist.
- using a gantry or ceiling hoist to lower the person.
- transferring a person into a special access bath, such as one with a front or side opening door.
- transferring person to wheeled shower chair and wheeling to a level access shower cubicle.
- using a shower trolley, which can be taken to the bed side for transfers then wheeled to the bathroom.
- rolling the person onto an inflatable shallow bath on their own bed, inflating and showering them in situ.

A person with little postural ability will require postural support in a domestic bath or shower chair for safety.

All of the above transfer methods (tasks one to eleven) could be used to access toilet or bath/bath seat. However, in each case an individual risk assessment will be necessary to plan for the need to undress the person, and for space to access the bathroom equipment. Care must always be taken when the person is wet as they may be slippery after bathing, and special care should be taken to dress them as quickly as possible to prevent excessive cooling.

Use of the toilet

Assisting a person to the toilet has long been considered as a very stressful task for staff *(Garg et al 1994)*. A reduction in staff injury rates was noted using belts with handles for light, weight bearing people and hoists and slings for heavy or non-weight bearing people and including environmental changes to the bathroom area. Their conclusion was that ergonomic changes reduced risk exposure more effectively than education programmes for staff. In this study, the use of the sanichair reduced the number of transfers from 6 to 2 per person for toileting and washing. As *Jensen (1990)* showed, the more transfers performed, the more staff injuries occurred.

The need to remove underwear from a person unable to weight bear may well cause problems. The person may wear adapted clothing to facilitate access, be able to rock from side to side to allow for removal of clothing or need to be returned to bed or a changing table to allow for safe access to clothing. Staff should ensure that people are well supported when having their incontinence pads changed.

For people able to weight bear, holding a grab rail whilst a handler assists may suffice, or another handler may be required. Staff should not assist a person to stand whilst removing the clothing at the same time. Another handler may be required to assist, or supplying a walking aid may help a person to remain standing whilst staff assist them with their clothing.

Seeing to cleansing after a person has used the toilet often presents a problem. If people are able to assist then clearly this operation should be facilitated, perhaps by use of toilet paper tongs or long handled devices, or with staff assistance. Staff should not be required to crawl under commodes to perform these tasks. If this cannot be achieved readily on the commode, then the person should be returned to bed or a changing table to enable this to be done. Alternatively, a height adjustable tilt in space commode/shower chair may facilitate this task.Use of a closimat toilet, with bidet function and a drying facility will ensure personal cleanliness in a dignified and comfortable way for many people requiring assistance.

Task Twelve

Transfer with slide/roll board with assistance of 1 onto bath seat

DEPENDENCY LEVEL

Mobility Gallery C
FIM 4

Person requires balance, good upper body strength, ability to support weight on arms, ability to move hips across to another seat, and motivation. Need not be weight bearing, but may initially require guidance across the board.

DESCRIPTION

- Transfer is easier if the chair is sideways on to the bath with armrests removed, but can be placed at right angles with fixed arms if curved board is used.
- The person reaches across to bathseat with outer arm, shuffles hips across and settles in new position. Handler ensures client remains on the board by placing hand on client's hips, with verbal instruction and minimal manual guidance, kneeling/ crouching in front of client. If person has good postural stability the handler's hands may be placed on or around the person's shoulders.
- The handler may need to lift the person's legs into the bath either before or after they are on the bath seat.

PERCEIVED EXERTION FOR HANDLER

Person requiring more than minimal assistance may require alternative method of transfer.

COMFORT FOR PERSON

Care should be taken not to "pinch" person's skin when inserting board.

SKILL LEVEL OF STAFF

Basic training required in communication and methods of selecting appropriate equipment and assisting people to move.

EVIDENCE AVAILABLE

1 Evidence *(Zhuang et al 1999)* shows that if assistance is required for this transfer by using a handling belt then the pushing forces are high, but this research described a supine lying to seated transfer to a chair with the person asked "not to assist", so may not be applicable. The sliding board used had a seat that slid along a groove in the board. The handler was recorded as pushing 81 Newtons, measured by pressure exerted by the feet on a force platform. Users perceived the board as being unsafe and uncomfortable, and staff stated that it was harder to use than the manual lift. It was, however, faster than hoisting.

2 Research by *Ulin et al (1997)* showed that with two assisting, the force required exceeded NIOSH levels of back compres-

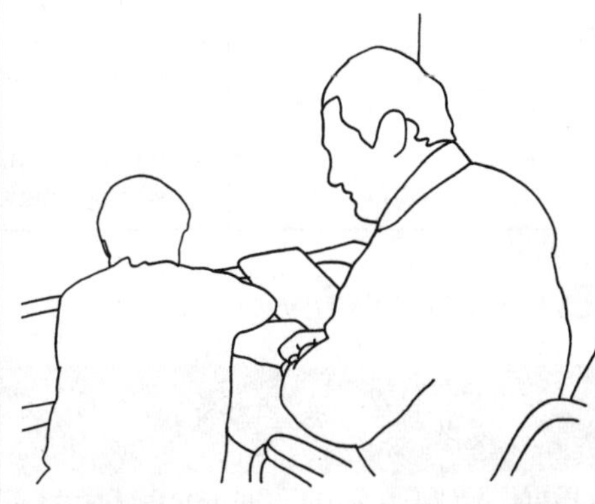

FIG 14.8a

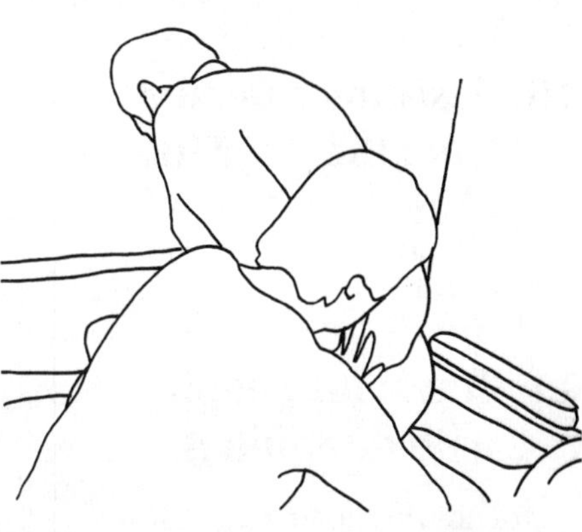

FIG 14.8b

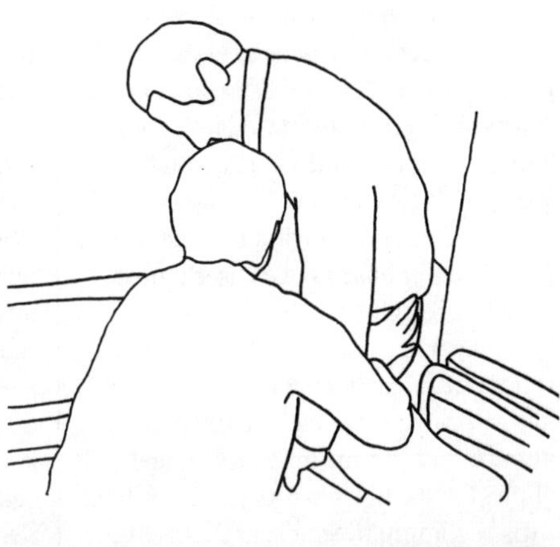

FIG 14.8c

	sion, but this was using a subject that was unable to assist at all, on a wooden board. 3 *DIAG (2001)* advice suggests that only minimal assistance from one or more carers should be required to achieve this transfer. *Safer Handling of People in the Community (1999)* cautions against using a roller slide sheet on top of a sliding board, as it may result in hazardous slipping.
DANGERS/ PRECAUTIONS	If client lacks balance or is unable to cooperate, then the handler may end up taking a great deal of their weight. The two surfaces must be adjacent to each other and similar in height. Not to be used in conjunction with a separate sliding sheet. The person may be wet and slippery.
FURTHER OPTIONS	• A turning disc under the feet, if the chairs are at right angles, to prevent the ankles twisting and feet catching on each other, may help. • If independent, the person may perform this transfer unaided. This method could be used to access a toilet, but bare buttocks do not always slide well on a board. • Use of a board with a round aperture may allow for the person to use the toilet with the board in situ. Care must be taken, when sliding onto a bath seat, that the person has good sitting ability, and is able to lift, or have their legs lifted into the bath.

Evidence review

Technique	REBA	Activity	Comfort	FIM	Mobility gallery	Skill level	Comment
TRANSFER WITH SLIDE/ROLL BOARD ONTO BATH SEAT WITH ASSISTANCE OF I HANDLER							
Figs 14.10 a–c	10	8	8	4	C	Novice	Putting legs into the bath and use of a slide board is a high risk activity.

10 Assisting a person from the floor to a chair

See chapter 17.

11 Travel for people with disabilities

Travelling in a vehicle for wheelchair users may involve either a transfer to the car seat or a way of accessing the vehicle to enable the person to travel in their wheelchair.

Some smaller mobile hoists will transfer a person unable to assist in their own transfer, and there are car top hoists and vehicle mounted hoists (see figures 14.9a – f and 14.10a and b) which will also achieve this transfer. Some car seats can swing out over the pavement for easier access (see figure 14.11a).

Some wheelchairs have a seat which slides onto a car seat chassis, others allow the person to elevate the seat to allow a sliding transfer. Some wheelchairs can be hoisted into the car intact, thus becoming the car seat themselves. If the wheelchair is parked on a sufficiently high kerb, a slide board may be used to allow access from a chair with removable armrests. Should the person be weight bearing they may be assisted into a car seat manually or using a handling belt. Alternatively, the use of a fabric swivel cushion may facilitate turning on the car seat to allow them to lift their feet or have their feet lifted into the foot well. If this cushion is affixed to the seat or has a non slip surface it may be acceptable to leave this under the person for the journey. People may wish to confirm this with their insurers.

Many wheelchair users stay in their wheelchair during transit. Of course it is important that both they and their wheelchair are restrained by safety straps/harnesses during travel. There are sources of information concerning the compatibility of wheelchairs and restraints *(Unwins 2001, Ricability 2002)* and as to the crash testing of wheelchairs restrained in a vehicle. In any case of doubt, the wheelchair manufacturer should be consulted. According to an article by the *Joint Committee on Mobility for Disabled People in Physiotherapy (1997)* 'Travelling in vehicles while in a wheelchair' there are risks inherent in both transferring into a vehicle seat to travel and in travelling in the wheelchair. Safety issues, person choice and reasonable practicability must all inform the method of travel selected. Advantages of reducing the number of transfers must be weighed against the problems associated with loading the occupied wheelchair into the vehicle. Methods may include the use of ramps, with or without a winch to assist, and passenger lifts, either rear or side mounted or free standing. The article concludes *"any debate on safety must be illuminated by an accurate assessment of risk and not based blindly on crash worthiness or imagined worst case scenarios"*.

Those people requiring access to community transport must have safe methods of access to the vehicle, and may require to stand on the passenger lift if they are unable to mount the steps unaided. Wheelchairs should enter the vehicle facing inwards on the lift and never travel facing sideways on, as the wheelchair restraints are not designed for this. There must be sufficient room between the seats for staff to access the restraint systems safely. Some staff may find restraining the wheelchairs and occupants involves working in a constrained space and entails stooping, stretching and twisting.

Task Thirteen

Transfer with hoist and sling, with 1 or 2 handlers from wheelchair to car seat

DEPENDENCY LEVEL

Mobility Gallery D
FIM 1

Person may be unable to assist with transfer.

DESCRIPTION

- Correct specified sling to be selected and applied in approved manner.
- This should then be connected to hoist and person raised from supporting surface and moved then lowered to receiving surface.
- Sling should be detached and either removed or tucked away to ensure comfort, dignity and safety.

PERCEIVED EXERTION FOR HANDLER

- Most exertion is usually felt when moving a mobile hoist with a person suspended, especially into such a confined space as a car interior.
- This is a very hard move to achieve.

COMFORT FOR PERSON

Correctly sized and fitted slings should not be uncomfortable, although some people may require special fabrics to ensure comfort, e.g. netting, fleece lined.

SKILL LEVEL OF STAFF

- Handler requires communications skills and ability to assist the person with specific equipment.
- Larger or inflexible staff may find this task very difficult.

EVIDENCE AVAILABLE

1 *Garg (1991)* showed that although some hoists required less effort than others, very heavy and totally dependent people should be transferred by well designed hoists, despite the longer time required.
2 *Marras et al (1998)* concluded that a non-weight bearing person of 50 kgs should be transferred by mechanical devices, not manually, due to excessive spinal loading, whether with the assistance of 1 or 2 handlers.

DANGERS/ PRECAUTIONS

- The car must have sufficient access for a hoist.
- A very small hoist should be used, to ensure the spreader bar will fit inside the car seat area.
- Mobile hoists should not be moved long distances with the person suspended.
- Risk assessment must inform the decision to transfer to a car seat from a wheelchair.
- Sling must be correct size/type/fit for purpose for each person.
- Due to space constraints the handler may be obliged to work in a stooped and twisted position and may need to place a foot inside

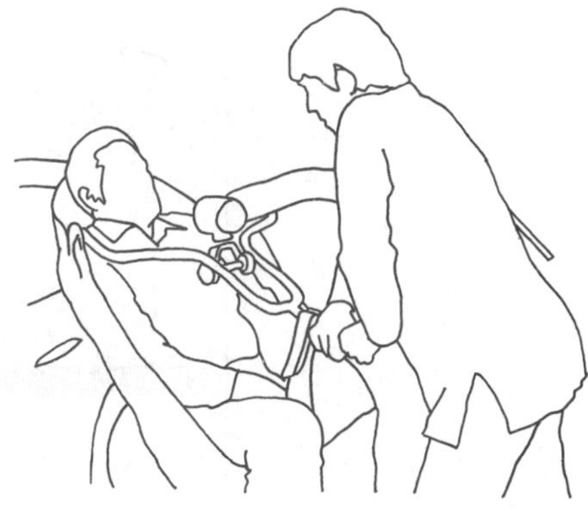
FIG 14.9a

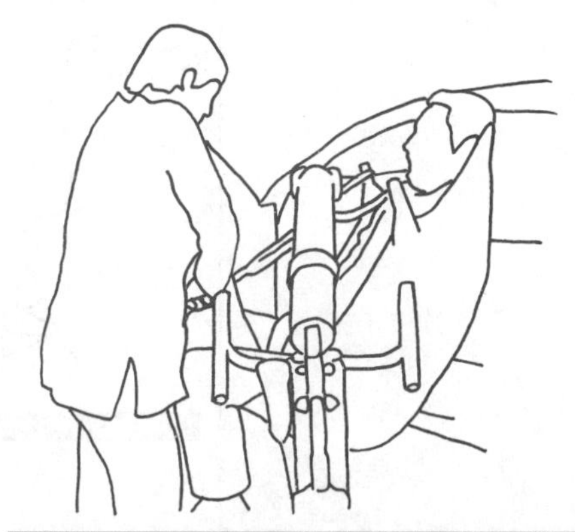
FIG 14.9b

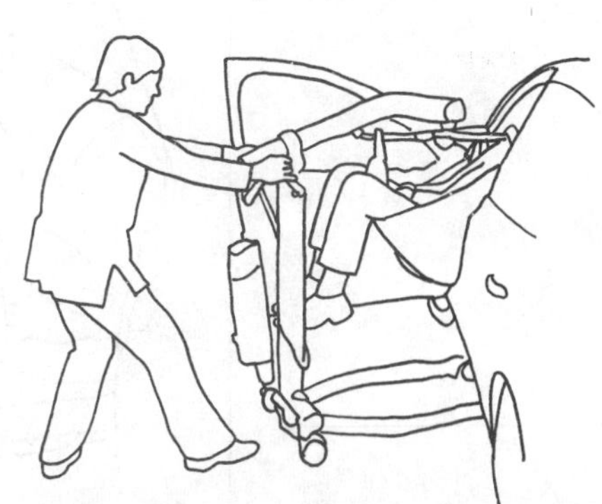
FIG 14.9c

the car or even kneel on the seat to position the person correctly in the car seat.

- There must be sufficient space for the handler to detach the sling from the hoist, and sufficient postural support to ensure that the person sits in the car safely and in comfort.

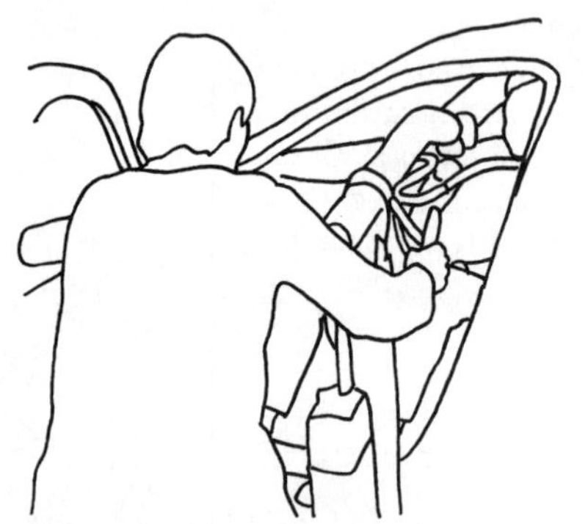

FIG 14.9d

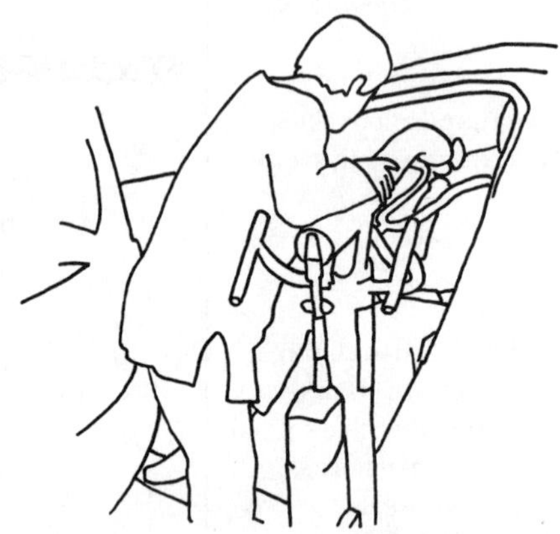

FIG 14.9e

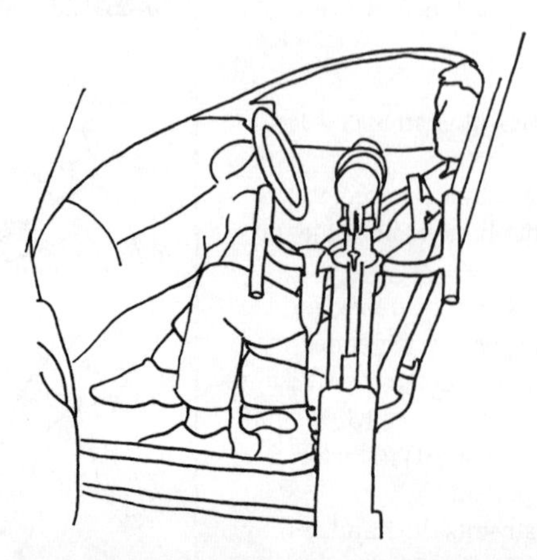

FIG 14.9f

Transfer with car mounted hoist

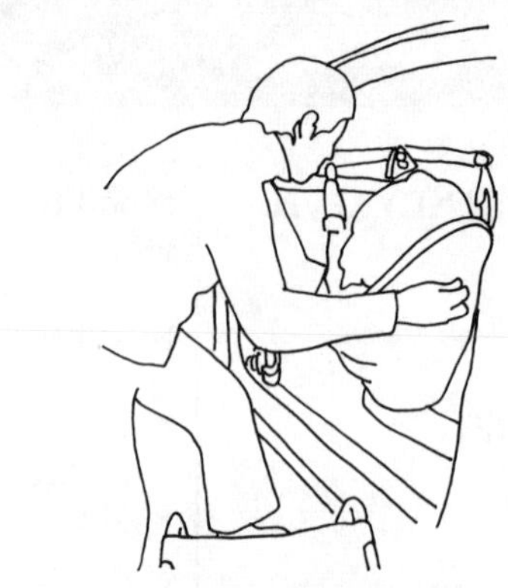

FIG 14.10a

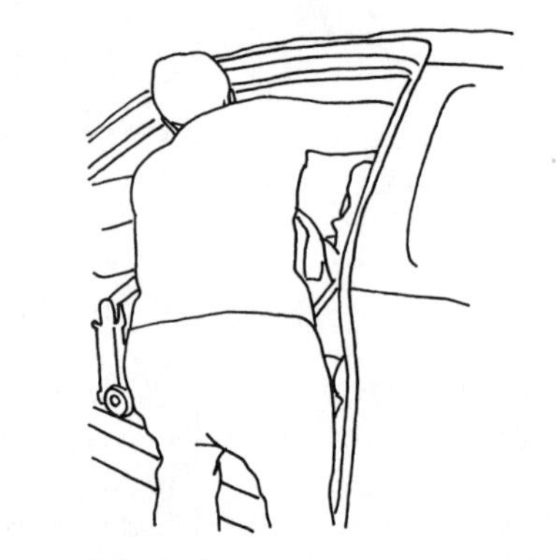

FIG 14.10b

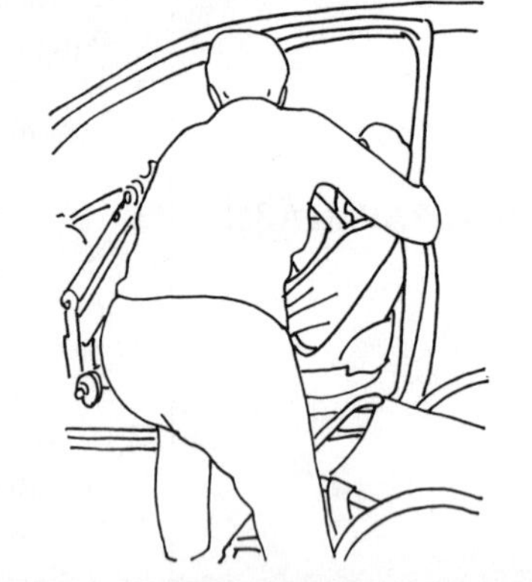

FIG 14.10c

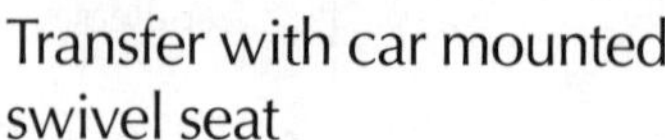

Transfer with car mounted swivel seat

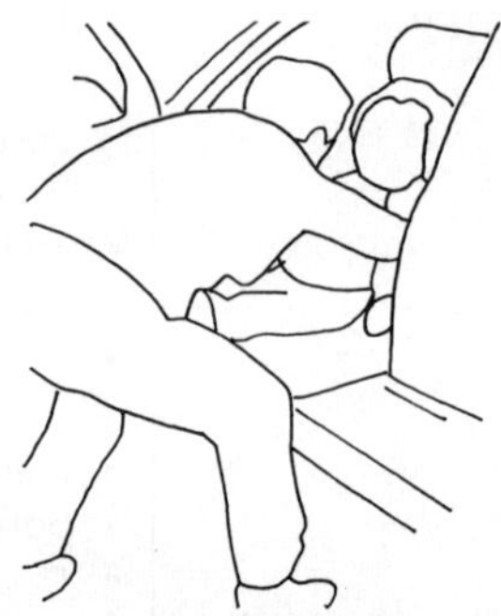

FIG 14.11a

Evidence review

Technique	REBA	Activity	Comfort	FIM	Mobility gallery	Skill level	Comment
TRANSFER WITH HOIST AND SLING WITH 1 OR 2 HANDLERS FROM WHEELCHAIR TO CAR SEAT							
Figs 14.9 a–f	11	2	8	1	D	Competent	Using a hoist for a car transfer is a very high postural risk.
TRANSFER FROM WHEELCHAIR TO CAR WITH A CAR MOUNTED HOIST AND 1 OR 2 CARERS							
Figs 14.10 a–c	6	2	8	1	D	Competent	The car mounted hoist gives a medium postural risk.
TRANSFER FROM WHEELCHAIR TO CAR WITH A CAR MOUNTED SEAT							
Figs 14.11 a	8	2	9	1	D	Competent	A car mounted seat gives a high postural risk.

Of course there is overlap in the above methods, depending on the individual capability and professional judgement of the handler, the equipment available and staff skill.

Children may also require help with walking, and there are several ways to assist this. If possible, the child should be encouraged to rise to their feet with as little help as necessary, as lifting from the floor is a hazardous occupation. Pulling a child up from the floor by their arms is potentially hazardous to their upper limb joints and puts the handler at risk of lifting from the floor and possibly slipping as they lean back to achieve this. An inflatable lifting cushion provides a safer method for a child with sitting balance (see chapter 17). Some children can be shown how to lean on strategically placed furniture to assist in rising. The above method of walking with a hoist and special harness, as detailed in chapter 13, could be used or a manually assisted lift with one or two handlers could be performed. Both handlers could crouch either side and assist a child with some weight bearing ability to their feet; use of a handling belt may assist with this task. Alternatively they could half kneel on one knee only, to each side and rise to their feet in a smoothly coordinated manner.

Task Fourteen

Assisting a child to their feet from the floor, with 1 or 2 handlers and a handling belt

DEPENDENCY LEVEL

Mobility Gallery B
FIM 2

- Child may be assisted to stand but requires some weight bearing ability when upright.
- Child should be able to assist with rising.

DESCRIPTION

- Child sits on floor, and one or two handlers crouch (see figures 13.9a–d) or half kneel (see figures 13.9e–g) at either side.
- Using a handling belt, the handlers assist child to his feet.

PERCEIVED EXERTION FOR HANDLER

- Some handlers may have problems rising from the floor themselves without using their hands to assist.
- This may be as much of a problem as the weight/dependency levels of the child.

COMFORT FOR PERSON

Care must be taken that the belt does not chafe, or pull on any feeding tubes or stoma.

SKILL LEVEL OF STAFF

- Handler requires communications skills.
- Use of this method requires special skill,

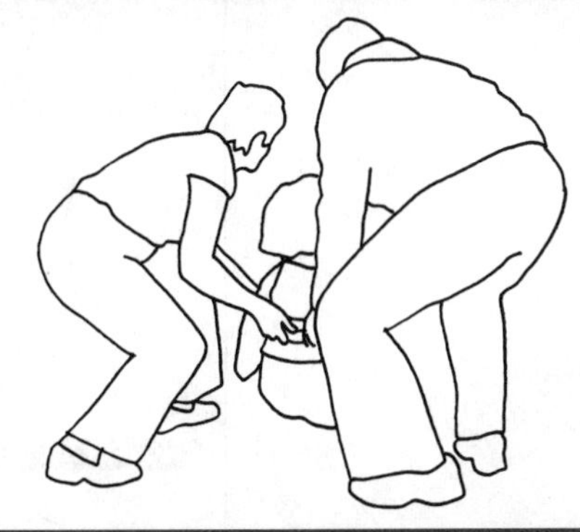
FIG 14.12a

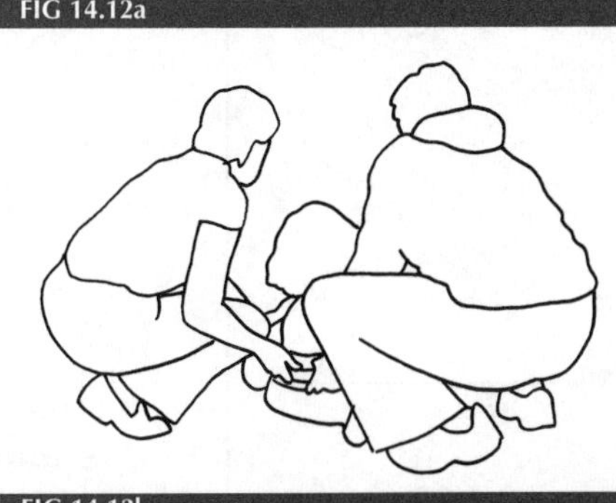
FIG 14.12b

and is usually confined to rehabilitation staff, or school support workers.

EVIDENCE AVAILABLE

DIAG (2001) suggests that independent transfers are encouraged, as the amount of physical force which handlers can apply in such a situation is very low.

DANGERS/ PRECAUTIONS

A heavy child, or one wearing calipers will present a greater risk to handlers.

FURTHER OPTIONS

- Some children can be encouraged to help themselves up from the floor, by turning onto all fours and using furniture to push up on.
- An inflatable rescue cushion could be used for a child with sitting balance.

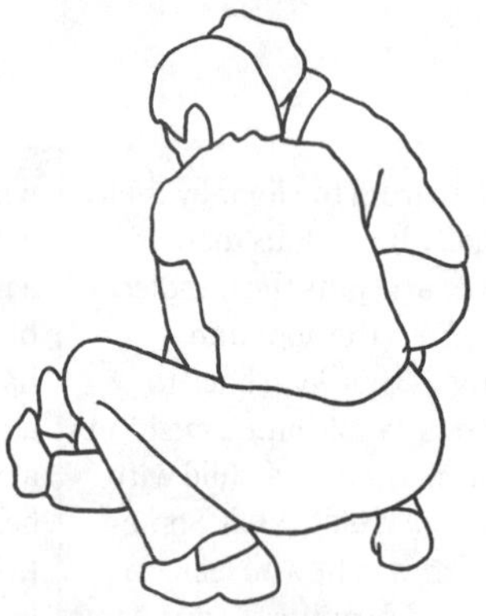

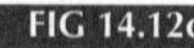

FIG 14.12c

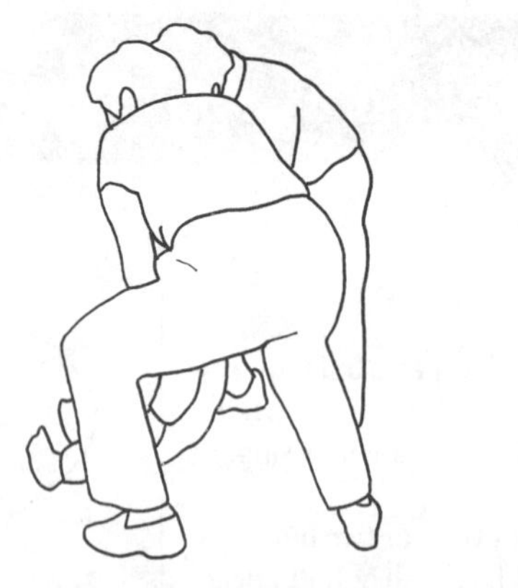

FIG 14.12d

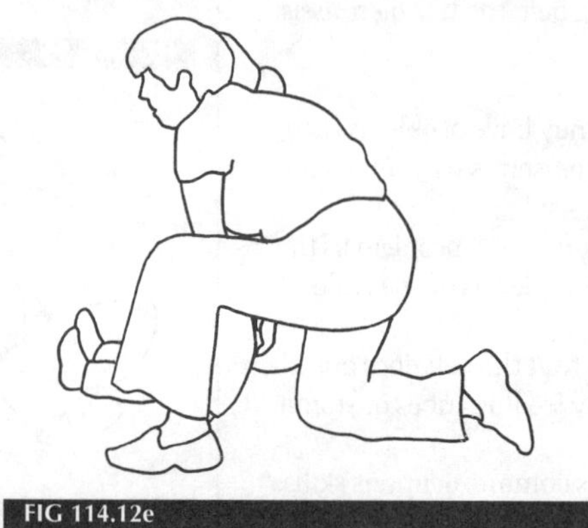

FIG 114.12e

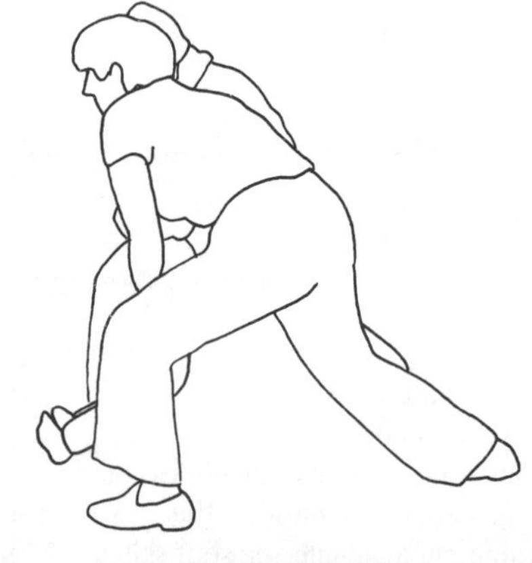

FIG 14.12f

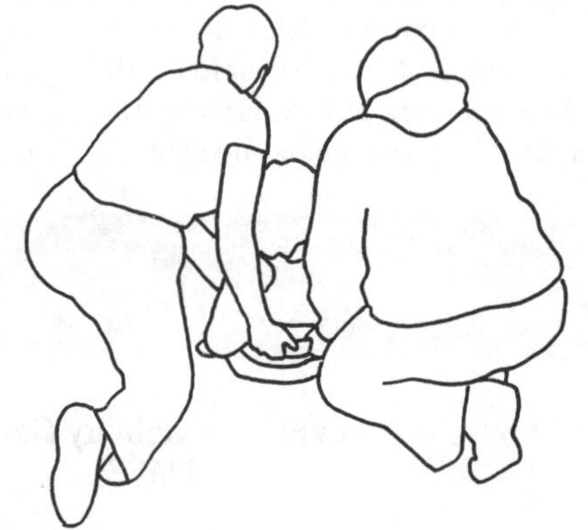

FIG 14.12g

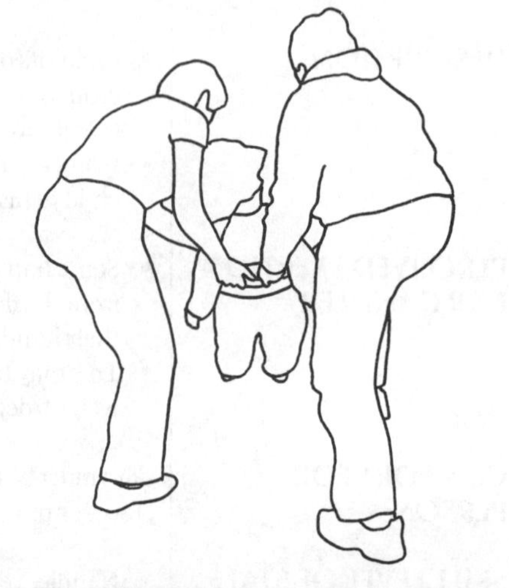

FIG 14.12h

Evidence review

Technique	REBA	Activity	Comfort	FIM	Mobility gallery	Skill level	Comment
ASSISTING A CHILD TO THEIR FEET FROM THE FLOOR WITH A HANDLING BELT							
Fig 14.12b	11	3	4	2	B	Advanced beginner	
Fig 14.12g	11	3	4	2	B	Advanced beginner	

12 Summary

The choice of method for a seated transfer must obviously be informed by many factors, including safety and wishes of person and handler, the abilities of both, the equipment available, the environment and the reason for the move. The legal requirement for a process of risk assessment should guide this decision, and the factors affecting it, clear to all who need to know. It is important that the clinical reasoning behind the choice is made clear, and that the situation is monitored and reassessed as necessary.

There is a variety of assistive equipment available, and staff must be trained and skilled in its selection and use in the relevant care setting. Training must be adequate in terms of content and duration to ensure understanding and familiarity with practical strategies *(Standards for training/trainers, National Back Exchange 2002).*

References

Alexander NB, Schultz AB, Warwick DN(1991). Rising from a chair: effects of age and functional ability on performance biomechanics. Journal of Gerontology: Medical Sciences, 46 (3)

Alexander P (1998). Risk management in manual handling for community nurses. In Hanson (ed) Contemporary Ergonomics.

Association of Paediatric Chartered Physiotherapist (1999). Paediatric Manual Handling, guidelines for paediatric physiotherapists. London: Chartered Society of Physiotherapy.

BackCare in Steed R (ed). Safer Handling of People in the community. London: BackCare

Benevolo E, Sessarego P, Zaliani A, Zelaschi G and Franchignoni F (1993). Ergonomic evaluation of five patient transferring techniques. Giornale Italiano di Medicini del Lavoro. 15:139 144

Bell F (1984). Patient-lifting devices in hospitals. London and Sydney: Croom and Helm

Bell F Dalgitty ME, Fennell M-J and Aitken RCB (1979). Hospital ward patient-lifting tasks. Ergonomics. Vol. 22, no. 11

Bell F (1987). Ergonomic aspects of equipment. Int.J.Nurs.Stud Gt Britain: Pegamon Journals

Busse M (2000). Effective rehabilitation and hoisting equipment: a case study. Nursing and Residential Care, 2, 4, 168–173

Care Standards Act 2000, Explanatory Notes. Norwich: The Stationery Office

Chan D, Laporte D, Sveistrup H (1999). British Journal of Occupational Therapy. Rising from sitting in elderly people, part 2. 62 (2)

Cherniak P, Caprio D, Fischer A, Tuckman J (1999). A novel device for walking training in elderly patients. Physiotherapy March. 85. (3) p.144–148

Dehlin O and Lindberg B (1975). Lifting Burden for a nursing aide during patient care in a geriatric ward. Scan Journal of Rehabilitation Medicine

Derbyshire Interagency Group (2001) Care handling for adults in hospitals and community settings. A code of practice. Southern Derbyshire NHS, Community Healthcare (North Derbyshire) NHS Trust, Derbyshire Local Education Authority, Derbyshire County Council Social Services, Chesterfield and North Derbyshire Royal Hospital NHS Trust and Work safe-work fit, Southern Derbyshire Acute Hospitals NHS Trust

Derbyshire Interagency Group (2001) Care handling of children in hospitals and community settings. A code of practice. Southern Derbyshire NHS, Community Healthcare (North Derbyshire) NHS Trust, Derbyshire Local Education Authority, Derbyshire County Council Social Services, Chesterfield and North Derbyshire Royal Hospital NHS Trust and Work safe-work fit, Southern Derbyshire Acute Hospitals NHS Trust

Duffy A, Burke C, Dockrell S (1999). The use of lifting and handling aids by hospital nurses. British Journal of Occupational Therapy Vol 6. No. 1

Fragala G (1993). Injuries cut with lift use in ergonomics demonstration project. Provider. October: 39-40

Gabbett J (1998). A pilot study to investigate the lifting and sliding of patients up in bed, unpublished M.Sc dissertation. University of Surrey

Gagnon M, Sicard C and Sirois JP (1986). Evaluation of forces on the lumbo-sacral joint and assessment of work and energy transfers in nursing aides lifting patients. Ergonomics 29, 3: 4007–21

Gagnon M and Lortie M (1987). Biomechanical approach to low back problems in nursing aides. In Asfour, S. (ed) Trends in Ergonomics/Human Factors IV, Holland: Elsevier Science Publishers BV

Gardner M, Holden M, Leikauskas Richard R (1998). Partial body weight support with treadmill locomotion to improve gait after incomplete spinal cord injury: a single subject experimental design. Physical Therapy. 78. (4). pp 36–1374

Garg A, Owen B (1991). A biomechanical and ergonomic evaluation of patient transferring tasks: bed to wheelchair and wheelchair to bed. Ergonomics, Vol 3, no. 3

Garg A, Owen B, Beller D and Banaag J (1991). A biomechanical and ergonomic evaluation of patient transferring tasks: wheelchair to shower chair and shower chair to wheelchair. Ergonomics, Vol 3, no. 4

Garg A, Owen B (1991). A biomechanical and ergonomic evaluation of patient transferring tasks. Designing for everyone. Y. Quiennec and F. Daniellon (eds) Vol 1. Proceedings of 11th Congress of IEA, Paris

Garg A and Owen B (1994). Prevention of back injuries in healthcare workers. International Journal of Industrial Ergonomics. 14. (1994) 315–331

Gingher M, Karuza J, Skulski M and Katz P (1996). Effectiveness of lift systems for long term care residents. Physical and Occupational Therapy in Geriatrics 14 (2): 1–11

Health and Safety Executive, (2001). Handling Home Care, Sudbury, HSE Books

Health Service Advisory Committee: (1998). Manual Handling in the Health Services. Sudbury: HSE Books

Hesse S, Konrad M, Uhlenbrock D (1999). Treadmill walking with partial body weight support versus floor walking in hemiparetic subjects. Archives of Physical Medicine Rehabilitation. 80. April 1999. pp 421–427

Holden JM, Feernie G and Lunau K (1988). Chairs for the elderly – design considerations. Applied Ergonomics 19.4.281–288

Jensen R (1985). Events that trigger disabling back pain among nurses. Proceedings of the Human Factors Society 29th Annual Meeting, Human Factors Society, Santa Monica, 799–801

Joint Committee on Mobility for Disabled People (1997). Travelling in vehicles while in a wheelchair. Physiotherapy. June 1997 vol. 83, no.6

Kane M and Parahoo K (1994). Lifting: why nurses follow bad practice. Nursing Standard. Vol.8. no.25

Kelley DL, Dainis A and Wood GK (1976). Mechanics and muscular dynamics of rising from a seated position. Biomechanics. 888 127–34

Kendrick C, Holt R, McGlashan K, Jenner JR and Kircher S (2001). Exercising on a treadmill to improve functional mobility in chronic stroke. Physiotherapy. 87.(5). pp 261–265

Kotake T, Dohi N, Kajiwara T, Sumi N, Koyama Y and Miura T (1993). An analysis of sit to stand movements. Archives of Physical Medicine and Rehabilitation. 74, 1095–99

Laporte DM, Chan D and Sveistrup (1999). Rising from sitting in elderly people, part 2: Implicationd of biomechanics and physiology. British Journal of Occupational Therapy. Jan 1999. 62 (1)

Lloyd P, Fletcher B, Holmes D, Tarling C and Tracy M (1998 revised). The Guide to the Handling of Patients (4th edition). National Back Pain Association/Royal College of Nursing

Malouin F, Potvin M, Prevost J, Richards CL, Wood-Dauphines S (1992). Use of an intensive task-orientated gait training program in a series of patients with acute cerebrovascular accidents. Physical Therapy. 72. (11) pp 781–9

Marras WS, Davis KG, Kirking BC and Bertsche PK (1999). A comprehensive analysis of low-back disorder and spinal loading during the transferring and repositioning of patients using different techniques. Ergonomics. Vol. 42, no.7, 904–926

McGuire T, Moody J and Hanson M (1996). A study into clients' attitudes towards mechanical aids. Nursing Standard. Vol. 11, no. 5

McGuire T, Moody J and Hanson M (1996). An evaluation of mechanical aids used within the NHS. Nursing Standard. Vol. 11, no. 6

McGuire T, Moody J and Hanson M (1997). Managers' attitudes towards mechanical aids. Nursing Standard. Vol. 11, no. 31

Moody J, McGuire T, Hanson M and Tigar F (1996). A study of nurses' attitudes towards mechanical aids. Nursing Standard. Vol. 11, no. 4

Munro BJ and Steele JR (1998). Facilitating the sit to stand transfer: a review. Physical Therapy Review. 3: 213–224

Munton JS, Ellis MI and Wright V. Use of electromyography to study leg muscle activity in patients with arthritis and in normal subjects during rising from a chair. Annals of Rheumatic Disease, 43, 63065

National Back Exchange, (2002). Standards for training and trainers. Essential Back Up revised 2002. Great Britain: National Back Exchange

Handley R (2004). Sling/hoist compatibility, risk assessment – the practical solution. The Column. August 2004.

Owen BD and Fragala G (1999). Reducing perceived physical stress while transferring residents. AAOHN Journal. 47:316–23

Ricability (2002). People lifters. A guide to devices which help wheelchair users get into a car. London: Ricability

Rodosky MW, Andriacchi TP and Andersson GBJ (1989). The influence of chair height on lower limb mechanics during rising. Journal of Orthopaedic Research. 7, 266–71

Roth P, Ciecka J, Wood E, and Taylor R (1993). Evaluation of a unique mechanical client lift. Efficiency and perspectives of nursing staff. AAOHN Journal 41 (5) 229–34

Ruszala S (2001). An evaluation of equipment to assist patient sit to stand activites in physiotherapy. Unpublished MSc dissertation, University of Wales: School of Health Care Studies

Schultz AB, Alexander NB and Ashton-Miller JA (1992). Biomechanical analysis of rising from chair. Journal of Biomechanics. 25 (12) 1383–91

Stevens C, Bojsen-Mollen F, Soames RW (1989). The influence of initial posture on the sit to stand movement. In: Chan D, Laporte D, Sveistrup H (1999). British Journal of Occupational Therapy. Rising from sitting in elderly people, part 2. 62 (2)

Tinetti ME, Richman D, Powell L (1990). Falls efficacy as a measure of fear of falling. Journal of Gerontology: Psychological Sciences 45(6)

Ulin S, Chaffin DB, Patellos C and Blitz S (1997). A biomechanical analysis of methods used for transferring totally dependent patients. Scientific Nursing 14 (10) 19–27

Unwins Safety Systems (2001). Passenger safety wheelchair guide. Yeovil: Unwins

Varcin-Coad L, and Barrett R (1998). Repositioning a slumped person in a wheelchair. A biomechanical analysis of the transfer techniques. AAOHN Journal 46,(11) 530–6

Weiner DK, Long R, Hughes MA, Chandler J, Studenski S (1993). When older adults face the chair-rise challenge: a study of chair height availability and height modified chair-rise performance in the elderly. Journal of the American Geriatrics Society, 41, 6–10

Zhuang Z, Stobbve TJ, Hsaio H, Collins J W and Hobbs GR (1999). Biomechanical evaluation of assistive devices for transferring residents. Applied Ergonomics 30:285–94

Zhuang Z, Stobbve TJ, Collins JW, Hsaio H and Hobbs GR (2000). Psychophysical assessment of assistive devices for transferring patients/residents. Applied Ergonomics 31: 35–44

15

Lying to sitting

Sheenagh Orchard RGN RNT CertEd(FE) DipNurs(Lond)
Manual Handling Training Consultant

1 Introduction

Altering position from lying to sitting is a common activity seen in most care settings. Many people can achieve this position change unaided or with minimal intervention such as verbal guidance or physical prompting. Handlers sometimes aid people with movement unnecessarily. There may be many reasons for this, for example, due to time pressures, and this can affect a handler's choice and method of intervention *(Brulin et al 2000)*. The first consideration should be 'can the person move themselves?' and secondly 'can they move themselves if given instruction or aids?'. Manual intervention should be considered as a final, and ideally short term, solution.

2 Factors affecting the choice of intervention

There are many factors which affect the choice of intervention and these can be considered using the TILE format of assessment (see chapter 9). The examples are intended to give an idea of the factors which must be considered but are a limited range of those actually seen in the workplace and assessors must consider more broadly the factors affecting their own work settings.

Task

Handlers will transfer a person from lying to sitting for positional change to aid aspects such as comfort, tissue viability, digestive and respiratory processes. The transfer may also be used prior to, or during, a secondary activity such as washing, dressing, feeding, therapy or administering medication. Moving people within the bed is considered a high risk in comparison to many other activities *(Bertolazzi and Saia 1999)* and this must be taken into account when considering whether a manual intervention can or should be used.

The risks and type of intervention used will alter depending on the circumstance. For example, time and speed can be a factor to relieve respiratory distress but will not be an issue if the person merely wishes to sit up to read or watch television.

If a secondary activity is involved, such as washing or dressing, account must be taken of the postural stresses and static muscle work seen in these activities *(Knibbe and Knibbe 1995, Lusted et al 1996)*. Therapists and midwives undertake tasks which affect their working postures and require musculoskeletal effort *(Fenety and Kumar 1991, Hignett 1996, Hignett 2001a)*.

Individual capability

All aspects that relate to an individual's capability must be considered as required under the Manual Handling Operations Regulations 1992 (as amended):

Regulation 4(3)

"...in determining the appropriate steps to reduce that risk regard shall be had in particular to:

a the physical suitability of the employee to carry out the operations;
b the clothing,footwear or other personal effects he is wearing;
c his knowledge and training etc."

In determining physical suitability there must be an understanding of the biomechanical stresses imposed by certain activities, for example studies show that in handlers the assisting of lying to sitting gave the most reactive force at L5/S1 *(Khalil et al 1987)*. It is important that there is adequate health screening and health support of handlers. Handlers should recognise their own responsibilities under the Health and Safety at Work Act 1974 of working within their own individual capability and reporting issues which affect their health and safety at work.

There are many instances where handlers cannot effectively and safely work on their own and therefore, a second handler is recommended *(Lusted et al 1996)*.

Studies show that *"Individual differences and preferences between nurses affect postural stress and time taken" (Knibbe and Knibbe 1995)*. A handler's knowledge and training will affect their skill level and there are some methods described for the manual assistance of lying to sitting which require high levels of knowledge and skill. It must be ascertained that the handler has the correct knowledge and training to implement the designated method of assistance. However, there is considerable evidence to support the view that training of handlers as a sole intervention does not reduce musculoskeletal injury *(Engkvist et al 2001, Fanello et al 1999)*. In departments with considerable levels of handling, training, in the absence of engineering controls, does not sufficiently reduce back pain *(Lynch and Freund 2000)*.

Where knowledge and training development are used as part of a multi-factor intervention there is an improvement in mental and physical aspects of work, particularly where problem solving and team work are included *(Pohjonen et al 1998)*. Sickness absence can also be seen to be reduced where multi-factor intervention is implemented *(Collins 1990)*. This has cost benefits to the organisation as well as personal benefits to the handler.

Staffing limitations and lack of time available for the activity affect the safe outcome of handling *(Brulin et al 2000, Scott 1995)*.

Load (person to be assisted)

The factors relating to the person requiring assistance are of paramount importance and must be considered in detail.

The assessment must include all their physical and behavioural needs. In addition, aspects such as religious and cultural beliefs, language, cognitive abilities and handling constraints such as intravenous infusion, catheters etc must be included in the assessment. Assessment of the person has been covered more fully in other chapters of this book.

In relation to assisting a person from lying to sitting a key factor is the ratio of their Body Mass Index (BMI) compared to that of the handler(s). The handler may consider that as they are only moving part of the person's body weight that their overall weight is not of importance. What might be an appropriate decision for a small child cannot necessarily be deemed safe and appropriate in an adult setting. Size is by no means the only key factor in deciding how to assist a person from lying to sitting but obviously the larger and more incapacitated an individual the more likely it becomes that equipment will be needed in order to avoid the hazardous handling. This is inherent in the requirement of the Manual Handling Operations Regulations 1992.

It is worth noting that some people's interpretation of 'avoiding hazardous handling' in lying to sitting is to leave the person lying. An appropriate intervention must be identified by assessment in order to meet the person's need. For example,

- **a** Do they genuinely need to sit, if not leaving them lying may be appropriate?
- **b** Could they be encouraged to sit independently?
- **c** If urgent, could this be best managed by two handlers with a third to adjust the backrest or give additional support?
- **d** Transfer the person by lateral transfer to a profile bed which assists them to sit.

The very heavy person cannot usually lie flat, therefore, it is a forseeable circumstance that they will need assistance to sit and this must have been taken account of by assessment and systems of work.

Environment (and equipment)

Care settings themselves present with their own particular issues.

- **a** In acute settings such as hospitals, GP practices and for ambulance crew, the equipment they use will affect their handling practice. The person may be on a trolley, bed, couch or plinth, all of which may have additional fixtures and fittings such as rails, oxygen or monitors and they may be fixed height or height adjustable.
- **b** Residential, nursing or home care settings may have divan beds, double beds *(Skarplik 1988)* or people being cared for on a mattress on the floor (the latter can now be replaced by height adjustable beds that lower to within 6 inches from the floor).
- **c** Emergency settings, sensory rooms, childcare settings and areas managing people with challenging behaviours may involve the person being on the floor.

Each brings with it particular influences to the activity of lying to sitting which have arisen not from the people involved but from the environment or equipment.

There are issues relating to environment and/or equipment that can be present in any setting. These include space constraints, poor physical working environments *(Brulin et al 2000)*, lack of equipment, inappropriate equipment that is not easily accessible. It is recognised that an adequate supply, or equipment that is suitable for the task, will assist in the overall risk management *(Bewick & Gardner 2000, Panciera et al 2000)*. However, for the most effective outcomes a combination of risk management strategies to include equipment provision, environmental adaptations, ergonomic and organisational measures, training etc. must be in place *(Garg & Owen 1992)*.

3 Choosing an intervention

Decisions on the type of intervention to be used to assist people from lying to sitting must be based on a full assessment which takes account of all factors. Only then can guidance be given to handlers on which approach is the most appropriate for each situation.

The following suggestions do not cover every possible approach but are a range, currently used by practitioners, and it is important to recognise that each has its own inherent handling risks when considering which approach to use.

Manual interventions always carry a degree of risk to both the handler and the person being assisted. The level of risk indicated in the evidence results alongside each intervention (see tasks one to nine) is one factor to be considered when assessing which intervention is most appropriate. However, it is also important to recognise that the scores relate specifically to the situation as it was assessed and this may differ in some degree to the 'real life' situations where the intervention is to be used. For example, there may be distractions in the workplace, pressure of time, varying levels of staff skill etc. which would affect the risk outcomes. It is, therefore, imperative that a choice of intervention is based on a detailed assessment of the 'actual' situation, not on an assumption that the evidence set out below, undertaken in controlled circumstances, will automatically be valid in other settings. The evidence results within this chapter should be seen as a guidance for the potential levels of risk not taken as the actual level of risk that would apply if that approach were used elsewhere and a review of evidence alone does not constitute any adequate risk assessment.

Adequate training is required as part of a safer handling strategy so that risks to the handler and the person can be reduced as far as is reasonable in the circumstances. Handlers must be competent and confident in the use of equipment if it is to be used successfully. Where any form of manual intervention is used the need for good training is vital as the risks are increased further for inexperienced or poorly skilled handlers.

4 Lying to sitting using equipment

Equipment plays a large part in creating quality of work and quality of care in handling. There is a wide range of equipment available to eliminate the manual transfer of people from lying to sitting, The use of such equipment is the optimum approach in all settings as there are benefits not only to the handler's health but also to the comfort and independence of the person being moved. Additionally there are cost benefits to the care provider. The cost benefits of the judicious introduction of equipment arise from areas such as reduced staffing levels *(Hampton 1998)*, reduced absence and injury cost and reduced costs relating to tissue viability/pressure area management *(Kings Reference Total Bed Management)*; and better rehabilitation with reduced lengths of stay in care.

The most beneficial profiling equipment is electric powered and height adjustable *(Dhoot & Georgieva*

1996, Mitchell et al 1998). Assessment must be made of the risks related to the controls, for example, in some settings these need to be isolated to handler use only. The wires can be a strangulation or trip hazard and can interfere with positioning of a hoist. If cot sides or bed rails are to be used these must have been considered within the assessment.

The adjustment of manual backrests may involve excessive forces, postural stress and arm/shoulder strain *(Birtles M, and Williams S, 2004)*.

Profiling equipment includes beds (adult, paediatric and cots), trolleys, examination couches and plinths. Specialist equipment with accessories is available for areas such as operating theatres, accident and emergency, clinics, therapy areas, daycare settings, surgeries and renal dialysis units. In some of these settings it is desirable and possible for the equipment to convert from lying to a fully seated 'chair' position. Additionally the facility for rapid release to a lying position for cardiac resuscitation is necessary for certain settings. Profiling equipment can be a simple raising backrest or more complex configurations with several sections e.g. to raise knees or elevate legs. Assessment of the individual will identify which is most appropriate. It is important to consider carefully the type of system used for very heavy people as it is important that the base of the backrest recedes as the person is raised to sitting in order to accommodate their hips and buttocks. The different profiling options are described as 2, 3, 4, 5 or 6 section profiling systems. These numbers refer to the range of position changes that can be achieved. One of the position changes is generally the high/low facility. It is possible for this facility to extend down to several inches from the floor and up to a full working height for handlers.

Other position changes can include:

- Raising and reclining back rest.
- Knee break to support the person's knees in a bent position.
- Elevation of the leg section while the person is sitting.
- Lowering of the leg section to create a 'chair-like' position.
- Tilt from head or foot end (Trendelenberg and reverse Trendelenberg).
- Lateral 30 degree tilt.

The more refined position changes include:

- Retractable raising back rest which allows space for the buttocks as the person is raised into sitting.
- Forward moving seat section as the back rest is raised and recedes, which reduces pressure on the abdomen ie the person is not just being 'folded in half'.

5 Height adjustable, profiling equipment

There is equipment suitable for most care settings and is tailored for the particular needs of each situation. Some examples are:

Table 15.1

Setting	Equipment	Features
Paediatric	Cots and cot-beds	Extra low/independent access, lowerable sides, folding doors, see-through sides, soft sides
Very heavy people	Beds, trolleys, couches and plinths	Increased safe working load, specialised profiling system to recede at base in order to accommodate the person's body, lateral tilt, integral bed rails, bed to chair conversion, standing bed conversion, extra wide, integral pressure relieving systems, integral lateral transfer systems
Clinics and therapy areas	Couches, plinths, examination and treatment tables	Static and wheeled versions, extra wide Prone profiling, conversion to seated positions, side bending and lateral tilt, positive and negative positioning, detachable head/foot sections, split and/or angular leg support, wide range of specialist attachments
Challenging behaviour	Beds	Floor level/low or independent access (this replaces caring for people on a mattress on the floor with its inherent handling risks)
	Cotsides/bed rails (Where these are assessed as required and suitable)	Netting sides Soft/Inflatable or padded sides
Community, elderly care and long term care	Beds	Folding for flat storage (see figure 15.1a) Collapsible for easy transport and assembly, floor level/low/independent access, aesthetic styling e.g. wood, integral cot-sides/hand assist rails, double beds, one side profiling in a double bed, integral pressure relieving systems, massage facility
Acute	Beds and trolleys	Emergency lowering e.g. for cardiac arrest, extra wide, integral pressure relieving systems Lateral tilt, Trendelenberg and reverse Trendelenberg

6 Supplementary equipment

It may be more appropriate to add equipment to an existing bed, for example, if a person in the community wishes to retain their own bed or they share a double bed. However, the costs are not necessarily less since it is now possible to purchase profiling, height adjustable beds including the extra low versions for between £600 and £1,000.

Bed raiser

Divan beds can be elevated on bed blocks but will give a fixed height. An electric bed frame raiser can be placed under a fixed height divan creating an electric height-adjustable system.

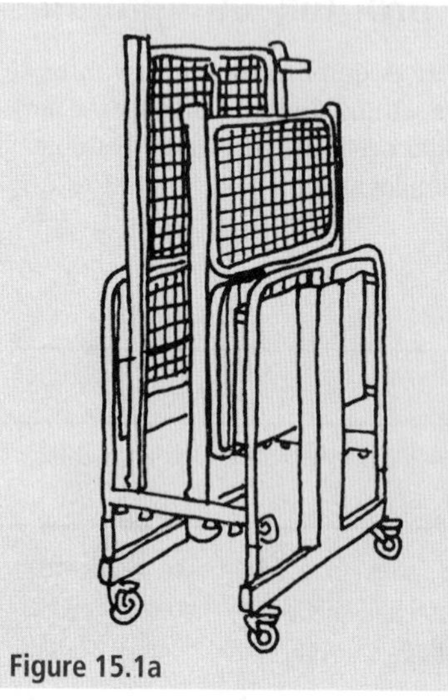

Figure 15.1a

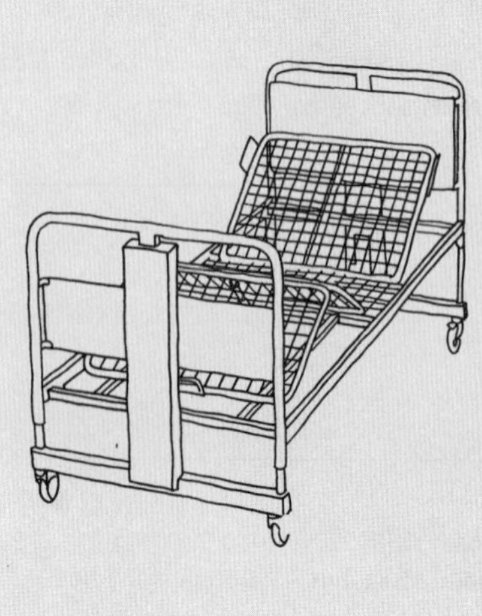

Figure 15.1b

Pillow lifter

These are placed under the pillows and elevate the person to a sitting position. These can be inflatable airbags or electric powered.

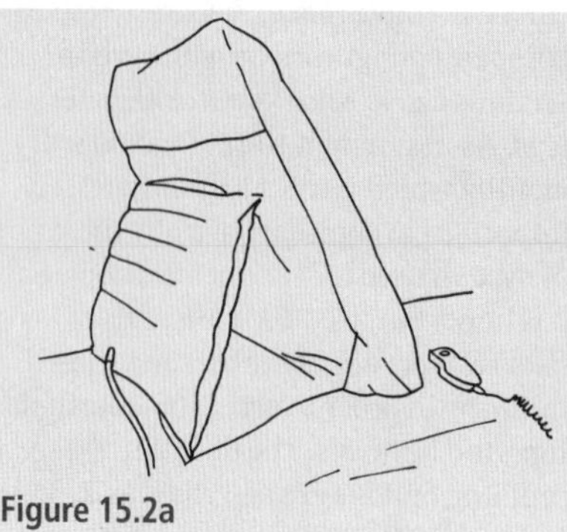

Figure 15.2a

Mattress elevator

These are placed under the mattress and elevate the person to a sitting position. These are usually an electric driven metal frame. The mattress must be suitable for use with this equipment and a foot board or mattress retainer used to prevent the mattress from slipping off the end of the bed.

7 Manual assisted lying to sitting

Tasks one, three, five and six achieve sitting for the person without the physical assistance of the handler. The person is either being assisted by verbal instruction, prompting and demonstration rather than direct hand support, or the handler is using the controls of the equipment and the equipment is producing the physical assistance to sit (FIM 5 – 7). These options would achieve lying to sitting with lower risk to the handler than other options and more independent function from the person.

Tasks two and four require some direct hand contact to enable the person to complete the sitting action but the person should be expending 75% or more of the effort (FIM 4). It is worth noting that the person may not 'consciously' feel that they are expending this level of effort because they will be benefiting from the 'unconscious' muscle effort or response as well as the psychological support of the handler's presence and encouragement. The positive effects of good communication and rapport between handler and person should not be underestimated when facilitating movement.

Tasks seven and eight should be used with considerable caution and should be considered as 'single instance' options to meet immediate need and replaced by an equipment aided move where possible, and as soon as possible. This is due to the fact that the person requiring this level of assistance has considerably reduced independent function. If they have the ability to assist tasks one to five would be more appropriate.

If they do not have the ability to assist then, task six using profiling equipment, is the most appropriate choice of intervention both from a quality of work and quality of care perspective. The decision to progress with a manual assisted lie to sit must come from detailed assessment with sound reasoning given for the retention of any risks to the handler or reduced comfort for the person being moved. Costs of equipment have reduced significantly and can no longer be considered as justification for not purchasing the equipment necessary to manage the risks.

The FIM will be 3 even where the person has head control and 2 where they have no head control. Therefore, the assistance given will be significant. The risks will increase if:

- The task is repeated substantially during a shift.
- The handlers are of different height, BMI or skill level.
- The person being moved is of different height or BMI to the handlers.
- The person is on the floor.

These moves have inherent risks to handlers as there are many factors which can adversely affect the postures or effort needed to achieve the move. Some of the factors being:

- Poor postural awareness of the handler.
- Inadequate space.
- No height adjustable bed or trolley.
- Time constraints.
- Staffing levels and/or skills.
- Behavioural attributes of the person being moved.
- Sudden unexpected movement of the person being moved.

If the change of position is rapid it can cause discomfort, pain or dizziness to the person being moved. A fully supported, gentle raise, using profiling equipment is a more appropriate solution. In the future, as equipment provision improves, these manually assisted methods (tasks seven and eight) should have been eliminated in all care settings. These methods would only then be used where the situation has arisen through an unforseen or emergency circumstance.

If the person requires repositioning in bed as well as assistance to sit the best option for this level of dependency of person is to move them up the bed supine on slide sheets and to assist them to sit at the end of the move (see chapter 16). Alternatively they should be repositioned using a hoist.

8 Hoists and slings

People can be repositioned in bed using a suitable hoist and sling. It should be remembered that adept use of such equipment can facilitate independence and dignity of the person as well as providing a safe means of transfer. Hoists provide a solution for some repositioning and transfers and have been found to aid in the reduction of back pain of handlers when introduced as part of a safer handling strategy *(Knibbe and Friele 1999)*. There have been significant advances, both in hoists and slings, in recent years. There are now lightweight transportable, mobile and overhead tracking systems; hoists designed for specific locations such as swimming pools, horse riding and boats; and hoists for specific situations such as moving the very heavy person.

This has improved the quality of working life for the handler and the comfort for the person being moved. However, use of hoists has its own risks and this must be taken into account when undertaking risk assessment. The postural stresses can be significant as can stresses acting on the spine whilst applying a sling or manoeuvering a hoist *(Dolan et al 1998)*.

There are problems in using hoists, but sometimes this rests with the handler's attitudes rather than a valid reason. Handlers often state that the person does not wish to be hoisted but this may not be the case *(McGuire et al 1996a)*. If handlers are inadequately trained and do not use the equipment regularly they will lack proficiency and confidence in the use of hoists and slings. They may, therefore, choose to avoid using the equipment, or they use it incorrectly or incompetently, all of which will lead to a reduction in quality of work and quality of care.

The art of successful hoisting, for both handler and person, is in the choice of equipment and its sensitive introduction. When a hoist is to be introduced into a person's own home there are particular issues which may need to be taken into account such as structural alterations, personal wishes of the person or family and all surrounding physical, social and psychological influences. This can make the introduction of a hoist a complex issue *(Conneeley 1992)*.

When choosing a hoist and/or sling account must be taken of:

- the tasks to be undertaken,
- the environments where it is to be used
- compatibility with other equipment such as the bed
- the handlers individual capability (physical as well as knowledge and skills)
- the needs of the person to be moved.

Many people need a sling designed specifically for their individual need, although manufacturers have increased their range of standard slings. All people need a sling of the correct size and type to give them suitable support.

The wide range of hoists and slings now available, whilst improving the quality of hoisting, does create issues for handlers, as they may meet many variations in their work. This may be a particular issue for those working in the community or for bank and agency staff.

It is not possible within this chapter to cover all the issues relating to the use of hoists and what is currently available, therefore, handlers should refer to other sources of information and guidance to ensure a full knowledge and understanding of hoists, slings and their use, such as:

- *The Guide to the Handling of Patients 3rd and 4th editions*
- *Safe Handling of People in the Community*
- *Handling Home Care*
- *Hoist and sling manufacturers – specialist advice and equipment instructions.*

There are many issues regarding hoists and slings and these must be considered within the whole safer handling strategy of an organisation and correct management applied equally and separately to the hoist and the slings. It is necessary, therefore, to be able to uniquely identify each hoist and sling, and reference must be made to relevant legislation e.g. *Provision and Use of Work Equipment Regulations (PUWER) 1998, Lifting Operations and Lifting Equipment Regulations (LOLER) 1998*. The following are some of the areas requiring consideration:

Purchase and provision

- Appropriate for purpose, task, environment, user
- Sufficient quantity available to ensure accessibility at all times
- Sufficient in range of type to meet all the requirements of that place of work
- Plan for replacements

(See also usability trials in chapter 4).

Insurance

- General – damage and replacement.
- Specific – compatibility issues.

Advice should be sought by people who purchase their own equipment for use in their own home or who have been given grants to purchase equipment.

Maintenance and servicing

There are specific requirements under *PUWER 1998* and *LOLER 1998* regarding maintenance and servicing, the general requirement in most circumstances being a 6 monthly inspection. This applies to the hoist and the slings (see also chapter 1).

All handlers should do a visual check of equipment,including slings, prior to each use and report defects and/or remove the item from use.

Reporting systems

Accident and incident reporting

These should not only include the reporting of equipment failures but also system failures such as insufficient quantity to allow care to be met adequately e.g. the only sling is in the wash.

Training

- This should be specific to the equipment used by the handler
- Instructions of use of equipment should be available to support training.

Supervision

Management systems should ensure:

- adequate supervision of those using equipment.
- enforcement of use of equipment where it has been assessed as required.

Risk assessment

This must cover all aspects of the hoisting situation:

- **Task** – e.g. bathing, lift height required, what type of hoist, spreader and sling are needed.
- **Individual capability** – e.g. the physical suitability, knowledge and skills of the handler.
- **Load** – e.g. the safe working load of the hoist, all the needs of the person being moved must be considered.
- **Environment** – e.g. turning circle required, floor surface, obstructions or space constraints.

The aim of the following information is to raise the awareness of the reader regarding products and their use. Having identified which product is potentially suitable for their own circumstances the reader should seek additional information relating to that equipment, and its use, prior to purchase/use. All equipment must be used in accordance with the manufacturers instructions.

9 The hoist

- Hoists may be powered by mechanical, electrical or hydraulic means.
- The number of handlers required to assist in hoisting depends on a detailed risk assessment. Some people use a hoist independently. Some organisations state in their policies that two handlers must be present.
- The safe working load of the hoist must be known.
- Many hoists have integral weigh scales or can have scales attached in order to weigh a person as they are lifted.
- The handler must be familiar with the manual emergency lowering system and emergency stop system of electric hoists.
- The hoist must be inspected according to Lifting Operations and Lifting Equipment Regulations 1998 – i.e. in most circumstances 6 monthly.

Types of spreader bar

There are different configurations of spreader bar, each with its own advantages. It is important for all hoists that the spreader bar is a safe distance from the persons face during all stages of a lift.

Rotating spreader

These facilitate manoeuvering of the person into a correct position or to ensure their knees are away from the mast during transfer. The person may have a tendency to 'swing' during transfer.

Tilting spreader

This is a Y shaped or wishbone spreader with a positioning handle to recline or tilt the person. This action can be difficult for handlers and some are now power assisted. The person has less tendency to 'swing' during transfer.

Spreader attachments

Some hoists have attachments such as stretcher attachments or side bars to convert two point attachment to a four point attachment. In some cases a hoist can be converted from a sling lifting to a standing aid hoist. This conversion can be a significant handling activity and should not be done repeatedly during a short working period.

Points of suspension

- **2 Point** – The leg and shoulder attachments (and additional attachments if present) all meet at two points either side of the person.
- **3 Point, Y or Wishbone** – The leg attachments are held in close proximity or on a single attachment while the shoulder attachments remain separate at either side of the person.
- **4 Point, H or X** – All attachment points are separated.

Increasingly 3 or 4 point attachments are used as they tend to improve the comfort for the person being lifted.

Categories of hoists

Fixed position/wall mounted

- These may be on a floor frame e.g. placed behind a bed for community settings or fixed to the wall/floor e.g. bedrooms, bathrooms, swimming pools.
- The range of the transfer is dictated by the length of the boom.

Mobile hoists

- These can be moved from one point to another.
- The size of the hoist affects the turning circle, lifting height and lift capacity.
- The floor surface, space, obstructions and other environmental issues will affect the ease of movement from one point to another.
- They must be compatible with other furniture e.g. bed.
- They are designed as lifters not transporters and are intended to transfer a person a short distance only.
- The hoist must be manoeuvered by the handle provided, not by pulling on the person or boom.
- Push and pull the hoist slowly. Rapid and jerky movement increases discomfort to the person being lifted and also raises the stresses to the spine of the handler.
- Only raise the person to the height required to clear the surface they are going to/from. Do not raise the person above the maximum lift height of the hoist.
- Lower the person to the lowest comfortable position before transfer.
- The chassis/legs can be adjusted for access.
- Brakes are generally left off during lifts, on flat surfaces, to allow the hoist to reposition when the person's weight is taken.
- Brakes should be applied when assessment indicates this is required e.g. if the person is likely to go into extensor spasm or if the person is being lifted from the floor and having the brakes off would increase risk to the person. Brakes should also be applied when lifting on slopes, or when the hoist is stored.

Mobile hoists are not usually the hoist of choice for lifting the very heavy person although there are mobile hoists designed with high safe working loads. In this circumstance the intention is for the mobile hoist to be brought to the person to be lifted, NOT to move once the person is lifted, e.g. raising a person for change of bed linen/hygiene care.

If the very heavy person is to be transferred from lying to sitting and requires to be moved:

Either hoist the person and move the bed and change the bed for a chair without moving the hoist.

Or use an overhead tracking system.

Mobile seat/stretcher hoists

There are mobile hoists which have a seat or stretcher attachment rather than a sling system. These are usually used to meet toileting/hygiene needs of an individual. The stretcher attachment increases the length of the hoist and makes it more difficult to manoeuvre.

Ceiling/overhead tracking hoists

These may be:

a Free standing e.g. a gantry, pillar mounted or a temporary/ mobile system.

b Non structural attachment e.g. supported by poles to the structure of the building, such as the floor and ceiling, but not fixed permanently into the structure of the building.

c Fixed permanently to the structure of the building.

The systems can be manual or power driven. The controls for power driven systems are usually on a cable but there are now wireless and infra red controls to aid independent use.

A portable unit allows detachment and use of the unit on a different area of tracking. Alternatively, some systems can transfer through doorways.

The tracking can be:

a straight line

b curved

c X/Y or H frame to cover a whole room or area.

Choice of tracking depends on the type of transfer and the room coverage required. Turntables can be built into the system to allow change of direction.

The main advantages of tracking systems are:

- Some people can use them independently.
- No storage problems.
- Environmental issues such as floor surfaces, obstructions and space are better managed.
- The manual handling during manoeuvering is reduced.

Sample checklist prior to using a hoist

Check :

- the safe working load and date of last inspection.
- for signs of general wear and tear, loose parts etc.
- the spreader is firmly attached to the lifting mechanism, particularly if the hoist has an interchangeable spreader facility.
- the sling retention clips on the spreader are intact and working.
- the wheels/castors move freely.
- the brakes are in working order.
- the emergency lowering and stop systems are functioning.
- there is no leakage of hydraulic fluid (hydraulic hoists).
- the battery is charged (electric hoists).
- the legs/chassis open and close correctly.
- the handlers are trained in its use.
- the manufacturer's instructions are available and being applied.

10 The sling

The key to successful and comfortable hoist transfers lies in a large part with having the correct sling both in size and type. Each person must be assessed individually for the size and type of sling suitable to meet their needs. This should be written in their individual care/handling plan. Additionally, if specific positioning/sling loops are to be used this should be identified to ensure consistency of handling. In most settings the person's needs will be met by a reasonable size range of standard slings. As this should be sufficient to take account of the people's physical and weight variation. The more complex the person's needs the more likely they will need a 'person specific' sling for their individual use.

Slings can be individually designed and tailored for particular requirements and manufacturers produce a range of standard 'specials' such as amputee slings. Ideally slings should be allocated for individual use. Where slings are used in a multi user setting there must be suitable and sufficient quantities to allow for rotation to washing. Additionally, consideration must have been given to cross contamination/infection issues. Disposable slings and slings which incorporate microbe resistant properties are now available.

Slings must be washed and dried according to the manufacturer's instructions – many cannot be washed in biological detergents or dried in tumble dryers. Slide sheets can be used to aid sling introduction for lying or seated people but must be removed prior to lifting. There are slings now available which use materials specifically designed to aid introduction.

The decision as to whether to leave a sling in situ after transfer has to be made by individual assessment. The assessment must take account of tissue viability, comfort, dignity, choice of the individual and the difficulty for the handler of removal and re-insertion. Skin damage can occur both from leaving a sling in situ and from constant removal/re-application. If a sling is to be left in situ this must have been taken into account when choosing the sling e.g. fleece lining, breathable material or even gel inserts to relieve pressure. Very thin 'parachute type' materials are available to aid with managing hoisting with complex seating.

Compatibility

Slings are designed for use with particular styles of spreader bar/point attachment. It is important, within the assessment, for the sling prescriber to ensure that a sling is suitable for use with a particular hoist/spreader. There is a requirement in BS EN 10535 (the British/European Standard for hoists), that the sling manufacturer states which hoists and spreader bars a sling is compatible with.

Some manufacturers raise concerns by suggesting that products are not compatible with no logical rationale provided to support incompatibility. It is important to identify whether or not there are specific incompatibility issues and this may best be decided through discussion with the relevant hoist and sling manufacturers. However, there are many circumstances where a range of different products can be used successfully together.

Selecting a sling type

Does the person require:

- Supine or seated lift
- Head support
- Back/shoulder support
- Full thigh/hip support
- Commode aperture
- Special materials or specific adaptations.

What transfer/activity is required:

- Toileting
- Bathing
- Transfer to chair/moulded seating
- Repositioning in bed

- Lateral/supine transfer
- Lift from the floor
- Transfer to specialist settings e.g. swimming pools, horse riding, boats etc.

Generally, the more heavy or dependent a person the greater the support necessary from the sling. The more supportive the sling, the more difficult it is usually to apply, and it may be necessary for the sling to be applied on a bed/couch.

The very heavy person will need a specific sling with an adequate safe working load.

Sample checklist prior to using a sling

Check:

- It has been assessed as suitable for that individual.
- It is the correct size, weight capacity and type.
- The handler is trained.
- The manufacturers instructions of use are available and applied.
- There are no obvious signs of general wear and tear e.g. loose/broken stitching, worn areas on attachment points, discoloured, frayed or torn material.
- The label is legible.
- The date of last inspection.

Standard sling types

Toileting/Dress/Access (fig 15.3a)

- Easy to fit.
- Allows good access for dressing, toileting, hygiene needs.
- Low level of support – can have additional head support.

If a person appears to be insufficiently supported by this type of sling and seems to be 'falling out' of the aperture they must be reassessed for sling type and size.

Figure 15.3a

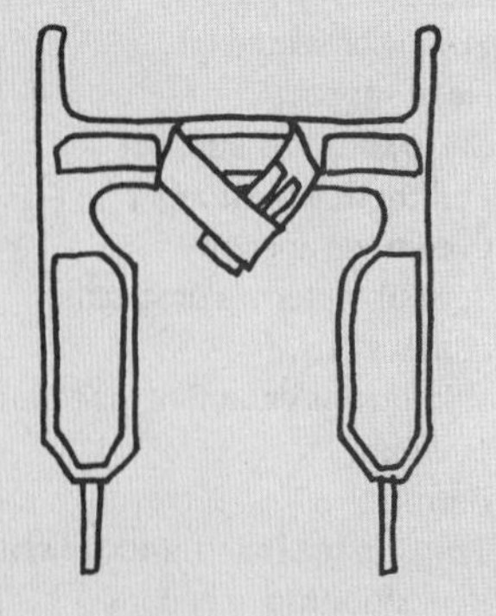

General purpose (figs 15.3b and c)

- Can be inserted while the person is seated or lying.
- Allows for toilet access but not for adjusting clothing whilst hoisted.
- Higher level of support – can have additional head support.

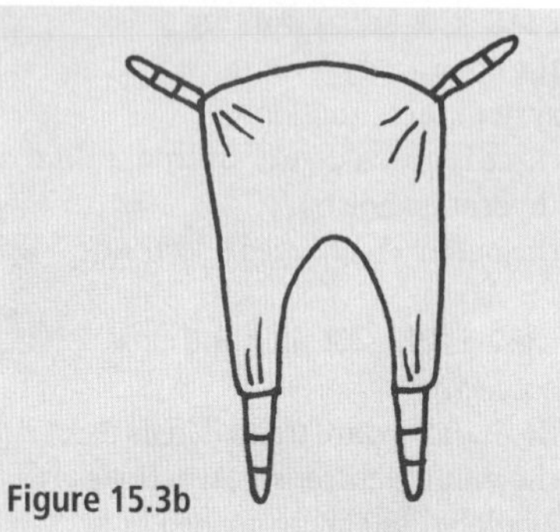

Figure 15.3b

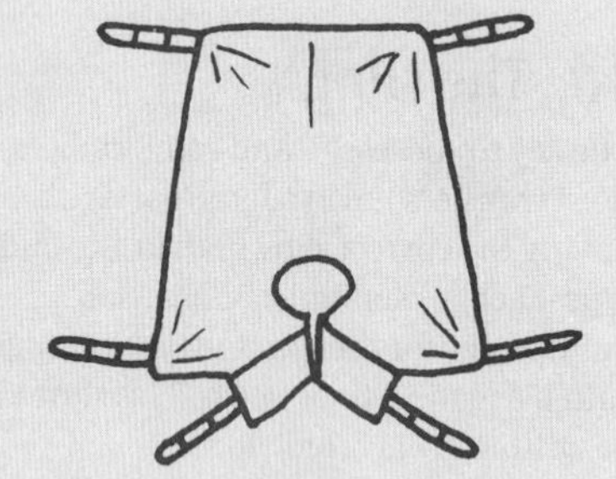

Figure 15.3c

Toileting and general purpose slings have divided leg bands. There are different ways of applying the leg bands.

a Pass a leg band under each leg, and **either** pass one through the strap designed to hold the legs together available on the other band **or** cross the loops from each leg band through each other and attach to the opposite side of the spreader. This conformation ensures the person does not slip out of the sling and their legs are held comfortably together in adduction and they retain some dignity (figure15.3d).

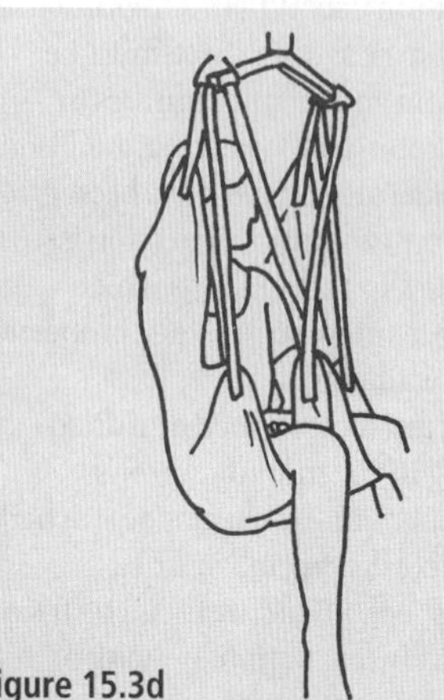

Figure 15.3d

b Pass the leg bands under each leg but not crossed over in the middle. This conformation leads to abduction of the legs, is less comfortable and less dignified, and can be unsafe as the person is not held into the sling. Additionally they may start to slip out of the commode aperture as this is not held to its designed size. (Not recommended).

c Pass both leg bands under both legs. This conformation keeps the legs together providing dignity and is useful for people wearing skirts. It is comfortable but the person can slip out of the sling particularly if they have extensor spasm or do not retain a good sitting position (figure 15.3e).

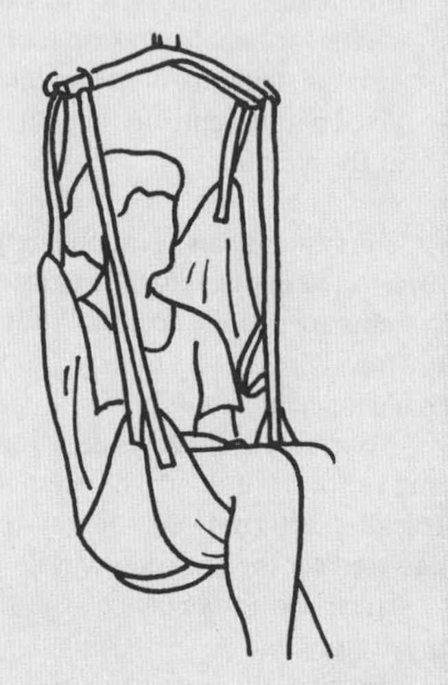

Figure 15.3e

Hammock (fig 15.3f)

- Needs to be inserted while the person is lying down.
- Less versatile than access or general purpose slings.
- Gives high level of support and can have additional hip support straps, head support and commode aperture.

Amputee (fig 15.3g)

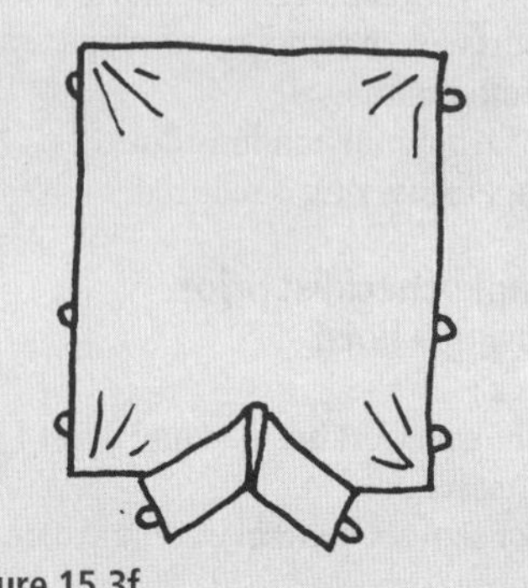

Figure 15.3f

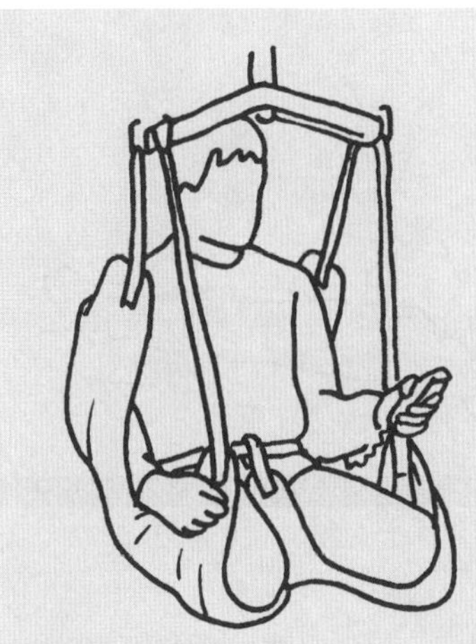
Figure 15.3g

- Necessary for most people with lower limb amputation.
- Allows for greater support and comfort.

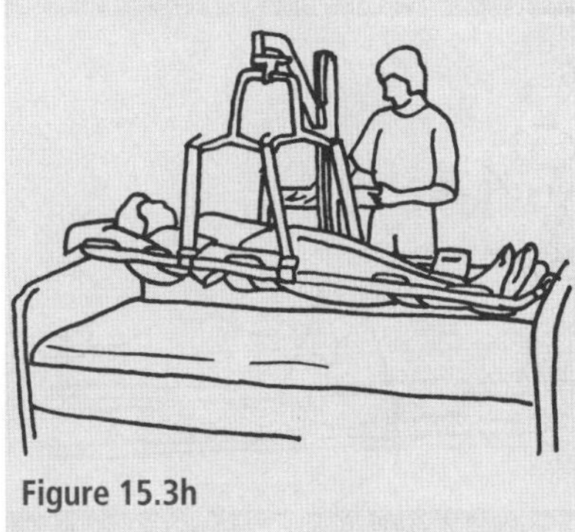
Figure 15.3h

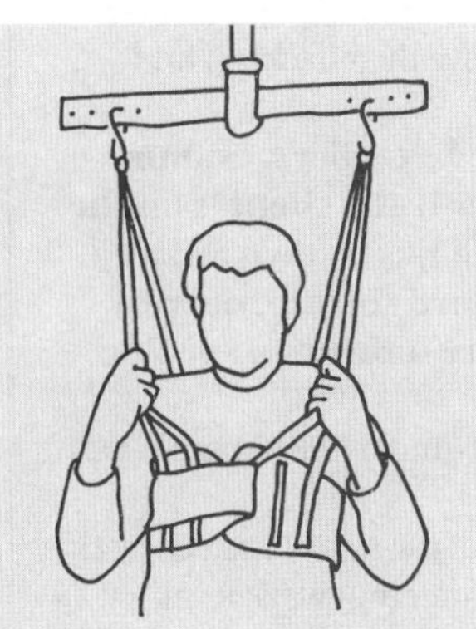
Figure 15.3i

Bathing
Made from mesh or specific water releasing material which allows water to drain out quickly and aids drying.

Stretcher (fig 15.3h)
- These may be fabric, rigid scoops or made up of flexible bands.
- The person is fully supported in the lying position.
- The hoist must be designed, or have attachments to accommodate this type of sling.

Walking harness (fig 15.3i)
(See also chapter 13 on assisted walking.)

Conclusion
With the considerable improvement in available equipment to assist with lying to sitting, in time, there will be less need for manual options, certainly in long term or high dependency situations. There will remain situations where manual options are necessary, or even desirable, and the approaches to the task given in this chapter are to assist assessors and handlers in making informed, evidence based decisions during assessments. Each approach has its own 'pros' and 'cons' and it is for each assessor to identify the most appropriate method for the situation and person they are assessing.

The assessor must be able to give the reasoning or justification for their choice and evaluate the situation regularly to ensure its continued safety. There is rarely a single correct approach for a specific situation or person, that is why decisions must be based on assessment. It is a matter of reviewing the options, understanding the reasoning behind the method, using the evidence available and coming to a decision which manages the risks within reasonable limits whilst achieving the task required to meet the need of the person being assisted (see also chapter nine).

Practical Techniques

Task One

Lying to sitting – with no physical help from another person

DEPENDENCY LEVEL

Mobility Gallery A, B
FIM 6 or 5

INSTRUCTION / EQUIPMENT

The person needs to have cognitive and physical ability to move themselves. The handler facilitates the person's movement by verbal prompt and providing any equipment identified by assessment.

- Assess person's ability to sit unaided
- **If they can** do this – proceed
- Some people will need additional assistance (see task two)
- **If they cannot lift their head from the pillow** consider an alternative method which gives more support e.g. electric profiling bed **either** the person can come up to a full sit **or** rest on their elbow to receive medication

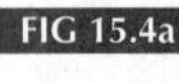

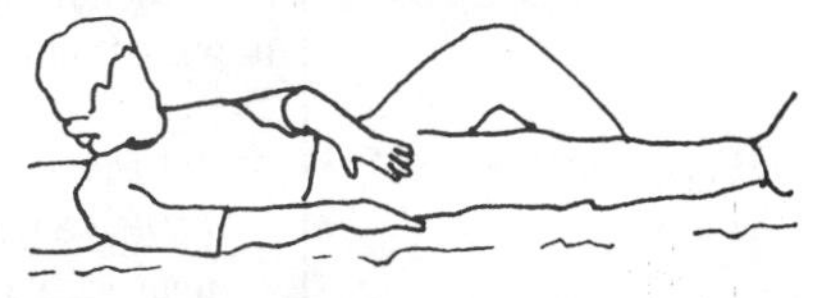
FIG 15.4a

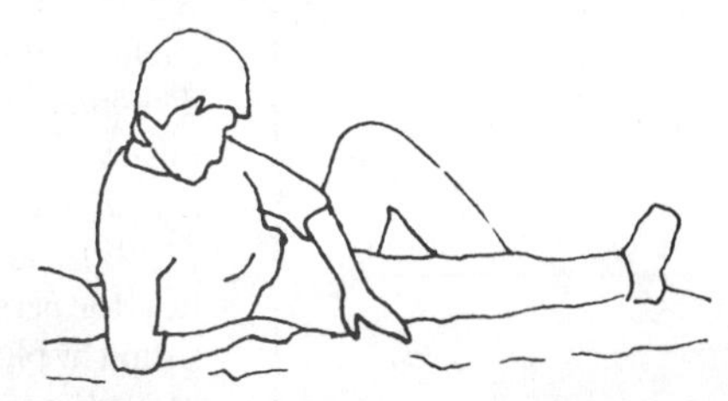
FIG 15.4b

or whilst they have their backrest and pillows adjusted.

- **Suitable for beds, trolleys, examination couches or if the client is on the floor – but each has its own risks eg. fixed height, hard surface, narrow, and will require individual specific assessment.**
- No equipment required (see options).

DESCRIPTION

- Handler stands at the side of the bed by the person, approximately at waist level, for safety and assurance
- The following sequence should proceed in a natural, free flowing manner.
- Ask the person to lift their head from the pillow bringing their chin forward to their chest, raise their far shoulder and reach across towards their opposite hip.
- At the same time they can flex their knees slightly.
- This will bring them to a sitting position or up onto their other elbow, where they can then push up to a sit or rest in that position (figures 15.4a–c).
- The same move can be achieved on a trolley (figures 15.5a–c).

OPTIONS / VARIATIONS

- Some people find it easier to turn completely onto their side prior to pushing themselves up into a sitting position.
- The person could use a bed lever, hand/rope ladder, overhead lifting pole to assist themselves up – these can be used in conjunction with a profiling bed/pillow lifter to reduce the effort and distance needed.
- Any such equipment should only be introduced following assessment.
- Profiling bed/pillow lifter/ mattress variator could raise the person to a reclining or sitting (figure 15.5d).

SKILL LEVEL

It may be necessary to instruct the person, and therefore knowledge of 'normal' movement may be required – as the person moving themselves.

EVIDENCE AVAILABLE

1. *The Handling of Patients 4th edition (1997/8)* describes that the common approach to sitting a person up is to bend them forward from a supine position as this is the easiest way of applying a force but it is not the natural way of sitting. To sit from supine without rolling places much greater demands on the person's abdominal muscles.
2. *Safer Handling of People in the Community (1999)* also describes this approach and how the person can support themselves in sitting by placing their hands on the bed just behind their hips.

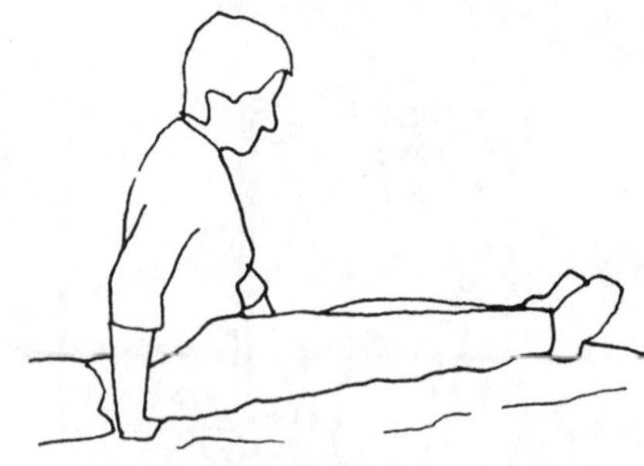

FIG 15.4c

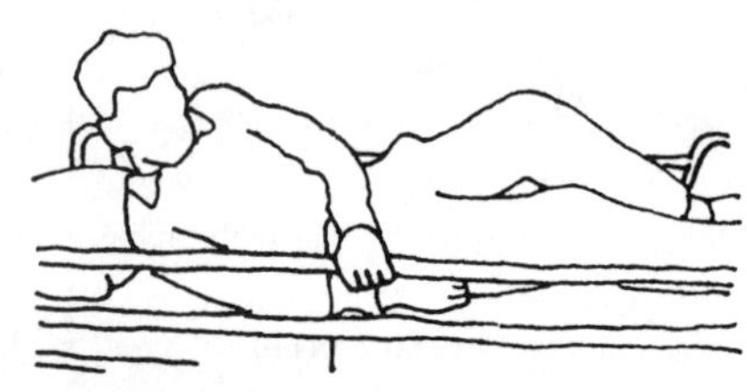

FIG 15.5a

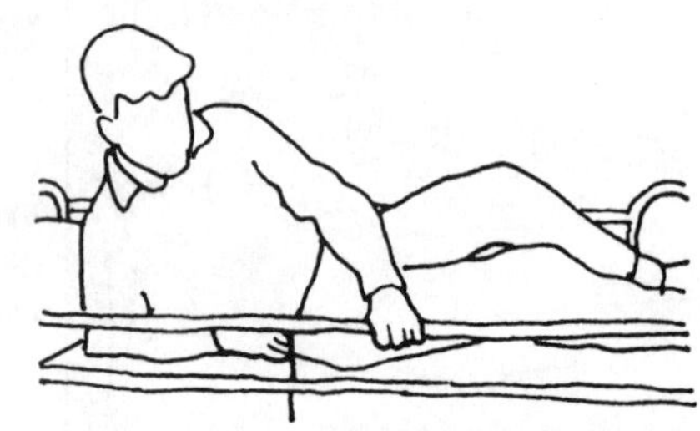

FIG 15.5b

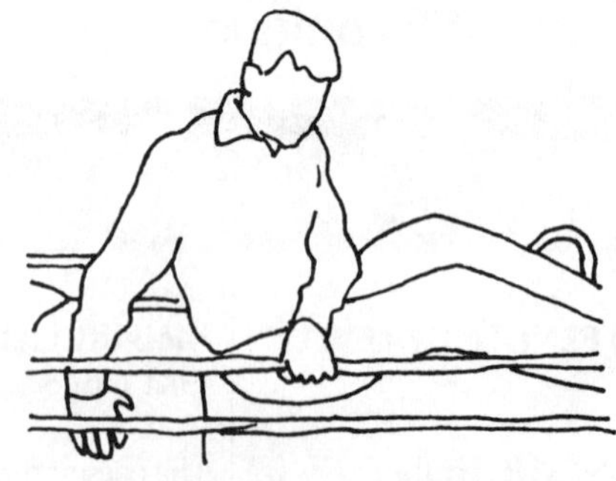

FIG 15.5c

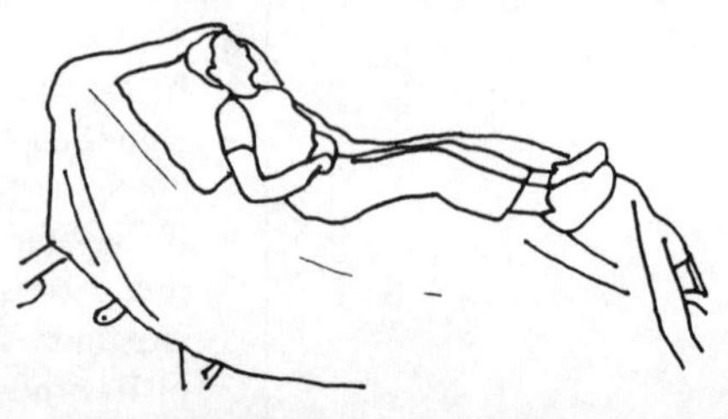

FIG 15.5d

DANGERS & PRECAUTIONS	• The person's ability must have been assessed correctly. • Consider safety of the handler's position if the person presents with challenging behaviour. • Consider the safety of the person as they turn to one side of the bed – is there sufficient room, larger people need wider beds/trolleys. • Consider any attachments to the person e.g. IV infusions, tubes etc.

Task Two

Lying to sitting – with some physical assistance by another person

DEPENDENCY LEVEL

Mobility Gallery B, E
FIM 1, 3

INSTRUCTION / EQUIPMENT

- The person needs to have cognitive and physical ability to give some assistance.
- Assess the persons ability by asking them to lift their head off the pillow and lay it back again.
- **If they can** do this – proceed.
  If they cannot consider an alternative method which gives more support e.g. electric profiling bed.
- Additional assistance is required from the handler due to the person's reduced independent function e.g. after abdominal surgery, pregnancy, weakness.
- **Suitable for beds, trolleys, examination couches or if the person is on the floor – but each has its own risks eg. fixed height, hard surface, narrow , and will require individual specific assessment.**
- No equipment required (see options).

DESCRIPTION

- The handler stands at side of the bed by the person, approximately at waist level, for safety and assurance.
- The handler must adjust the bed height where possible and position themselves taking account of their own posture.
- The handler should stand facing the person with some flexion in both hips and knees, having the nearside leg back and the outer leg forward helps to avoid twisting.
- The following sequence should proceed in a natural, free flowing manner (figures 15.6a–b).
- Ask the person to lift their head from the pillow bringing their chin forward to their chest.
- At the same time the person can flex their knees slightly.
- The person turns towards the handler, the handler guides the person's shoulder across and down the bed. Using the arm nearest to the person (i.e. handler's right hand reaches to person's left shoulder or vice versa) and allows space for the

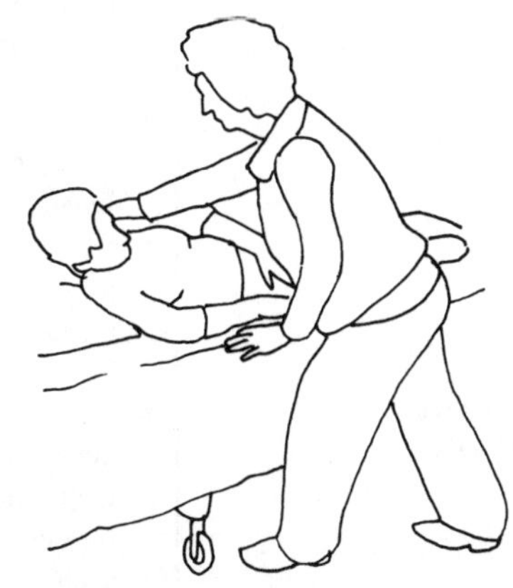

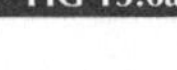

FIG 15.6a

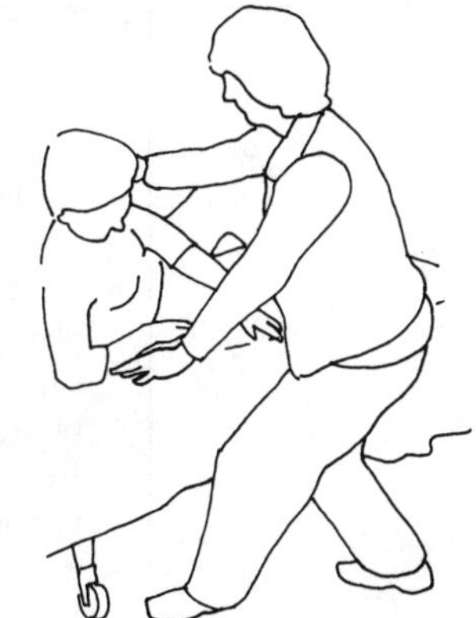

FIG 15.6b

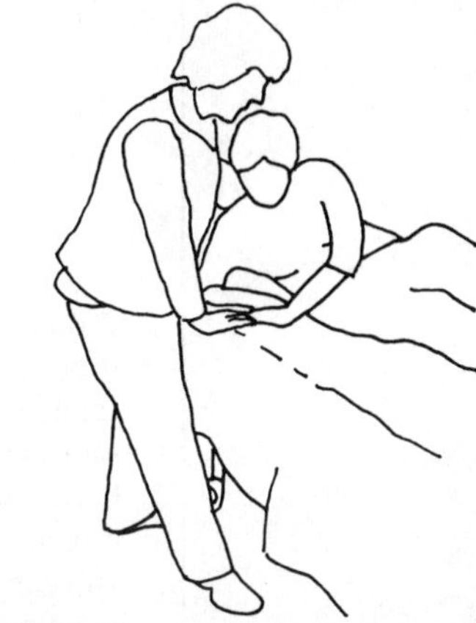

FIG 15.6c

DESCRIPTION (continued)

person's head to move forward easily.

- Encourage the person to also reach with their hand towards their opposite hip to aid the movement of their shoulder.
- The handler should achieve this transferring their body weight without pulling with their arm.
- This will bring the person to a sitting position or up onto their other elbow, where they can then push up to a sit or rest in that position (**figures** 15.6c–d).
- This manoeuvre can also be used to assist people who are on the floor - the handler should protect their knee with a kneeler/padding (**figures** 15.7a–c).
- The handler transfers their body weight by sitting back onto their heel from a high kneel position.
- Some people have not got the flexibility and joint range to achieve this comfortably and should not attempt this move.

OPTIONS / VARIATIONS

a The handler can place their left hand on the person's left shoulder (or vice versa), which allows the person to place their hand on the handler's shoulder. This approach requires skilled handlers with appropriate specialised training, the risks to the less skilled handler being:

- Twisting, over reaching, person 'pulling' on handler's shoulder. If the handler does not move appropriately they will occupy the space the person intends to move into and the person cannot then raise to their elbow.

b The person could roll onto their side completely prior to pushing themselves up to a sit, or the handler could assist them to roll onto their side, and then bring the person's shoulders up into a sitting position as the person assists.

- To roll the person the handler should ask the person to look in the direction they are turning, reach over with their far arm, position their near arm so that they do not roll onto it and either bend their far knee, both knees or cross their ankles. The handler should place a hand at the person's shoulder and hip or knee and guide the person over. The movement is achieved the by transferring their body weight, not by pulling with their arms.

Either transfer weight from a forward foot to back foot with both feet placed firmly on the floor (**figures** 15.8a–b)
or transfer weight from a knee on the bed back to the foot on the floor (**figure** 15.9a).

c A profiling bed/pillow lifter/mattress variator could raise the person to a reclining or sitting position (**figures** 15.10a–d).

- The handler can then guide the person's

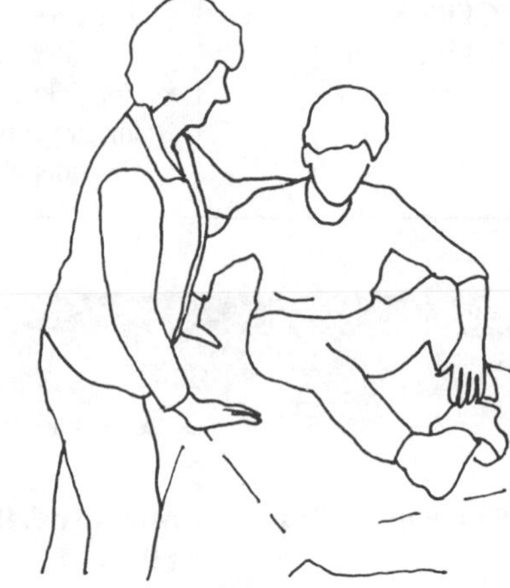
FIG 15.6d

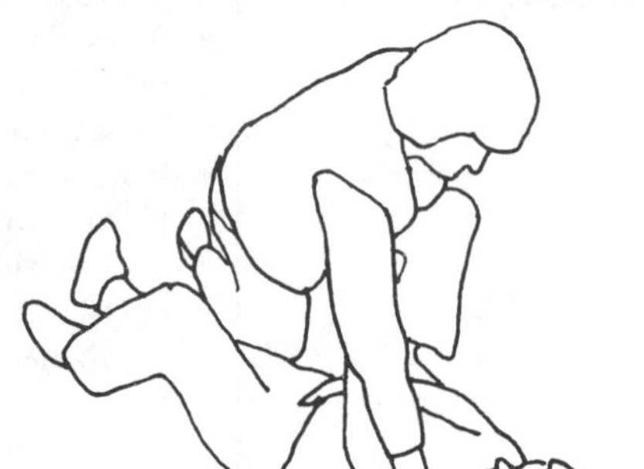
FIG 15.7a

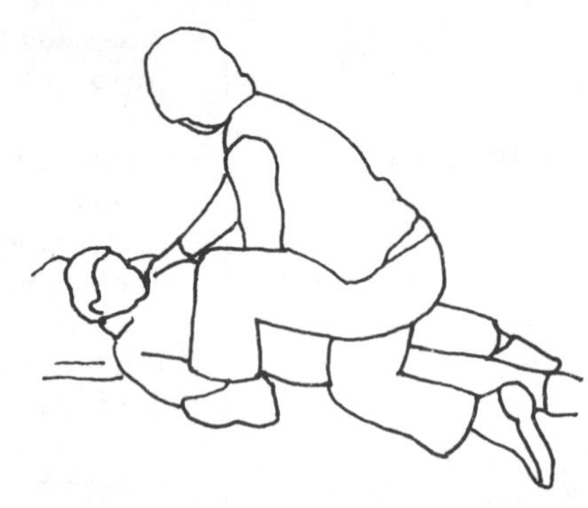
FIG 15.7b

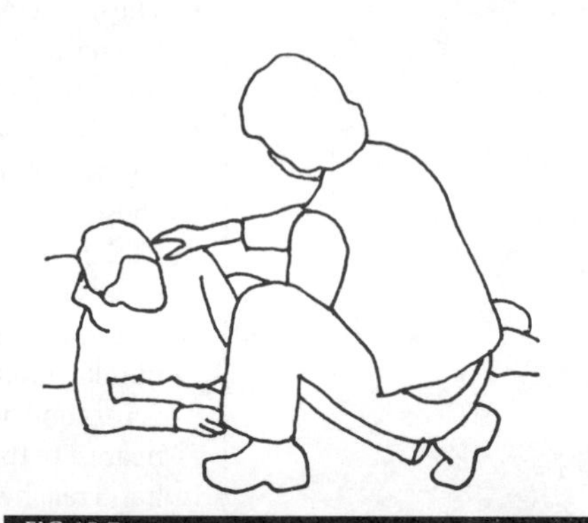
FIG 15.7c

shoulders forward if necessary e.g. to insert an X-ray plate or adjust pillows. This forward assistance should be achieved by transferring the body weight forward with the person whilst supporting their shoulders.

This guidance, where the handler transfers their weight forward with the shoulders, cannot be used to raise a person from supine, as the effort required is considerable and places an unnecessary force through the shoulders and/or neck. The person must be in a partially raised position, supported by the bed or trolley prior to forward assistance.

EVIDENCE AVAILABLE

The Handling of Patients 4th edition (1997/8) recommends that the person should always be allowed to move themselves where possible and to use simple aids such as rope ladders to hold themselves forward once they are sitting.

DANGERS & PRECAUTIONS

- As for task one, and
- Incorrect assessment of the person's ability could lead to the handler 'lifting' the person forward to a sitting position instead of the sit being achieved substantially by the person.
- Twisting or over reaching by the handler when bringing the person's far shoulder towards their opposite hip or when rolling the person onto their side, particularly if the bed height is not adjusted prior to the move.
- Shoulder/neck strain to handler if inappropriate level of assistance given and/or transfer of weight is not used to achieve the sit or roll.
- Do not use this manoeuvre if the person resists forward movement.
- Ensure there is no medical reason why the person cannot roll onto one side e.g. post hip replacement,

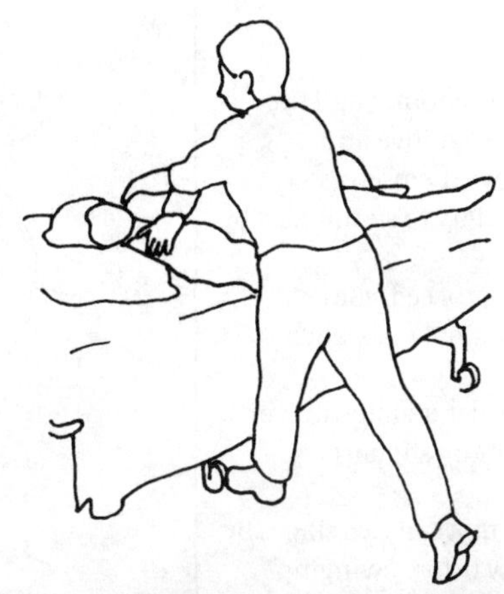

FIG 15.8a

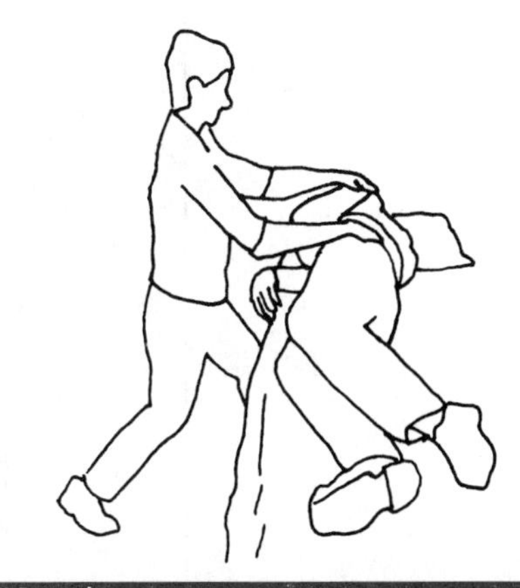

FIG 15.8b

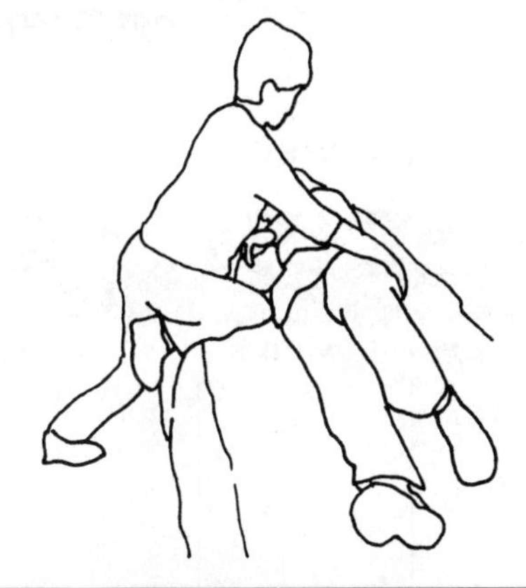

FIG 15.9a

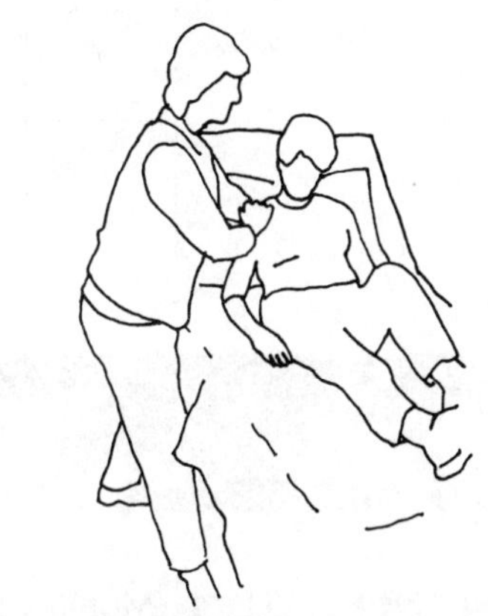

FIG 15.10a

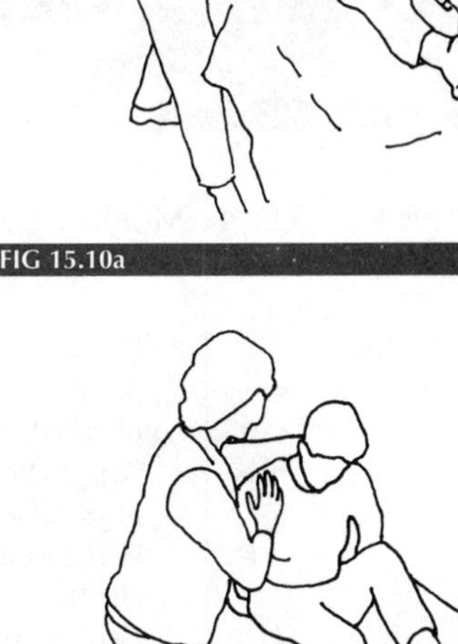

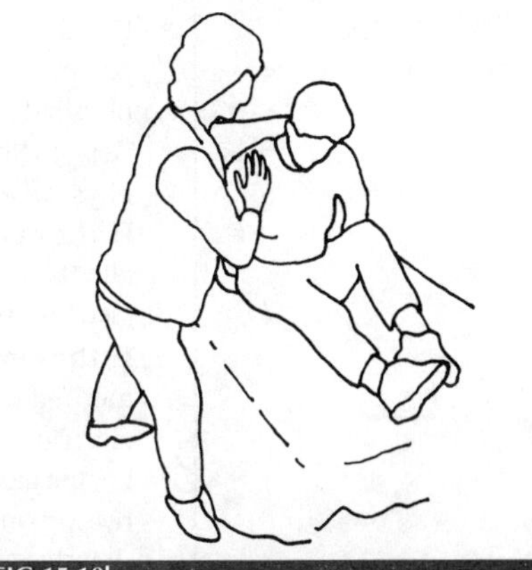

FIG 15.10b

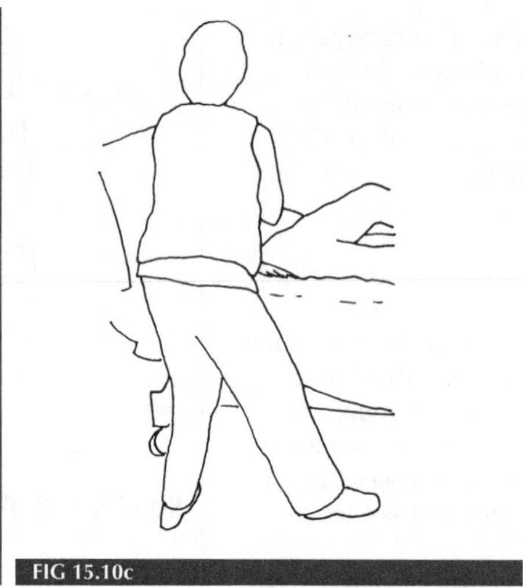
FIG 15.10c

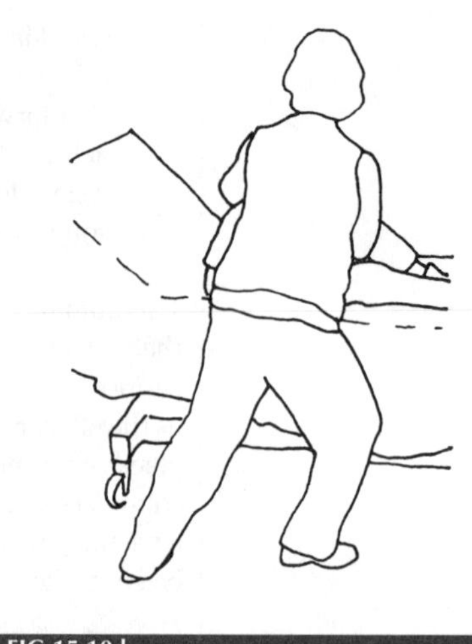
FIG 15.10d

Evidence review

Technique	REBA	Activity	Comfort	FIM	Mobility gallery	Skill level	Comment
LYING TO SITTING WITH SOME PHYSICAL ASSISTANCE BY ANOTHER PERSON							
Fig 15.6a	9	8	8	3	B	Novice	
Fig 15.6d	10	7	4	3	B	Advanced beginner	
Fig 15.8a	9	1	7	1	E	Advanced beginner	
Fig 15.8b	3	1	7	1	E	Advanced beginner	
Fig 15.9a	9	1	7	1	E	Advanced beginner	

Task Three

Lying to sitting on the side of the bed – no physical assistance from another person

DEPENDENCY LEVEL

Mobility Gallery C
FIM 7

INSTRUCTION / EQUIPMENT

- Handler uses verbal prompting and the person needs to have cognitive and physical ability to move themselves.
- Assess the person's ability to sit unaided by physical assistance.
  If they can do this – proceed. some clients will need additional assistance (see task two).
  If they cannot consider an alternative method which gives more support e.g. electric profiling bed.
- People can make the move in two stages by resting on their elbow before swinging their legs over the side of the bed to sit up.

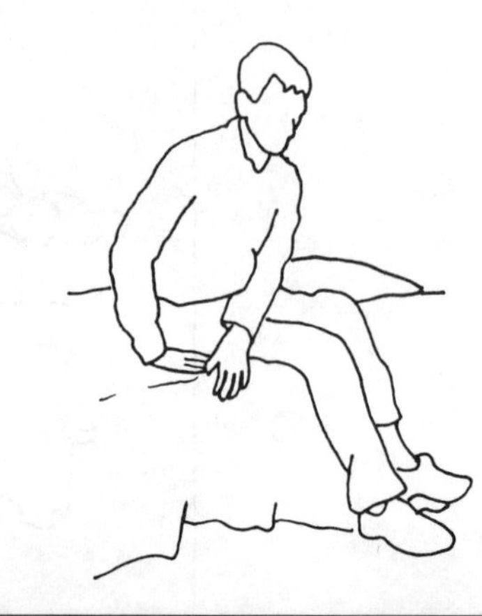
FIG 15.11a

- Suitable for beds, trolleys, examination couches – but each has its own risks e.g. fixed height, hard surface, narrow, and will require individual specific assessment.
- Additional care must be taken if there is also a pressure relieving mattress or mattress overlay.
- No equipment required (see options).

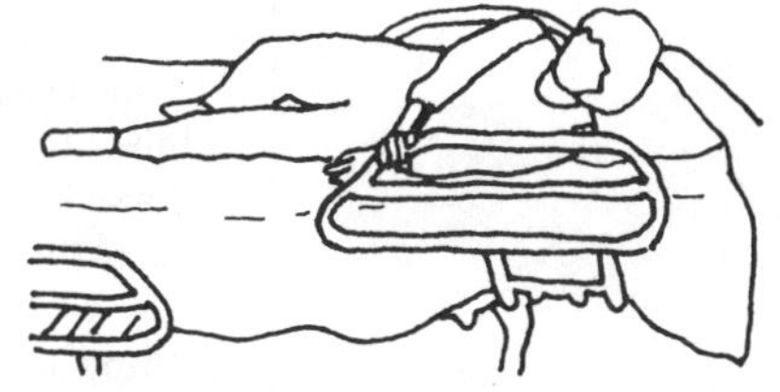
FIG 15.12a

DESCRIPTION

- Handler stands at side of the person, approximately at waist level, for safety and assurance.
- The handler must adjust the bed height, where possible taking account of the need for the person to end the move with their feet on the floor.
- The following sequence should proceed in a natural, free-flowing manner.
- Proceed as for task one (figures 15.4a–c and figure 15.11a) – This will bring the person to a sitting position or up onto their other elbow, where they can then push up as they swing their legs off the side of the bed. A slide sheet under their legs will aid this but the handler must ensure this does not fall to the floor and become a slip hazard.

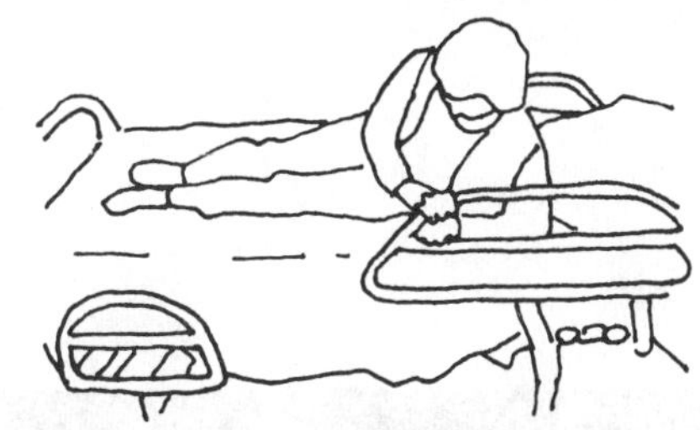
FIG 15.12b

OPTIONS / VARIATIONS

- The person could roll onto their side completely prior to pushing themselves up to a sit whilst bringing their legs off the side of the bed – a bed lever/ rail or hand/rope ladder could also be used to assist themselves up (figures 15.12a–d).
- A flexible turn disc can be used under the person's hips to assist the person to rotate in order to sit on the side of the bed.
- A profiling bed/pillow lifter/mattress variator could raise the person to a reclining or sitting position prior to bringing their legs off the bed – a leg lifter can be used (figures 15.13a–b).

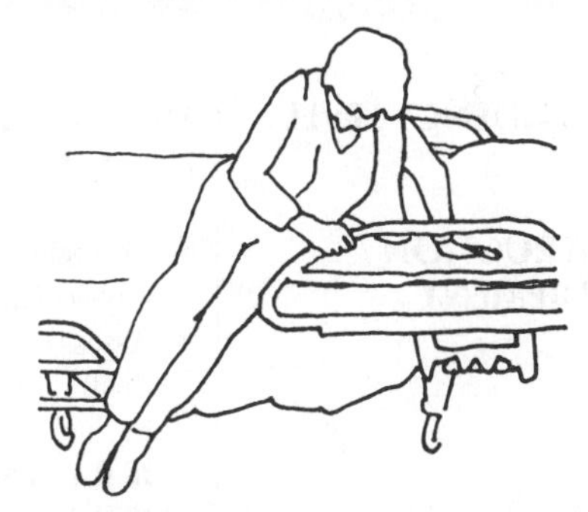
FIG 15.12c

SKILL LEVEL

It may be necessary to instruct person and therefore knowledge of 'normal' movement may be required as client moving themselves.

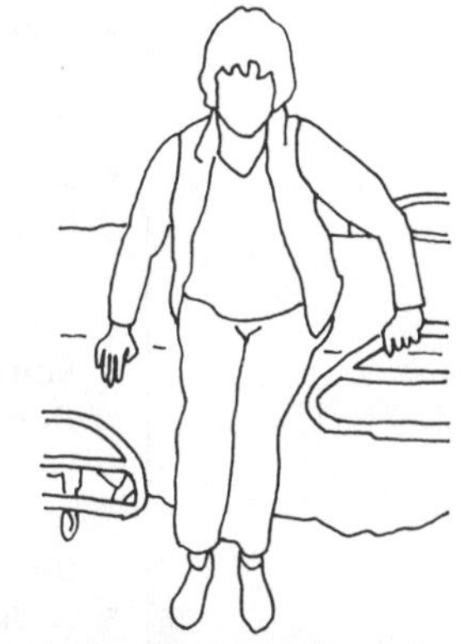
FIG 15.12d

EVIDENCE AVAILABLE

1 The *Handling of Patients 4th edition (1997/8)* suggests the use of a slide sheet in place of a flexible turn disc with the caution that there is risk that a person could slide off the edge of the bed.

2 *Safer Handling of People in the Community (1999)* recommends that the person has upper limb strength and good sitting balance.

DANGERS & PRECAUTIONS

- As for task one, and if there is a mattress overlay or pressure relieving mattress this may 'dip' or tend to cause the person to slide off the side of the bed.

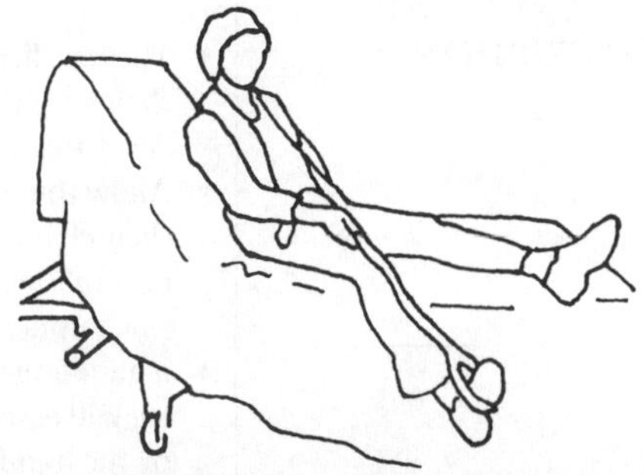
FIG 15.13a

- Assess the risks to the person's legs e.g. tissue viability, oedema, pulling a catheter tube.
- If a slide sheet is used ensure it does not fall to the floor and become a slip hazard.
- Incorrect assessment of the person's sitting ability – potential to fall off the side of the bed if unbalanced.

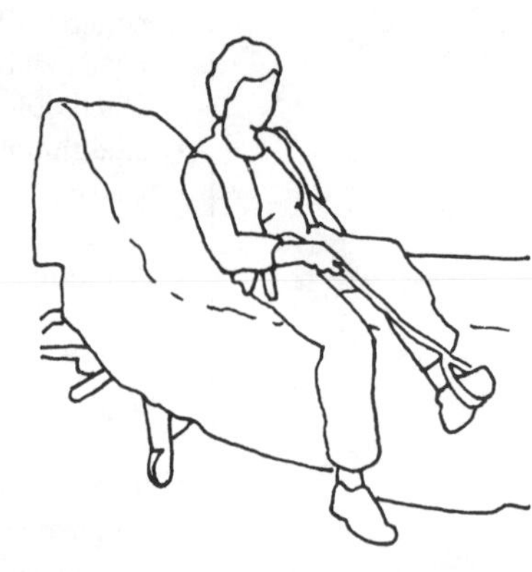
FIG 15.13b

Task Four

Assisting a person to sit on side of bed

DEPENDENCY LEVEL

Mobility Gallery B, D
FIM 3, 4

INSTRUCTION / EQUIPMENT

- The person needs to have cognitive and physical ability to give some assistance.
- Assess the person's ability by asking them to lift their head off the pillow and lay it back again.
  If they can do this – proceed.
  If they cannot, consider an alternative method which gives more support e.g. electric profiling bed.
- People can make the move in two stages by resting on their elbow before swinging their legs over the side of the bed to sit up.
- Additional assistance is required from the handler due to the person's reduced independent function e.g. after abdominal surgery, pregnancy, weakness.
- **Suitable for beds, trolleys, examination couches – but each has its own risks e.g. fixed height, hard surface, narrow and each will require individual specific assessment.**
- Additional care must be taken if there is also a pressure relieving mattress or mattress overlay.

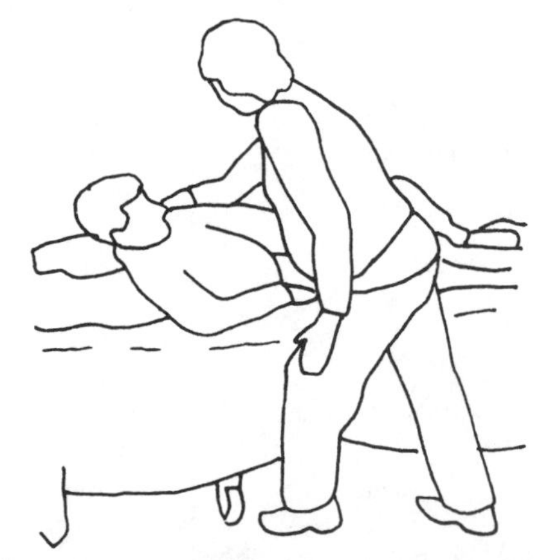
FIG 15.14a

DESCRIPTION

- The handler assists the person up onto their elbow as in task two (figure 15.14a).
- Allow the person to support themselves on their elbow while the handler assists the person's legs off the side of the bed (a slide sheet under the person's feet and calves or a handling strap under the person's lower leg will assist this).
  or the handler can assist the person's shoulders (figures 15.15a–b) to an upright

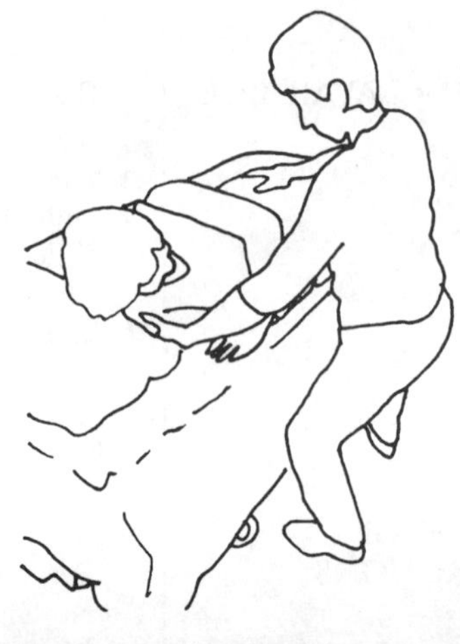
FIG 15.15a

position as the person simultaneously pushes themselves up. The handler must achieve this by transferring their weight from side to side.

- Two handlers can assist (figure 15.16a) – one at the person's shoulders and the other guiding the legs, ideally with a slide sheet.

OPTIONS / VARIATIONS

- The person could roll onto their side completely prior to being assisted up to a sit.

EVIDENCE AVAILABLE

1 *The Handling of Patients 4th edition (1997/8)* stresses that caution must be used when assisting legs as these can weigh 30% (*Pheasant 1996*) or more of the body weight of the person and there is the danger of stooping.

2 *Safer Handling of People in the Community (1999)* describes the handler assisting by holding both the person's shoulders and stresses that the movement must be well co-ordinated.

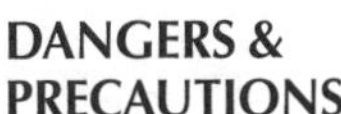

DANGERS & PRECAUTIONS

- As for task three, and the following:
- Handler over reaching by trying to assist the person's legs and shoulders at the same time.
- Handler taking excessive weight by lifting the person's legs off the bed.
- Inappropriate bed height for handler or person e.g. too high off the floor for the person, too low for the handler.
- Do not use this manoeuvre if the person resists forward movement.

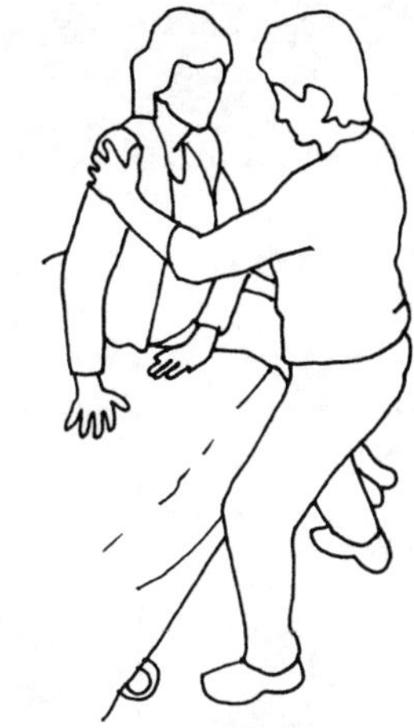

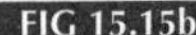

FIG 15.15b

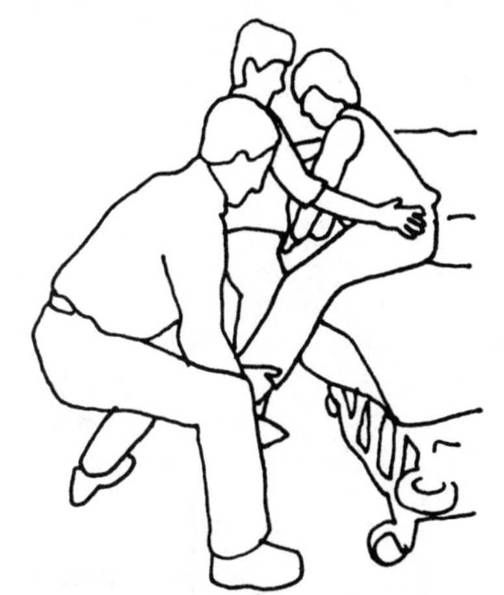

FIG 15.16a

Evidence review

Technique	REBA	Activity	Comfort	FIM	Mobility gallery	Skill level	Comment
ASSISTING AN INDEPENDENT SIT TO SIDE OF BED							
Fig 15.14a	6	3	8	4	B	Competent	Postural risk is less with no hands on the bed
Fig 15.16a	8	5	8	3	D	Advanced beginner	
as Fig 15.16a plus sling	3	5	8	3	D	Advanced beginner	Postural risk is less with handling sling (see fig 15.22a)
Fig 15.21a	4	5	8	3	D	Advanced beginner	Legs onto bed half kneeling

Task Five

Lying to sitting using aids

DEPENDENCY LEVEL

Mobility Gallery A, B, C, D
FIM 6 or 5

INSTRUCTION / EQUIPMENT

- Use of rope/hand ladder (figures15.17a), grab rail or bed lever.
- The person should be assessed prior to introducing this equipment to ensure it meets their need and there are no contra-indications of use (see dangers and precautions).
- This equipment should be specifically designed to attach to the bed in order to assist a person to move within, in or out of bed. It must be correctly attached following the manufacturer's instructions of use.
- This type of equipment is available for divan, community, nursing care and hospital beds – some can also be used with trolleys and examination couches.

DESCRIPTION

- Rope/hand ladder – the person 'walks' their hands up the ladder by pulling with each hand in turn (figures15.17b).
- Bed lever and grab rails – must be firmly fixed in place to enable the person to grip the object and pull themselves up to a sitting position (figures15.18a–b).
- The above equipment can be used in conjunction with a profiling bed/pillow lifter to reduce the effort needed and distance travelled.

SKILL LEVEL

It may be necessary to instruct the person, therefore knowledge of 'normal' movement may be required as the person is moving themselves.

EVIDENCE AVAILABLE

1 *The Handling of Patients 4th edition (1997/8)* identifies that even if a person cannot pull themselves up to a sitting position with a rope ladder they may be able to maintain the position by holding on once sitting. These aids may be of particular use in long term care in the community.
2 In a survey of handling devices rope ladders were found to be rarely used. The common problems with use being time to use the device, staff experience and lack of availability *(Owen 1988)*. It is likely that for rope ladders the lack of availability was the major factor.

DANGERS & PRECAUTIONS

- The person must have a reliable grasp.
- Injury to person's arms, shoulder, neck through inappropriate assessment or if the equipment is not attached correctly

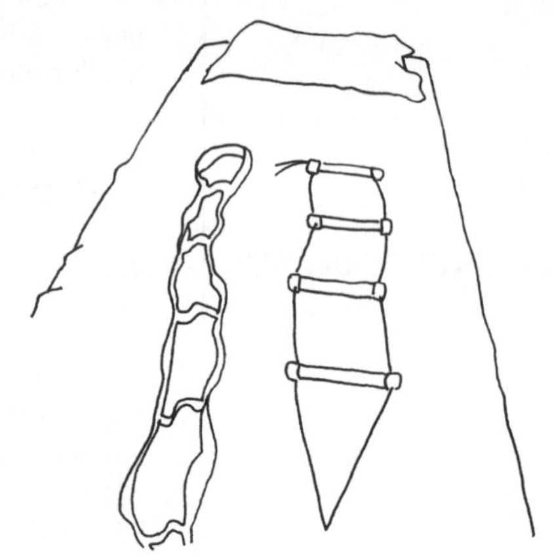

FIG 15.17a

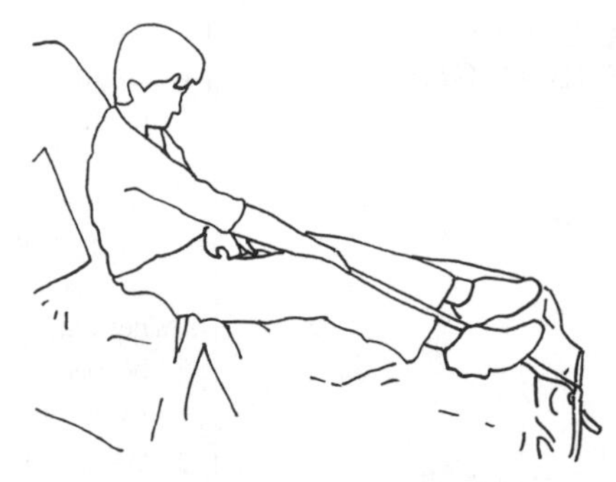

FIG 15.17b

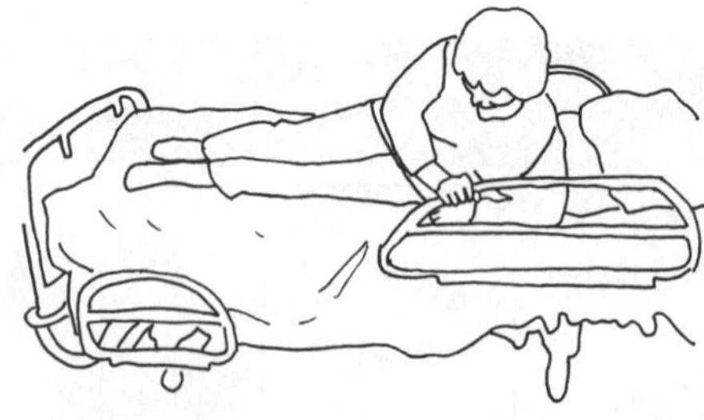

FIG 15.18a

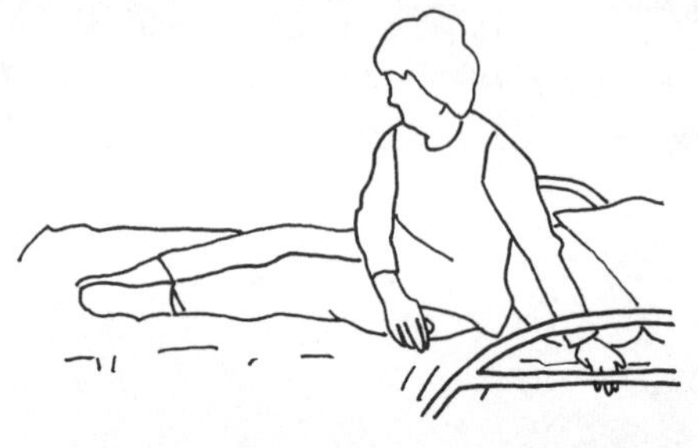

FIG 15.18b

DANGERS & PRECAUTIONS (continued)

and/or checked regularly.

- The elbow to elbow method described in *The Handling of Patients 4th edition (1997/8)* can be replaced by the above described aids. This reduces the likelihood of injury to handler if used and the person is too heavy, does not use their abdominal muscles to aid the sit or if they 'pull' on the handler.
- All equipment should be assessed as suitable for that individual person, particularly where the person's physical, mental or behavioural state could put them at risk with equipment with leads or moving parts. Be aware of particular strangulation risk and/or self-harm.

Task Six

Lying to sitting using equipment

DEPENDENCY LEVEL

Mobility Gallery A, B, C, D
FIM 6, 3, 2, 1

INSTRUCTION / EQUIPMENT

- Electric profiling bed , trolleys, couches (figures 15.19a–b).
- Pillow lifter – e.g. electric, air-filled.
- Mattress elevator/variator – to prevent the mattress slipping off the bed there should be a foot board to the bed frame or a mattress retainer fitted.
- There is also specifically designed equipment which converts from chair to stretcher, wheelchair to stretcher, bed to chair, which will allow the persons position to be changed with no manual assistance.

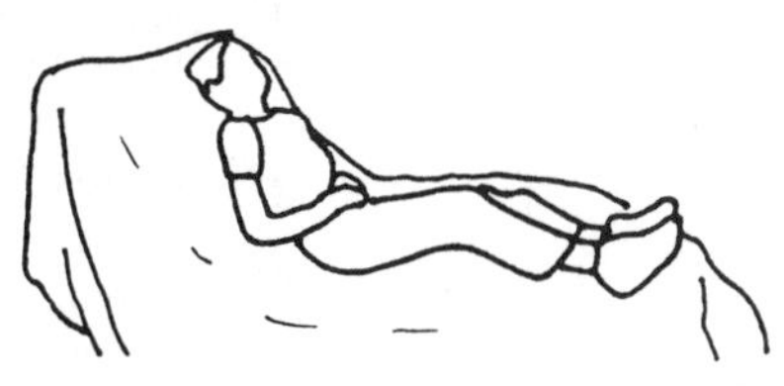

FIG 15.19a

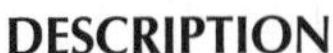

DESCRIPTION

- This type of profiling equipment can be used by the person to allow them independence, despite reduced ability, if they have the ability to use the controls.
- The equipment can be used to gradually increase the person's ability and function by reducing the position of elevation and requiring the person to 'complete' the sit using their own muscle effort.
- It should also be considered in paediatric settings when a more gradual or better supported change of position/less direct hand contact to child is required.
- This is the optimum method for the very heavy person, high dependency situations and areas of work where the handlers repeat this type of manoeuvre regularly, whether in acute/long term/community care settings:
  e.g. ITU, Coronary Care, Terminal Care, High Dependency Units, people with significant loss of function etc.

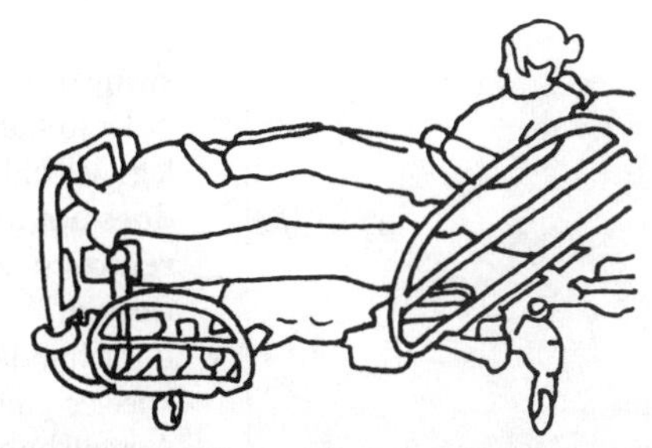

FIG 15.19b

Use of profiling equipment is the method of choice for:
People with limited function and ability – particularly if they have poor head control or poor cognitive ability.

OPTIONS/ VARIATIONS

- Profiling equipment can also be used to

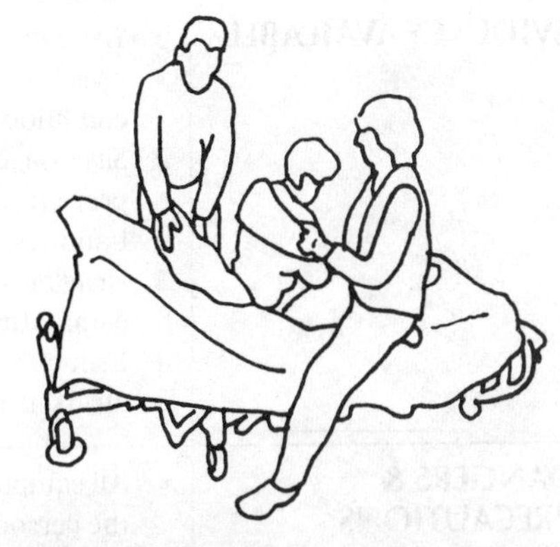

FIG 15.20a

assist the person to sit independently to the side of the bed by elevating them to a sitting position. They can then bring their legs off the side of the bed (see task three options).

- Following assessment other equipment can be used by the person in conjunction with the profiling system depending on their ability e.g. rope ladder, monkey pole, bed lever/rail, hand blocks.
- If the person needs to assist themselves further forward once the bed is fully profiled e.g. to have pillows adjusted, (figure 15.20a) encourage them to reach towards their opposite hip or assist them by guiding their shoulder towards their opposite hip (see task one and two) or use a handling aid e.g. handling strap to support them forward while a second handler adjusts the pillows.

Many handlers do not find this 'knee on the bed' approach comfortable and should not attempt it. Additionally the Safe Working Load of the bed should be assessed.

- Profiling equipment can be used to sit the person prior to the handler assisting them to the side of the bed.
- Once in the sitting upright position the person can then be encouraged/assisted to swing their legs over the side of the bed in order to stand – a slide sheet under their legs will aid this. **Ensure the slide sheet does not fall to the floor and is removed as soon as the legs are positioned.**
- If the handler kneels it is preferable to use a kneeler/pad or similar (figure 15.21a).
- A small handling aid such as a handling strap can be used to support the persons legs allowing the handler to lower the legs without excessive bending or reach (figure 15.22a).

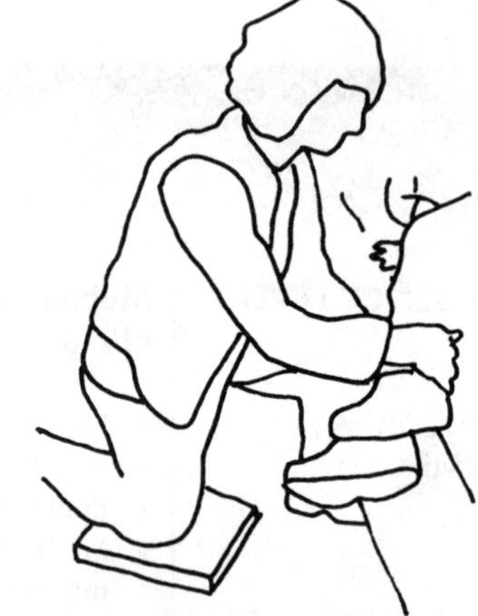

FIG 15.21a

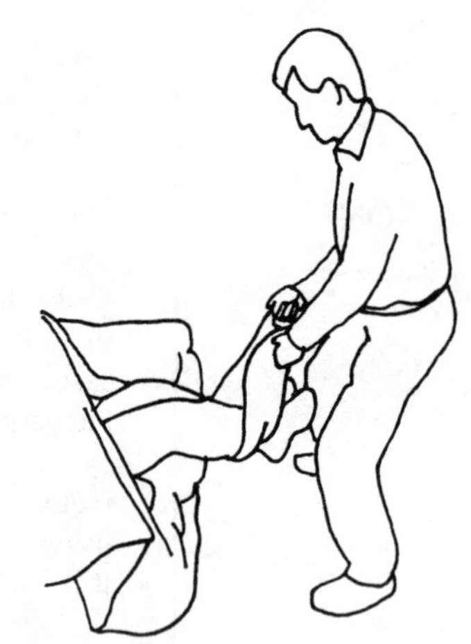

FIG 15.22a

SKILL LEVEL	The handler must have knowledge of the use and application of the equipment.
EVIDENCE AVAILABLE	1 *The Handling of Patients 4th edition (1997/8)* suggests that tilting the bed combined with the use of a slide sheet will assist in moving the person in the bed (the person's medical condition must be assessed prior to using this method e.g. cardiac status). 2 *Safer Handling of People in the Community (1999)* identifies that use of profiling beds can prevent slipping down the bed, reduce the time required for care and the numbers of handlers. 3 *Handling Home Care (2001)* refers to reducing handlers poor postures by raising the bed and eliminating a 'drag lift to sitting' by use of a mattress variator. 4 Reduction of injury to handlers is also identified by *Dhoot & Georgieva (1996)* and for paediatric settings using height adjustable cots by *Kitson (2000)*.
DANGERS & PRECAUTIONS	• All equipment should be assessed as suitable for that individual person, particularly where the persons physical, mental or behavioural state could put them at risk with equipment with leads, Be aware of particular strangulation risk and/or self-harm.

DANGERS & PRECAUTIONS (continued)

- It may be necessary to ensure the controls can be 'isolated' for handler use only, to prevent inappropriate use by the person.
- Profiling beds vary in the way they 'profile' this must be taken into account when purchasing/leasing where the method of 'profile' could affect the final sitting position of the person (see previous reference to the heavy person).
- Some people will need a profiling system that has a 'knee break' which raises the knees as the person is raised to sitting.
- The complete range of positions that a bed can offer must be taken into account when assessing a person's need.
- For manual profiling systems it may be necessary for the person to be sitting forwards whilst a second handler raises the profiling system.
- **Manual profiling systems do not necessarily reduce the effort or likelihood of injury to the handler who may be tempted to sit the person up at the same time as profiling the equipment. This can be a considerable effort/musculoskeletal stress – electric options are preferable both from quality of person's independence/care and for quality of work.**

Evidence review

Technique	REBA	Activity	Comfort	FIM	Mobility gallery	Skill level	Comment
LYING TO SITTING USING EQUIPMENT							
Fig 15.20a	4	5	7	3	B	Competent	Handling sling sitting on bed is the best technique for promoting person activity and reducing postural risk for the handler

Task Seven

Manual assisted lying to sitting – one knee on the bed

DEPENDENCY LEVEL

Mobility Gallery B, C
FIM 3

INSTRUCTION / EQUIPMENT

One limitation of this manoeuvre is 'for what purpose is the move being done?' – if the handlers are required to support the person in the sitting position they cannot also do secondary activities such as adjusting pillows, pulling out a backrest etc.

Assessment must identify whether:

- The person could support themselves forward with a rope ladder/bed rail
  or the person can be supported by one handler while the other changes position and carries out the secondary activity (figure 15.23a).
  or a third handler is needed to undertake the secondary activity.
- Use of profiling equipment can be more cost effective as well as reducing potential risks to handlers – producing Quality of Care and Quality of Work.
- The change of position from lying to

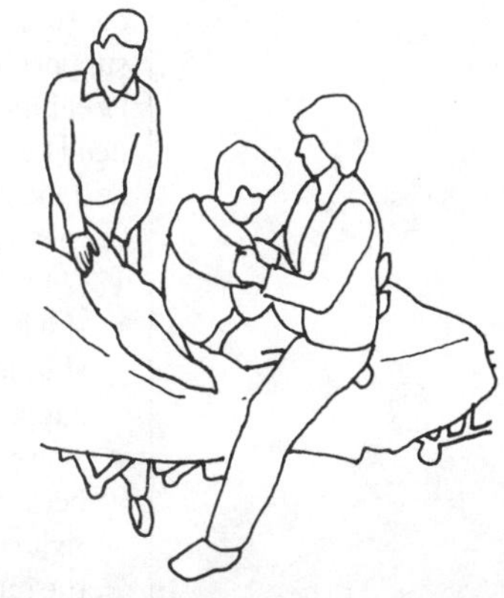

FIG 15.23a

sitting is fairly rapid for the person which is not desirable in many circumstances/ conditions and it is less comfortable – again this rapid postural change is eliminated by the use of appropriate profiling equipment.

- Two handlers required for adult situations.
- Generally equipment will reduce the REBA score for the handler as it will reduce reach and potential twisting, e.g. handling strap, handling netting, handling sheet with or without handles.
- One handler could consider this approach if:

a the assessment of the handler's and person's BMI and the ability of the person clearly identify that neither would be compromised by the use of one handler e.g. if the person is a small child. It would be essential in most cases for the handler to be using equipment e.g. handling strap/netting to assist in the manoeuvre to reduce the reach across to the person's far shoulder and to give adequate support.

b if the person is already in a semi-lying/ reclining position and has the ability to provide most of the effort for the sit, they should not be 'leaning their weight' making the handler do all the work.

- The bed must be an appropriate height for the comfort and balance of the handlers.
- This method cannot be used on certain fixed height equipment e.g. trolleys/examination couches if the handlers cannot achieve an aligned pelvis with one foot firmly on the floor.
- Safe working load of the bed must be sufficient to support the combined weight of the person and handlers. Some beds can tip up when handlers kneel on them.

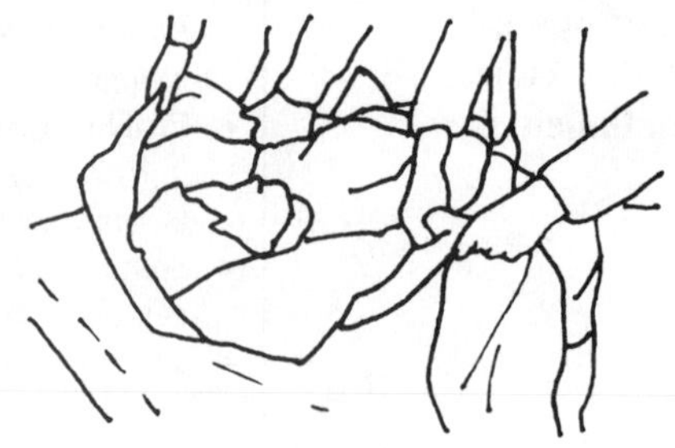

FIG 15.24a

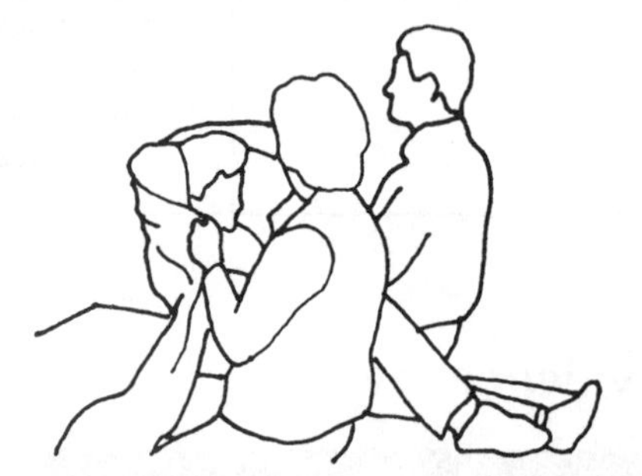

FIG 15.24b

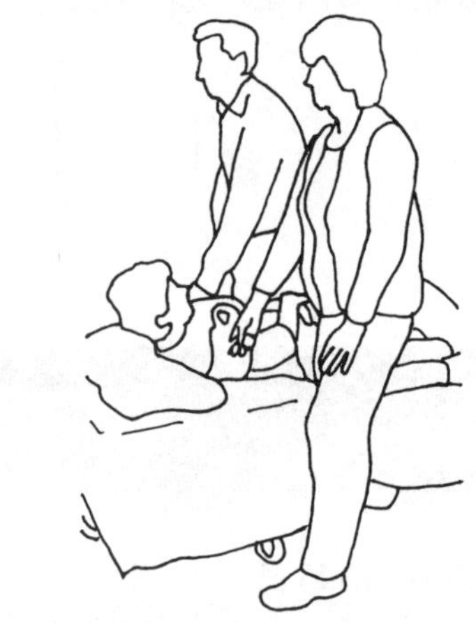

FIG 15.25a

DESCRIPTION

The basic manoeuvre is described below using a handling strap – the assessment will identify which 'hold' or equipment should be used to support the person.

However, if the person has poor head control, handling netting can be used to support across the person's shoulders as well as behind their pillow, to assist in bringing the head forward at the time of the sit – this must be done with great caution so as not to pull the head forward during the move (figures 15.24a–b).

- If a handling aid is used e.g. strap, it should be placed behind the person to support their shoulders (figures 15.25a).
- The strap must not be placed too low behind the person's back as this will reduce the mechanical leverage making the manoeuvre considerably more difficult.

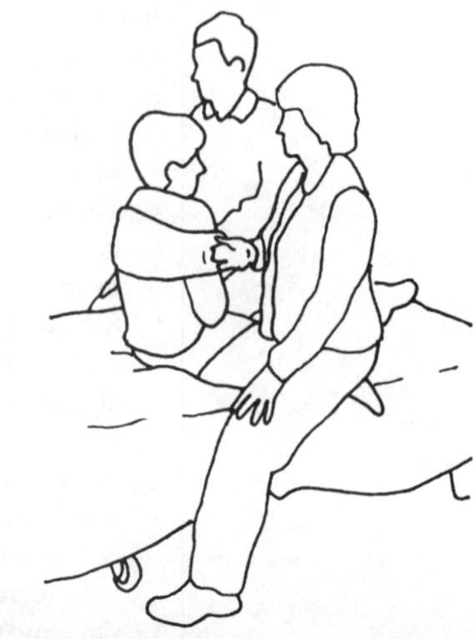

FIG 15.25b

- The strap must be held taut to avoid slipping, some straps have a non-slip surface.
- The handlers place one knee on the bed, one each side of the person, with their supporting foot flat on the floor.
- The handler's knees should be beside the person's waist/hips (if the handler's knees are placed too far forwards, the person will end up behind them at the end of the manoeuvre with twisting or strain on the handler's shoulders and loss of any counterbalance to support the sit).
- The handler's raise themselves to a 'high kneel' creating a space between their buttocks and heel, with their spines in a naturally upright position.
- Hold the handling strap taut with the inside hand, close to the person's shoulders. Ensure the aid gives good, even support across the person's shoulders and is not pulling behind their neck.
- Ask the person to bring their chin towards their chest and to bend a knee.
- Use a command such as **'ready, steady sit'** not '1,2,3'.
- On 'Sit' the handlers, in unison, move their body weight back towards their heel.

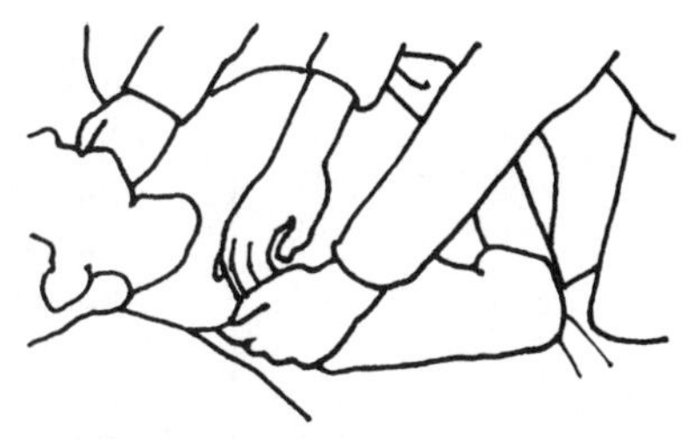

FIG 15.26a

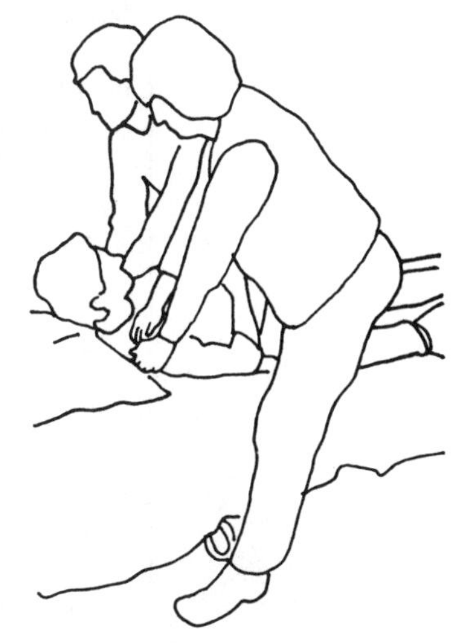

FIG 15.26b

OPTIONS / VARIATIONS

Support of the person's shoulders with:

a Scapula hold
The handler's 'cup' the person's shoulder. The reach required may eliminate this as a choice for some handlers (figures 15.26a–c).

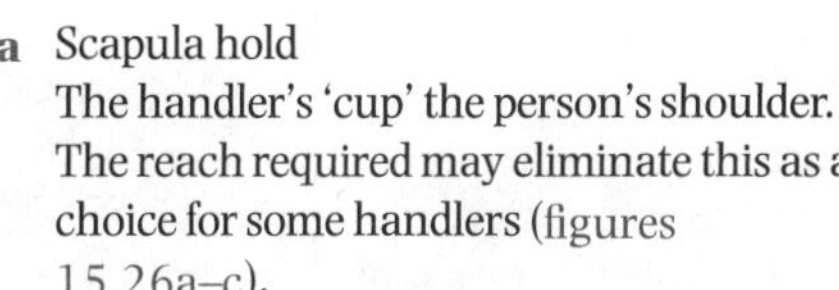

b Designated handling netting or handling sheet
This can reduce reach and twist, allows two hands to be used by the handlers and gives additional support to the person (figures 15.27a–b).

c Single handler for child
The handler takes the handling strap/netting in each hand beside each of the child's shoulders – the breadth of the child's shoulders must not cause the handler to over reach (figures 15.28a–b).

If this method is used for an adult or larger child the person should already be in a semi-reclined position to reduce the distance brought forward (figures 15.29a–b).

d Elbow to elbow hold described in *The Handling of Patients 4th edition (1997/8)* The risks related to this manoeuvre are that the person is very likely to 'pull' themselves up using the handler's arm/s as a lever. It would be more appropriate to give them

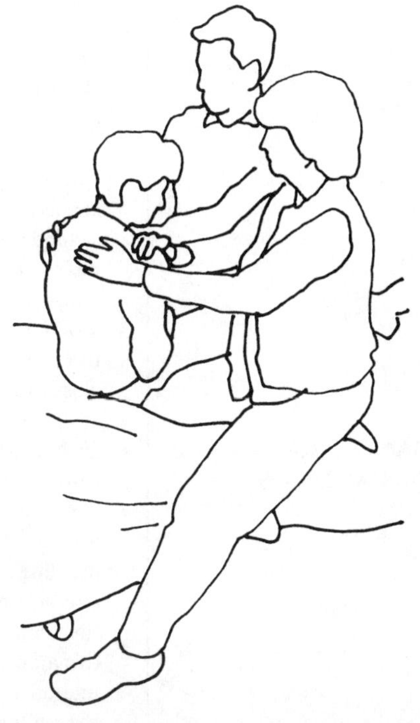

FIG 15.26c

equipment designed for this such as a rope ladder, bed lever/rail.

- If a person has the ability to achieve this move without pulling on the handlers they are likely to be able to use task one avoiding the potential risks to the carer.
- The handler should not provide more than 10kg of force (*The Handling of Patients 4th edition 1997/8*) and this is difficult to ascertain in most situations.

This is an option if the risk assessment justifies its use and no other appropriate method could be used.

e Adapted for assisted sit when the person on the floor (account must be taken of the pressure on the handler's knees – knee padding/kneeler should be available.)

- The handlers kneel next to the person's hips – their outside leg is raised forward with their foot flat on the ground
- On the command 'sit' they move their body weight back until they are resting or almost resting on their heel.

If additional head support is needed a third handler must assist behind the person's head, transferring their weight forward by raising themselves up off their heel on the command 'sit' (figure 15.30a–c).

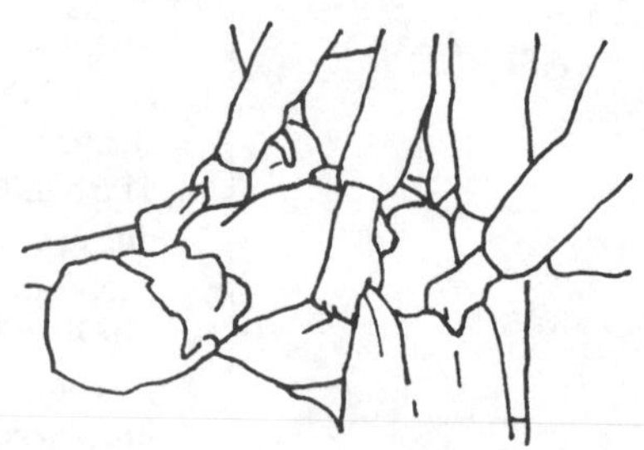
FIG 15.27a

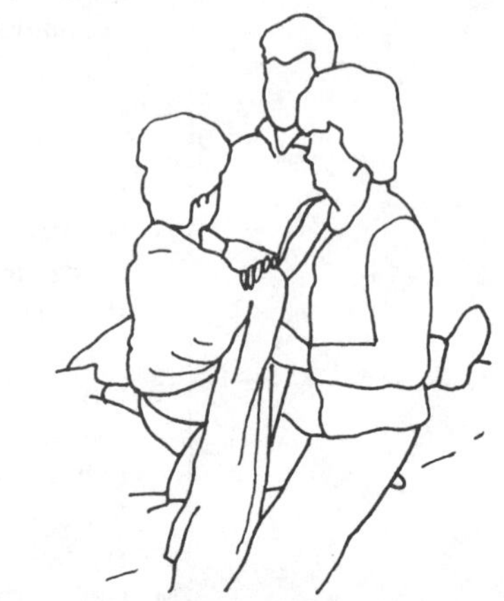
FIG 15.27b

EVIDENCE AVAILABLE

1. *Safer Handling in the Community (1999)* suggests this manoeuvre as an interim procedure in the absence of mechanical devices and recommends ideally the use of a non-slip sling.
2. *The Handling of Patients 4th edition (1997/8)* refers to the use of sheets/draw sheets to support the person to a sit, although it is stressed that this must be used with caution as they can tear. Nowadays the use of designated handling sheets or other equipment would be considered more appropriate particularly now it is so much more readily available and cheaper.
3. *HOP4* also raises the caution of reaching too far forward to hold the equipment close to the person's shoulders.

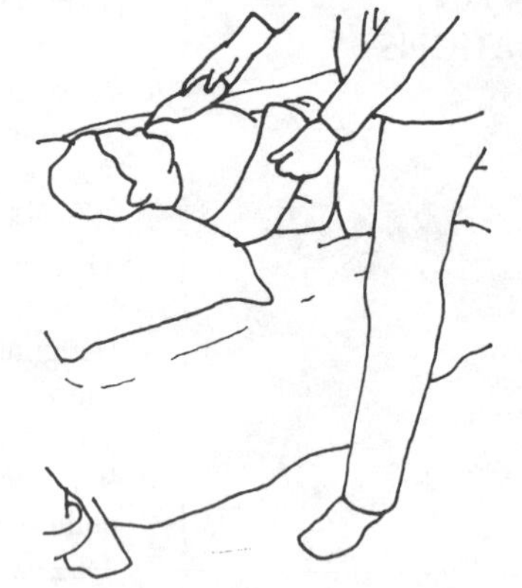
FIG 15.28a

DANGERS & PRECAUTIONS

- Do not use this manoeuvre if the person resists forward movement.
- Assessment should always consider avoidance of this manoeuvre – using profiling bed systems/pillow lifters/profiling trolleys/profiling examination couches will eliminate the need for this manual manoeuvre, therefore, this manual approach should be considered as a short term intervention.
- **Where the person has poor head**

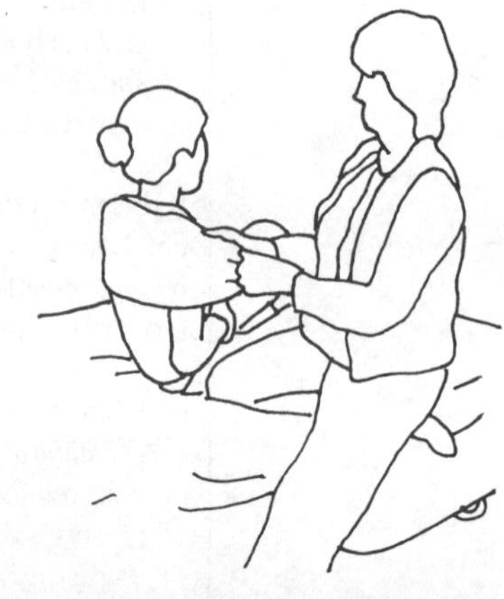
FIG 15.28b

control a profiling system should be considered a priority – this method should only be used as an immediate temporary intervention and great care must be taken not to pull the head forward during the assisted sit (an additional handler may be required to support the head while the other handlers achieve the sit). The 'sit' must be created by bringing the shoulders forward, the head is merely brought up at the same time.

- Ensure any equipment is supporting the shoulders and not pulling across at the person's neck – injury to the person could occur if equipment pulls the neck to assist the sit.
- Non designated handling aids such as bed sheets/draw sheets/towels cannot be recommended for this manoeuvre as they will not have been tested for the stresses which build up in the materials and are likely to rip with potential harmful effects on both handlers and person. As the need for this manoeuvre is a forseeable care activity the necessary equipment should be provided.
- Some manufacturers now produce linen sheets which are specifically designed and sold as 'handling sheets' which could be used. These will have a designated life span as a handling aid which will be found on the sheet and manufacturers instructions.
- If the person is taller than the handlers this can raise the effort required to complete the manoeuvre and the handler's hands will end up higher than their shoulders making support of the person difficult.
- If the person is larger than the individual handlers there will be additional effort required by the handlers. Depending on the ability of the person, generally one should consider avoiding this manoeuvre for any situation where the person's BMI is greater than either of the handler's. The less able the person, the more you need the individual handler's BMI to be greater than the persons.
- Not all handlers will have the range of movement in their knee joint and the flexibility to achieve this move comfortably – they should not attempt it, particularly if the person is on the floor.
- Take account of the SWL of the bed/trolley and also any attachments such as bed rails which may compromise the handler's posture or stability.
- Some beds can tip up when handlers kneel on them.

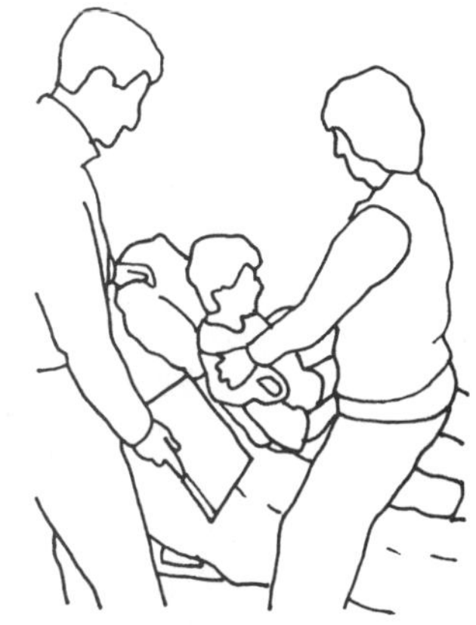

FIG 15.29a

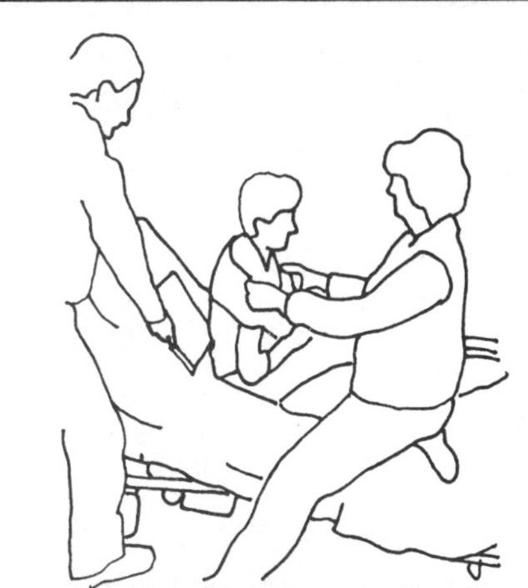

FIG 15.29b

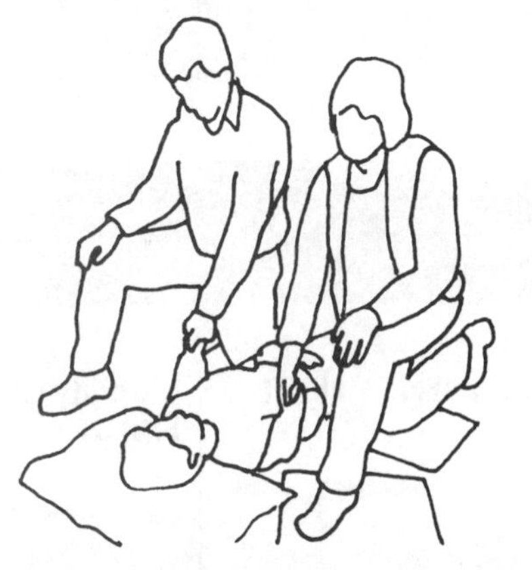

FIG 15.30a

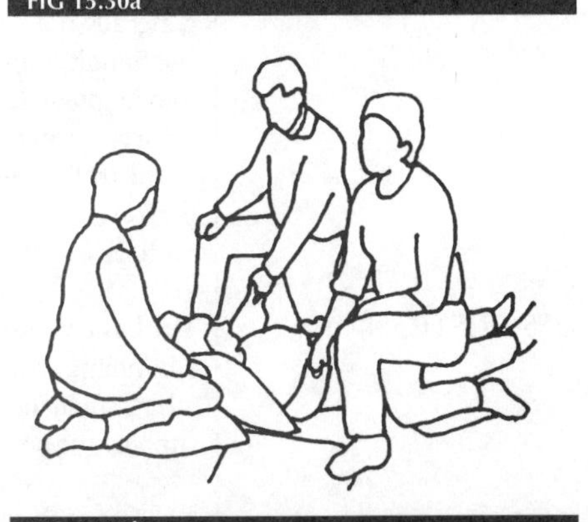

FIG 15.30b

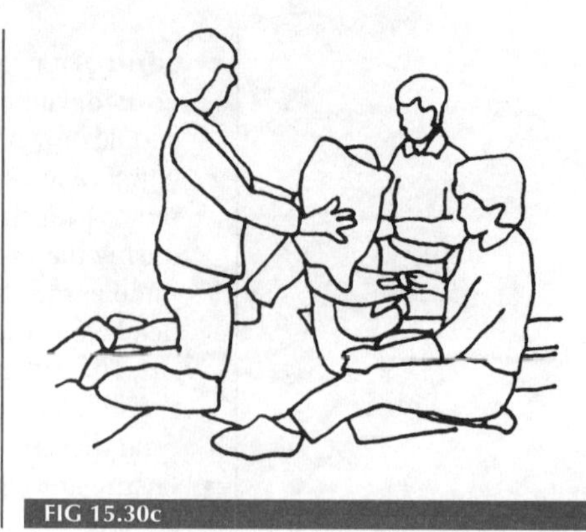
FIG 15.30c

Evidence review

Technique	REBA	Activity	Comfort	FIM	Mobility gallery	Skill level	Comment
MANUAL ASSISTED LYING TO SITTING – ONE KNEE ON THE BED							
Fig 15.24b	4	5	7	3	B	Competent	2 people may decrease the postural risk to handlers slightly
Fig 15.25b	4	5	7	3	B	Advanced beginner	
Fig 15.26b	10	8	3	3	B ,C	Proficient	Less secure hold for handler, with greater postural risk
Fig 15.27b	4	5	7	3	B	Competent	

Task Eight

Manual assisted lying to sitting –'standing weight transfer'

DEPENDENCY LEVEL

Mobility Gallery C
FIM 3

As for task seven and eight

The scapula hold to support the person is generally not suitable for this approach where the handlers are standing beside the bed. It may be possible to use where the person is on a narrow trolley, depending on the assessment of the trolley height, height and weight of the person and the arm length/reach of the handlers.

DESCRIPTION

The basic manoeuvre is described below using a handling strap – the assessment will identify which 'hold' or equipment should be used to support the person (figures 15.31a–c).

- The handlers should stand beside the

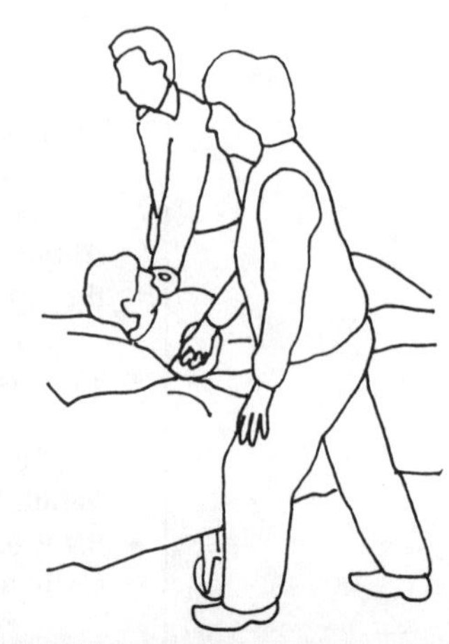
FIG 15.31a

person's hips facing the head of the bed.

- A handling strap is placed behind the person to support their trunk and shoulders.
- If the person has poor head control handling netting can be placed behind their shoulders and pillow to assist in bringing the head forward at the time of the sit – this must be done with great caution not to pull the head forward.
- The handler's feet are placed firmly on the floor, with one foot ahead of the other. Generally the outer foot is placed forward of the foot nearest the bed as this reduces the likelihood of twisting during the manoeuvre and allows for free movement of that leg if the handler needs to step back.
- Hold the handling strap close to the person's shoulders with the inside hand. Ensure the strap is taut and gives good and even support across the person's shoulders and is not pulling behind their neck.
- It is important that the bed is not raised too high prior to this manoeuvre or the 'sit' is hard to achieve since the person's shoulders will end up higher than the handlers.
- The bed/trolley height should allow the person's shoulders to end up just below the shoulders of the handlers with the person still slightly in front of the handlers at the end of the move.
- Ask the person to bring their chin towards their chest and to bend one knee if this is more comfortable.
- On the command **ready, steady, sit** the handlers transfer their body weight from their front foot to their back foot.
- Some people prefer to transfer their weight by stepping back to achieve the move – people must be given the opportunity during training to identify the movement pattern that suits their individual capability.

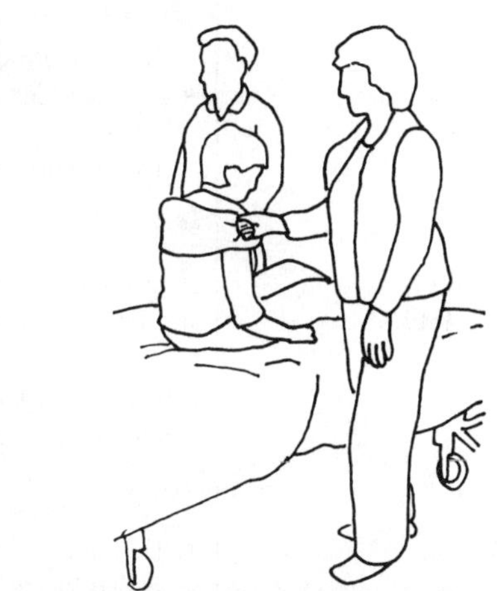

FIG 15.31b

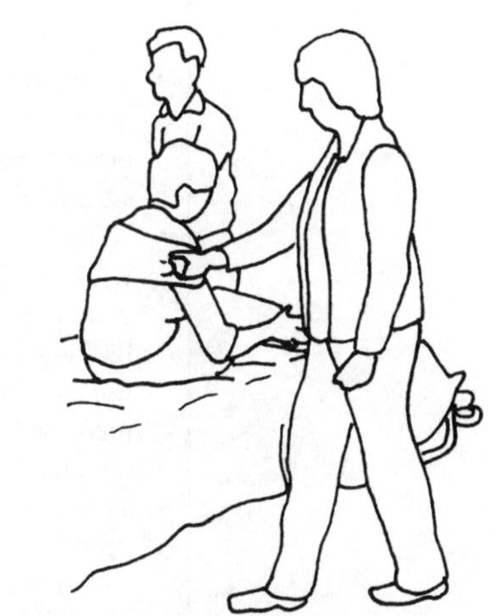

FIG 15.31c

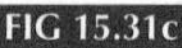

Two handlers working together need to be working in coordination with the same depth of 'travel' when they transfer their weight. This means that handlers need to be fairly well matched in height and weight or else one person 'travels' further than the other which can affect the stresses of this manoeuvre. It will affect the coordination and depth of 'travel' if one handler steps back and the other merely transfers their weight from the front to the back foot.

OPTIONS / VARIATIONS

- Designated handling netting/sheet (figures 15.32a–b).
- The handling netting is held as for task seven supporting the person's head if necessary.

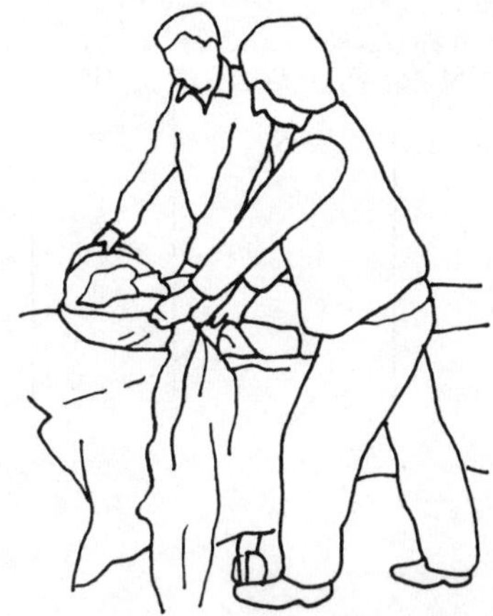

FIG 15.32a

Lying to sitting

- Single handler for child – the child needs to be positioned close to the side of the bed that the handler is standing.
- The handler takes the netting in each hand beside each of the child's shoulders – the breadth of the child's shoulders must not cause the handler to over reach.

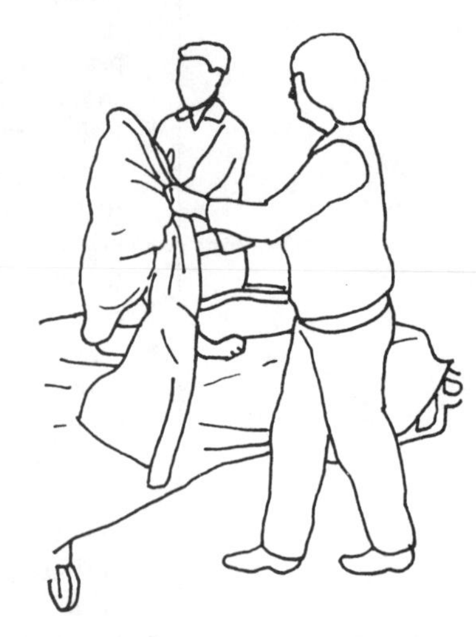

FIG 15.32b

DANGERS & PRECAUTIONS

If a person has poor head control this method should only be used as an immediate temporary intervention and they should be transferred as soon as possible to a profiling bed or provided with a pillow lifter.

- As for task seven.
- Do not use this manoeuvre if the person resists forward movement.
- The handlers are further away from the person and can give little or no support if the person leans forward at the end of the move.
- The position of the handlers can lead them to twist or over reach if they have inadequate equipment or are unskilled.
- If the person is taller than the handlers this can raise the effort required to complete the manoeuvre and the handlers hands will end up higher than their shoulders making support of the person difficult. This can be avoided by ensuring the bed is at a height where, on sitting, the person's shoulders are slightly lower than the handler's shoulders.
- As for the 'knee on the bed option' If the person is larger than the individual handlers there will be additional effort required by the handlers. Depending on the ability of the person, generally one should consider avoiding this manoeuvre for any situation where the person's BMI is greater than either of the handler's. The less able the person the more necessity for the individual handler's BMI to be greater than the persons. The risks are additionally increased due to the handlers being further away from the person than for the 'knee on bed option'.
- This manoeuvre is very 'sensitive' to a variation in height of the two handlers as they will 'travel' different distances as they transfer their weight and therefore one handler could use more effort. It is important that the assessment takes account of the handler's individual capabilities and how this will affect the smooth achievement of the move.

Evidence review

Technique	REBA	Activity	Comfort	FIM	Mobility gallery	Skill level	Comment
MANUAL ASSISTED LYING TO SITTING – STANDING WEIGHT TRANSFER							
Fig 15.31c	5	3	8	3	C	Advanced beginner	This technique slightly increases the postural risk and decreases the activity level of the person when compared to knee on bed. However it is better for the novice. Scores are the same using strap or netting.

Task Nine

Repositioning using a hoist and sling

DEPENDENCY LEVEL

Mobility Gallery E
FIM 1

INSTRUCTION / EQUIPMENT

- Appropriate hoist – mobile, free standing/wall mounted, overhead tracking.
- Appropriate sling size and type.
- Pair of flat slide sheets to introduce the sling if necessary.

DESCRIPTION

- Overhead tracking will reduce the risks associated with manoeuvring mobile hoists under beds.
- These do not have to be built into the structure of the building as there are now many 'free-standing' and gantry systems which allow for temporary use or to allow the system to be moved as the requirement changes.
- Where mobile hoists are used the purchasing decision and assessment prior to use must ensure that it can be used safely with all other equipment such as the bed e.g. sufficient clearance under the bed, adequate space around the bed, sufficient height clearance and lifting height.
- Wall mounted hoists can eliminate risks associated with manoeuvring a hoist under a bed.
- For comfortable and safe transfers using hoists and slings it is vital that the correct size and type of sling is used for each individual person so that they have the support they require.
- Where turning a person to insert a sling on the bed is uncomfortable for the person or causes musculoskeletal strain to the handlers, flat slide sheets can be used eliminating the need for the person to be turned.

Inserting a sling in bed with flat slide sheets

- The slide sheets are generally inserted as a pair, however, one can be inserted using the described method and the second sheet introduced afterwards by sliding it in under the first sheet.
- The two sheets can be rolled together or turned as a panel of approximately a hand width (figures 15.35a–c).
- The sheets can be introduced from the person's feet or head end – for inserting a sling it is more appropriate to start at the head as there is no need for the sheets to be under the feet.
- It is generally more comfortable, and

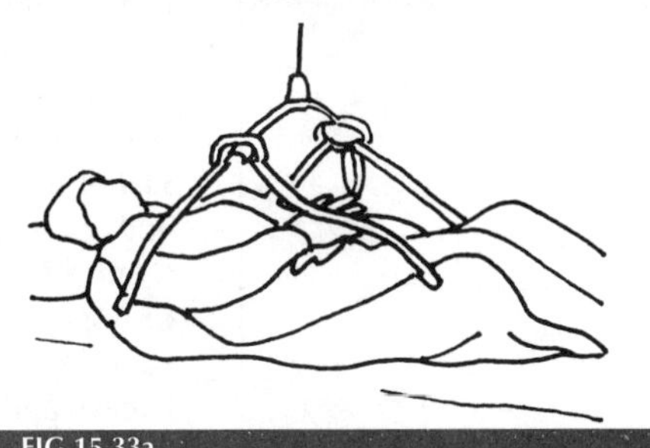

FIG 15.33a

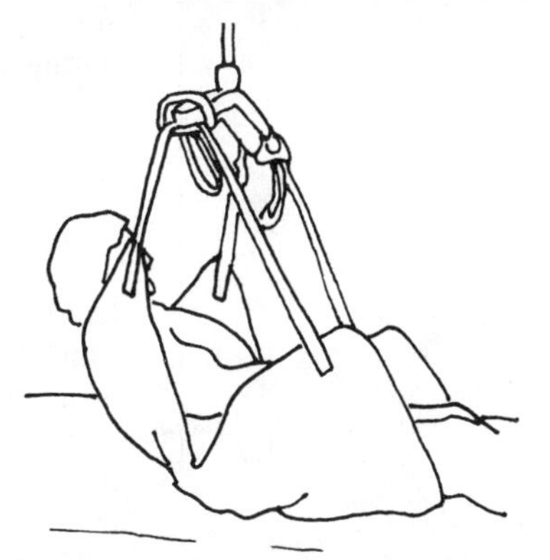

FIG 15.33b

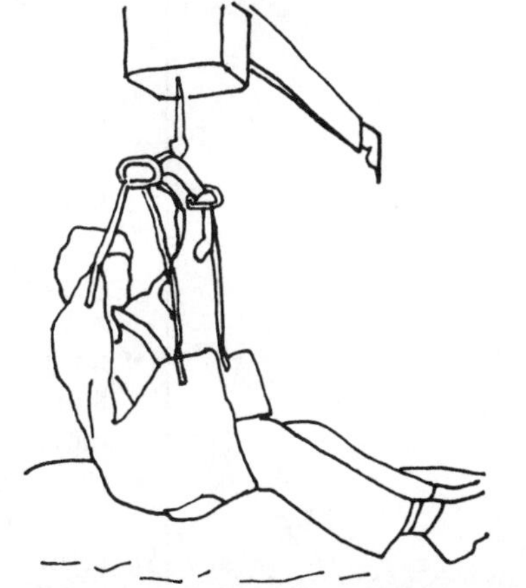

FIG 15.33c

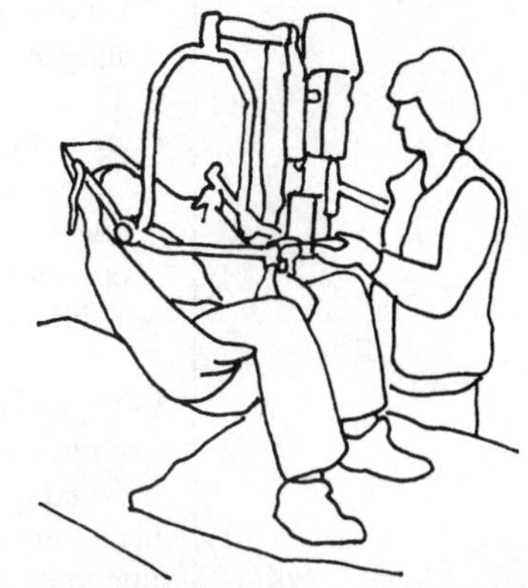

FIG 15.34a

reduces the effect of noise from the sheets as they are inserted, if the sheets are introduced with the pillow between the slide sheets and the person's head – the roll or panel next to the bottom sheet.

- The slide sheets are introduced by 'turning' them down towards the foot of the bed (see also chapter 16).
  Either by grasping the corner of the panel and bringing it down and back (figures 15.36a–b)
  or by grasping the whole top edge of the panel/roll with the palm up and bringing it down and back (figures 15.37a–b). The choice depends on the comfort and strength of the handler's wrist and grip during the manoeuvre.
- It is important that the handlers work together keeping the slide sheets taut, flat to the bed and turned in unison as they are inserted down the persons back.
- The handlers should be positioned comfortably either with one knee on the bed or standing beside the bed with the bed height adjusted appropriately. The handler should be in a 'tug of war'(see figures 15.38a–c) position thus drawing the sheets towards themselves, not positioned sideways which will necessitate wrist rotation and pulling from the shoulder. As with all slide sheet manoeuvres the handler must use transfer of body weight to achieve the task, not just pull with their arm as this could cause musculoskeletal stress to the shoulder and or cervical spine. If there is a resistance from the slide sheets and the handler feels they have to 'pull' significantly an alternative approach e.g. rolling the person should be considered.
- It will help, particularly at the person's hips, if the mattress is pushed down slightly as the panel is turned back (figure 15.37b).
- Once the slide sheets are in situ the sling can then be introduced by sliding it between the two slide sheets until it is in position (figures 15.39a–b). Again, the handlers must work with the sling taut, flat to the bed and in unison pulling the sling towards themselves (figures 15.40a–e).
- Once the sling is in position the slide sheet closest to the person is removed by turning one bottom corner under itself to the opposite side of the bed and gradually sliding it on itself up and out.

A sling specifically designed to assist the turning of a person in bed is now available. Insertion does not require the person to be turned and this can then be used to turn and support them while their lifting sling is put in position (see task two, chapter 16).

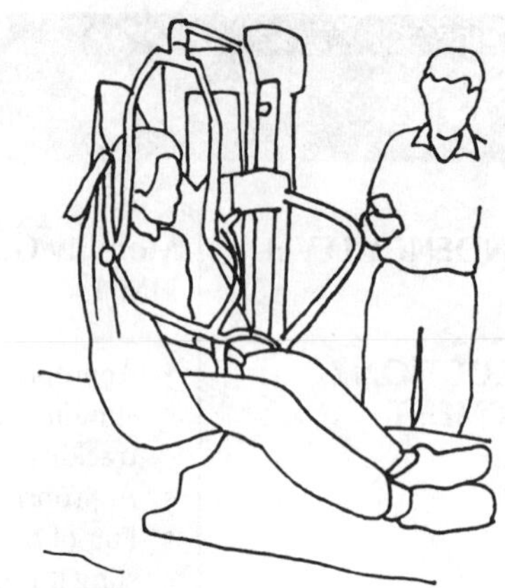

FIG 15.34b

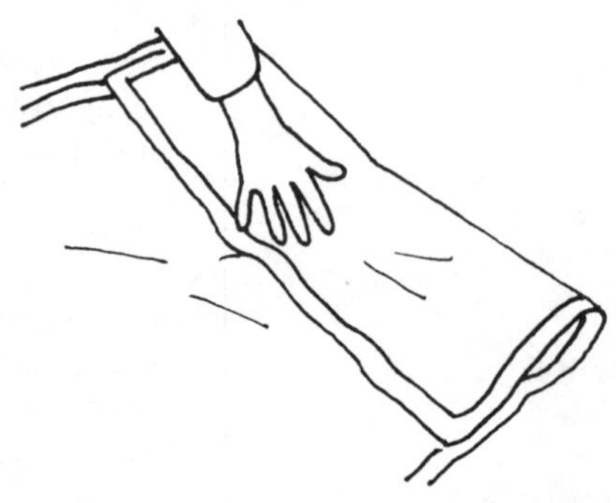

FIG 15.35a

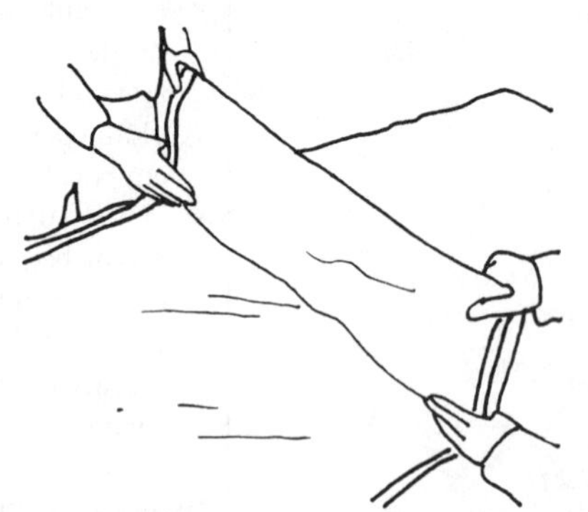

FIG 15.35b

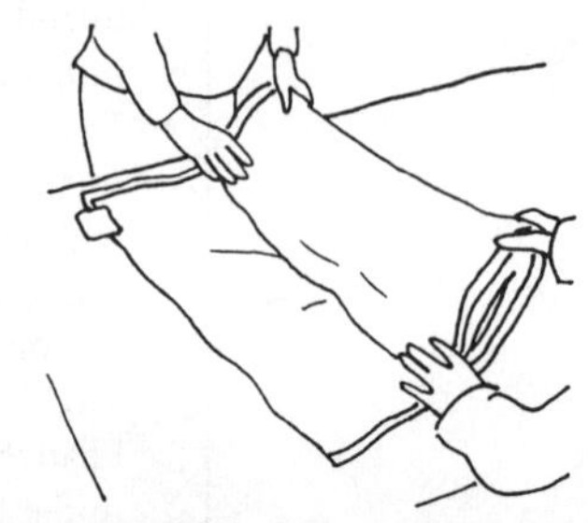

FIG 15.35c

EVIDENCE AVAILABLE

1 Staff attitudes may be the reason for not using hoists *(McGuire et al 1996a)*.
2 Training that uses a problem solving approach and is equipment specific would increase usage *(Moody et al 1996)*.
3 Overhead lifters can reduce the biomechanical loads to a handlers back *(Zhuang et al 1999)*.

DANGERS & PRECAUTIONS

- Musculoskeletal strain from manoeuvring a mobile hoist.
- Stresses/discomfort to the person and/or handler from inserting a sling, particularly by rolling the person.
- Caution must always be used to ensure the person's safety whilst they are on the slide sheet.
- The method of inserting a sling and the size and style of the sling must take account of all the person's needs including support, head support, tissue viability, cross infection etc.
- The manufacturer's instructions of use must be adhered to and agreement made by the relevant manufacturers over compatibility of slings and hoists.

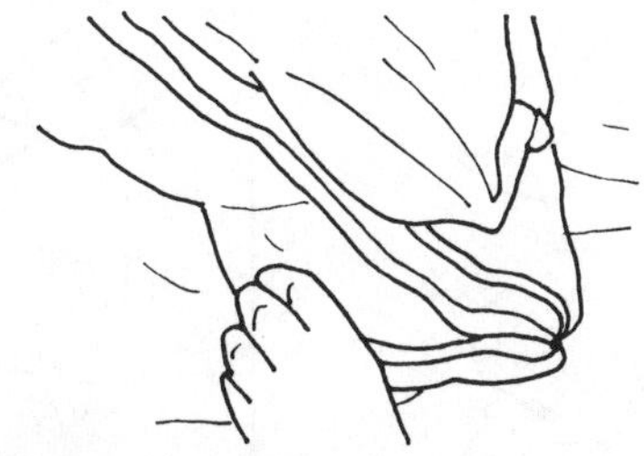
FIG 15.36a

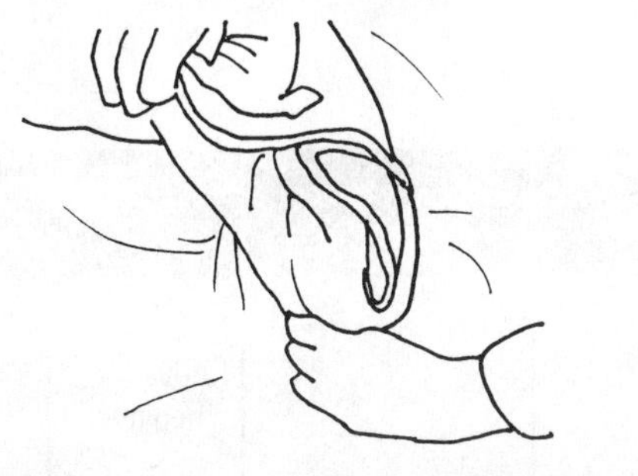
FIG 15.36b

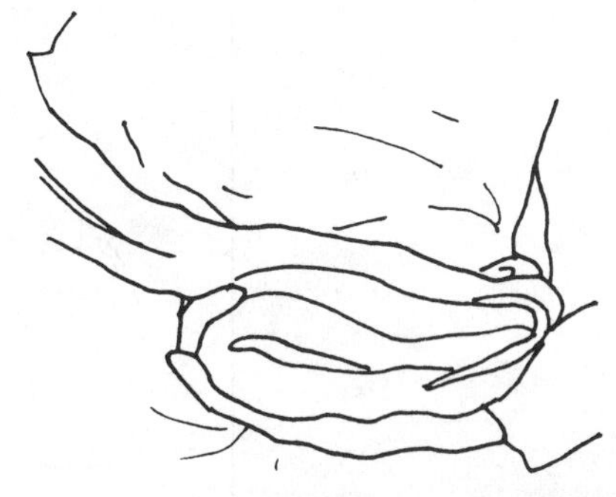
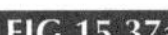
FIG 15.37a

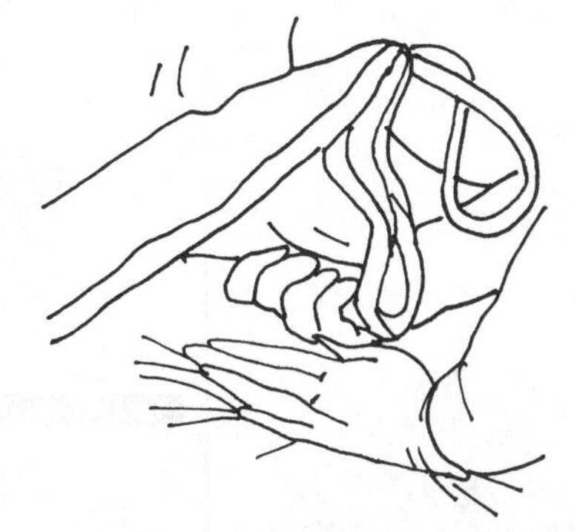
FIG 15.37b

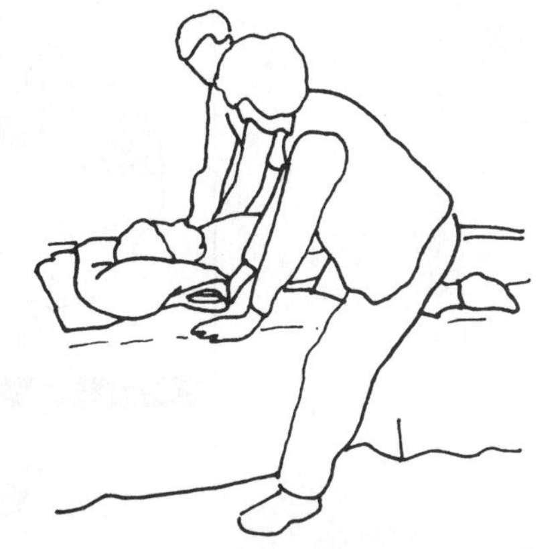
FIG 15.38a

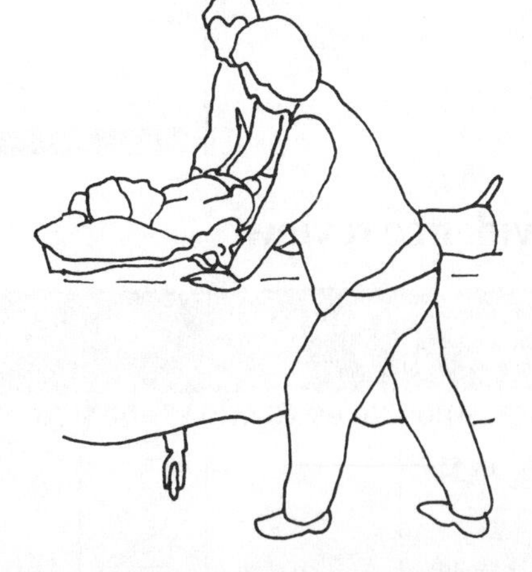
FIG 15.38b

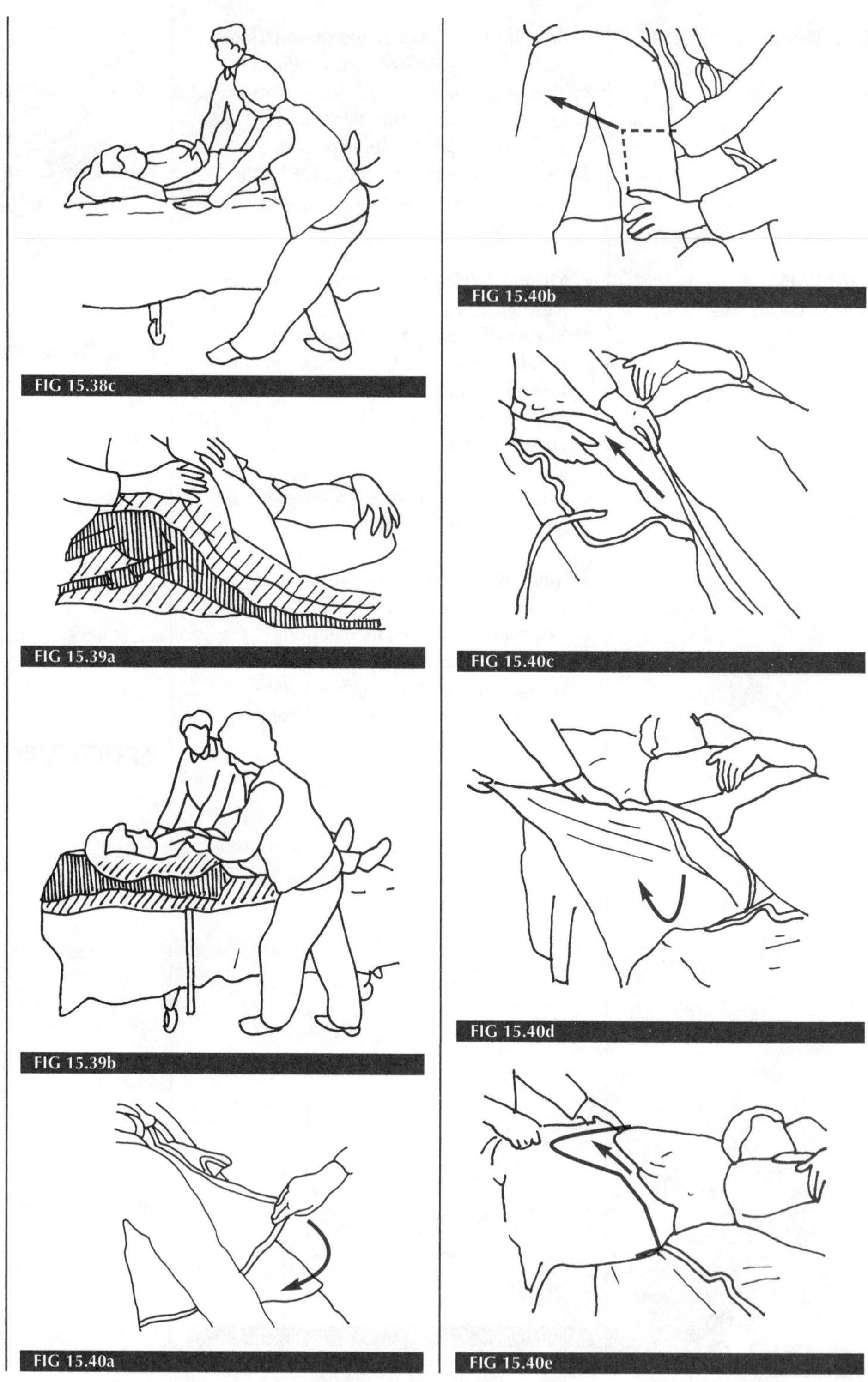

FIG 15.38c

FIG 15.39a

FIG 15.39b

FIG 15.40a

FIG 15.40b

FIG 15.40c

FIG 15.40d

FIG 15.40e

Evidence review

Technique	REBA	Activity	Comfort	FIM	Mobility gallery	Skill level	Comment
REPOSITIONING USING A HOIST AND SLING							
Fig 15.34a	2	1	9	1	E	Advanced beginner	Tipping hoist
Fig 15.39a	5	1	9	1	E	Competent	Inserting sling

References

Bertolazzi M, and Saia B (1999). 'Risk during manual movement of loads', Giornale Italiano do Medicina del Lavoro 21 (2): 130–3

Bewick N, and Gardner D (2000). 'Manual handling injuries in health care workers', International Journal of occupational Safety and Ergonomics 6 (2): 209–21

Birtles M, and Williams S (2004). 'An ergonomics evaluation of hospital bed backrests', The Column vol 16.2 18–20

Brulin C, Winkvist A, and Langendoen S (2000). 'Stress from working conditions among home care personnel with musculoskeletal symptoms', Journal of Advanced Nursing 31 (1): 181–9

Collins M (1990). 'A comprehensive approach to preventing occupational back pain among nurses', Journal of Occupational Health & Safety – Australia & New Zealand 6 (5): 361–8

Conneeley AL (1992). 'The impact or the manual handling operations regulations on the use of hoists in the home: the patient's perspective', British Journal of Occupational Therapy 61 (1): 17–21

Dhoot R, and Georgieva C (1996). 'The evolution bed in the NHS hospital environment', unpublished report, Lancaster University: The Management School

Dolan P, Standell CJ, Adams GG, Mannion AF and Adams MA (1998). 'Spinal loading during manual handling procedures in nursing', Proceedings of the International Society for the Study of the Lumbar Spine, Belgium: Brussels, 80

Engkvis I-L, Kjellberg A, Wigaeus HE, Hagberg M, Menckel E, and Ekenvall L (2001). 'Back Injuries among nursing personnel – identification of work conditions with cluster analysis', Safety Science 37: 1–18.

Fanello S, Frampas-Chotard V, Roquelaure Y, Jousset N, Delbos V, Jarmy J and Penneau-Fontbonne, D (1999). 'Evaluation of an educational low back pain prevention program for hospital employees', Revue Du Rhumatisme (Eng. Edn) 66 (12): 711–16

Fenet A, and Kumar S (1992). 'An ergonomic survey of a hospital physical therapy department', International Journal of Industrial Ergonomics: 161–70

Garg A, and Owen B (1992). 'Reducing back stress in nursing personnel: an ergonomic intervention in a nursing home', Ergonomics 35 (11): 1353–75

Hampton S (1998). 'Can electric beds aid pressure sore prevention in hospitals?' British Journal of Nursing 7(17): 1010–17

Hignett S (1996a). 'Manual handling risks in midwifery: identification of risk factors', British Journal of Midwifery 4 (11): 590–6

Hignett S (2001a). 'Manual handling risk assessments in occupational therapy', British Journal of occupational Therapy 64 (2): 81–6

Khalil TM, Asfour SS, Marchette B, and Omachonu V (1987). 'Lower back injuries in nursing: a biomechanical analysis and intervention strategy' in Asfour SS (ed). Trends in Ergonomics/Human Factors IV, Holland: Elsevier Science Publishers BV, 811–21

Kitson J (2000). 'Mind your back: variable height cots', Paediatric Nursing 12 (4): 26–7

Knibbe JJ, and Friele RD (1999). 'The use of logs to assess exposure to manual handling of patients, illustrated in and intervention study in home care nursing', International Journal of Industrial Ergonomics 24: 445–54

Knibbe N, and Knibbe JJ (1995). 'Postural load of nurses during bathing and showering of patients', Internal Report, Locomotion Health Consultancy, The Netherlands.

Lusted MJ, Carrasco CL, Mandryk JA, and Healey S (1996). 'Self reported symptoms in the neck and upper limbs in nurses', Applied Ergonomics 27 (6): 381–7

Lynch RM, and Freund A (2000). 'Short-term efficacy of back injury intervention project for patient care providers at one hospital', AIHAJ : Journal for the Science of Occupational & Environmental Health & Safety 61: 290–4

McGuire T, Moody J, Hanson M, and Tigar F (1996). 'A study into clients; attitudes towards mechanical aids', Nursing Standard 11 (5): 35–8

Mitchell J, Jones J, McNair B, and McClenahan JW (1998). Better Beds for Health Care: Report of the King's Fund Centenary Bed Project, London: King's Fund

Moody J, Mcguire T, Hanson M, and Tigar F (1996). 'A study of nurses' attitudes towards mechanical aids', Nursing Standard 11 (4): 37–42

Owen BD (1988). 'Patient handling devices: an ergonomic approach to lifting patients', in Aghazadeh F (ed). Trends in Ergonomics/Human Factors V Holland: Elsevier Science Publishers BV, 721–8

Panciera D, Menoni O, and Ricci M, (2000). 'Hoists; selection criteria and standards', Proceedings of the IEA2000/HFES 2000 Congress, The Human Factors and Ergonomics Society of California: Santa Monica, 5: 797–800

Pheasant S (1996). Bodyspace Anthropometry, Ergonomics and Design – Second Edition. Taylor and Francis, London

Pohjonen T, Punakallio A, and Louhevaara, V (1998). 'Participatory ergonomics for reducing load and strain in home care work', International Journal of Industrial Ergonomics, 21 (5): 327–41

Scott A (1995). 'Improving patient moving and handling skills', Professional Nurse 109 (11): 105–6

Skarplik C (1988). 'Patient handling in the community', Nursing 3 (30): 13–16

Tracey C (1998). 'Cashing in on the benefits offered by total bed management concept' British Journal Healthcare Management 4 (12) 598–600

Zhuang Z, Stobbe TJ, Hsiao H, Collins JW, and Hobbs GR (1999). 'Biomechanical evaluation of assistive devices for transferring residents', Applied Ergonomics 30: 285–94

16

Lying to lying transfers and associated manoeuvres

Jacqui Hall MSc (Health Ergs) MSc (Health & Social Research) Cert in Patient Handling & Moving NMA (Advanced) NEBOSH Cert RNT RGN Cert Ed NNEB
Senior Lecturer Northumbria University

1 Introduction

This chapter will describe the circumstances and environments in which lying to lying supine manoeuvres and transfers may take place and the equipment available to facilitate them. In addition, some factors that may affect the extent of the risk to the handlers involved in these transfers and associated manoeuvres will be discussed and some of the procedures described, together with their evidence base where it is available.

Historically, a lying to lying transfer was often achieved by the use of canvas and poles or manual lifts with three or more persons. These methods have long been proscribed (see chapter 18 for more detailed information on controversial techniques and hazardous postures) and over the past 25 years equipment to facilitate the sliding, lying to lying (lateral) transfer has come increasingly into use. In addition, as fabric technology has advanced, materials with lower coefficients of friction have been developed, which has seen the introduction of low friction rollers and low friction flat, padded or tubular sheets (see chapter 6 for further information on friction and its effects). However, it should not be assumed that the adoption of any sliding transfer manoeuvre in preference to a manual lift would necessarily significantly reduce any risk of musculoskeletal injury to the handlers *(Marras et al, 1999)*. Whilst compressive loading on the lumbar spine may be reduced, it is possible that shear force/strain may be increased and other soft tissues placed under stress (see section 7 of chapter 5). Anecdotally, injury to the handlers involved in lateral sliding transfers, has also been reported to include musculoskeletal damage to the upper back and neck, shoulder girdle and upper limbs, including the wrists and hands, as well as the low back.

Ideally, due to technological advances, mechanical aids should now be used to move a non weight bearing person, wherever possible. However, it is recognised that there are still some areas where this is not practicable, such as some emergency retrievals by the *Ambulance Service (Hall, 2004)*.

2 Equipment

The first consideration when embarking on lateral transfers in controlled environments is the type of equipment from which, and to which, the person is to be transferred. Depending upon the circumstances the equipment could include a bed, ambulance stretcher trolley, A&E stretcher trolley, theatre table, radiography table, examination/treatment plinth or mortuary table. More detailed information on types of beds is available in chapter 15 but, in respect of lateral transfers, it is advantageous for both transfer surfaces to be adjustable in height.

As stated above, the range of hard and soft transfer systems have increased significantly, particularly over the last decade. Hard equipment would include traditional full length but slightly flexible boards, some with handholds and some that fold. These boards have a much higher frictional coefficient than the modern fabrics used for sliding sheets and they should now be considered only as bridging devices for use in association with soft transfer devices such as single, double and/or padded slide sheets which come in various designs, lengths and widths, some with integral straps, some with detachable straps and some without straps altogether. *Garg, Owen and Beller (1991)* found that pulling the load/person, produced less strain on handler's backs, than lifting the load. Also, *Garb and Dockery (1995)*, reported that there was increased pressure on the intervertebral discs, when the handler stretched to reach over the bed (a common fault), to take hold of the canvas/bed sheet which is often used in the lateral transfer. Long handles on the slide sheets, can reduce the effort exerted when reaching for the slide sheet in order to pull the person across the bed/trolley during a lateral transfer.

Tissue viability is a necessary consideration when using these boards. Flesh can stick to hard transfer boards, causing discomfort or potential skin injury to the person being transferred. Wet sheets and canvasses can also stick, increasing the force required to transfer the person and placing stress on the fabric so that it can tear, potentially resulting in injury to the handlers or the person being transferred. More recently, inflatable and mechanised transfer devices have become available. Lateral transfers can also be achieved by using mobile or gantry hoists with stretcher attachments (see figure 16.1).

Additional care should be taken when transferring from one surface to another as the depth and type of the mattress used on the bed can make a noticeable difference. Consideration must be given to ensuring that the use of low air loss mattresses (for pressure area care) have the pressure raised prior to the transfer, to provide a firmer surface, therefore facilitating a more efficient transfer.

Up to date information and training on the range of equipment, including beds, mattresses, trolleys, hoists and sliding transfer systems, can be accessed through the *Disabled Living Foundation*, (2001) or on their web site at www.dlf.org.uk

3 Environment

Lateral transfers routinely take place in a variety of mainly hospital based settings such as hospital wards, accident and emergency departments, theatres, radiography, the mortuary etc. On occasions, lateral transfers can be made in a less controlled environment, giving rise to high risks of musculoskeletal damage and early retirement as seen in the Ambulance Services (*Lavender et al, 2000*).

Within operating theatres, *Garb and Dockery (1995)* identified several types of activities that they believed were responsible for back injuries to staff working there. One of these activities included moving patients in theatres, where the patients were rolled on their sides and rolled back onto a short roller board. One handler would reach over the stretcher to lift and pull patients from the theatre table to the stretcher trolley, and as many as three handlers would push the person being transferred from the opposite side of the theatre table. *Garb and Dockery (1995)*, suggested that the force exerted in this position varied between 375kg and 795kg, which exceeded the recommended limit as set by *Chaffin and Park (1973)* and the revised NIOSH equation by *Waters et al (1993)*. *Spencer et al (2001)* found consistently lower force measurements in relation to the use of full length slide sheets with a transfer board over the use of a canvas with a transfer board, although their research methods included a somewhat crude measuring system. *McFarlane (1998)*, also found evidence to suggest that two flat slide sheets, used in conjunction with a full length sliding board, produced a lower force measurement than a bed sheet and transfer board, or using a roller board (i.e. a full length transfer board with an integral roller sheet attached).

Ambulance crews may find themselves in a variety of less controlled situations in which two or more personnel may have to retrieve a poorly or injured person from a car or some more complex situation and then transfer using a scoop stretcher/spinal board to a stretcher trolley. *McFarlane (1998)* describes the methods used in Australia by ambulance staff and found the weights carried by staff to be in excess of the recommendations given in the revised NIOSH equation *(Waters et al, 1993)*, and the revised recommendations given by the *HSE (2004)*. Newer methods are being introduced to reduce the effort required to initiate this lift (see task 5).

Alternatively, ambulance personnel might need to retrieve a casualty from a bed in a person's bedroom or nursing/care home to a carry chair/scoop stretcher/spinal board and then onto a stretcher trolley/trolley cot *(Hall, 2004)*. Some complex retrieval methods are covered in chapter 17. After transfer to hospital the injured/poorly person will be transferred again to the A & E examination trolley, and this is the environment with which the general public would most readily associate lateral transfers.

4 Developing protocols

Within each healthcare setting lying to lying transfers are likely to take place in substantially the same way. In such situations a standard or generic protocol can be devised and implemented based on relevant local circumstances following an adequate generic manual handling risk assessment (see chapter 9). This should include equipment specification and the method to be adopted; *Marras and Davis (1998)* highlight the problems associated with lifting, with regard to one versus two hands being used. Lateral transfers between horizontal surfaces need to be initiated by two or more handlers working as a team. Team handling has also been addressed by the *HSE (2003)* with the introduction of the Manual Handling Assessment Chart *(HSE 2004)*, Any protocol should therefore include the minimum number of handlers and their relative roles and positions during the transfer.

It should also be recognised that the standard protocol may not be appropriate to every transfer, in which case consideration must be given to the potential need for alternative equipment and/or strategies *(DIAG, 2003)*. For instance, if the person to be transferred is very heavy, which is entirely foreseeable, it will be necessary to have a system for accessing heavy duty beds, trolleys and possibly mechanised lateral transfer systems. This would include heavy duty hoists with stretcher attachments as shown in figure 16.1 *(DLF 2001)*.

Alternatively, if the transfer were for a child to be moved, consideration of the child's disability, unpredictability, and general diagnosis, as well as the weight and mass of the child, would need to be assessed. In all cases an individual assessment is required to ensure that a safe system of practice is in place, which is designed to protect the handlers as well as the person to be transferred.

The protocol may reflect the generic protocol within the context of moving the person, but could be adapted to the person's-specific/individualised needs/requirements.

Figure 16.1a

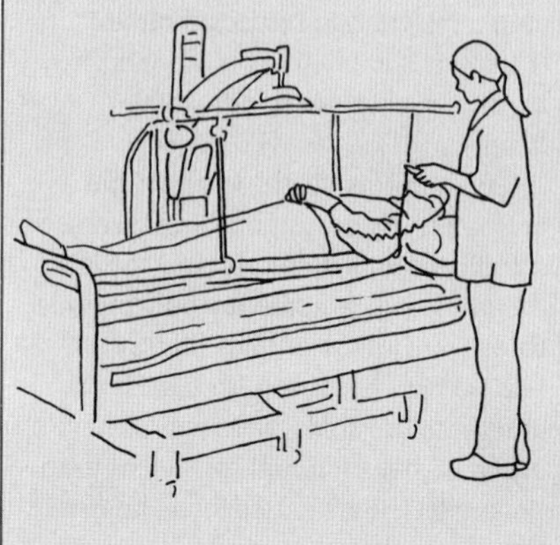

5 Person being transferred

It is assumed throughout this chapter that the person being transferred is entirely passive during the transfer procedure, usually because they are injured, very poorly, and unconscious or under anaesthetic. However, handlers must recognise the full potential of what the person can do for themselves in the particular circumstances. Where a person is able to transfer independently they should be asked to do so, possibly by undertaking a weight bearing transfer through standing, or a long sitting transfer with the assistance of hand blocks or a seated or supine transfer with a sliding/transfer aid to facilitate the process.

A simple request to ask the person to turn their head in the direction of movement, prior to rolling onto their side, can make a significant difference to the efficiency of the procedure, *(Aitchison, 1999)*. Alternatively, first moving the person's head in the direction of movement (for the passive person), will give the same promotional effect, prior to rolling. This then aids the positioning/placing of the sliding aids after the person is rolled onto their side, prior to the transfer (see task one).

6 Methods of transferring from lying to lying

Wherever possible, the person being moved will be encouraged to assist in the procedure. However, within the nature of a lateral transfer of lying to lying, it is expected, as previously stated, that the person being transferred is entirely passive throughout the transfer procedure. The handlers will be expected to be involved in an element of pushing and pulling during the transfer procedures *(NBE, 2003)*. Care must be taken regarding the weight/load involved in the transfer. Ideally, mechanical aids should be used to move a non weight bearing person, where this is practicable.

Within the limits of the equipment available to transfer a person using low friction rollers and sliding boards, the stance and movements adopted by the handlers will be described in the following methods. These tasks form the basis of the generic protocol, which is involved in lateral transfers.

The following tasks are described and discussed to aid in the procedure of the lateral transfer:

Task 1

Inserting a slide sheet

(see also chapter 15)

- Inserting a slide sheet by rolling the person from side to side.
- Inserting 2 large slide sheets (or a tubular slide sheet), under the person by placing them under the head or waist and unravelling the sheets to the person's feet or head and feet.
- Inserting 2 large slide sheets under the person by placing them under the head and unravelling the sheets to the person's feet.
- Supine slide up the bed.

Task 2

Turning and supporting using overhead tracking, a turning sling and hoist prior to the lateral transfer

- Inserting the turning sling (see also the procedure for inserting a slide sheet, task one).
- Turning a person with the use of overhead tracking, a turning sling and a hoist.

Task 3

Use of a lateral transfer using an inflatable transfer mattress between bed and stretcher trolley

- Insertion of an inflatable transfer mattress (see also the procedure for inserting a slide sheet, task one).
- Lateral transfer using an inflatable transfer mattress to move a person from bed to trolley.

Task 4

Lateral transfers between bed and stretcher trolley

- Lateral transfers using a hard transfer board and 2 slide sheets
- Lateral transfer using a hard transfer board and slide sheet with handles
- Lateral transfer using a hard transfer board and padded fabric slide
- Lateral transfers using a transfer roller board and a intergral slide sheet.

Task 5

Scoop stretcher to stretcher trolley transfer

- Transfer to an ambulance stretcher trolley using a scoop stretcher or spinal board.

Practical techniques

Task One

Inserting a slide sheet by rolling the person from side to side

DEPENDENCY LEVEL

Mobility Gallery E
FIM 1

Totally dependent. Assuming the person to be transferred is passive.

DESCRIPTION

- Handler 1 prepares the sliding sheet(s) by rolling it until it is half its width.
- With the person lying supine (flat and face up), their head is positioned facing in the direction of movement.
- Depending on the size and medical condition of the person, this task would require a minimum of two handlers.
- The handlers need to be on either side of the bed for the person to be rolled, with the bed/trolley etc adjusted to a median height in respect of the handler's waist/pelvic crest height.
- To roll the person to the left, the person's left arm should be placed with palm uppermost resting on the bed and elbow bent upwards in a natural position.

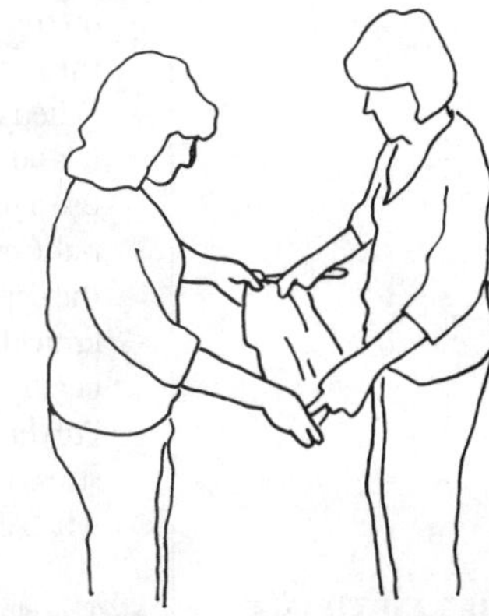

FIG 16.2a

- The right arm is positioned across their chest (see figure 16.2b).
- The person's right knee is raised with the foot flat to the bed, allowing handler 2 on the receiving side of the bed, to use the shoulder and knee as levers to roll/turn the person onto their side towards this handler.
- With the command **ready, steady, turn**, Handler 2 gently turns the person towards them, warning others of the intended manoeuvre.
- While the person is on their side Handler 1 inserts the slide sheet by ensuring that the rolled up part of the slide sheet is placed down the length of the person.
- The person is then allowed to return gently onto their back.
- Handler 2 now unravels the rolled up part of the slide sheet by gently easing it out to lie flat under the person.
- If this is not possible, the person may be rolled onto their other side, using the same method described above, to unravel the slide sheet.
- The person is now ready to be moved.

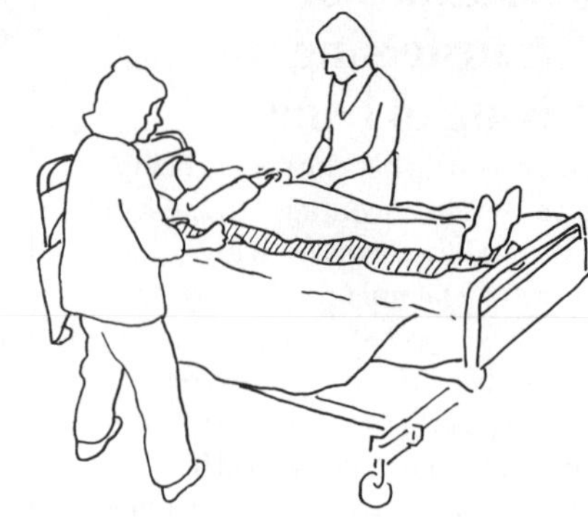
FIG 16.2b

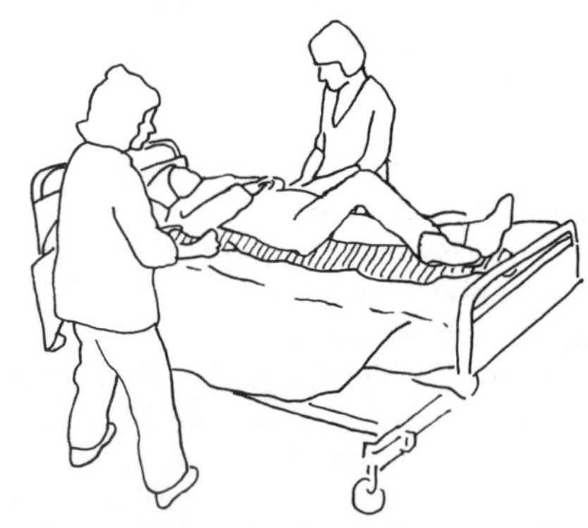
FIG 16.2c

COMFORT FOR PERSON

- Care must be taken, as the unconscious person will have no protective reflexes.
- Also, the less the person is rolled from side to side, the less risk of pain or discomfort will be endured.
- Reduction in rolling from side to side of a person returning from surgery after an anaesthetic will reduce the possibility of vomiting.

SKILL LEVEL OF STAFF

This method is easily learned.

EVIDENCE AVAILABLE

Lloyd et al (1997/8), Guide to the Handling of Patients 4th edition.

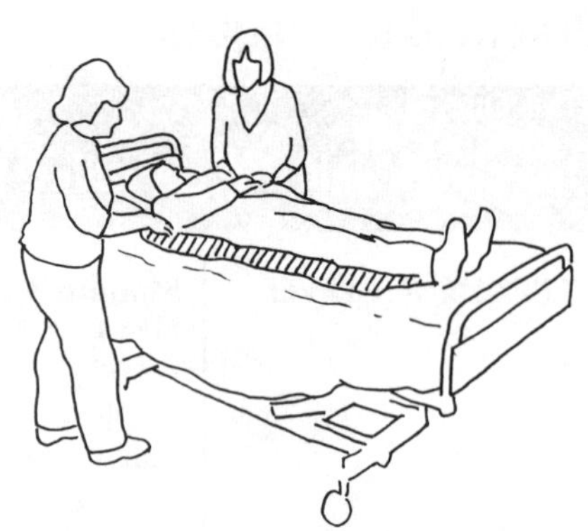
FIG 16.2d

DANGERS/ PRECAUTIONS

- Consideration must be given to whether the generic system is appropriate in each circumstance. If not then an alternative system must be devised and appropriate equipment used.
- More handlers will be needed depending on the medical condition and disability of the person e.g. Multiple fractures etc.
- When unravelling/unrolling the slide sheet, it is advisable to ensure that the handlers use a palm uppermost approach, which reduces the risk of injury or discomfort to the person. This prevents the handler's knuckles from being in contact with the person being moved.
- Further dangers include the risk of postural stress due to lateral flexion and/or rotation when carrying out these manoeuvres.

FURTHER OPTIONS

- The slide sheets can be rolled using a concertina effect, length ways and inserted

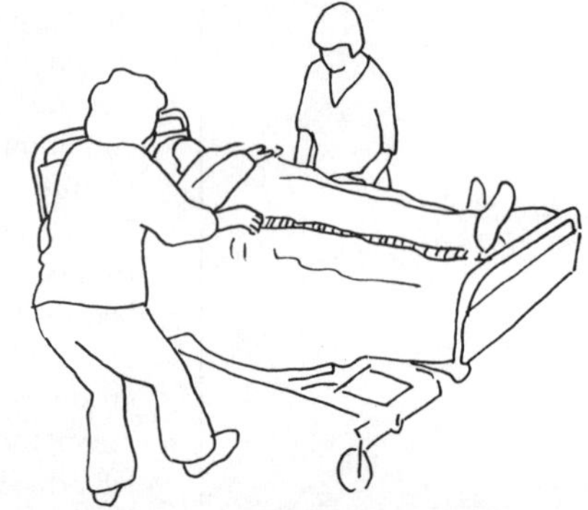
FIG 16.2e

under the cervical spine or the waist. Then one end is gently pulled upwards (using a see-saw action) from the waist towards the head and the other end downwards from the waist towards the feet.

- Alternatively the slide sheets are folded/rolled lengthways from top to bottom and are inserted under the head. The slide sheets can be placed under the person's pillow, if they have one, to prevent catching their hair (see figures 16.3a-c). The sheets are then gently unravelled (using a see-saw action) from head to toe rather than from side to side.
- Using two flat slide sheets in this manner, aids the insertion of a sling, which can be slid between the slide sheets like a sandwich and eased under the person. Once the sling is in the appropriate position for attachment, the top slide sheet is then removed allowing the sling to be attached to the hoist (see task nine, chapter 15).
- Moving a person who is supine, up the bed can be performed by using the above procedures to insert two sliding sheets or a long/full length low friction roller. With the slide sheet(s) in place and ensuring that the open ends of the slide sheet are in the direction of movement (if using a tubular sheet), the move up the bed can take place. Two handlers move to the top of the bed behind the pillows. They both stand forward on one leg ready to transfer their weight to the other leg backwards. Alternatively, they can stand balanced on both legs with knees relaxed and be ready to take a step backwards. Using a slide sheet with integral handles, they each take a hold of two handles, (one handler on one side of the person's head and the other handler on the other side. Using the commands **'ready, steady, slide'**, the handlers pull in unison, while transferring their weight backwards or taking a step back. If necessary, the handlers can pull by standing either side of the bed e.g. if there are space constraints (figure 16.2e), but they must face the bottom of the bed as they pull back, to reduce the strain of lateral flexion or rotation, which could result in spinal injury.

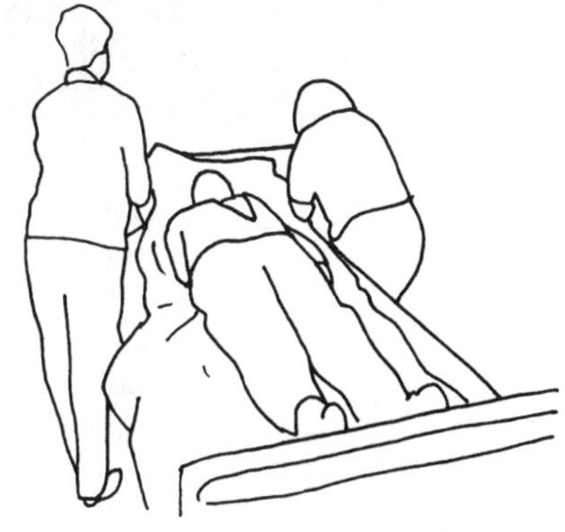

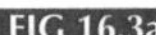

FIG 16.3a

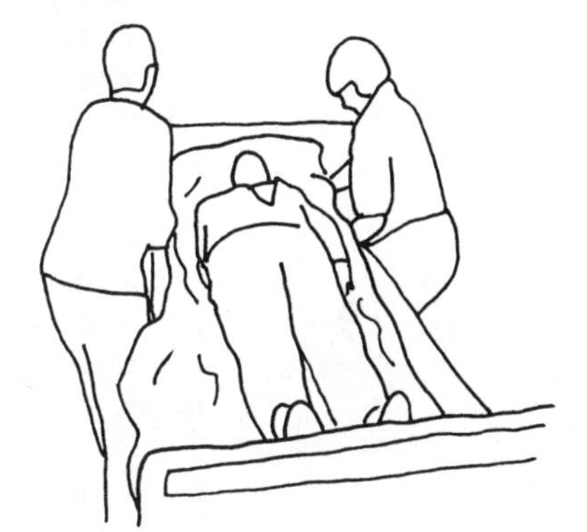

FIG 16.3b

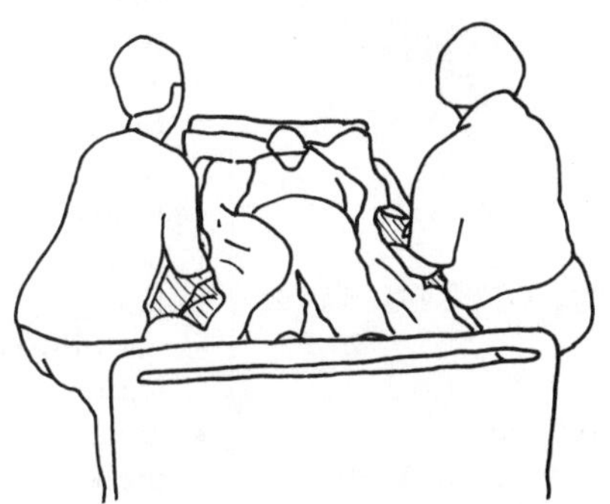

FIG 16.3c

NB On no account should the handlers on each side of the bed face each other during a supine slide up the bed. This will lead to rotation of the spine and possibly lateral flexion while pulling a load.

Evidence review

Technique	REBA	Activity	Comfort	FIM	Mobility gallery	Skill level	Comment
INSERTING A SLIDE SHEET							
Fig 16.1	6	1	10	1	E	Competent	

Task Two

Turning and supporting using overhead tracking, a turning sling and hoist, prior to a lateral transfer

DEPENDENCY LEVEL

Mobility Gallery E
FIM 1

Totally dependent. Assuming the person to be transferred is passive

DESCRIPTION

- This task requires the handler to prepare the person by explaining what they will be doing.
- A sling and hoist is used to turn this person onto their side.
- This is a specifically designed Turning sling.
- Overhead tracking hoist, or sling and manufacturer's own mobile hoist.
- This type of sling is very new to the market-place in the UK and it would be essential to carefully assess a person, prior to its use and to evaluate the assessment continuously to ensure its use remains beneficial and appropriate.
- Ideally, the sling could be positioned under the person using slide sheets (see task 1 above and chapter 15) to insert it or by using an air loss inflatable mattress (a pressure relief mattress) to press down on, when inserting the sling under the lumbar region of the person.
- Position the person in the bed so that when they turn they will not be too close to the side of the bed and bed rails.
- If necessary place a pillow between the person and the bed rail, away from their face.
- Ensure the two velcro surfaces are stuck together.
- The strap can then be passed underneath the person's back at the lumbar region.
- The strap is then gently pulled through and attached to the bed frame.
- The sling loops are attached to the spreader bar and the hoist raised slowly. This gently turns the person towards the bed rail.
- The person can then be supported at a 30 degree angle or more, with support from pillows, or fully onto their side, depending on the activity to be achieved and their comfort.
- If the person needs to be turned in the opposite direction at a later stage, the hoist is lowered, sling removed and replaced as before on the opposite side of the bed.

PERCEIVED EXERTION FOR HANDLER

There should be little or no effort required for this task.

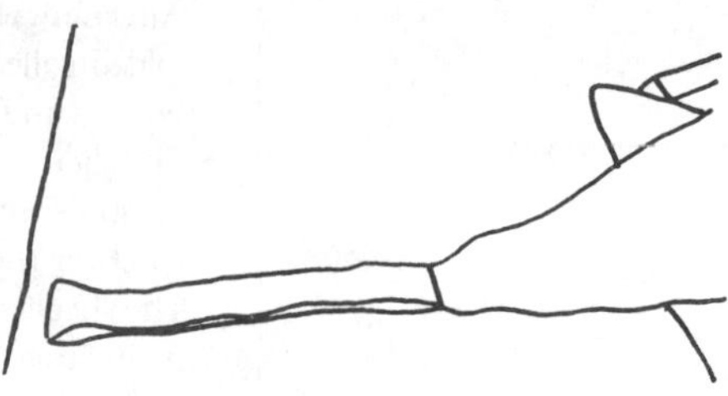

FIG 16.4a

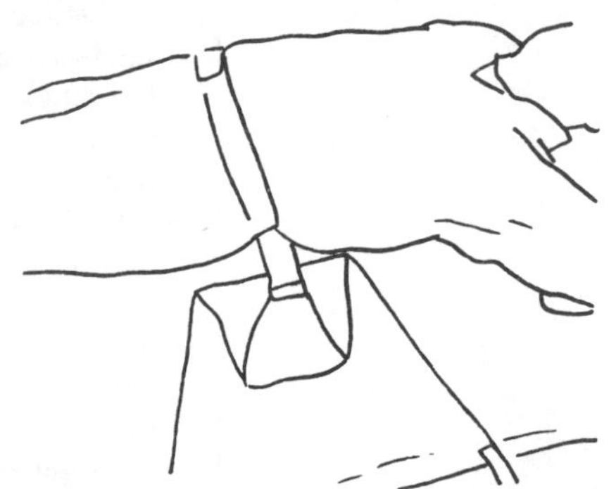

FIG 16.4b

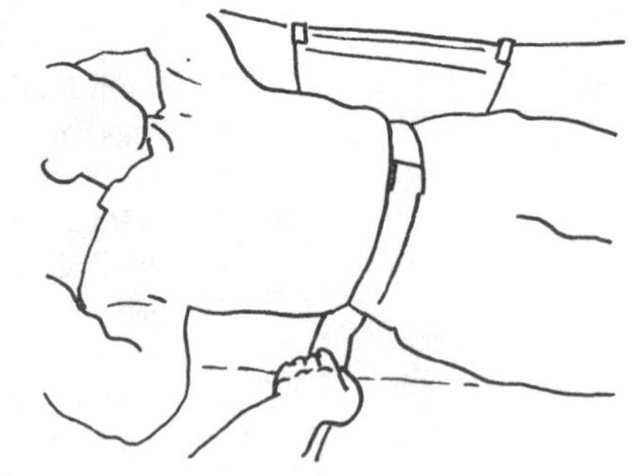

FIG 16.4c

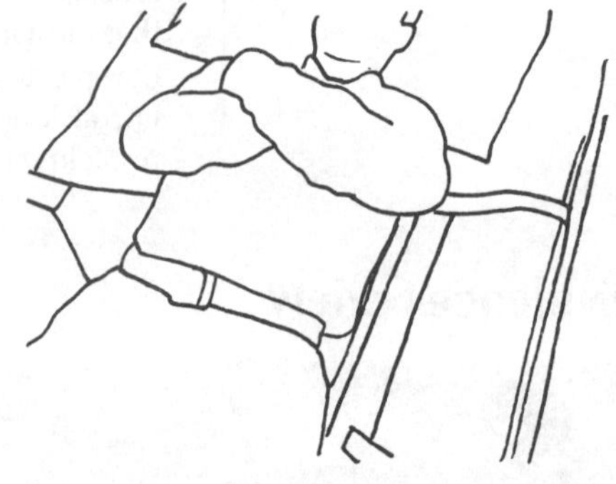

FIG 16.4d

COMFORT FOR PERSON

- Comfort and tissue viability for the person, should be monitored closely. However, there should be little discomfort for the person being turned.
- Comfort will be entirely person specific and, therefore, will require continuous assessment.
- For comfort and security two handlers may be required for this activity.

SKILL LEVEL OF STAFF

Some prior knowledge and specific training will be required to carry out the task safely but it is uncomplicated.

EVIDENCE AVAILABLE

New equipment. However, feedback from users suggests that it assists in the reduction of static loading and overreaching for care activities, such as supporting a person to turn over whilst hygiene needs are met or wound dressings changed. Therefore, it does meet with the needs to reduce the risks of manually handling a load, *(HSE, 2004)*.

DANGERS/ PRECAUTIONS

- Ongoing assessment of the person will identify whether the continued use is appropriate.
- There may be some people with particular chest, spinal or abdominal conditions that would preclude the use of this sling for medical reasons.
- It may be more appropriate to use the sling for short periods only in order to relieve Handler's static loading and extended reach, rather than for it to be used as the sole means of turning and support throughout a care activity.
- The manufacturers instructions of use should be followed.They recommend that the person be always turned towards a bed rail for safety.
- The recommendation not to use one manufacturers sling on another manufacturers hoist without prior knowledge and consent of both companies is of particular importance with this sling.
- When a mobile hoist is used, the direction of 'lift' on the joint between spreader bar and hoist boom is not the same as with a standard sling. This could adversely affect the integrity of this joint and the manufacturers advice must be sought.This may also be true for some overhead tracking systems.

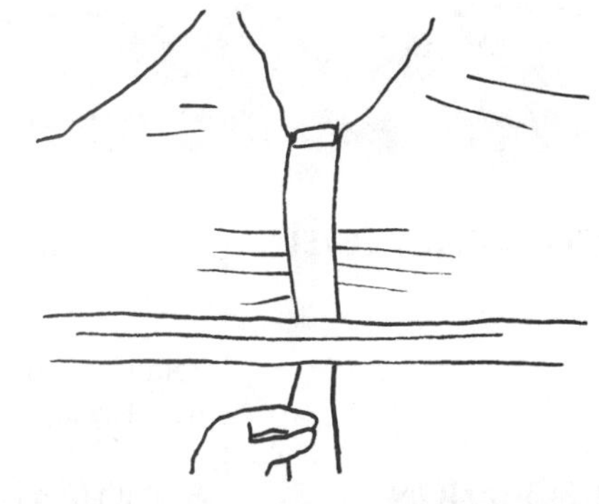

FIG 16.4e

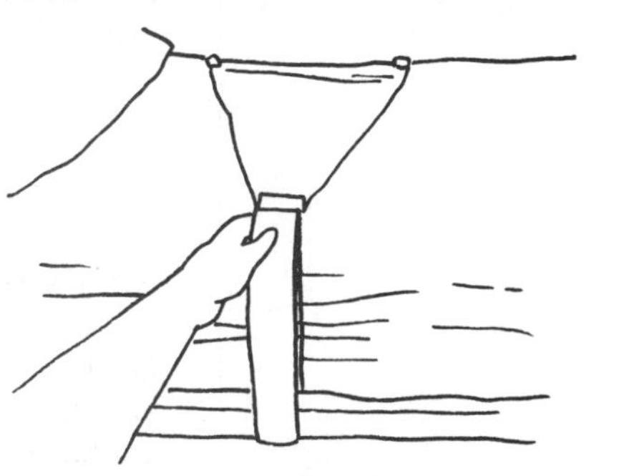

FIG 16.4f

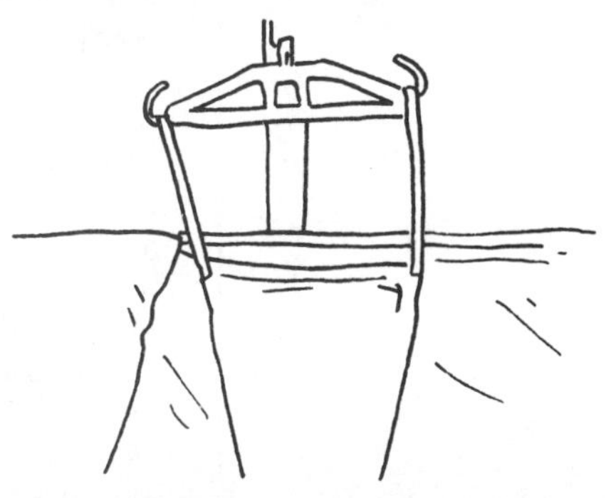

FIG 16.4g

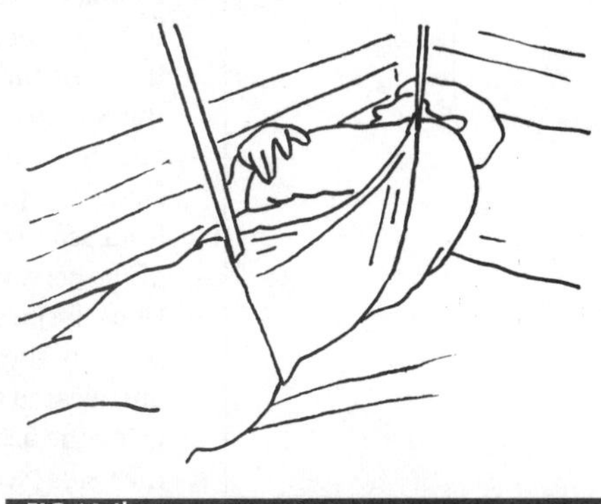

FIG 16.4h

FURTHER OPTIONS

The person can also be rolled onto their side by the help of a bed sheet, which should be positioned under the person. Lying with their head turned in the direction they are moving, the arm and leg closest to the handler is allowed to lie flat while the other leg has the knee flexed up. If possible the arm is gently placed over the person's body. The person should then be in a position to roll gently in the direction of movement assisted by the bed sheet and handler (see task one, figure 16.5a).

Task Three

Use of a lateral transfer using an inflatable transfer mattress between bed and stretcher trolley

DEPENDENCY LEVEL

Mobility Gallery E
FIM 1

Totally dependent. Assuming the person to be transferred is passive/unconscious.

DESCRIPTION

- With the person positioned lying supine (flat and face up), on a bed, preferably a profiling bed with variable height adjustment.
- An inflatable Mattress is positioned under the person prior to its inflation, (see insertion of slide sheet for method or chapter 15).
- A Trolley with adjustable height facility is positioned close to the bed.
- This task requires a minimum of two handlers, depending on the person's size and medical condition.
- The handlers need to be on either side of the bed for the person to be moved.
- The inflatable transfer sheet at this stage is in a deflated state. Once the mattress has been placed under the person to be moved, the mattress is secured to the person by straps held together by Velcro fasteners. The mattress is inflated using an electrical appliance, which inflates the mattress with air. Once filled, the mattress is ready to be used to transfer the person across the bed to the trolley.
- The bed and trolley are adjusted to a median height in respect of the handler's waist/pelvic crest height.
- The trolley and bed are positioned alongside each other.
- Handler 1 **pushes** the mattress across the bed starting at the foot end, then moving to the head end and ending at the middle of the person being moved, to ensure a safe and satisfactory position onto the trolley. Handler 2 **pulls** the mattress gently across from bed to trolley ensuring a safe delivery of the person onto the trolley.
- Once the person is in a satisfactory position, the mattress is deflated, the straps are released and the mattress is removed using the bed sheet to roll the person onto their side (see task 1 and chapter 15).

PERCEIVED EXERTION FOR HANDLER

The use of an inflatable mattress makes the transfer of a person so easy that this method comes highly recommended *(Hall, 2004)*.

COMFORT FOR PERSON

The amount of effort required is negligible for all concerned.

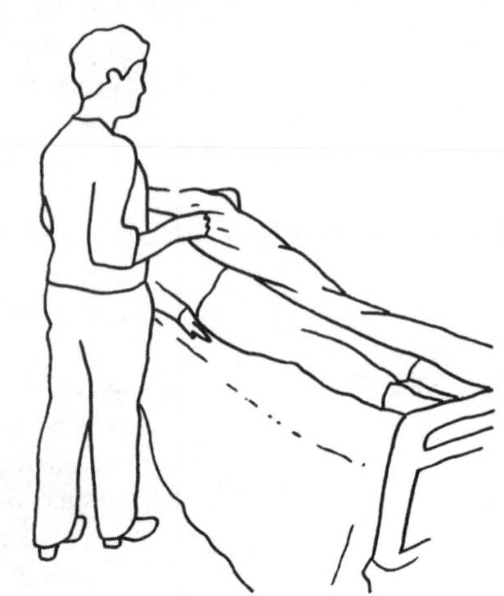

FIG 16.5a

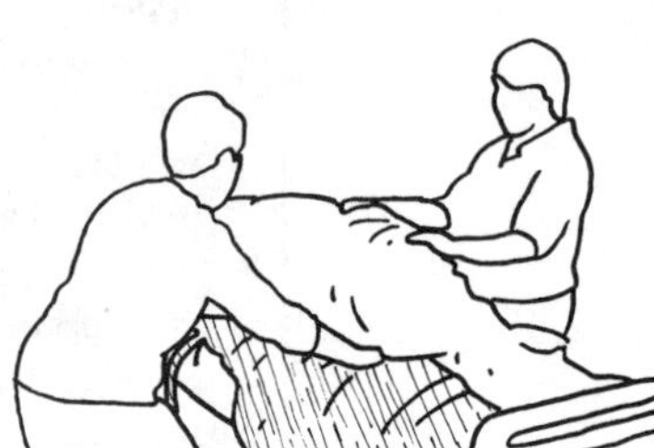

FIG 16.5b

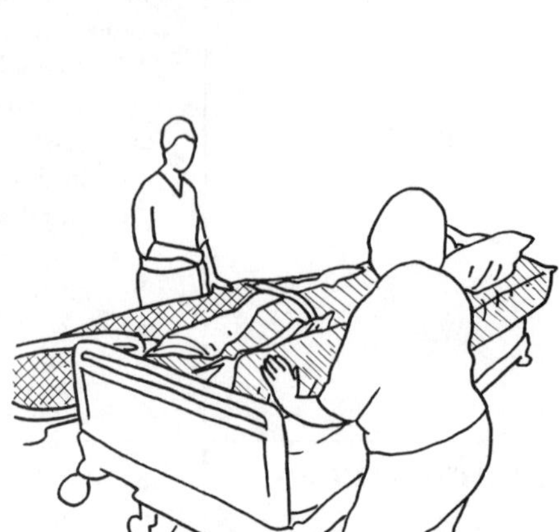

FIG 16.5c

There appears to be no discomfort for the person being moved.

SKILL LEVEL OF STAFF

- These handlers used the Neuromuscular Approach *(Crozier and Cozens 1998)*, however, this task takes little effort no matter which handling approach is used.
- As this mattress is a relatively new product some prior knowledge and specific training will be required to carry out the task safely but it is uncomplicated.

EVIDENCE AVAILABLE

1. A discomfort rating used by *Hall (2004)*, found this method of moving a patient was by far the least effort required.
2. National Back Exchange, Theatre Interest Group *(NBE, 2003)*, found this to be the greatest comfort for the person being transferred from bed to trolley.

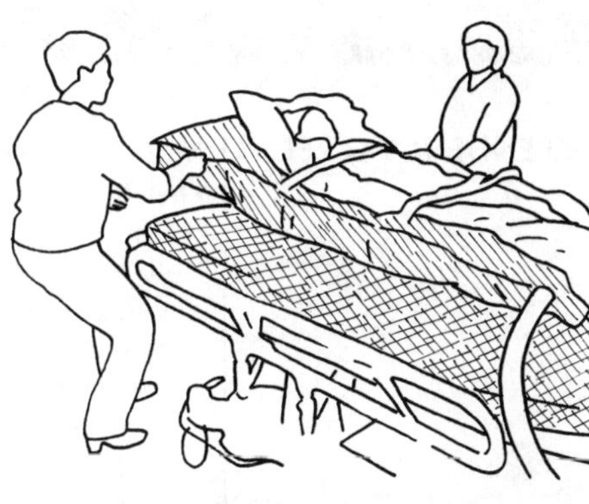

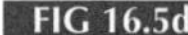

FIG 16.5d

DANGERS/ PRECAUTIONS

- Care needs to be taken that the handlers use the equipment correctly according to the manufacturer's instructions.
- It is the method of inserting the mattress, which poses the most problem. Even so, using the previous methods suggested, this is low risk

FURTHER OPTIONS

The use of other mechanical options would reduce the risk of injury to the people involved. These include hoisting with stretcher attachments and transfer trolleys with integral transfer facilities.

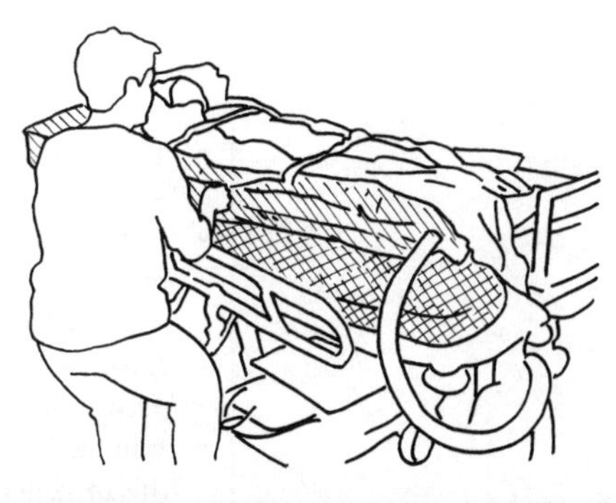

FIG 16.5e

Evidence review

Technique	REBA	Activity	Comfort	FIM	Mobility gallery	Skill level	Comment
INSERTING INFLATABLE TRANSFER MATTRESS							
Fig 16.5b	8	1	8	1	E	Advanced beginner	
USING INFLATABLE TRANSFER MATTRESS							
Fig 16.5c	5	1	10	1	E	Competent	Inflatable transfer mattress lowers postural risk but is a more complex technique. Very comfortable for the person

Task Four

Lateral transfers between bed and stretcher trolley, using a hard transfer board and 2 slide sheets

DEPENDENCY LEVEL

Mobility Gallery E
FIM 1

- In most cases these manoeuvres are carried out on an unconscious person who is totally dependent, or on a person who has limited ability to assist, who is usually going to or returning from the operating theatre. For those people that can assist to transfer from surface to surface, verbal instructions may be all that is required.
- In this task it is assuming the person to be transferred is passive.

DESCRIPTION

- With the person positioned lying supine (flat and face up), on a bed, preferably a profiling bed with variable height adjustment.
- The trolley should also have a height adjustable facility.
- The bed and trolley are adjusted to a median height in respect of the handler's waist/pelvic crest height.
- A transfer board and two slide sheets are used to aid this transfer.
- A minimum of 4 handlers is required for this task, depending on the person's size and medical condition.
- The person is prepared by rolling over onto their side (as described in task 1 above and chapter 15).
- Once the client has rolled over onto their side, the slide sheets are inserted.
- After the slide sheets are in place the transfer board is inserted halfway under the person forming a bridge between the bed and trolley.
- Careful positioning of the trolley alongside the bed requires enough space for the 4 handlers to move around the bed and trolley to prevent the handlers from reaching over them both.
- Having placed the trolley and bed along side each other, the slide sheets are positioned so that one is above the flat transfer board and the other is below it.
- The slide sheet placed on top of the transfer board, but under the person, is the slide sheet that will be pulled to transfer the person across from bed to the trolley.
- Handler 1 on the side of the bed at the head and shoulders of the person with their feet in stable base, with one foot forward and knees relaxed. Their arms have one hand placed on the person's shoulder and their other hand placed on the bed.
- Handler 2 is also on the side of the bed at

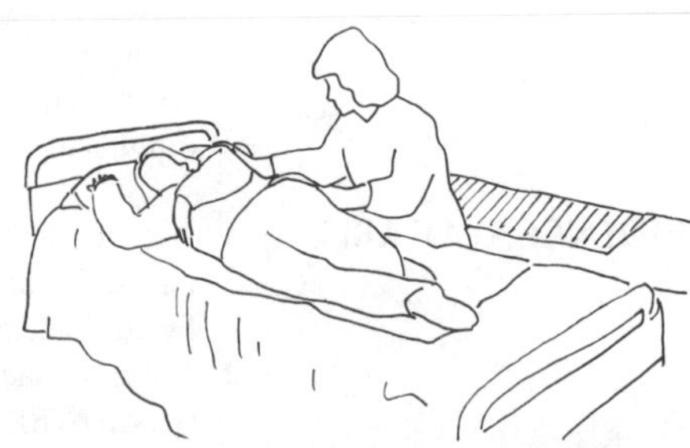

FIG 16.6a

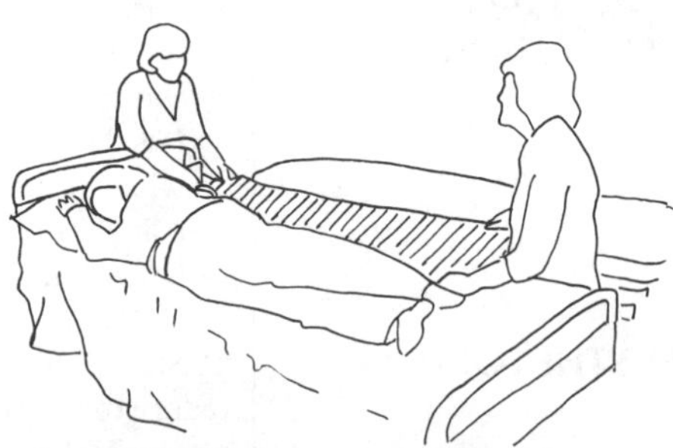

FIG 16.6b

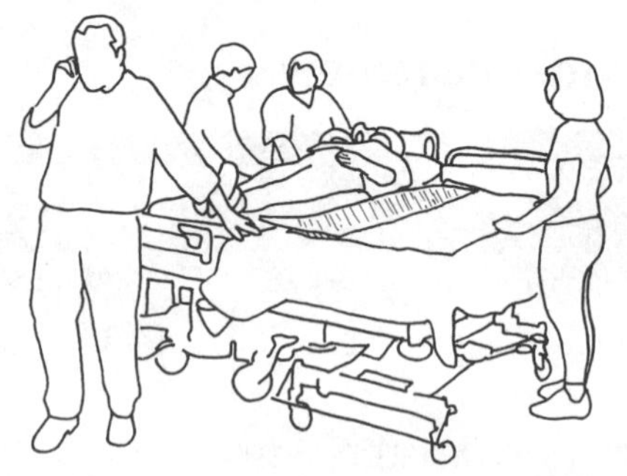

FIG 16.6c

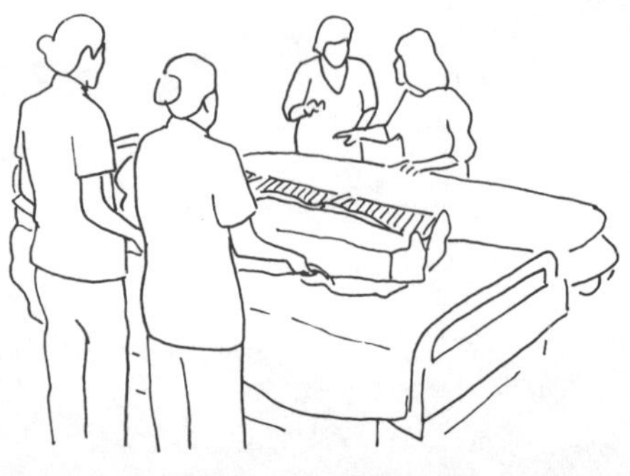

FIG 16.6d

the hip and legs of the person. Again the handler has their feet in a stable position as for handler 1. This handler also has one hand on the bed in front of them and the other hand in contact with the person's hip.

- Handler 3, is at the head end of the receiving side of the trolley, one foot forward with knees relaxed in an upright stance. Hands ready to hold the slide sheet at trolley height.
- Handler 4 is on the receiving side at the foot end of the trolley. One foot forward, knees relaxed. Both hands reaching across the trolley to take hold of the sliding sheet handle with overhand grasp (see figure 16.6e).
- On the command **'ready steady, slide'**, the handlers 1 and 2 push the person gently initiating the move, while handlers 3 and 4 pull the person across the bed to the trolley.
- Once the transfer is completed, the handlers remove the slide sheets and transfer board by rolling the client from side to side, (as previously described in task 1 and chapter 15).
- The trolley rails/sides are raised to prevent the person falling from the trolley.
- A similar procedure is followed to transfer the person back from the trolley onto the bed.
- Alternatively, the slide sheets can withdrawn by hander 3 by placing their hand under the person's neck (natural hollow) then withdraws the slide sheet towards the person's waist with an underhand grip (hands palm up). Meanwhile handler 4 withdraws the foot end of the slide sheet in a similar manner (see figure 16.6f).

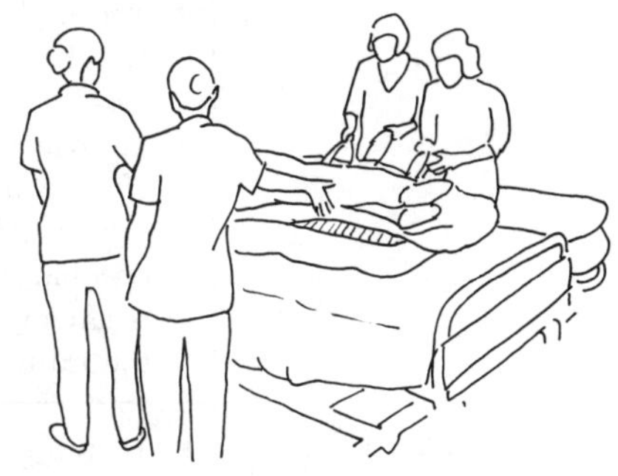

FIG 16.6e

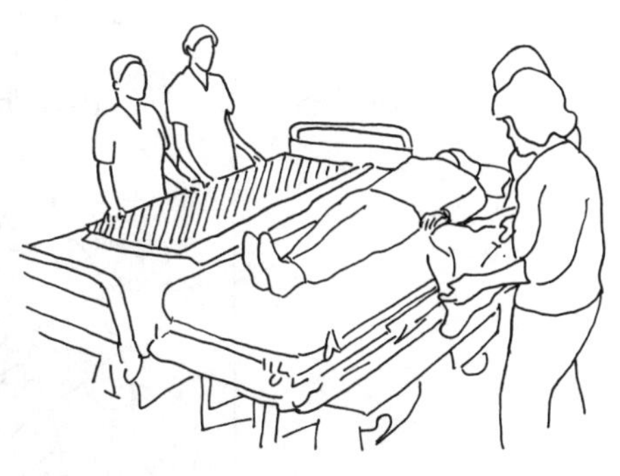

FIG 16.6f

PERCEIVED EXERTION FOR HANDLER	The Handlers recorded "low" to none in terms of discomfort during this procedure.
COMFORT FOR PERSON	For the person being moved this method was rated as having no discomfort. Although depending on the medical condition of the person care would need to be taken to avoid any discomfort especially when rolling the person from side to side.
SKILL LEVEL OF STAFF	Some prior knowledge and specific training will be required to carry out the task safely.
EVIDENCE AVAILABLE	**1** This method was indicated by *McFarlane (1994)* as being the method with the least effort and forces. **2** *Hall (2004)* found that this approach was subjectively assessed as having a low discomfort rating. However, the REBA score for the receivers was particularly high. **3** The roller-boards are another option but still require force to push and/or pull the patient across the bed/trolley, *McFarlane (1998)*. **4** The use of the lateral transfer board and padded mattress is generally more acceptable to the person being moved rather than the handlers *(DIAG 2003)*. **5** The single slide sheet with long handles and lateral transfer board reduces the reach required by slide sheets without the long handles. There is still a large amount of effort required to pull the patient across the bed/trolley but *MacFarlane (1998)*, recommended this method as one using less force.
DANGERS/ PRECAUTIONS	• The use of the brakes on the bed and trolley are of particular note, as the person could fall if the brakes are not applied when transferring the person. • Using two slide sheets has made this task easier, as less force is required, however, some people can be over-zealous in their approach and end up sliding the person completely off the bed/trolley. • Positioning of the handlers bodies against the bed or trolley will make a difference to the

	forces required. • The height of the bed can create less effort if it is raised in respect to the handler's waist/pelvic crest height. This reduces the stooping and therefore postural stress exerted when stooping over the bed/trolley. • The relaxing of the shoulders and knees prior to carrying out this task will also reduce the effort required. • A manual handling risk assessment must be completed that is specific to the handlers operating these manoeuvres and the person requiring care. Care also needs to be taken regarding the manufacturer's recommendations for use of the equipment. **NB** Kneeling on the bed/trolley during this manoeuvre is actively discouraged as there are safer options.
FURTHER OPTIONS	• There are a number of variations and options available, as indicated above. • Lateral transfer using a hard transfer board and slide sheet with handles • Lateral transfer using a hard transfer board and padded fabric slide/mattress. • Lateral transfers using a transfer roller board and a slide sheet. • The transfers of lying to lying (lateral transfers) all require a similar generic approach as described above. The slight variations require specialist training to carry out the task.

Lateral transfer (bed to bed) canvas/hard transfer board

✘ HAZARDOUS POSTURE FOR HANDLERS KNEELING ON THE BED

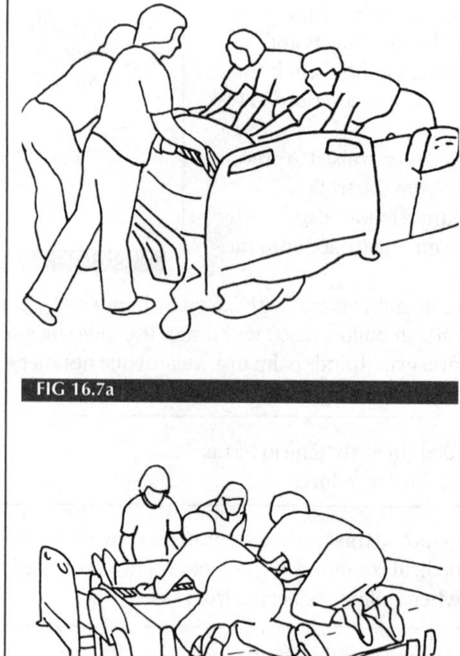

FIG 16.7a

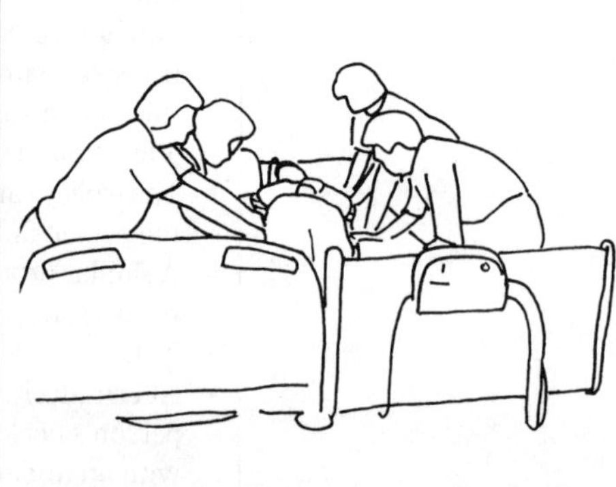

FIG 16.7b

FIG 16.7c

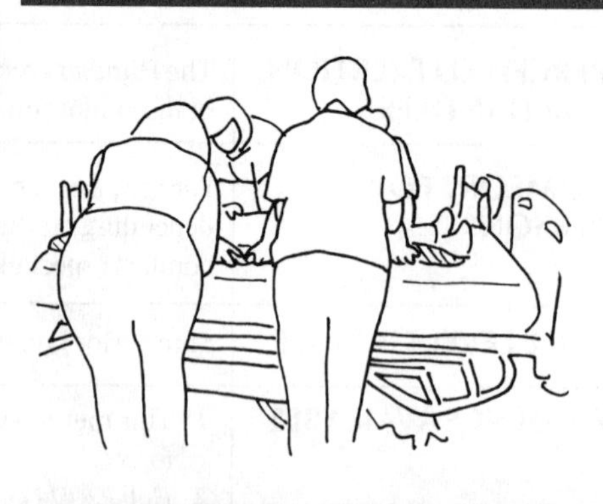

FIG 16.7d

Evidence review

Technique	REBA	Activity	Comfort	FIM	Mobility gallery	Skill level	Comment
LATERAL TRANSFER (BED TO BED) WITH CANVAS/HARD TRANSFER BOARD (PUSHING)							
Figs 16.7a-b	5	1	7	1	E	Advanced beginner	A wider sheet would give similar results to using handles 1A
LATERAL TRANSFER (BED TO BED) WITH CANVAS/HARD TRANSFER BOARD (PULLING)							
Figs 16.7c-d	12	1	7	1	E	Advanced beginner	A wider sheet would give similar results to using handles 2A

Lateral transfer (bed to bed) sheet with hand holds/hard transfer board

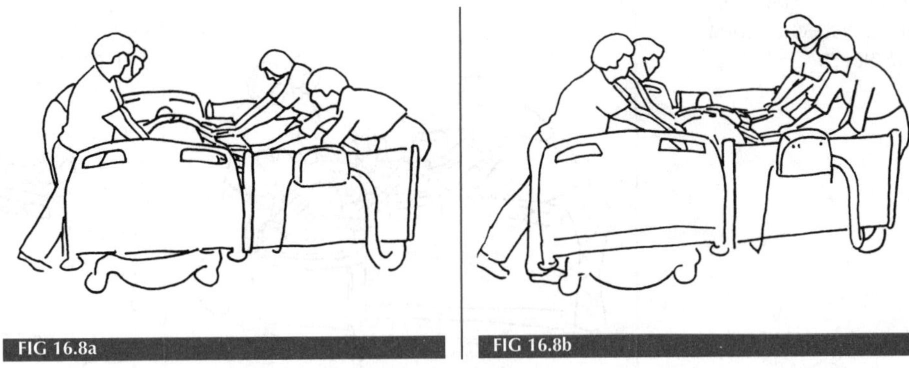

FIG 16.8a

FIG 16.8b

Evidence review

Technique	REBA	Activity	Comfort	FIM	Mobility gallery	Skill level	Comment
LATERAL TRANSFER (BED TO BED) WITH SHEET WITH HANDLES/HARD TRANSFER BOARD (PUSHING)							
Fig 16.8a	4	1	7	1	E	Advanced beginner	A wider sheet would give similar results to using handles
LATERAL TRANSFER (BED TO BED) WITH SHEET WITH HANDLES/HARD TRANSFER BOARD (PULLING)							
Fig 16.8b	8	1	7	1	E	Advanced beginner	Reba score increases if knee on the bed whether pushing or pulling. It is better to use a sheet with handles when performing lying to lying transfer

Lateral transfer (bed to trolley) hard transfer board, slide sheets with handles

✘ HAZARDOUS POSTURE FOR HANDLERS KNEELING ON THE BED

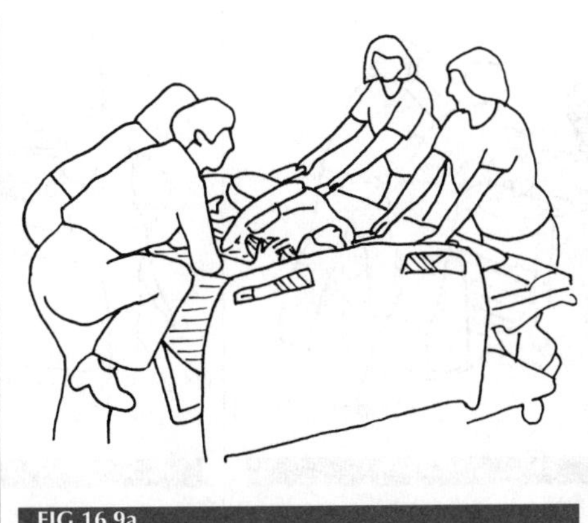

FIG 16.9a

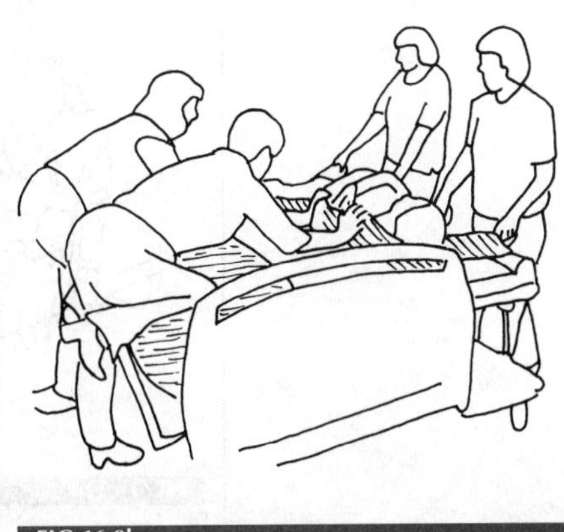

FIG 16.9b

Evidence review

Technique	REBA	Activity	Comfort	FIM	Mobility gallery	Skill level	Comment
BED TO TROLLEY (HARD TRANSFER BOARD, SLIDE SHEETS + HANDLES) PUSHING							
Fig 16.9a	11	1	7	1	E	Advanced beginner	Measurements taken at point when load is taken
BED TO TROLLEY (HARD TRANSFER BOARD, SLIDE SHEETS + HANDLES) PULLING							
Fig 16.9b	6	1	7	1	E	Novice	Decreased score as not over-reaching or kneeling on the trolley

Lateral transfer (trolley to bed) hard transfer board, slide sheets with handles

✗ HAZARDOUS POSTURE FOR HANDLERS KNEELING ON THE BED

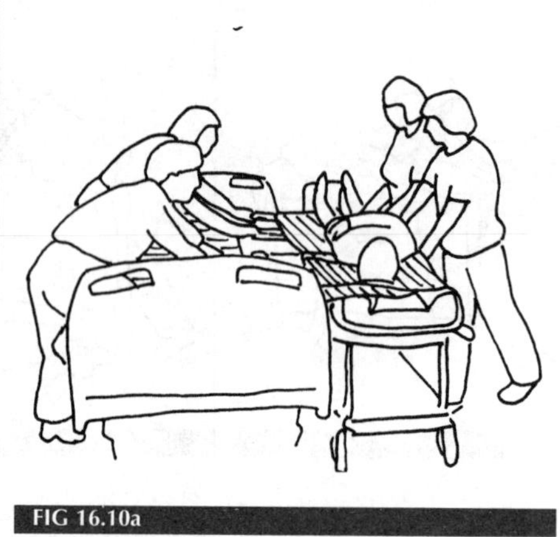
FIG 16.10a

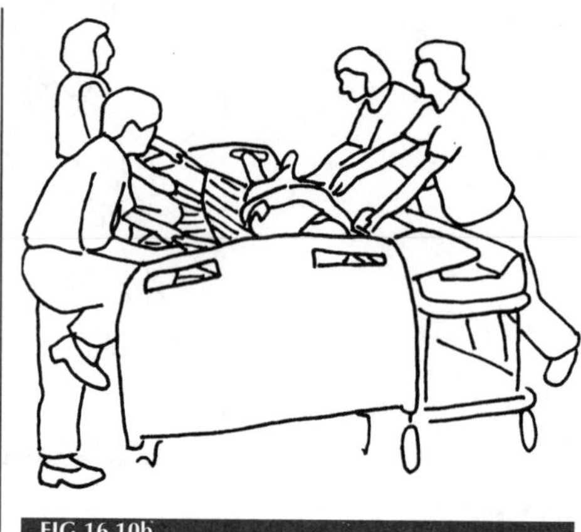
FIG 16.10b

Evidence review

Technique	REBA	Activity	Comfort	FIM	Mobility gallery	Skill level	Comment
TROLLEY TO BED (HARD TRANSFER BOARD, SLIDE SHEETS + HANDLES) – HANDLER ON LEFT AT FOOT END							
Fig 16.10b	6	1	7	1	E	Novice	Measurements taken at point when load is taken
TROLLEY TO BED (HARD TRANSFER BOARD, SLIDE SHEETS + HANDLES) – HANDLER ON LEFT AT HEAD END							
Fig 16.10b	2	1	7	1	E	Advanced beginner	Decreased score as not over-reaching or kneeling on the trolley

Lateral transfer (bed to bed) hard transfer board and slide sheet with long handles

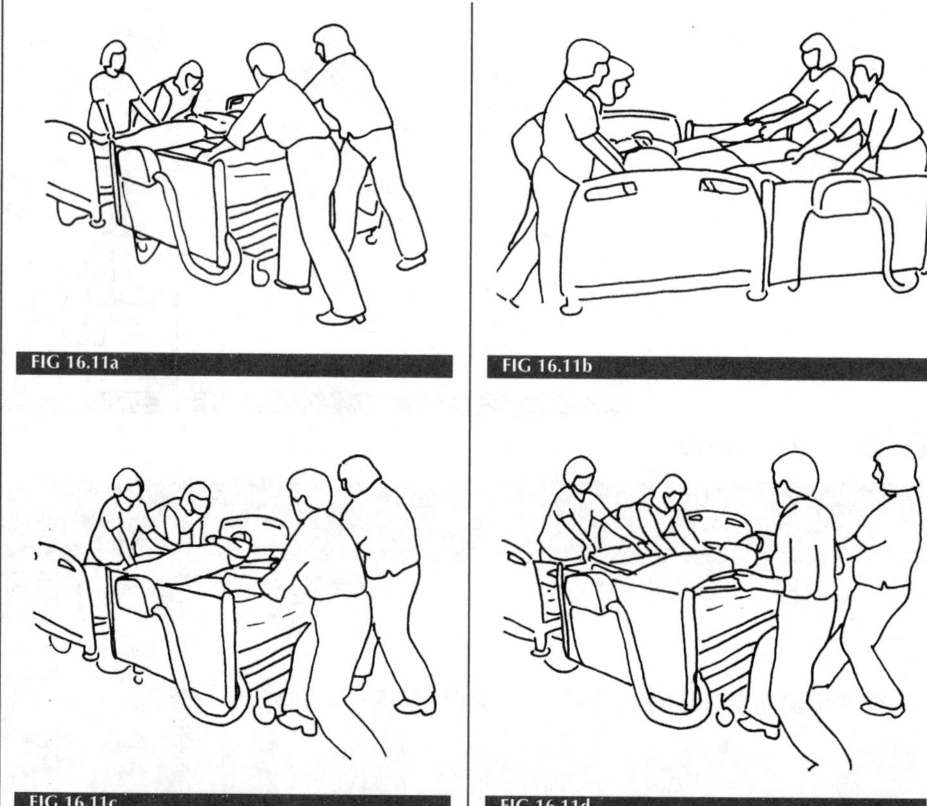
FIG 16.11a
FIG 16.11b
FIG 16.11c
FIG 16.11d

NB
No separate evidence gathered but postures much improved with the use of long handles

Lateral transfer (bed to bed) with wide slide mattress

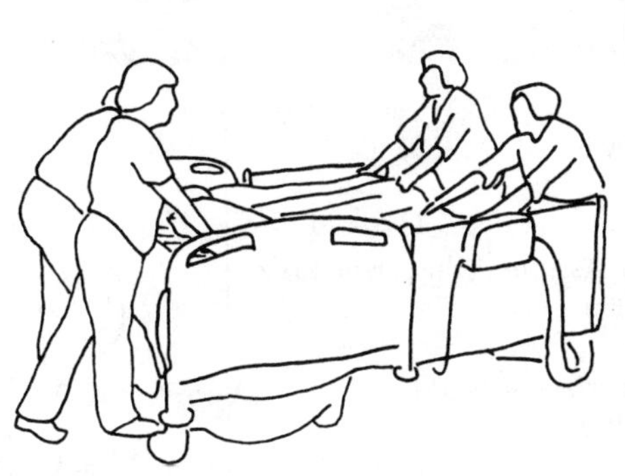

FIG 16.12a

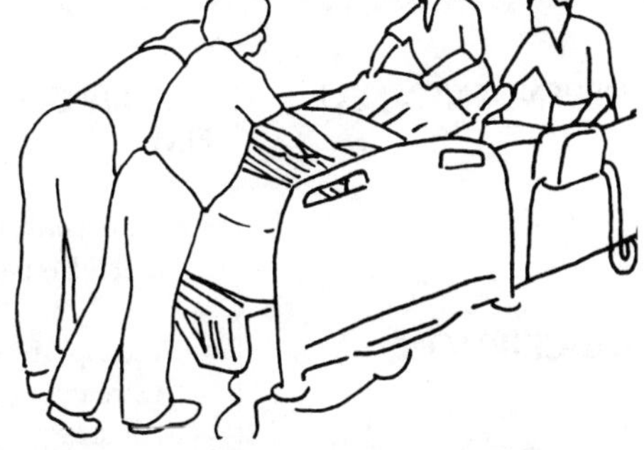

FIG 16.12b

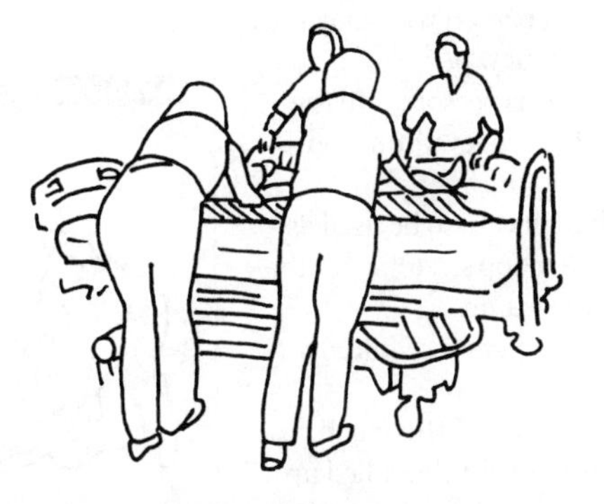

FIG 16.12c

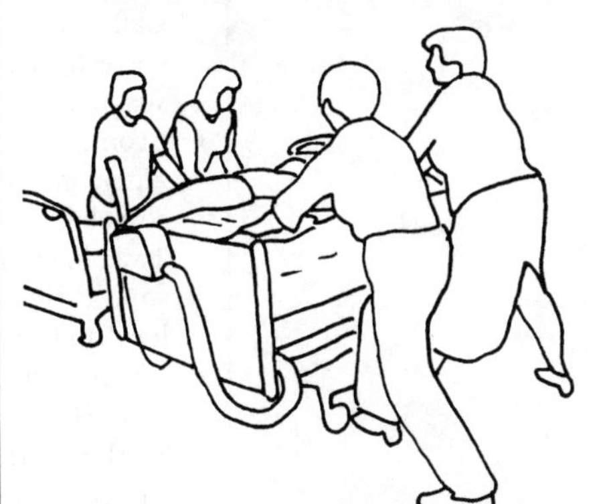

FIG 16.12d

NB

- No separate evidence gathered but postures much improved with the use of wide slide mattress
- Note should be taken of the effect on their posture of height differences between the handlers (see figure 16.12b)

Task Five

Transfer to an ambulance stretcher trolley using a scoop stretcher or spinal board

DEPENDENCY LEVEL	**Mobility Gallery E** **FIM 1** Totally dependent. Assuming the person to be transferred is passive	FIG 16.13a
DESCRIPTION	— A scoop stretcher/spinal board — A stretcher trolley — Blankets • The person is scooped onto the spinal board or scoop stretcher by experienced staff ensuring that the handlers are correctly handling a person who may have sustained a spinal injury. • In order to transfer this person onto the ambulance stretcher trolley, the scoop stretcher is placed on the floor. • Two rolled-up blankets are to be used as supports under the scoop stretcher, at the head and foot of the frame. • A minimum of 2 handlers is required for this task. • The handlers lift one end of the scoop stretcher at a time to insert the rolled up blankets one at either end. • The handlers then adopt a power lifting position in order to raise the scoop stretcher, with a firm grasp of each end. • Using the commands "Ready, steady, lift", the handlers lift together and take a sideways step to lower the scoop stretcher on to the ambulance trolley, which has been positioned close to the scoop stretcher. • The trolley should be positioned in such a way to reduce the distance and effort required by the handlers to transfer the person from the floor onto the trolley. • The stature and size of the handlers will indicate how high the trolley needs to be raised.	FIG 16.13b
PERCEIVED EXERTION FOR HANDLER	This is a difficult task which requires a lot of effort.	FIG 16.13c
COMFORT FOR PERSON	There should be little discomfort for the person, although any jerking/sudden movements could cause pain.	
SKILL LEVEL OF STAFF	This task needs practice and specific training.	
EVIDENCE AVAILABLE	Postures are not good according to *Hignett and McAtamney (2001)*	
DANGERS/ PRECAUTIONS	Care needs to be taken with a person with a potential spinal injury. The handlers are using a quite stressful posture.	
FURTHER OPTIONS	If a person does not have a spinal injury, an elevator cushion could be centralised under the scoop stretcher to raise it to a more manageable height in order to transfer the person onto a stretcher trolley, please contact the manufacturer for detailed guidance.	

7 Postural constraints

Operating theatre procedures will require further adaptations and attachments to the theatre bed/operating table in order to transfer some people. Also the medical condition/surgical procedure will dictate how and when a person can be moved. Some methods of moving the anaesthetised person on the operating table can utilise slide sheets and pillows strategically placed, in order to reduce lifting the load.

Care needs to be taken to reduce the time any handler has to stand in a position where they endure a static posture holding a load.

Transfers in X-Ray Departments and Diagnostic/investigation suites, all need to be aware of the problems associated with transferring a person. In certain circumstances the attachments to the person being transferred can be problematic. In other areas it is the specialised equipment that causes the obstruction to a safer handling procedure.

As with many transfers, it is the need to avoid postural stress that is paramount when pushing or pulling. Therefore, consideration should be taken of the lateral flexion and/or rotation, adopted by some handlers that need to be avoided *(Birtles and Williams, 2004)*.

Acknowledgements

I would like to take this opportunity to convey my special thanks and apreciation to the many people who contributed so kindly in a variety of ways. They include Jacqui Smith, Sheenagh Orchard, Simon Love, Nicky Hunter (for suppling photographs for task 5), Aileen Hunter, Deborah Southworth, Gary Maltby, Jenny Ross, Elaine Thynne,Tracey Carrott and all the other people who helped to formulate the illustrations and text included in this chapter.

References

Aitchison L (Editor) (1999). Safer Handling of People in the Community. Back Care: Middlesex

Chaffin, DB and Park KS (1973). A longitudinal study of low back pain as associated with occupational weight lifting factors. American Industrial Hygiene Association 34 513–525

Crozier L and Cozens S (1998). Chapter 6. The Neuromuscular Approach to Efficient Handling and Moving. In NBPA/RCN (1998) The Guide to the Handling of Pateints. 4th Ed Revised. National Back Pain Association in collaboration with the Royal College of Nursing. Middlesex.

Birtles M and Williams S (2004). An ergonomics evaluation of hospital bed backrests. The Column16.2 18-20.

Derbyshire Inter-Agency Group (2003). Specific handling procedures for theatre environments. Southern Derbyshire NHS Trust (Community Health), Northern Derbyshire NHS Trust (Community Health), Derbyshire Royal Hospital NHS Trust, Southern Derbyshire Acute Hospitals NHS Trust.(DIAG). (unpublished)

Disabled Living Foundation (2001). Handling People. Advice, Equipment and Information. www.dlf.org.uk [accessed on 17.01.05]

Garb JR and Dockery CA (1995). Reducing employee back injuries in the perioperative setting. AORN Journal 61(6) 1046–1052

Garg A Owen B and Beller D (1991). A biomechanical and ergonomic evaluation of patient transfer tasks. Ergonomics . 34 (3) 289-312

Hall J (2004). Ergonomic aspects of patient transfers between Paramedics and Accident and Emergency Department Nursing Staff. MSc thesis. Surrey University. (unpublished)

Health and Safety Executive (2003). Manual Handling Assessment Charts. Health and Safety Laboratory. HSE Books: Suffolk

Health and Safety Executive (2004). A Guide to the Manual Handling Operations Regulations 1992. L23. HSE Books: Suffolk

Hignett S and McAtamney L (2000). Rapid Entire Body Assessment REBA. Applied Ergonomics 31 201–205

Hunter N (2004). Handle with Care. A guide to backcare and manual handling for Ambulance Staff. East Anglian Ambulance Service NHS Trust.

Lavender SA, Conrad KM, Reichelt PA, Meyer FT and Johnson PW (2000). Postural analysis of paramedics simulating frequently performed strenuous work tasks, Applied Ergonomics 31 (1) 45–57

Marras WS, Davis KG, Kirking BC and Bertsche PK (1999). A comprehensive analysis of low-back disorder risk and spinal loading during the transferring and repositioning of patients using different techniques. Ergonomics 42 (7) 904–926

Marras WS and Davis KG (1998). Spinal loading during asymmetric lifting using one versus two hands. Ergonomics 41 (6) 817–834.

McFarlane, D (1998). A Survey of Aids for Sliding Transfers of Patients for the South East Sydney Area Health Service. Work Cover New South Wales. (unpublished report)

McFarlane D (1998). A Survey of Aids for Sliding Transfers of Patients for the South East Sydney Area Health Service. Work Cover New South Wales. (unpublished report)

National Back Exchange (2003). Equipment Evaluation. NBE Theatre Interest Group Minutes 1st Dec 2003 at Loughborough University (unpublished)

Spencer J, Denton D and Smith J (2001). Lateral Transfers. The Column 13.2 19–21

Waters TR, Putz-AndersonV, Garg A and Fine LJ (1993). Revised NIOSH equation for the design and evaluation of manual lifting tasks. Ergonomics 36 (7) 749–776

Lying to lying transfers and associated manoeuvres

17

The falling and fallen person and emergency handling

Mike Betts LPD RGN
Back Care Adviser Luton & Dunstable Hospital NHS Trust
Claire Mowbray LPD RGN
Back Care Specialist Nurse
Chiltern & South Bucks NHS Primary Care Trust

1 Introduction

Evidence shows that falls are a common occurence. Over 60% of those living in nursing homes will fall, while a third of people over 65 years and fifty percent of those over 80 years living in the community will fall, *(Cryer, Patel 2001)*. Approximately 5% of falls will result in fractures, *(Tinetti et al 1988)*. The handling of the falling or fallen person presents a high risk of injury to both persons and handlers.

Recent unpublished figures from the Health and Safety Executive (HSE) identified that in the two-year period ending in March 2003 there were 137 reported injuries to staff resulting in over three day absences. These figures include incidents where a staff member has tried to save/support a person who has fallen, or where the person grabs the staff member for support or falls onto them, causing injury.

Of the above incidents, 15 of the reported injuries occurred when a member of staff was assisting the fallen person, *(HSE 2004)* these figures are dependent upon the terminology used by the individual reporting the incident.

It is generally perceived by many health and social care professionals that allowing a person to fall to the ground is unacceptable and is a direct infringement of that individual's duty of care. This subject is a particularly emotive one, creating an ethical dilemma. On the one hand individuals feel they must protect those under their care, whilst on the other, they realise they have a responsibility to protect themselves. However, it has long been considered that to catch or control the descent of a falling person is inherently unsafe for the handler, *(RCN/NBPA 1997; BackCare 1999; Fray et al 2001; Resuscitation Council (UK) 2001)*. The extent of the risk of 'catching' the falling person is significant, (see force calculation at the end of this chapter).

Whether the handler is able to lower the falling peson will be dependent upon the handler's position at the start of the fall, i.e. close assisted walking, (see section 3 below).

There are considerable risks to the falling person if they are allowed to fall without intervention from the handler, particularly the elderly or frail, e.g. fractured hip and possible complications.

2 Causes and prevention

The causes of falls are multi-factorial and diverse, and include both intrinsic and extrinsic factors, (table 17.1).

Most falls can be successfully managed by preventing their occurrence in the first place.

Risk assessment is the key to successful management. A comprehensive risk assessment will consider both the intrinsic and extrinsic factors, which may place the person at higher risk of falls.

For example, a risk assessment may identiy the need to wheel a patient to the toilet if there is a sense of urgency and walk back to reduce the risk of a fall. Alternatively, it may identify the need for walking aids or a chair positioned halfway. The risk assessment will also consider the potential injuries should a person fall, which will determine the handling strategies adopted.

Organisations must have a documented policy or set of guidelines on the management of the falling or fallen person. This would include aims and objectives, a policy statement that emphasises the need for balanced

Table 17.1 Prevention of Falls Risk Assessment *(adapted from Cryer & Patel 2001)*

Intrinsic	Extrinsic
• Underlying medical condition e.g. postural hypotension. • Strength, balance, gait and physical performance e.g. dizziness, use of walking aids, lack of gait symmetry and step continuity. • Physical functioning e.g. difficulty walking 400m, urinary urgency • Foot problems and footwear • Sensory decline e.g. vision problems, peripheral neuropathy • Medical conditions e.g. acute illness, history of stroke • Psychological factors e.g. fear of falling • History of previous falls, particularly 3 or more in the last year or previous fall with injury. • Cognitive decline e.g. Alzheimer's disease	• Hurrying • Medicine use e.g. polypharmacy • Altered environmental conditions • Variations in floor surfaces • Space, furniture and layout • Frictional variations between shoe and floor • Ill fitting shoes • Poor housing and lighting

decision making, and training requirements.

Training in the practical aspects of managing the fallen person and some emergency situations may expose the candidates to techniques which have an inherent risk. These situations must be discussed even if they are not demonstrated or practised.

3 Management of the falling person

Previously advocated methods for controlling a person's descent, which may result in a reduced risk of injury to the person, are set out in task one. These methods assume that:

- The handler is standing by the side of the person and slightly behind, before the person starts to fall. If not, they will be unable to get behind the person to be able to control the descent.
- The person is falling backwards or directly downwards
- There is sufficient space with no obstructions e.g. beds, commodes
- The person is not resisting
- There is no significant height difference. A particularly small handler may have difficulty controlling the descent of a particularly tall person and vice versa.
- The person is not significantly heavier than the handler.

These techniques would not be appropriate if the person was falling away from the handler or was any significant distance away. In these situations the handler may have to release their hold of the person and allow them to fall. The handler may need to move obstructions out of the way, to prevent an increased risk of injury to the person.

4 Management of the fallen person

There are a number of options for assisting a fallen person from the floor.

- The person gets up from the floor independently, without any assistance from the handlers.
- The person is instructed by the handler to get up from the floor using the backward chaining method.
- The use of an inflatable cushion.
- The use of a hoist / other mechanical or electrical equipment.
- Manual lifting of small children.
- Manual lifting in an emergency or exceptional circumstances (This is a high risk activity).

The fallen person should be examined for any injuries, before moving her.

There may be times when a person, providing they are not in immediate danger, should be left on the floor. Such times include individuals who intentionally place themselves on the floor for attention and known epileptic sufferers having a seizure.

Backward chaining (task three)

There may be a number of reasons why a fallen person is not able to get up from the floor without assistance. The person may panic and adopt ineffective strategies, such as rising directly from supine *(Tinetti et al 1993)*. Reduced muscle strength and joint mobility may render a person unable to get up independently. Persons who have a history of falls can be taught backward chaining.

Backward chaining involves training an individual to get to the floor from a standing or sitting position. This will enable the person to get up from the floor, in the event of a fall, unaided or with minimal supervision.

It has been suggested that a person may need between 4 and 15 training sessions, before they are able to successfully adopt this approach *(Reece and Simpson 1996)*.

The use of mechanical equipment

If a person cannot get up from the floor even with verbal prompting, mechanical equipment must be used. The type of equipment used is dependant upon a comprehensive risk assessment of the person, environment and the individual capabilities of the handlers.

The person's weight must be within the safe working load of the equipment used.

5 Emergency situations

Emergency or life-threatening situations may occur at any time and may not be foreseen. Wherever possible, equipment should be used, to minimise the risk of injury. However, if there is not sufficient time to get the equipment, a manual manoeuvre may be necessary.

Scenarios covered in this chapter are:

- Moving a collapsed person from chair to floor
- Evacuating people down stairs, in the event of a fire
- Evacuation from a pool
- Evacuation from a confined space
- Manual lifting from the floor
- Lowering a patient from a complete / incomplete strangulation

If an emergency occurs in an area without suitable equipment or sufficient staff, a risk assessment must be completed after the event and suitable control measures established.

Practical techniques

Task One

Lowering the falling person

DEPENDENCY LEVEL

Mobility Gallery B
FIM 3

DESCRIPTION

Method

- Release hold of the person and move behind.
- Both hands open and take a step backwards, to maintain a stable base. Keep in close (figure 17.1a).
- Avoid holding the person's arms but hold around the trunk (figure 17.1a).
- Bend both knees.
- Lower the person to the floor (figures. 17.1b – d).

SKILL LEVEL

High level of skill and physical fitness of the handler.

EVIDENCE AVAILABLE

1 *(National Back Pain Association/Royal College of Nursing 1997/8).* The Guide to the Handling of Patients: Introducing a safer handling policy, 4th Edition, National Back Pain Association.
2 *(BackCare 1999).* Safer handling of people in the community, National Back Pain Association.

DANGERS/ PRECAUTIONS

- As the handler bends his knee, the person may place all of her weight onto the handler's leg causing a musculoskeletal injury.
- May cause the handler to lose his balance
- The person may fall onto the handler.
- The person may grab the handler's arms.
- At some stage during the move, the handler will be taking the majority of the person's weight.
- The force required to support a falling person can be calculated *(Fray 2003)* (see force calculation at end of chapter).

DANGERS TO THE PERSON

- There is a risk of musculoskeletal or other injury.
- The person may develop a fear of falling, which may result in reduction of independence.

PRECAUTIONS

- The risk of injury will increase with the weight of the person.
- The handler must hold the person in such a way that he can release his hold in the eventuality of a fall.
- This move must be undertaken immediately the person starts to fall.

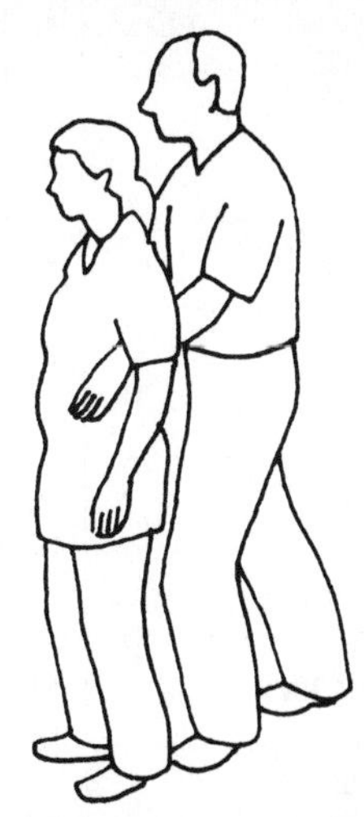

FIG 17.1a

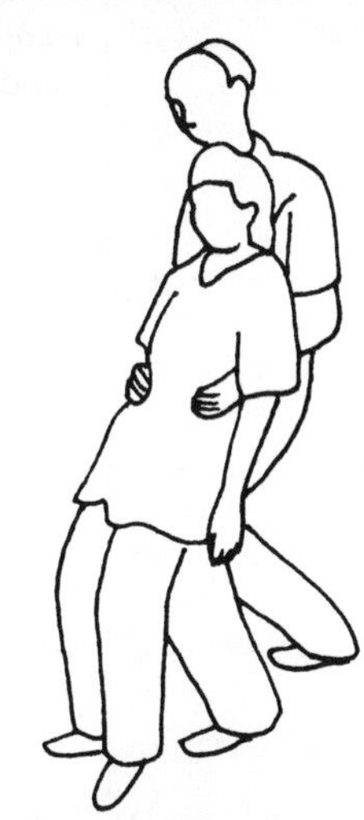

FIG 17.1b

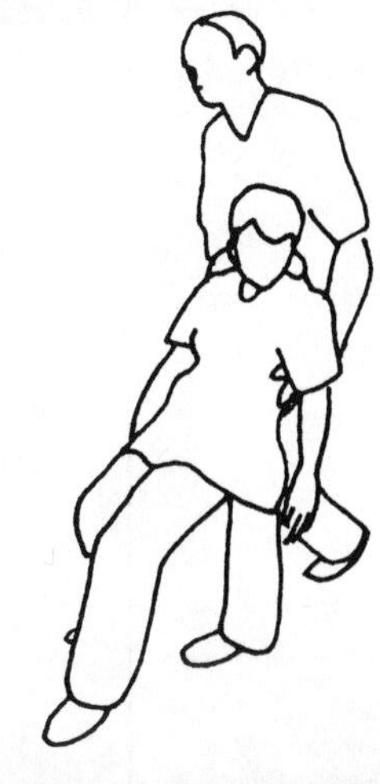

FIG 17.1c

FURTHER OPTION

Option
The task name and level of person independence remain the same. The only difference is that the forward leg is straight.

- Release hold of the person and move behind.
- Both hands open and take a step backwards, to maintain a stable base. Keep in close (figure 17.2a).
- Avoid holding the person's arms but hold around the trunk.
- Keep the forward leg extended (figure 17.2a onwards).
- Lower the person to the floor (figure 17.2a onwards).

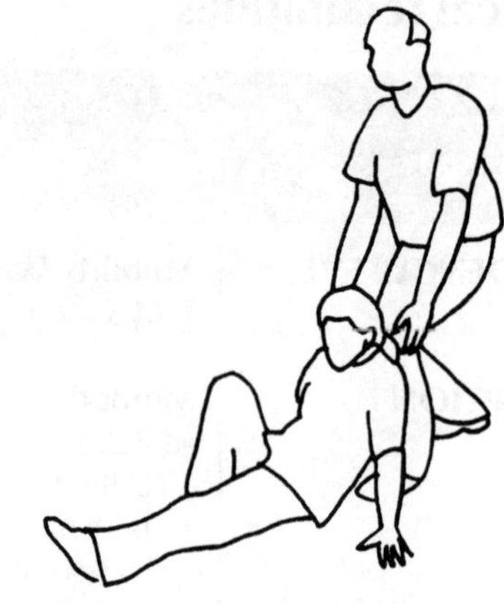
FIG 17.1d

SKILL LEVEL

High level of skill and physical fitness of the handler.

DANGERS/ PRECAUTIONS

As with method, but with the addition of a higher risk of injury to the forward leg due to the hyperextension.

NB
A manual handling risk assessment must be completed that is specific to the person and handlers.

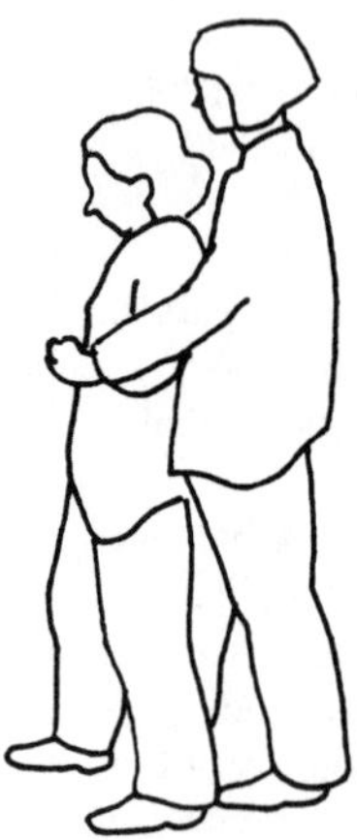
FIG 17.2a

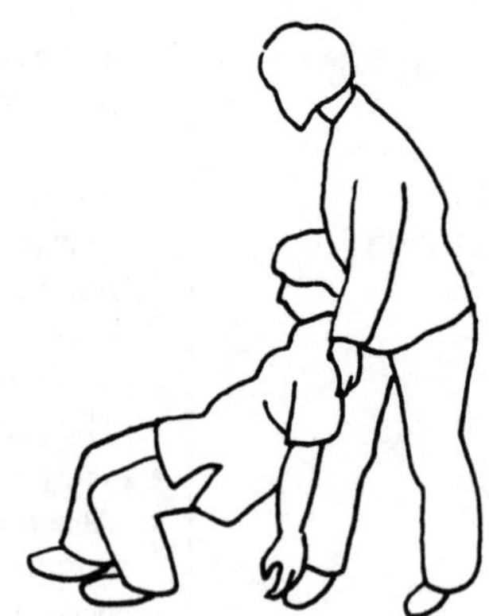
FIG 17.2c

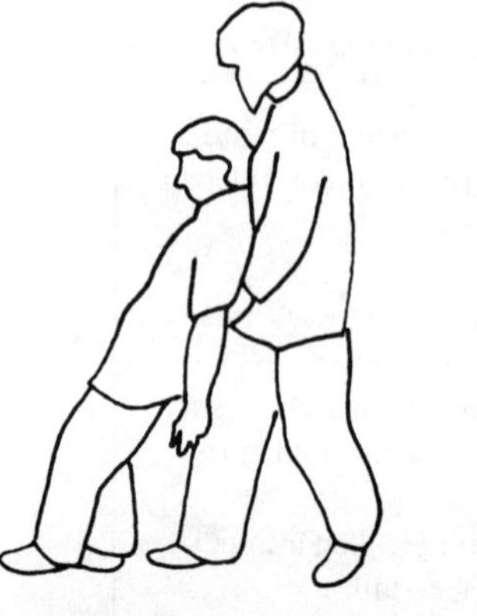
FIG 17.2b

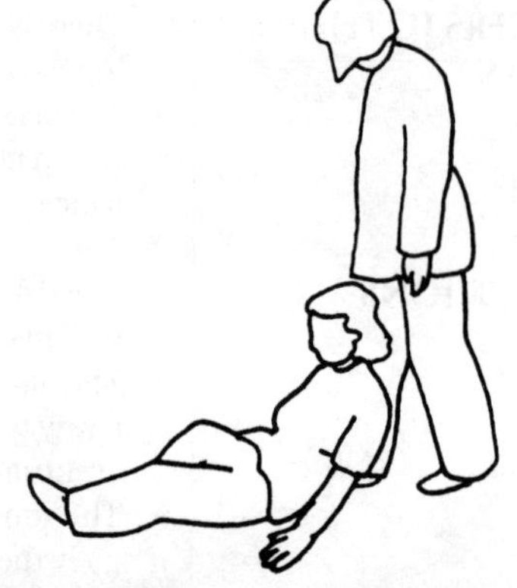
FIG 17.2d

Evidence review

Technique	REBA	Activity	Comfort	FIM	Mobility gallery	Skill level	Comment
LOWERING THE FALLING PERSON							
Fig 17.1c	10	1	5	3	B	Proficient	High postural risk
Fig 17.1d	7	1	3	3	B	Proficient	Medium postural risk but slightly less comfortable for the person

Task Two

Allowing a person to fall

DEPENDENCY LEVEL	**Mobility Gallery** A **FIM** 6
DESCRIPTION	• As the person begins to fall, the handler releases his hold and allows the person to fall to the floor, without physical intervention. • Wherever possible, the handler must move away any objects, which may cause injury to the person. • The handler may need to redirect the person's fall, away from any dangerous or immovable objects.
FALLING ON STAIRS	If the person falls on steps or stairs, the handler may be able to redirect the person's fall towards the higher stair.
SKILL LEVEL	The handler needs to be able to assess the situation quickly and with confidence
EVIDENCE AVAILABLE	1 *(BackCare 1999)* Safer handling of people in the community, National Back Pain Association. 2 *(Resuscitation Council (UK) 2001)*. Guidance for Safer Handling during Resuscitation in Hospitals, Resuscitation Council (UK).
DANGERS/ PRECAUTIONS	**Dangers to the handler** • Potential loss of balance, when on stairs. • Potential musculoskeletal injury, when redirecting the fall. **Dangers to the person** • There is a risk of serious musculoskeletal or other injury including fractures. Fractured hips are the most common serious injury to older people. • The person may develop a fear of falling, which may result in reduction of independence.
FURTHER OPTIONS	A comprehensive risk assessment may identify the need for an additional member of staff, walking behind the person with a wheelchair. In the event of the person falling, their descent can be redirected into the chair.
SKILL LEVEL	The handler needs to be able to assess the situation quickly and with confidence.
DANGERS AND PRECAUTIONS	**Dangers to the handler** Potential musculoskeletal injury when redirecting the fall. **Dangers to the person** • There is a risk of serious musculoskeletal or other injury. • The person may develop a fear of falling, which may result in increasing dependence. **NB** A manual handling risk assessment must be completed that is specific to the person and handlers.

Task Three

Instructing a person to get up from floor, using minimal supervision (Backward Chaining)

DEPENDENCY LEVEL

Mobility Gallery A
FIM 7

DESCRIPTION

Position a chair at the head end of the person.

- Encourage the person to roll onto her side, (figures 17.3a and b).
- Bend both knees and then raise up onto lower elbow, (figure 17.3c).
- Press down with lower elbow and upper hand to raise onto all fours, (figure 17.3d)
- Lean on the chair using both hands, (figure 17.3e).
- Instruct the person to raise one leg and place one foot on the floor, (figure 17.3f).
- Push up to straighten legs and turn to sit onto the chair, (figure 17.3g).

SKILL LEVEL

The handler needs to be able to confidently instruct the person.

EVIDENCE AVAILABLE

1 *(BackCare 1999)* Safer handling of people in the community, National Back Pain Association
2 *(Adams, Tyson 2000)* 'The effectiveness of physiotherapy to enable an elderly person to get up from the floor' Physiotherapy April 2000, 86. 4
3 *(Reece, Simpson 1996)* 'Preparing older people to cope after a fall' Physiotherapy, April 1996, 82, 4

DANGERS TO THE PERSON

If assessed inappropriately, the person may lose her balance.

FURTHER OPTIONS

Option 1

For a taller person, position the chair to the side of the kneeling person (figure 17.4a). Mobility Gallery and FIM remains the same.

- The person holds the arm or the seat of the chair with her nearest hand (figure 17.4b).
- The person raises her nearest leg so that her foot is flat on the floor (figure 17.4c).
- The person slides her bottom onto the chair (figure. 17.4d).

Option 2

The person could lean against an upturned chair to orientate herself before she stands (figure. 17.4f).

The handler needs to be able to confidently instruct the person.

(National Back Exchange Oxford Region Group, 1999). Generic safe systems of work for

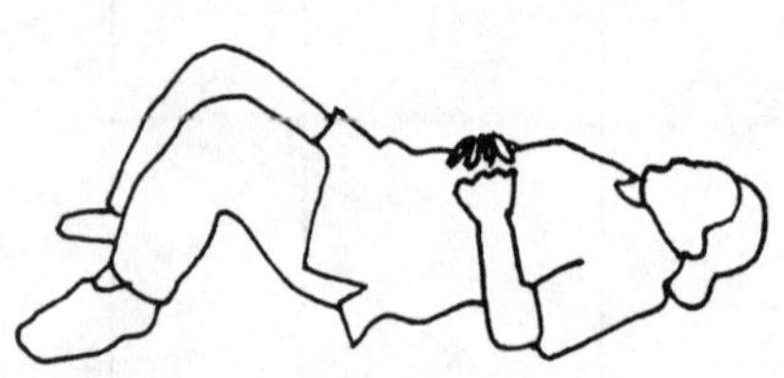
FIG 17.3a

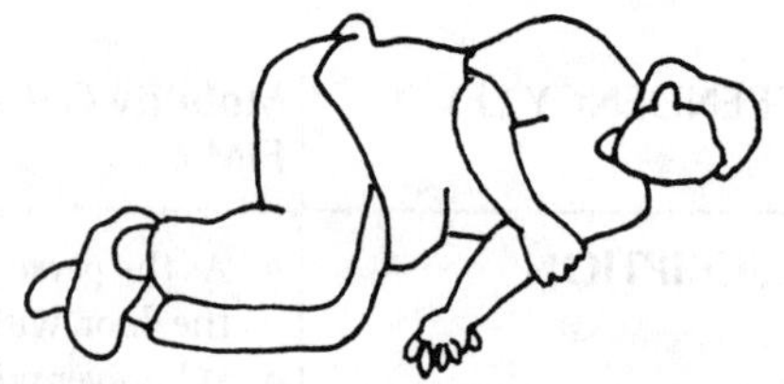
FIG 17.3b

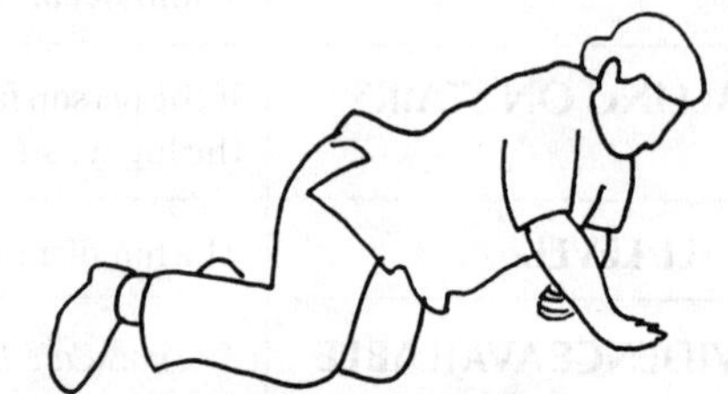
FIG 17.3c

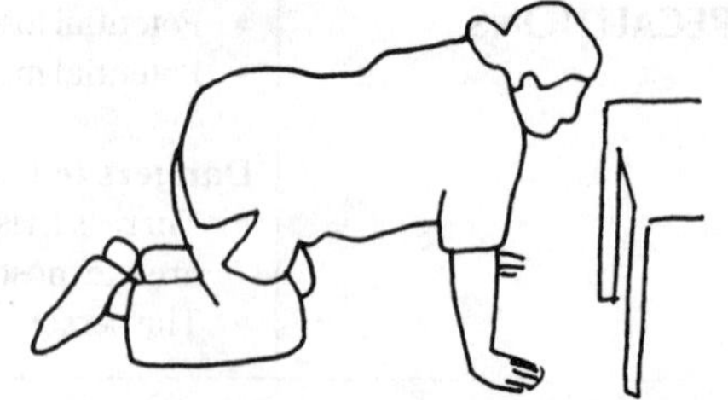
FIG 17.3d

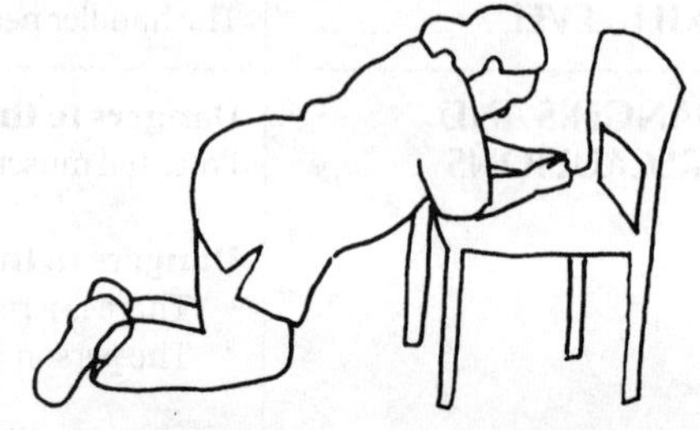
FIG 17.3e

person handling and inanimate load management.

Option 3

Mobility Gallery remains the same,
FIM 5
If the person in unable to kneel, the handler should:

- Instruct the person to sit forward on the floor.
- Place a foot stool/chair cushion behind her.
- The person places their hands behind their and onto the sides of the stool/cushion.
- She must bend her knees and dig in with her heels to push up onto the stool/cushion.
- This must be repeated onto gradually higher surfaces until she is in a position to be able to stand.
- Alternatively, the stairs could be used in the same way, particularly in a domestic environment (figures 17.5 a – d).

The handler needs to be able to confidently instruct the person.

NB

A manual handling risk assessment must be completed that is specific to the person and handlers.

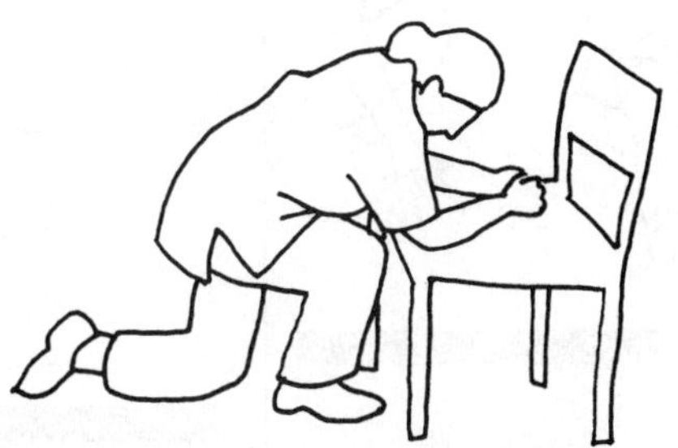

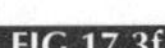

FIG 17.3f

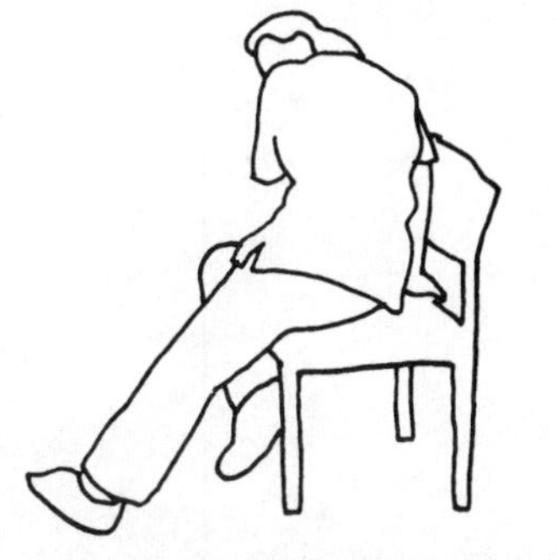

FIG 17.3g

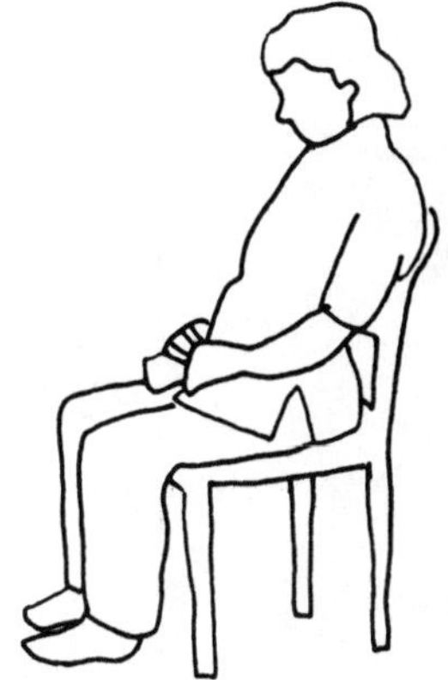

FIG 17.3h

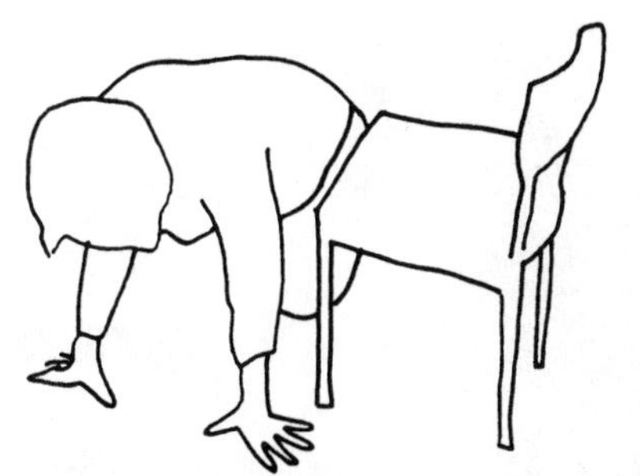

FIG 17.4a

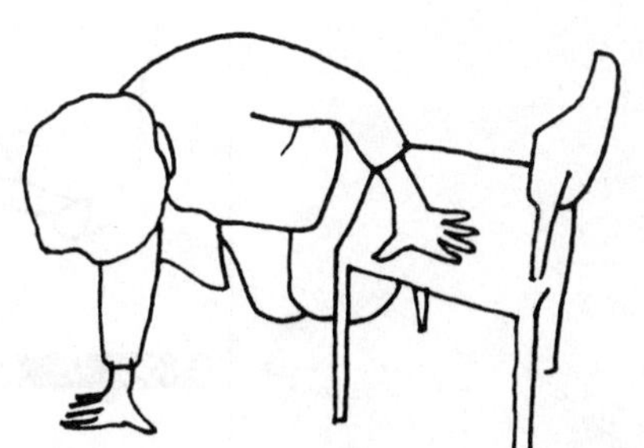

FIG 17.4b

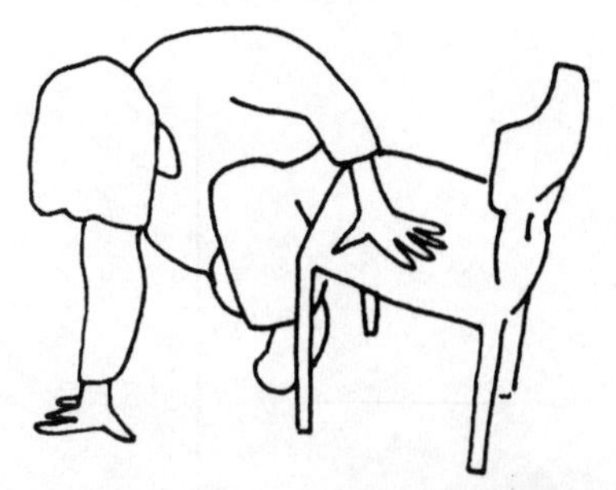

FIG 17.4c

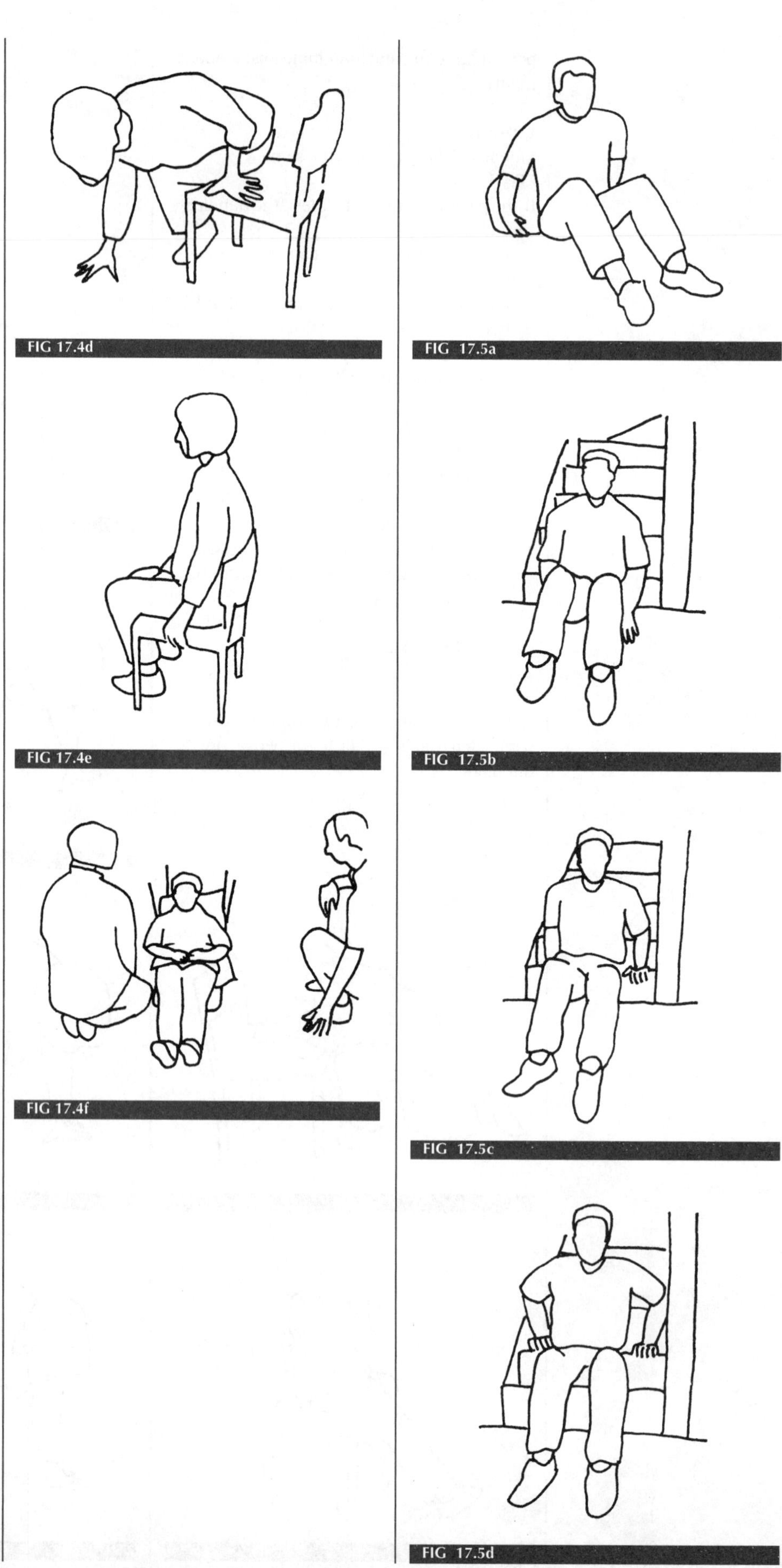

FIG 17.4d

FIG 17.4e

FIG 17.4f

FIG 17.5a

FIG 17.5b

FIG 17.5c

FIG 17.5d

Task Four

Rolling a person on the floor, to position handling equipment

DEPENDENCY LEVEL

Mobility Gallery B, C, D, E
FIM 1

DESCRIPTION

- Position the person's furthest arm across her chest and the nearest arm away from the body, to prevent the person rolling onto it.
- Bend the furthest knee or cross the ankles.
- Ask the person to turn her head in the direction of the intended movement.
- Hold the person's far shoulder and hip (figure 17.6a).
- The handler needs to start in a high kneeling position and rock back onto his heels, using a weight transfer technique, to roll the person (figure 17.6b).

SKILL LEVEL

The handler needs to be physically fit and must be able to kneel on the floor and rock backwards.

EVIDENCE AVAILABLE

1 *(BackCare 1999)* Safer Handling of People in the Community, National Back Pain Association
2 *(National Back Pain Association/BackCare 1997/8)* The Guide to the Handling of Patients, 4th Edition, National Back Pain Association

DANGERS/ PRECAUTIONS

- This method of rolling should not be used on people with suspected spinal injuries (see further options).
- The person should never be rolled away from the handler.
- People who are confused may resist the movement, so caution should be taken.

FURTHER OPTION

Rolling a person with suspected spinal injuries, to insert a split spinal stretcher
Mobility Gallery E;
FIM 1

- A minimum of five members of staff are required.
- The lead handler kneels at the head end of the person and supports the person's head and neck for the duration of the transfer.
- Three members of staff start off in a high kneeling position on one side of the person, approximately level with the person's shoulders, hips and thighs.
- If the person's condition permits, their nearest arm is positioned away from the body to prevent them rolling onto it.
- The fifth member of staff kneels on the opposite side of the person, to position one half of the split stretcher as the person is turned.

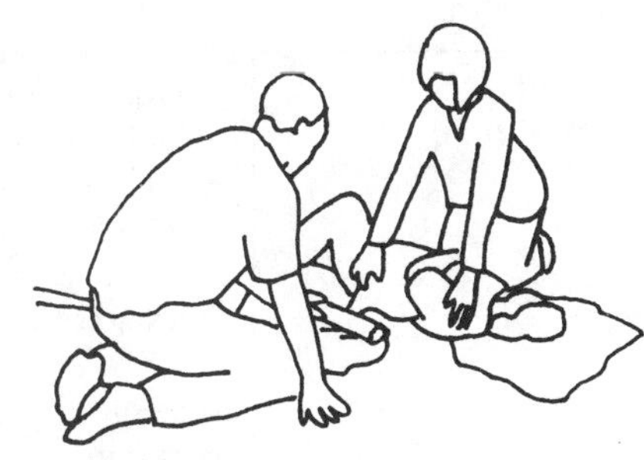
FIG 17.6a

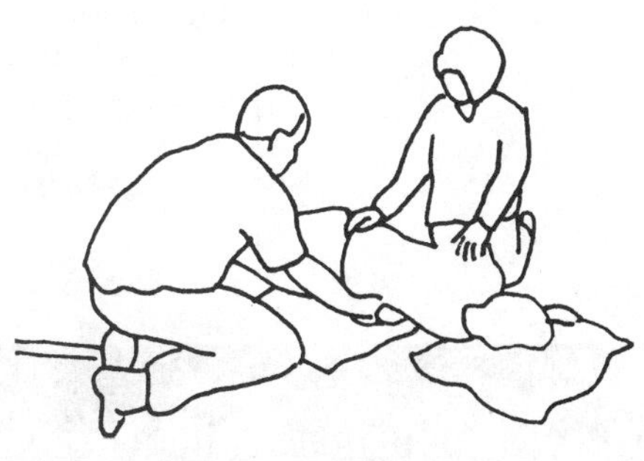
FIG 17.6b

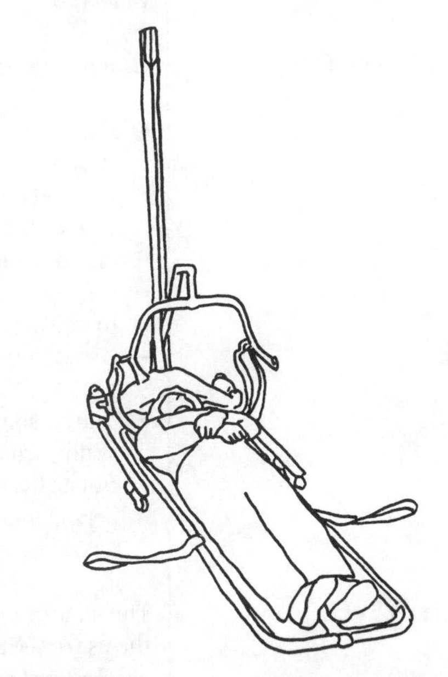
FIG 17.7a

	• The lead handler controls the move and gives the agreed commands. On the final command, the three handlers at the side of the person rock slightly back, tilting the person slightly to allow insertion of the stretcher. • This is repeated on the other side and the two parts of the stretcher are joined together. • The stretcher is connected to the hoist and the person is transferred onto a bed or trolley, (see option 2 in task 8, figures 17.16a-e).
SKILL LEVEL	The handlers need to be physically fit and must be able to kneel on the floor and rock backwards. This method involves a high level of skill and experience.
EVIDENCE AVAILABLE	*(Resuscitation Council (UK) 2001)*. Guidance for Safer Handling during Resuscitation in Hospitals, Resuscitation Council (UK).
DANGERS/ PRECAUTIONS	• The lead handler will control the turn and any instructions should be given by that person only, *(McCarthy 1998)*. • The holds and position adopted by the staff will depend on an individual assessment of the person. • The height and reach of the handlers may dictate which position, in relation to the person, they are allocated. Even slight flexion, extension or twisting of the spine may cause irreversible cord damage. The person must be moved as a single rigid movement *(Watson, Royle 1987)*. The handlers are in a full kneeling position for a short period of time. This means that the centre of gravity is behind the handler, increasing the force on their hamstrings, gluteal muscles and lumbar spine. This can be reduced by adopting a half kneeling position, where one foot is on the floor. However, if the handler's hips are not level, there is a risk of rotation of the lumbar spine. This posture also reduces the handler's reach. **NB** A manual handling risk assessment must be completed that is specific to the person and handlers.

Task Five

Use of an inflatable cushion to assist a person up from the floor

DEPENDENCY LEVEL	**Mobility Gallery A, B, C** **FIM 3**
DESCRIPTION	• Roll a person onto her side, as described in task four. • Roll up the side of the cushion, opposite to the air pipes, until it is rolled halfway. • Position the rolled up cushion so that the whole of the person's bottom is supported (figure 17.6b). • Roll the person onto her other side in order to unfurl the cushion (figure 17.8a). • Assist the person to sit forward (figure 17.13). • The person may need to be supported in sitting, from behind (figure 17.8b). • Inflate the cushion (figure 17.8c) until the person is in a position to safely stand or transfer.
SKILL LEVEL	The handler needs to have received training in the use of the equipment and to be physically able to kneel on the floor.

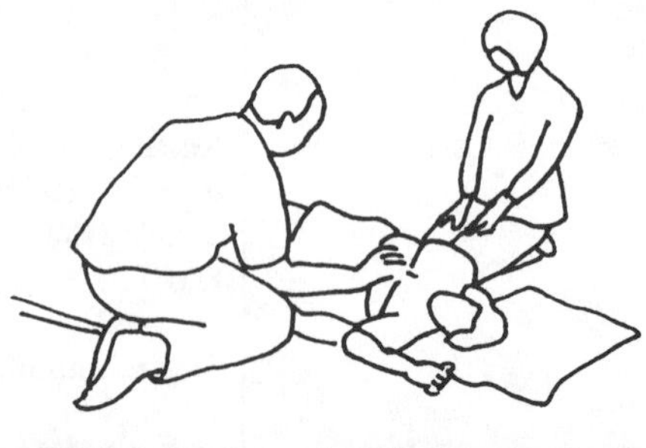

FIG 17.8a

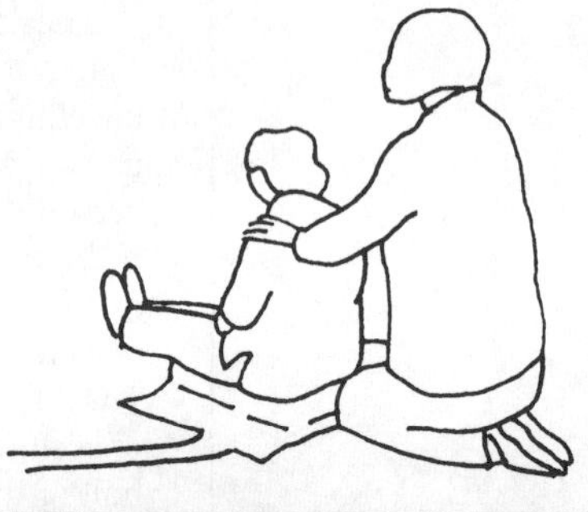

FIG 17.8b

EVIDENCE AVAILABLE

1 *(National Back Pain Association / Royal College of Nursing 1997/8)* The Guide to the Handling of Patients, 4th Edition, National Back Pain Association.
2 *(BackCare 1999)*, Safer Handling of People in the Community, National Back Pain Association.

DANGERS/ PRECAUTIONS

The person must have sitting balance and upper body control and be able to understand and follow instructions. This device cannot be used without the assistance of a handler.

FURTHER OPTIONS

Option 1 (Preferred)

Mobility Gallery A, B, C
FIM 5

- As an alternative to rolling the person onto the cushion, a slide sheet (either a loop or folded flat sheet) should be positioned under the person's bottom and on top of the cushion (figure 17.9a).
- The person should slide herself onto the cushion, in small stages (figure 17.9b).
- The slide sheet should be removed before the person is elevated.

Option 2

Mobility Gallery A, B, C
FIM 3

- The slide onto the cushion can be assisted by a handler kneeling behind the person.
- The handler holds the top layer of the slide sheet with both hands and starts off in a high kneeling position (figure 17.10a).
- The person slides backwards onto the cushion, as the handler rocks back onto their heels (figure 17.10b).

SKILL LEVEL

The handler needs to have received training in the use of the equipment and to be physically able to kneel on the floor and rock back on their heels.

DANGERS AND PRECAUTIONS

The person must have sitting balance and upper body strength and be able to understand and follow instructions.

NB
A manual handling risk assessment must be completed that is specific to the person and handlers.

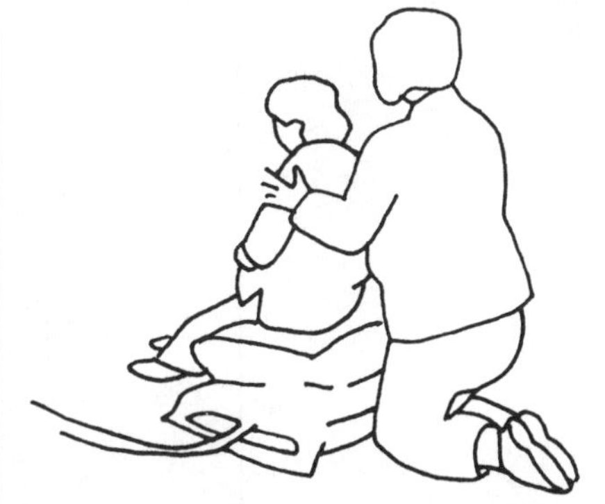

FIG 17.8c

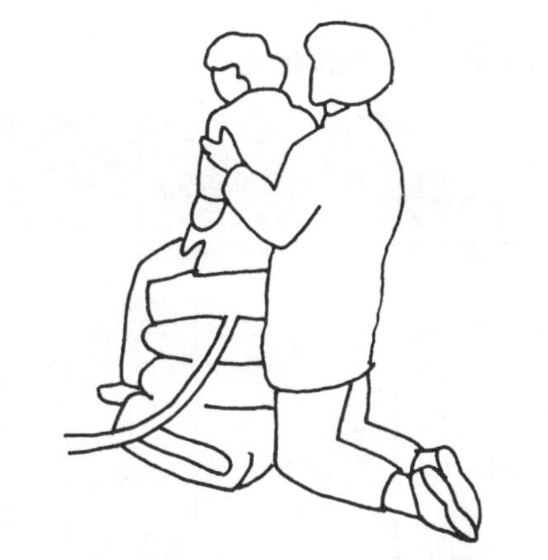

FIG 17.8d

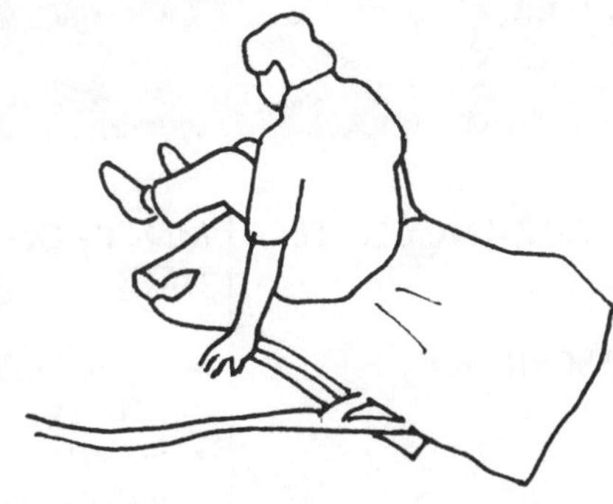

FIG 17.9a

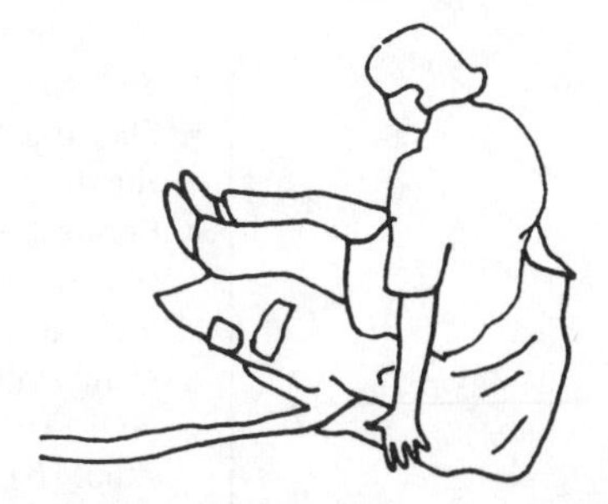

FIG 17.9b

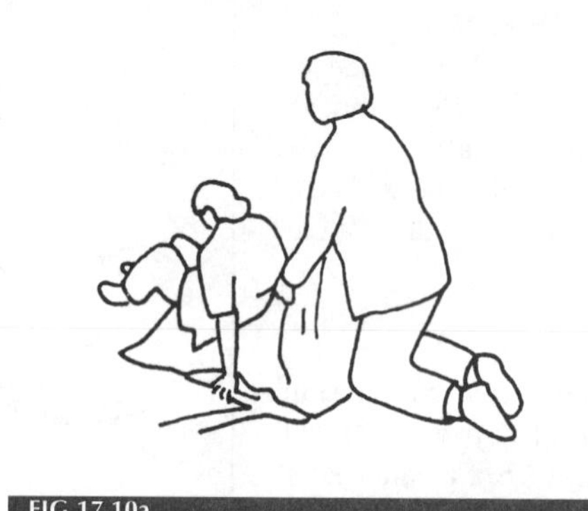
FIG 17.10a

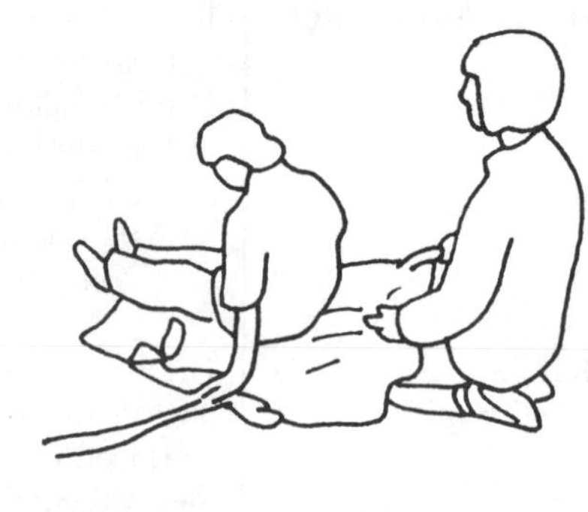
FIG 17.10b

Evidence review

Technique	REBA	Activity	Comfort	FIM	Mobility gallery	Skill level	Comment
USE OF AN INFLATABLE CUSHION TO ASSIST A PERSON UP FROM THE FLOOR							
Fig 17.8d	9	1	3	3	B	Competent	Inflatable cushion appears to have a lower REBA score but also requires a higher skill level
Fig 17.10a	10	2	9	3	C	Competent	Use of slide sheet to position person on an inflatable cushion – this method gives greater comfort and has a slightly higher risk level

Task Six

Use of an electric raiser

DEPENDENCY LEVEL

Mobility Gallery C
FIM 3

DESCRIPTION

- Roll the person onto her side and into the recovery position (see task four).
- Place the raiser behind the person, making sure there is sufficient space for it to roll and ensure the straps are easily accessible and free to slide under the person, (figure 17.11a).
- Slide the chest strap under the person's axilla using the extension strap, (figure 17.11b).
- Slide the thigh straps under the person.
- Slide the raiser against the person and pull the straps fully through.
- Connect the lower straps to the corresponding straps on the top of the raiser and tighten them so that the person is comfortable but cannot move, (figures 17.11 c and d). NOTE – the thigh straps should be secured diagonally across the person.
- Insert the roll bar into the square hole by

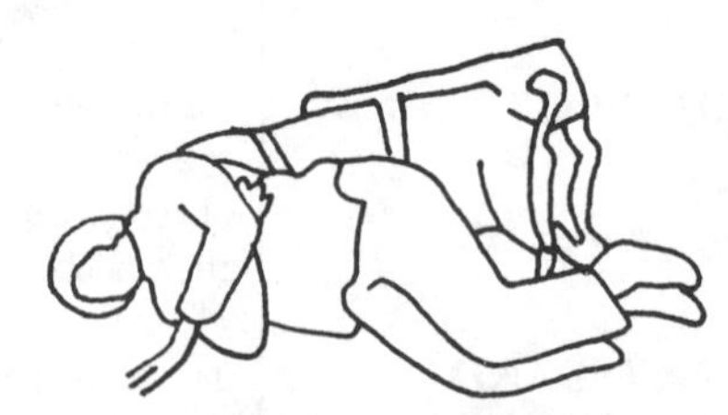
FIG 17.11a

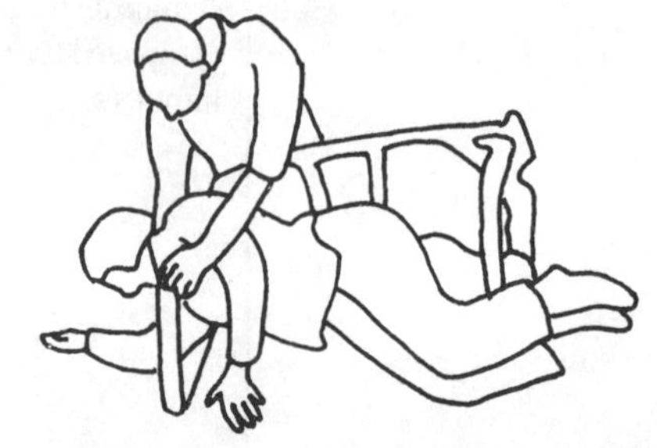
FIG 17.11b

the shoulders. The bar should face over the person.

- The handler should hold the lever and roll the person toward himself, ensuring he rocks back onto his heels as he does so, (figure 17.11e).
- Once the person is on her back, raise the person into a sitting position (figures 17.11f and g).

SKILL LEVEL

The handler must have had training in the use of this equipment.

DANGERS/ PRECAUTIONS

- As can be seen from figure 17.11c (below), inserting the straps may require the handler to lean over the person. It is preferable to insert the straps and then go around to the front of the person, assuming there is sufficient room, and attach and secure them from that position.
- As the equipment assists the person into a sitting position, the person needs to have the ability to stand or to have sitting balance to facilitate a lateral transfer.
- Additional assistance may be identified from the assessment.

NB

A manual handling risk assessment must be completed that is specific to the person and handlers.

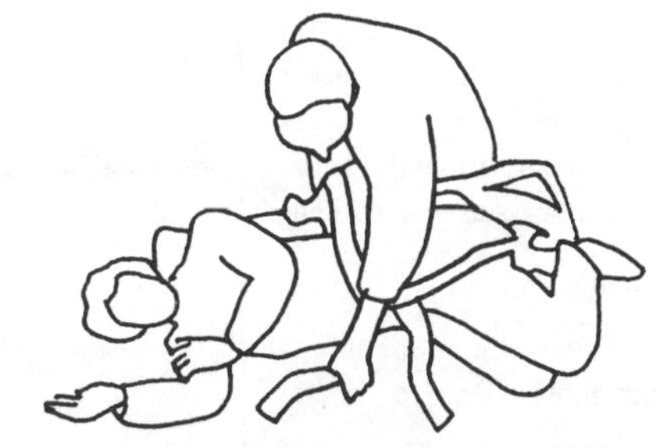

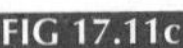

FIG 17.11c

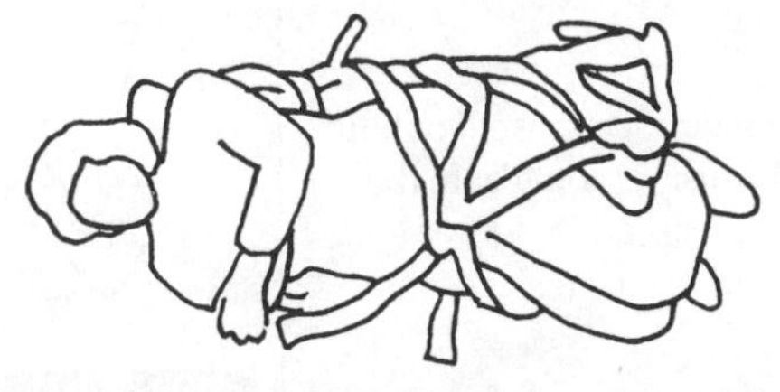

FIG 17.11d

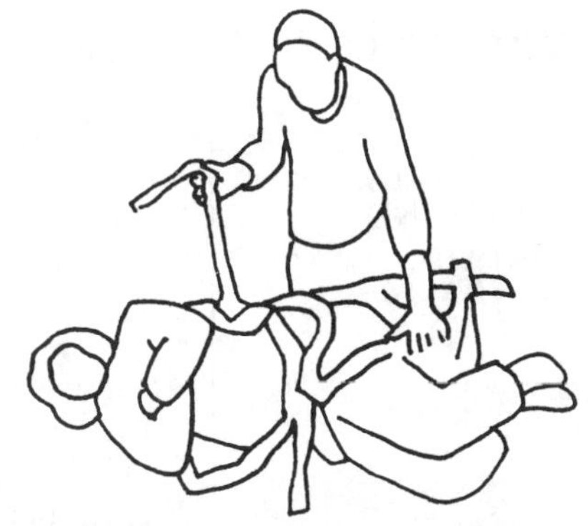

FIG 17.11e

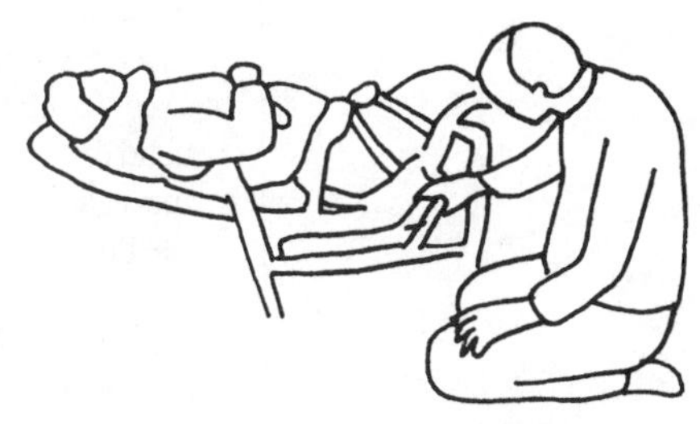

FIG 17.11f

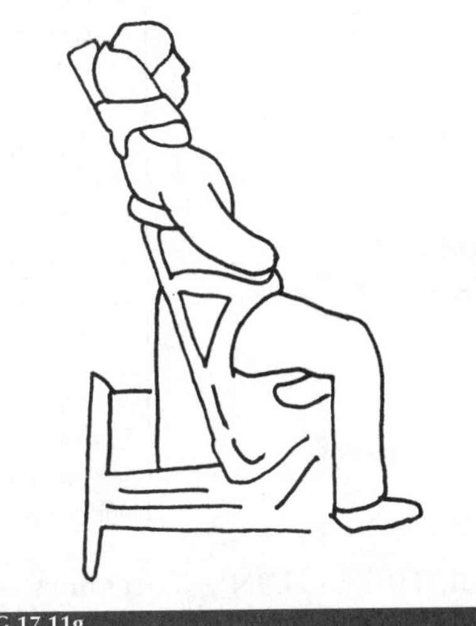

FIG 17.11g

Evidence review

Technique	REBA	Activity	Comfort	FIM	Mobility gallery	Skill level	Comment
USE OF AN ELECTRIC RAISER							
Fig 17.11c	12	–	–	3	C	Proficient	

Task Seven

Inserting a fabric sling under a person

INDEPENDENCE

Mobility Gallery B, C, D, E
FIM 1, 2

DESCRIPTION, OPTIONS AND VARIATIONS

Method

Inserting the sling – The person is unable to sit forward.

- If the person is able to roll, roll the person onto their side and insert a rolled up sling halfway under them. Roll back onto the sling and turn in the other direction, completely unfurling the sling, (see task four for rolling technique).
- If the person is unable to roll the sling can be inserted from the head, neck or waist.
- A handler must be on each side of the person.
- Insert two rolled up flat slide sheets / loop sheets under the person, either from the head or foot end and gently unroll them.
- Insert a sling between the two sheets, from the head end and pull them towards the person's sacrum, ensuring the sling is even both sides. As the sling is slid between the sheets, the handlers must rock back on to their heels, (figure 17.12b).
- This will need to be repeated until the sling is in place. The handlers will need to move down each time.
- Once the sling is in place, remove the top sheet by turning it under itself and slide it out.

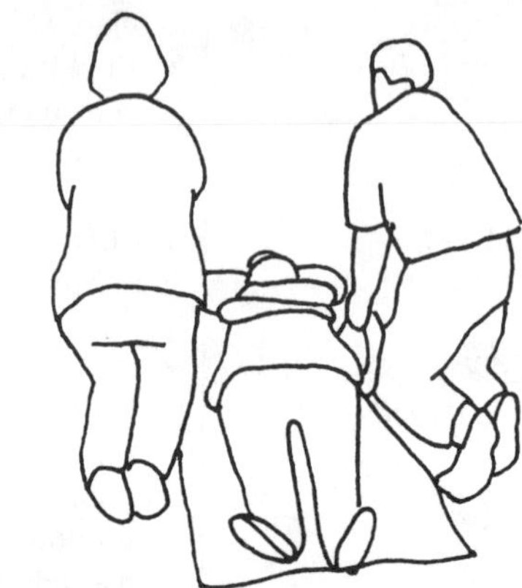

FIG 17.12a

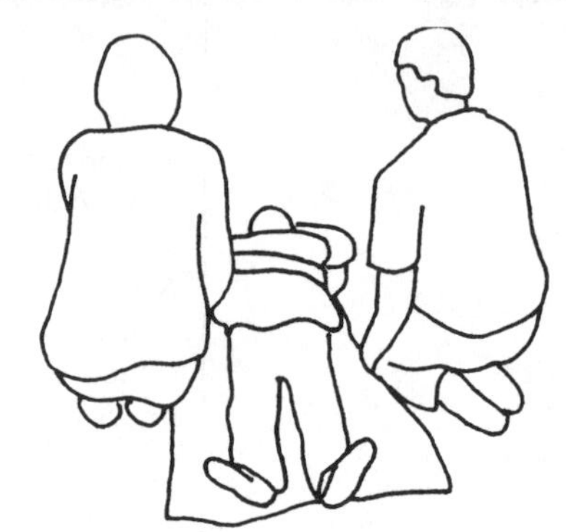

FIG 17.12b

SKILL LEVEL

Medium level of skill – The handlers must be able to sit back on their heels.

DANGERS TO THE HANDLER

The handlers must ensure that they minimise the amount of spinal rotation, when inserting the sling.

When unrolling the slide sheets, avoid pulling upwards as this will cause discomfort to the person and increase the amount of force and effort required to carry out the task.

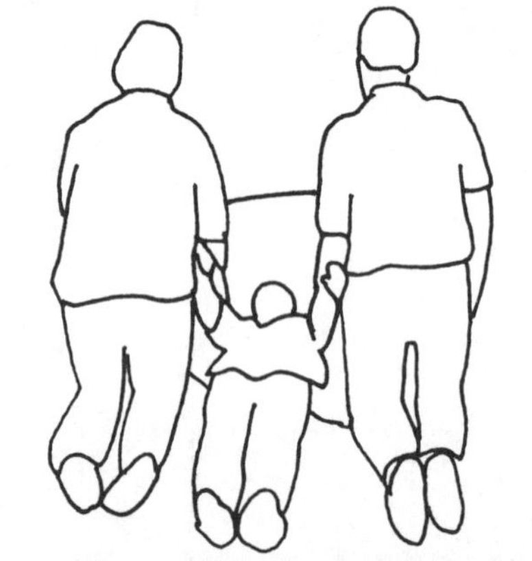

FIG 17.13a

FURTHER OPTION

Option

Sitting the person forward to insert the sling using the elbow to elbow grip, (the person must have strength in both arms).

Mobility Gallery remains the same
FIM 3

- If the person is able, their knees should be in a slightly flexed position to reduce possible abdominal discomfort.
- With a handler at each side of the person,

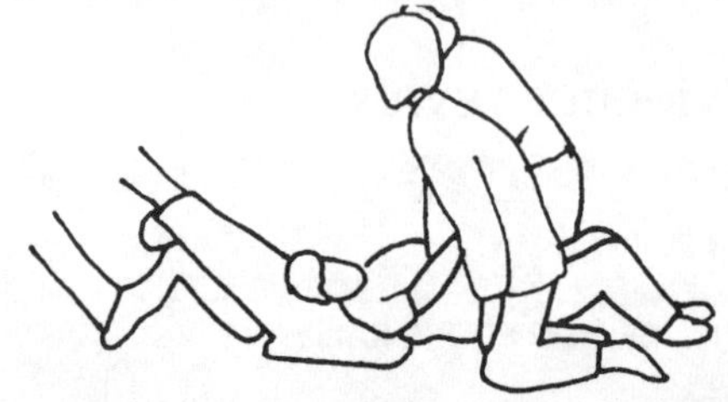

FIG 17.13b

the handlers take hold of the person's nearest arm at the elbow, using their nearest arm. (figures 17.13 a and b)

- The handlers will start in a high kneeling position.
- Each handler rocks back on to their heels, as the person sits up, (figures 17.13 c and d).
- One of the handlers supports the person by kneeling beside the person with the shoulder nearest to the person supporting them, (figure 17.13e).
- The hoist sling is placed behind the person
- An upturned chair can then be used to support the person whilst a hoist is being collected (figure 17.13f).

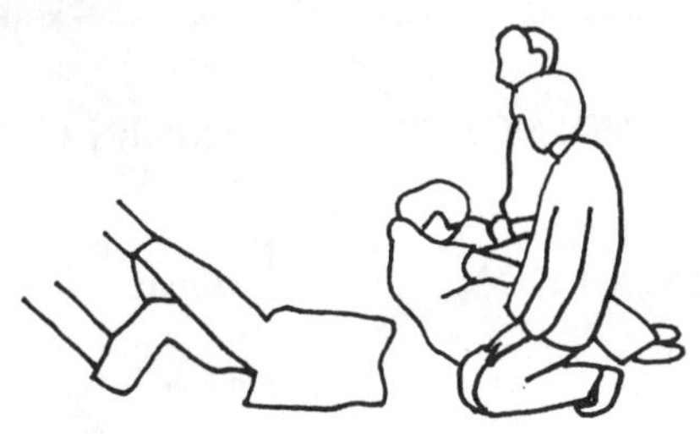

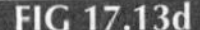

FIG 17.13d

SKILL LEVEL

Medium level of skill – The handlers must be able to rock back on to their heels.

DANGERS TO THE HANDLER

- If the person falls back, this may result in an injury to the handler(s). The person may also injure the handlers when pulling up on their arms.
- Once in the seated position, if the person falls back or moves, this may result in an injury to the handlers.

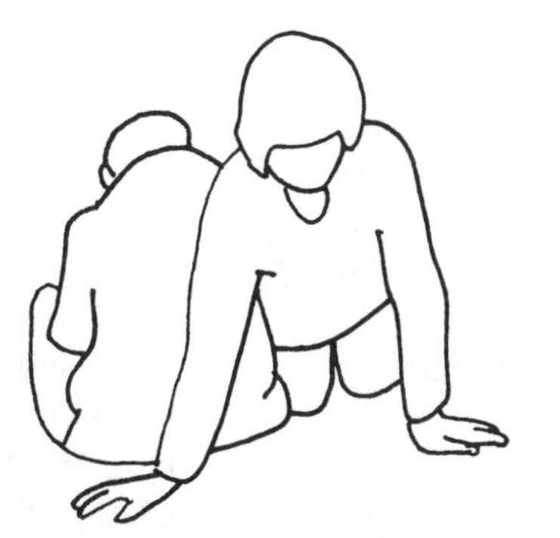

FIG 17.13e

NB

A manual handling risk assessment must be completed that is specific to the person and handlers.

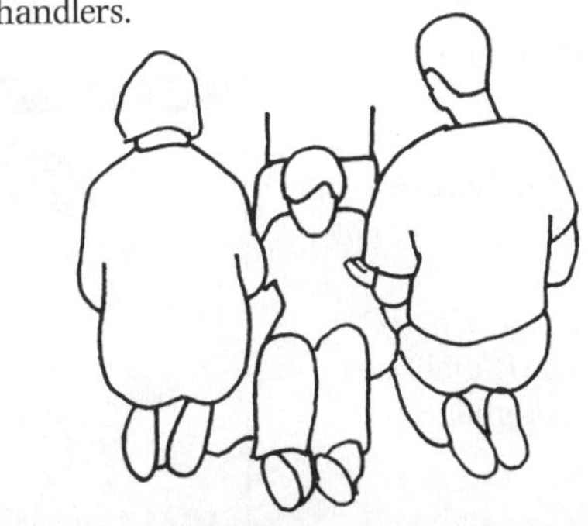

FIG 17.13c

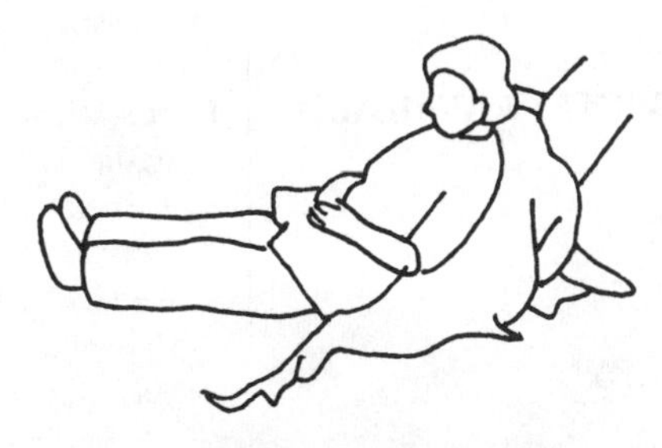

FIG 17.13f

Evidence review

Technique	REBA	Activity	Comfort	FIM	Mobility gallery	Skill level	Comment
INSERTING A FABRIC SLING UNDER A PERSON							
Fig 17.12b	9	5	8	2	C	Advanced beginner	There is not a big difference between these techniques. Sitting the person forward requires greater activity and has slightly lower postural risk. Slide sheet is used with a less able person.
Fig 17.13d	8	1	7	1	E	Advanced beginner	

Task Eight

Hoisting from the floor

DEPENDENCY LEVEL

Mobility Gallery B, C, D, E
FIM 1

DESCRIPTION

Hoisting from a sitting position

- Position the hoist sling under the person, as described in task seven.
- If the person has the ability to sit forward, against an upturned chair, (refer to task three), the hoist can be brought in from the side.
- One leg of the hoist is positioned under the chair. The other is under the person's bent knees, (figure 17.14a).
- If using hoists with looped slings, the sling needs to be connected using shorter loops at the shoulders and longer loops at the legs. This enables the person to be transferred in a sitting position.
- If using hoist slings with clip connectors, once the person has been raised, the spreader bar can be used to adjust the person's position.
- The person can then be lifted and transferred into a bedchair.

SKILL LEVEL

The handler must have had training in the use of a hoist.

EVIDENCE AVAILABLE

1 *(BackCare 1999)* Safer Handling of People in the Community, National Back Pain Association.
2 *(National Back Pain Association/BackCare 1997/8)* The Guide to the Handling of Patients, 4th Edition, National Back Pain Association.

DANGERS/ PRECAUTIONS

- There must be sufficient space available at the side of the person to position the hoist.
- The person needs to be able to bend their knees.
- The person must have sitting balance.
- This technique should not be used following successful resuscitation on the floor. The sitting position may increase chest and gastric pressure, resulting in reduced efficiency of ventilation (*Resuscitation Council (UK) 2001*).
- The brakes of the hoist need to be off during the hoisting procedure. This will enable the hoist to maintain its balance.

FURTHER OPTIONS

Option 1
Hoisting from a lying position

Mobility Gallery and FIM remain the same

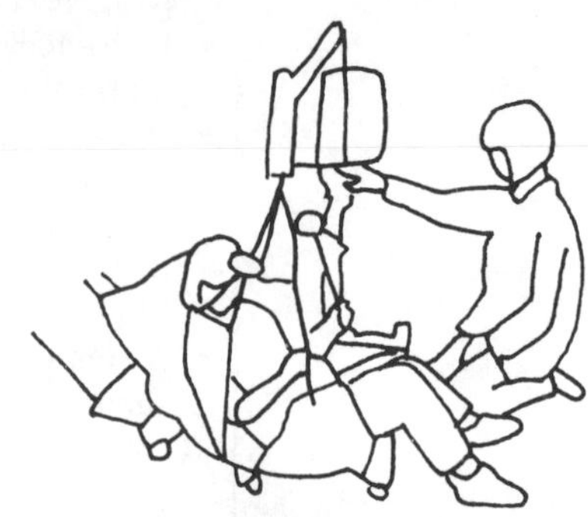

FIG 17.14a

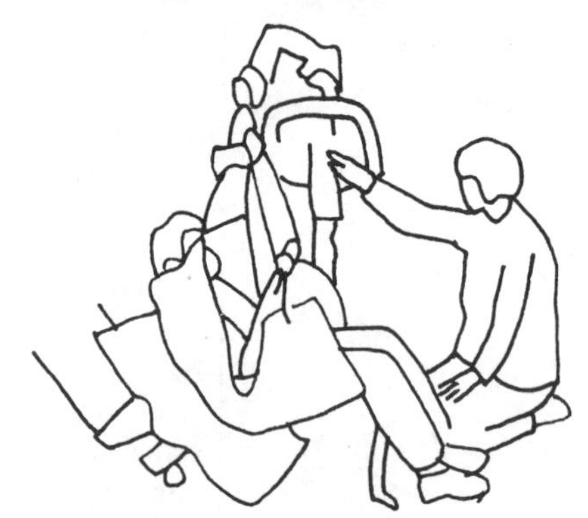

FIG 17.14b

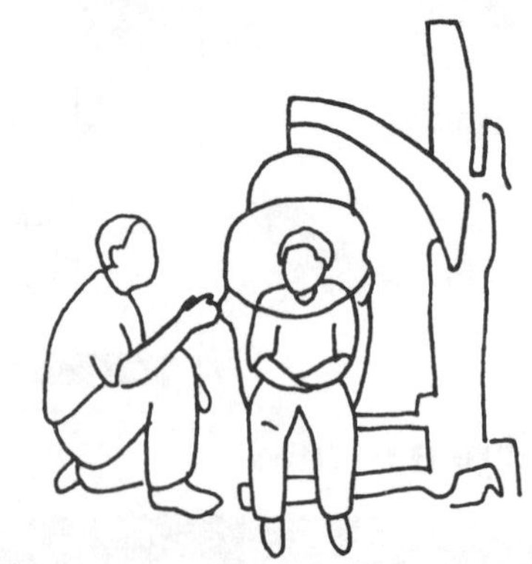

FIG 17.14c

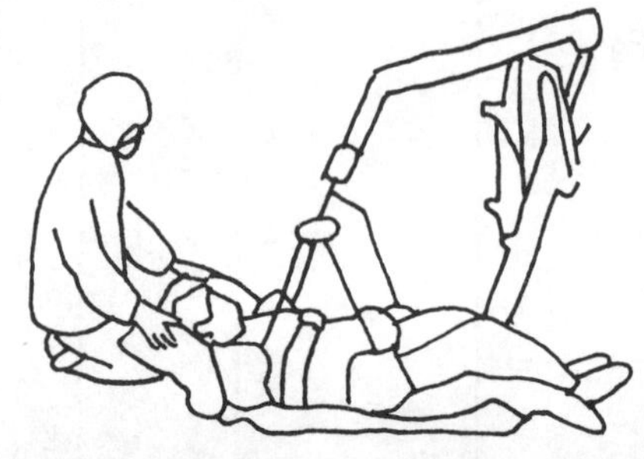

FIG 17.15a

DESCRIPTION

- Position the hoist sling under the person as described in task seven.
- The hoist is brought in from the person's foot end.
- The person's legs will need to be lifted over one side of the base (a pillow should be placed between the person's legs and the base to prevent discomfort).
- If using hoists with looped slings, the sling needs to be connected using long loops at the shoulders and legs.
- The person can then be lifted and transferred into bed.

SKILL LEVEL

The handler must have had training in the use of a hoist.

EVIDENCE AVAILABLE

1 *(BackCare 1999)* Safer Handling of People in the Community, National Back Pain Association
2 *(National Back Pain Association/BackCare 1997/8)* The Guide to the Handling of Patients, 4th Edition, National Back Pain Association.
3 *(Resuscitation Council (UK) 2001).* Guidance for Safer Handling during Resuscitation in Hospitals, Resuscitation Council (UK).

DANGERS/ PRECAUTIONS

- The handler must check that the sling is compatible with the hoist.
- If the sling has no head support, the handler may need to support the person's head (figure 17.15a).

Option 2
Use of a stretcher hoist

Mobility Gallery and FIM remain the same.

- The assessment of the person will dictate the number of handlers required, when using the stretcher hoist. There must be a minimum of two, regardless of the person's condition.
- The person must be rolled to position the stretcher attachment, (see task four), except when using a slat stretcher.
- For a slat stretcher, the slats can be inserted without moving the person.
- The hoist is positioned at the head end and the head straps are connected to the hoist, (figure 17.16c).
- The hoist is raised until there is sufficient clearance to position the hoist fully under the stretcher, to connect the remaining straps, (figure 17.16d).
- The person is then lifted and transferred onto a bed or trolley, (figure 17.16e).

A scoop stretcher is depicted above. There are,

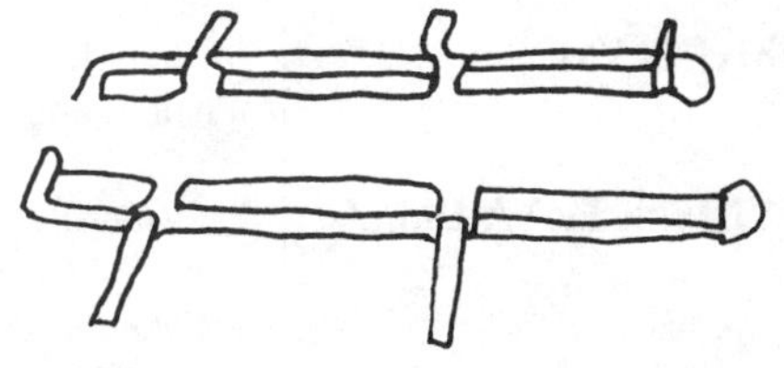

FIG 17.16a

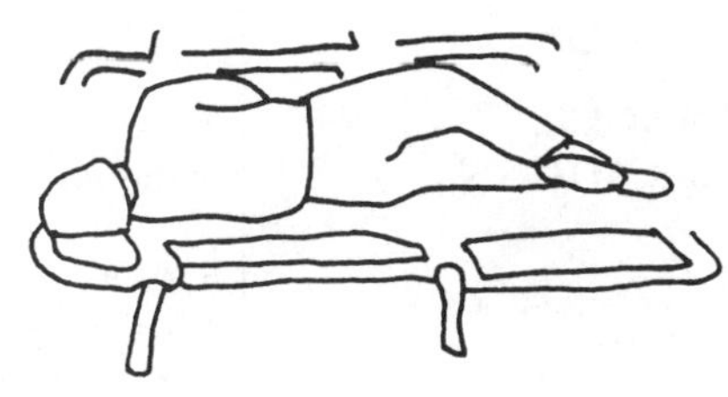

FIG 17.16b

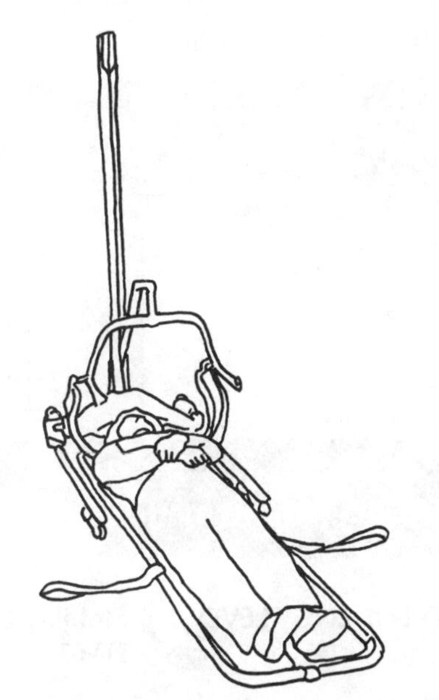

FIG 17.16c

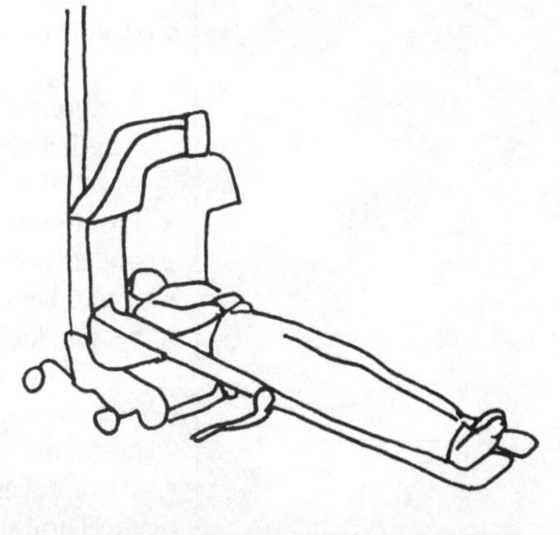

FIG 17.16d

however, fabric and slat stretchers available.

SKILL LEVEL

The handler must have had training in the use of a hoist and any particular attachment.

EVIDENCE AVAILABLE

1 *(National Back Pain Association/BackCare (1997/8)* The Guide to the Handling of Patients, 4th Edition, National Back Pain Association.
2 *(Resuscitation Council (UK) 2001)*. Guidance for Safer Handling during Resuscitation in Hospitals, Resuscitation Council (UK).

DANGERS/ PRECAUTIONS

The handlers must ensure that the two parts of the scoop are connected securely.

NB
A manual handling risk assessment must be completed that is specific to the person and handlers.

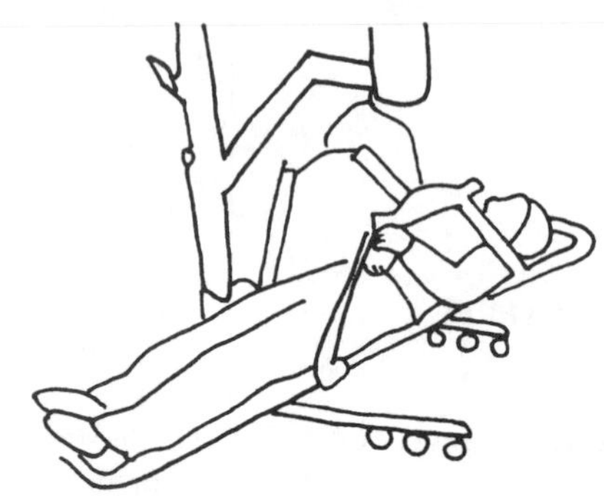

FIG 17.16e

Evidence review

Technique	REBA	Activity	Comfort	FIM	Mobility gallery	Skill level	Comment
HOISTING FROM THE FLOOR							
Fig 17.14b	10	1	5	1	E	Proficient	
Fig 17.15a	9	1	5	1	E	Proficient	

Task Nine

Hoisting from a mattress on the floor

DEPENDENCY LEVEL

Mobility Gallery B, C, D, E
FIM 1

DESCRIPTION

Persons at a high risk of falling may be nursed on a mattress on the floor, as a temporary measure until a bed can be provided which adjusts to a very low level. The following procedure can be used to raise the person.

- Position either two flat slide sheets or full length loop sheets under the person, (see task seven).
- Position the hoist sling under the person and on top of the slide sheet.
- A handler must be on either side of the person, facing the head end with their inner knee placed on the mattress at the person's hip level, in a high kneeling position, (figure 17.17a).
- The handlers hold the top layer of the slide sheet and slide the person down the mattress in small stages, by rocking back

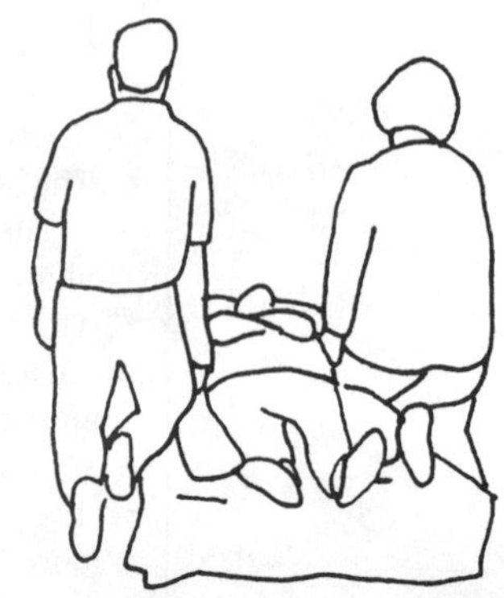

FIG 17.17a

onto their heels. At each stage, the handlers must move down the mattress and reposition themselves.

- The movement must finish with the person's buttocks positioned at the foot end of the mattress, (figure 17.17b).
- The hoist is brought in from the foot end of the mattress, with one hoist leg parallel to one side of the mattress and the other hoist leg just under the other bottom corner of the mattress. The legs of the hoist must be at their widest, (figure 17.17c).
- If using hoists with looped slings, the sling needs to be connected using long loops at the shoulders and legs.
- The person can then be lifted and transferred.

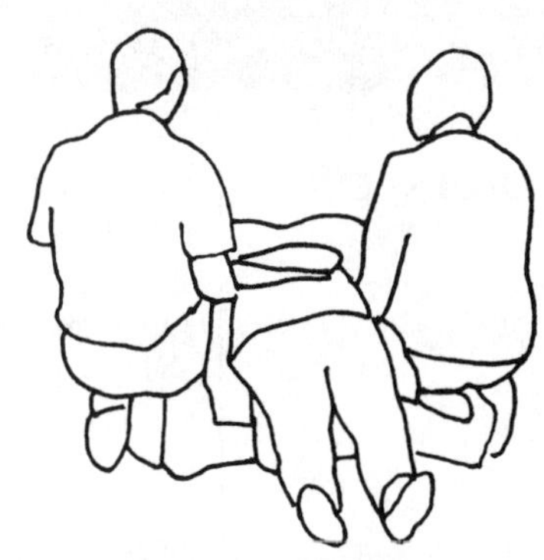

FIG 17.17b

SKILL LEVEL

The handlers must have received training in the use of a hoist.

DANGERS/ PRECAUTIONS

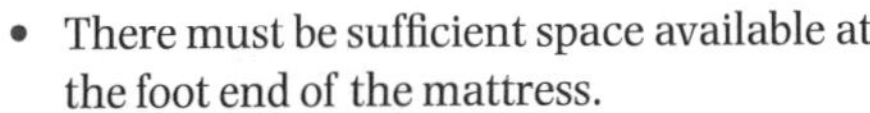

- There must be sufficient space available at the foot end of the mattress.
- Caring for people on a mattress on the floor, creates a high risk of injury to staff due to the fixed postures staff are forced to adopt.
- The brakes of the hoist need to be off during the hoisting procedure. This will enable the hoist to maintain its balance.

NB
A manual handling risk assessment must be completed that is specific to the person and handlers.

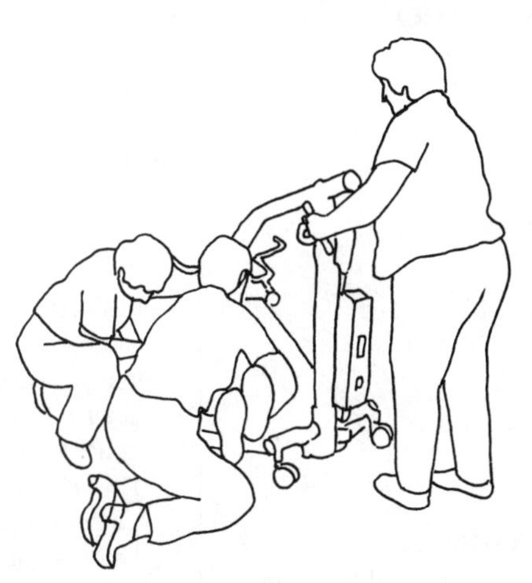

FIG 17.17c

Evidence review

Technique	REBA	Activity	Comfort	FIM	Mobility gallery	Skill level	Comment
HOISTING FROM A MATTRESS ON THE FLOOR							
Fig 17.17c	12	1	8	1	E	Advanced beginner	Inserting a sling with a mattress on the floor gives a higher REBA score.

Task Ten

Management of a person who has fallen in a confined space

INDEPENDENCE

Mobility Gallery A, B, C, D, E
FIM 1

Although independent people may have the ability to get up from the floor with minimal supervision, if they have fallen in a confined space, there is unlikely to be sufficient room for the person to roll over and get up onto all fours.

DESCRIPTION, OPTIONS AND VARIATIONS

It is relatively common for people to fall by the side of a toilet or bath, for example, and become wedged between fixed furniture. The handler should examine the person for any injuries and check that the person has not suffered a cardiac or respiratory arrest. If the person has not arrested, the following procedure should be undertaken.

- Roll the person as far as the space allows, to insert a full length loop slide sheet or two flat slide sheets. Alternatively, place a folded slide sheet(s) under the person's head or feet and unfurl the slide sheet(s) under the length of the person's body.
- The person's head will need to be supported by one handler (figure 17.18a). This may necessitate the handler kneeling or sitting on the toilet lid, if the person has fallen by the toilet.
- Depending on the assessment of the person and environment, one or two handlers should kneel at one end of the person, nearest the open space, holding the top layer of the slide sheet, in a high kneeling position (figure 17.18b)
- On the commands, the handler(s) rock back on their heels, to slide the person out of the confined space, in small stages. The other handler should continue to support the person's head (figure 17.18c)
- Once the person is in an open area, the person can be instructed to get up from the floor or a suitable mechanical device can be used.

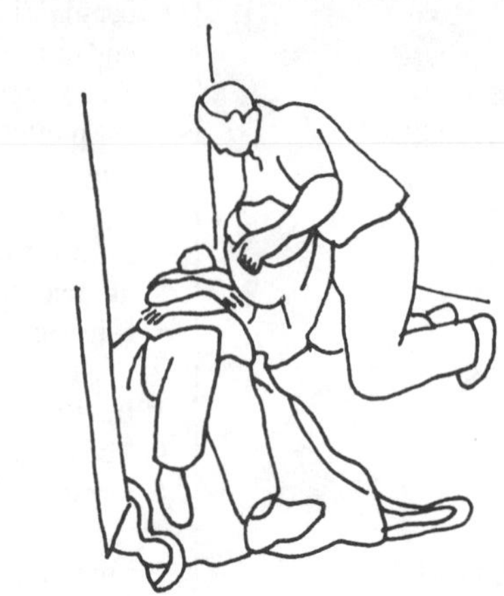

FIG 17.18a

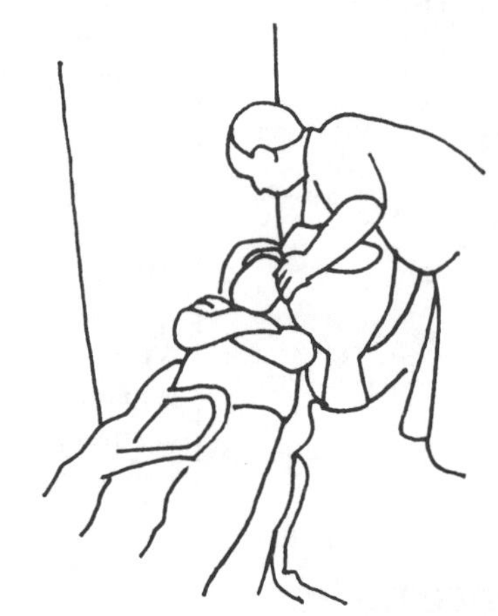

FIG 17.18b

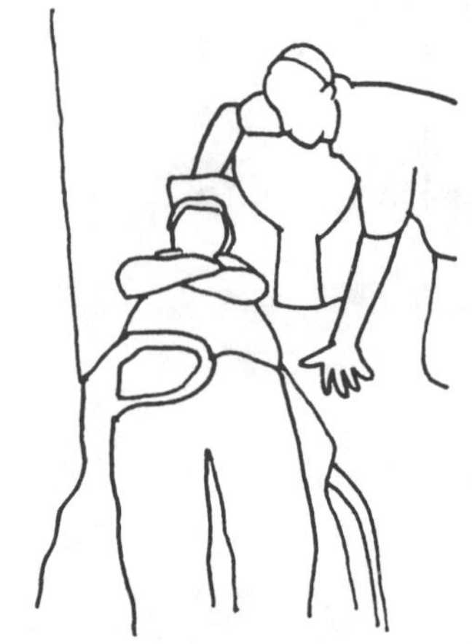

FIG 17.18c

SKILL LEVEL

The handlers need to have received training in the use of the slide sheet(s) and have the physical ability to kneel on the floor and rock back on their heels.

EVIDENCE AVAILABLE

(Resuscitation Council (UK) 2001). Guidance for Safer Handling during Resuscitation in Hospitals, Resuscitation Council (UK).

DANGERS/ PRECAUTIONS

The handler supporting the person's head is unlikely to be in the optimum position. This

handler should ensure that they adopts the best position possible, in the space available.
NB
A manual handling risk assessment must be completed that is specific to the person and handlers.

Evidence review

Technique	REBA	Activity	Comfort	FIM	Mobility gallery	Skill level	Comment
MANAGEMENT OF PERSON WHO HAS FALLEN IN A CONFINED SPACE							
Fig 17.8a	11	1	4	1	E	Novice	

Task Eleven

Manual lifting of small children from the floor

DEPENDENCY LEVEL

Mobility Gallery A, B, C, D, E
FIM 1

DESCRIPTION

- A small child may be manually lifted from the floor by one handler.
- The handler starts in a kneeling position on one or both knees, to one side of the child.
- One hand is placed under the child's hips. The other hand is placed under the child's neck and shoulders, (figure 17.19a).
- The child is lifted towards the handler's chest or onto their lap and the handler then stands, (figure 17.19b).

SKILL LEVEL

Low level of skill. The handler must be physically able to kneel on the floor.

EVIDENCE AVAILABLE

(Royal College of Nursing/National Back Pain Association 1997/8) The Guide to the Handling of Patients, 4th Edition, National Back Pain Association.

DANGERS/ PRECAUTIONS

- The child may be unpredictable and should be handled with care.
- The assessment needs to be continually reviewed, as the child becomes older and heavier. The numerical guidelines for lifting and lowering *(HSE 2004)* should be used as an indicator to determine when mechanical equipment should be used e.g. hoist, inflatable cushion.

FURTHER OPTION

Option
Mobility Gallery and FIM remain the same

- A transfer scoop can be used to facilitate an improved handhold, particularly with

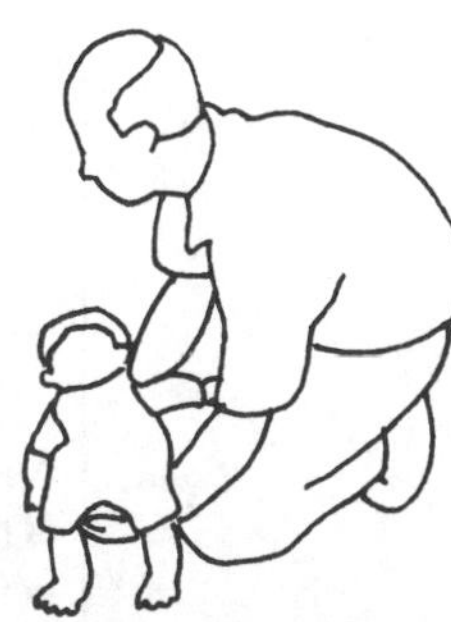

FIG 17.19a

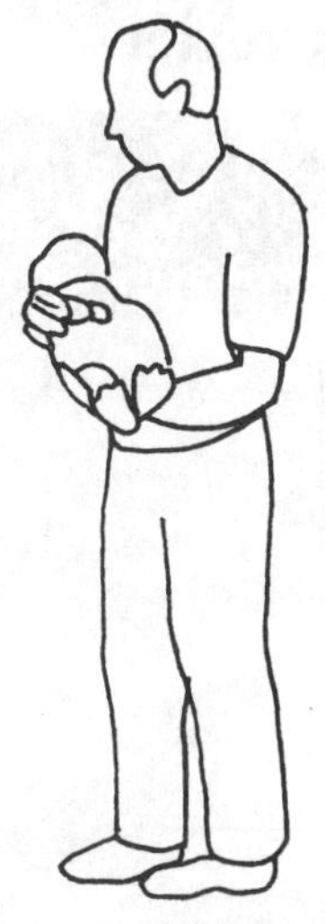

FIG 17.19b

The falling and fallen person and emergency handling

children with low muscle tone.
- The scoop can provide head support and options include firmer leg support.
- The person will be rolled into the scoop, (see task 4).
- The chest strap should be fastened securely.
- The leg supports should be passed underneath both legs, in order to support the thighs, (figure 17.20a).
- A handler should crouch on each side of the child, holding the back and leg handles of the scoop, (figure 17.20b).
- The handlers' starting position will be with one leg in front of the other, to maintain a stable base, (figure 17.20b).
- On the command, the handlers will stand, lifting the child from the floor.

SKILL LEVEL

The handlers should have knowledge and training in the use of the equipment and be able to stand from a crouched position.

DANGERS/ PRECAUTIONS

- The child may be unpredictable and should be handled with care.
- The assessment needs to be continually reviewed, as the child becomes older and heavier. The numerical guidelines for lifting and lowering *(HSE 2004*–see appendix 4*)* should be used as an indicator to determine when mechanical equipment should be used e.g. hoist, inflatable cushion.
- If the child hyperextends, or has a seizure or erratic movements, and the chest strap is not securely fastened, there is a risk that they may slide out of the scoop.

NB
A manual handling risk assessment must be completed that is specific to the person and handlers.

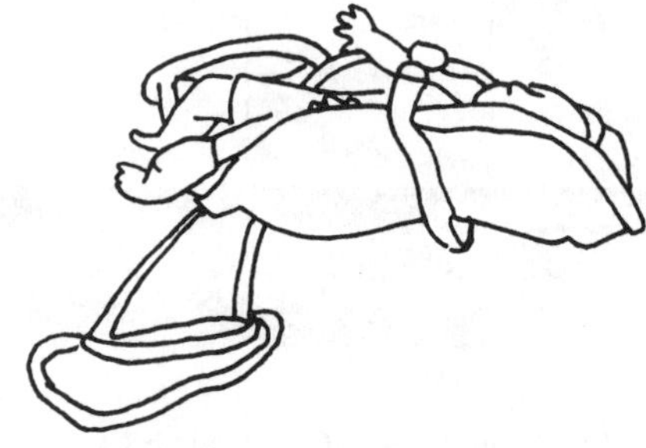

FIG 17.20a

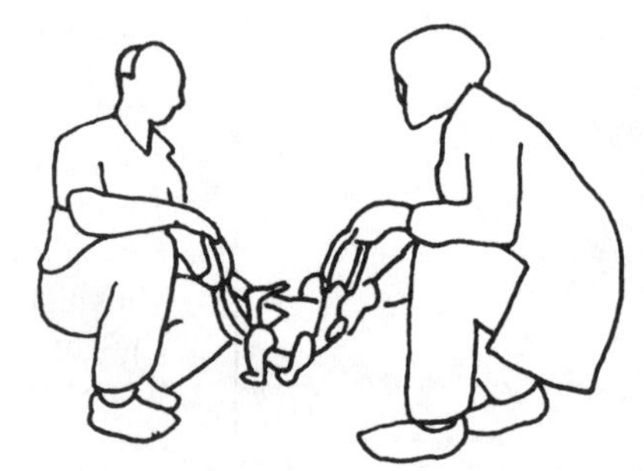

FIG 17.20b

Evidence review

Technique	REBA	Activity	Comfort	FIM	Mobility gallery	Skill level	Comment
MANUAL LIFTING OF SMALL CHILDREN FROM THE FLOOR							
Fig 17.19a	11	1	10	1	E	Novice	
Fig 17.20b	6	1	8	1	E	Novice	Less postural risk when using a scoop

Task Twelve

Manual lifting of an adult in an emergency

DEPENDENCY LEVEL	**Mobility Gallery** A, B, C, D, E **FIM 1**
DESCRIPTION	This is a high risk activity and should only be undertaken in life threatening or exceptional circumstances, where no other option is available. • The person should be rolled, (see task four) to position a transfer or lifting sheet underneath them a wider sheet will improve the handler's posture at the start of the lift. • There must be a minimum of seven staff for this procedure. • Three members of staff are positioned on each side of the person and hold the edge of the transfer sheet with both hands. • The seventh member of staff will bring in the trolley from the foot or head end of the person. • The handlers' starting position will be with one leg in front of the other, to maintain a stable base. • On the command, the six handlers will stand, in unison, keeping the person as close to them as possible. • The seventh handler will then bring in the trolley.
SKILL LEVEL	High level of physical fitness.
EVIDENCE AVAILABLE	*(Resuscitation Council (UK) 2001)*. Guidance for safer handling during resuscitation in hospitals, Resuscitation Council (UK).
DANGERS/ PRECAUTIONS	• A bed should not be used, as this will cause the handlers to hold the person at arms length, increasing the risk of injury. • The handlers will be taking all of the person's body weight, increasing the risk of injury to the handlers. The handlers are also lifting from below mid lower leg height. • The safe working load of the transfer / lifting sheet should be checked, to ensure that the weight of the person does not exceed it. • Following this procedure, a full risk assessment should be undertaken, as it is foreseeable that a similar incident will occur. Suitable mechanical equipment must be provided. **NB** A manual handling risk assessment must be completed that is specific to the person and handlers.

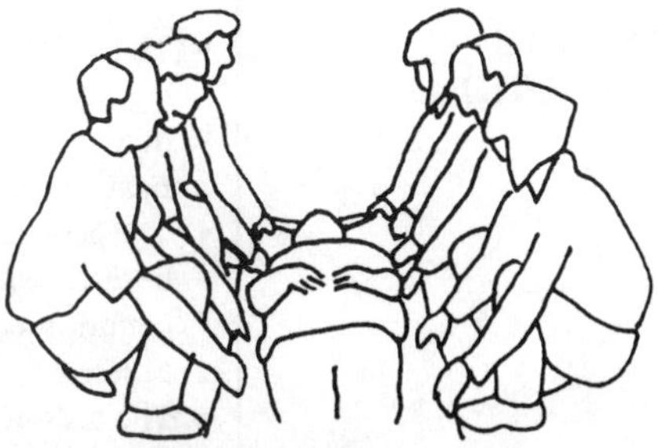

FIG 17.21a

Evidence review

Technique	REBA	Activity	Comfort	FIM	Mobility gallery	Skill level	Comment
MANUAL LIFTING OF AN ADULT IN AN EMERGENCY							
Fig 17.21.a	10	1	9	1	E	Proficient	

Task Thirteen

Emergency evacuation down stairs

DEPENDENCY LEVEL

Mobility Gallery A,B,C,D,E
FIM 1

DESCRIPTION

These are high risk activities and should only be undertaken in life threatening or exceptional circumstances, e.g. fire, where horizontal evacuation is not possible.

- Transfer the person onto an evacuation chair using the appropriate manoeuvre, (see chapter 14).
- Strap the person into the chair and tilt the chair back, (figure 17.22a)
- A second handler is required to support the foot end of the chair, as the person is taken down the stairs.
- The evacuation chair should be slowly rolled off of each step, controlling the speed of the descent.

There are other versions of this chair, including ones with tracks or skis.

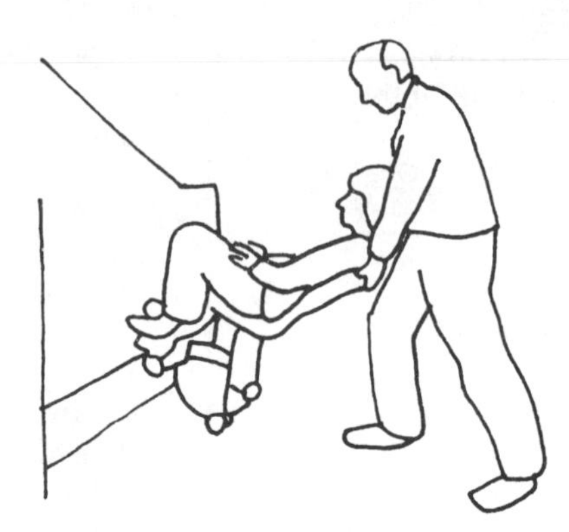

FIG 17.22a

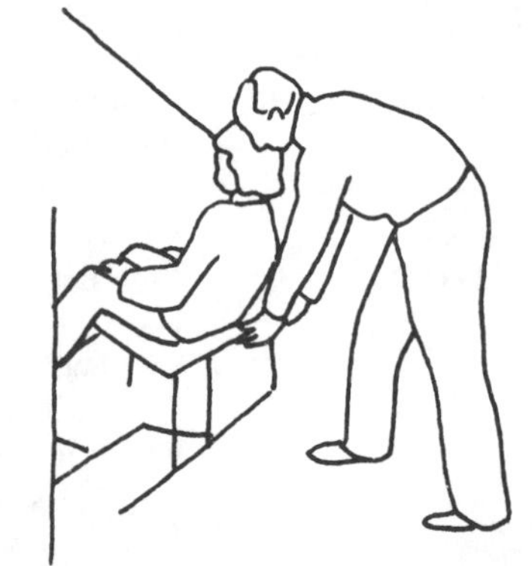

FIG 17.22b

SKILL LEVEL

The handler must have received training in this manoeuvre and be physically fit.

EVIDENCE AVAILABLE

(Royal College of Nursing/National Back Pain Association (1997/8) The Guide to the Handling of Patients, 4th Edition, National Back Pain Association.

DANGERS/ PRECAUTIONS

- The speed of the descent needs to be carefully controlled. It will be more difficult to control the speed with a heavier person.
- The person may find this manoeuvre to be distressing and the handler must communicate with the person at all times.
- The person must not exceed the safe working load of the chair.

FURTHER OPTION

Option

Carrying a supine person up or down stairs

- The person should be rolled, (see task four) to position a transfer or lifting sheet underneath them.
- The number of staff required for this manoeuvre will be dependant on the available space. However, there must be an absolute minimum of four staff.
- The positioning of the handlers will depend on the angle of ascent / descent and the available space.
- The handlers' starting position will be with one leg in front of the other, to maintain a stable base.

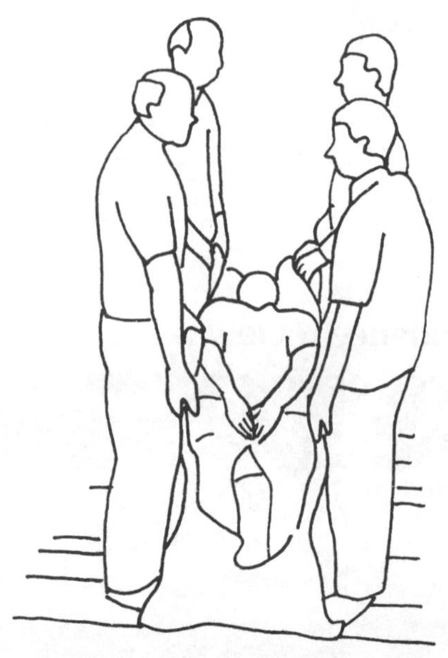

FIG 17.23a

- On the command, the handlers will stand, in unison, keeping the person as close to them as possible.
- The handler at the front, (in the direction of travel), should control the manoeuvre.
- This manoeuvre should be planned so that the person is only carried a minimal distance.

SKILL LEVEL

The handler must have received training in this manoeuvre. The handler must be physically fit.

EVIDENCE AVAILABLE

(Meek 2004). Manual Handling. Solutions, Training and Advisory Ltd.

DANGERS/ PRECAUTIONS

- The handlers will be taking all of the person's body weight, increasing the risk of injury to the handlers.
- The safe working load of the transfer / lifting sheet should be checked, to ensure that the weight of the person does not exceed it.
- Following this procedure, a full risk assessment should be undertaken, as it is foreseeable that a similar incident will occur. Suitable mechanical equipment must be provided.

NB
A manual handling risk assessment must be completed that is specific to the person and handlers.

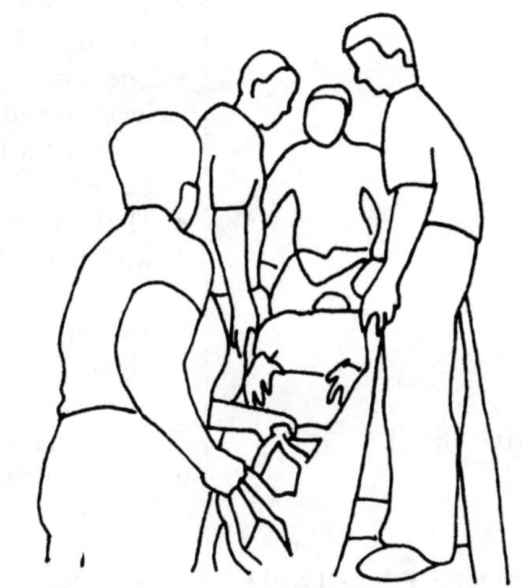

FIG 17.23b

Evidence review

Technique	REBA	Activity	Comfort	FIM	Mobility gallery	Skill level	Comment
EMERGENCY EVACUATION DOWN STAIRS – USING A FIRE BLANKET							
Fig 17.23a	5	1	–	1	E	Advanced beginner	

Task Fourteen

Chair to floor in an emergency

DEPENDENCY LEVEL

Mobility Gallery A, B, C, D, E
FIM 1

DESCRIPTION

This is a high risk activity and should only be undertaken in life threatening or exceptional circumstances, e.g. cardiac arrest, seizure.

- The handler must kneel to one side of the person.
- The person's nearest arm is placed across her chest (figure 17.24a).
- The handler pushes against the person's nearest thigh with both hands, in order to position the person's hips at the front of the chair (figure 17.24b).
- The handler holds the person's furthest hip with one hand, while the other hand is on the person's nearest thigh (figure 17.24c).
- The person is pushed/pulled to the floor (figure 17.24 d and e).

SKILL LEVEL

The handler must have received training in this manoeuvre. The handler must be physically able to kneel on the floor.

EVIDENCE AVAILABLE

(Morton, Parry 2001). Transfer to the floor. Paper presented at National Back Exchange Conference, by Hilary Morton, North East Wales NHS Trust.

DANGERS/ PRECAUTIONS

- If the person is on a lightweight chair, a second handler will be required to hold the chair.
- During the final stage of the manoeuvre, the person's head should be supported to prevent injury.

FURTHER OPTION

Option

- The handler must kneel to one side of the person.
- The handler positions the person's feet away from him.
- The handler's near hand holds the person's furthest shoulder and pulls the person towards them until the person's head is resting against the handler (figure 17.25a).
- The handler's nearest hand holds behind the person's waist. The handler's other hand presses against the person's knees, (figure 17.25b).
- The handler pulls / slides the person towards him, until the person's hips are on the edge of the chair. In a continuous movement, slide the person over the side of the chair, onto the floor (figure 17.25c).
- The handler moves back slightly to allow the person's head and shoulders to be lowered to the floor.

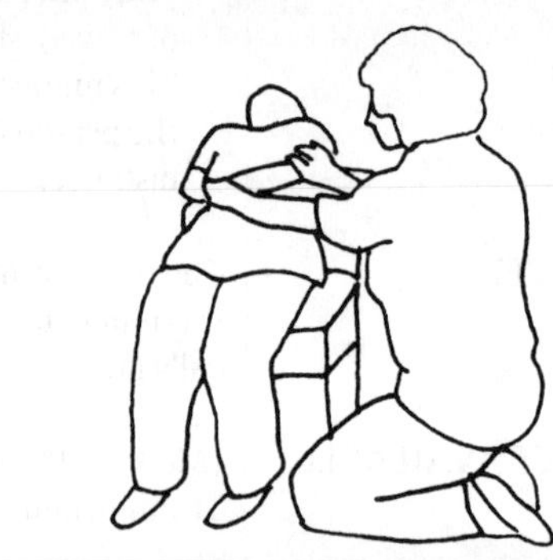

FIG 17.24a

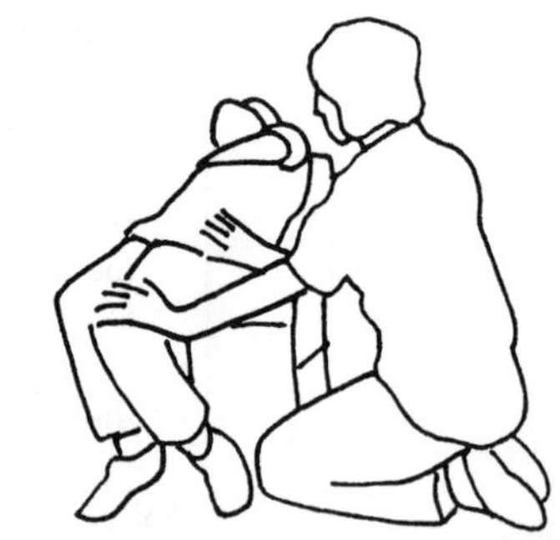

FIG 17.24b

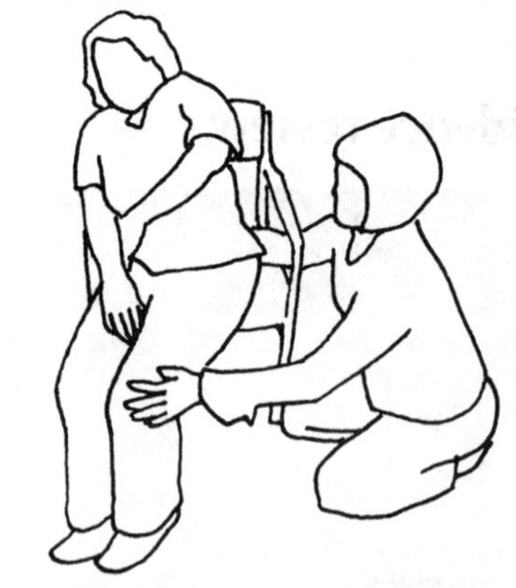

FIG 17.24c

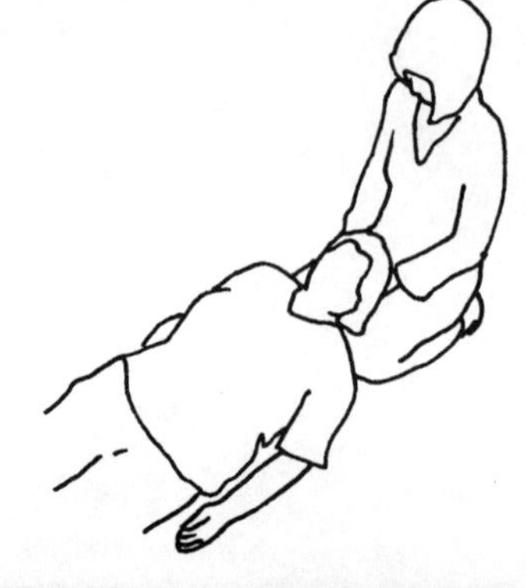

FIG 17.24d

SKILL LEVEL

The handler must have received training in this manoeuvre. The handler must be physically able to kneel on the floor.

EVIDENCE AVAILABLE

(Meek 2004). Manual Handling. Solutions, Training and Advisory Ltd.

DANGERS/ PRECAUTIONS

- If the person is on a lightweight chair, a second handler will be required to hold the chair.

NB
A manual handling risk assessment must be completed that is specific to the person and handlers.

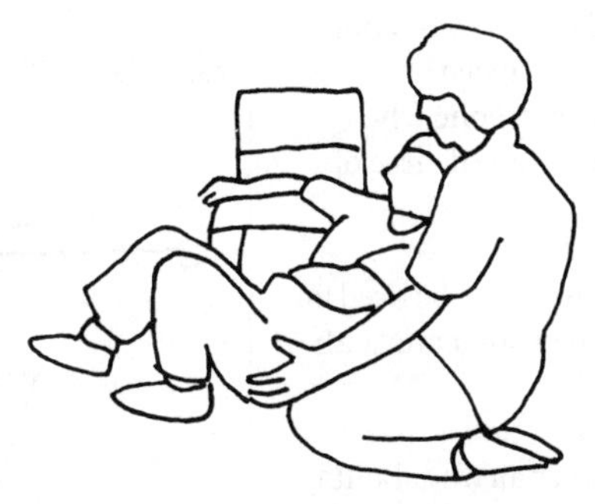

FIG 17.24e

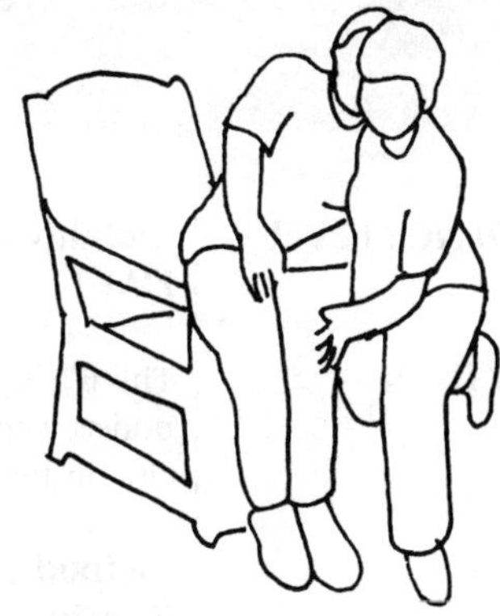

FIG 17.25a

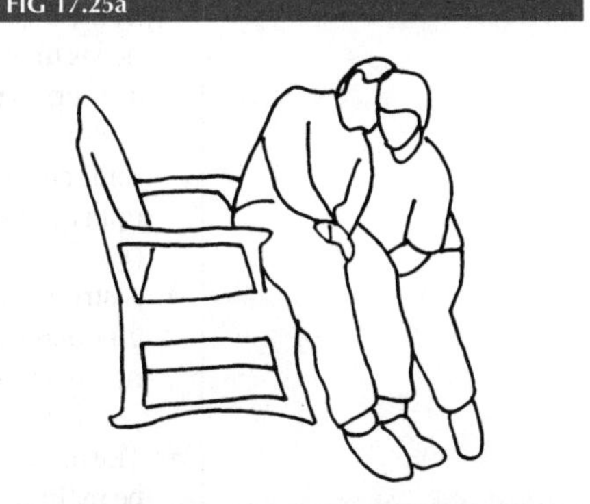

FIG 17.25b

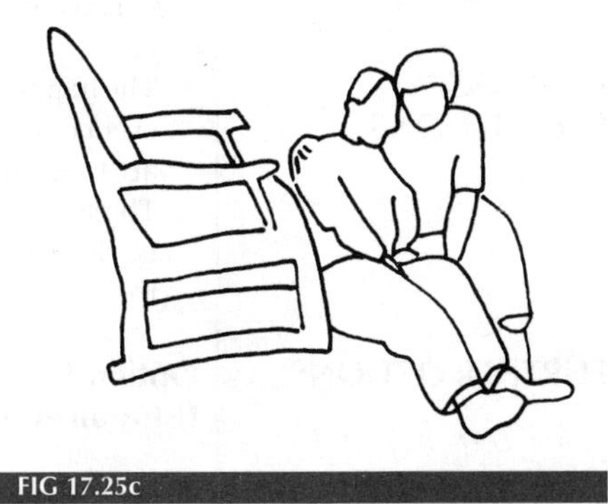

FIG 17.25c

Evidence review

Technique	REBA	Activity	Comfort	FIM	Mobility gallery	Skill level	
CHAIR TO FLOOR IN AN EMERGENCY							
Fig 17.24a	11	1	2	1	E	Competent	

Task Fifteen

Evacuation from pools

DEPENDENCY LEVEL

Mobility Gallery A, B, C, D, E
FIM 1

DESCRIPTION

This is a high risk activity and should only be undertaken in life threatening or exceptional circumstances.

Method
Hoisting

- In the event of an emergency, the person needs to be positioned on the hoist chair, as soon as possible and strapped in.
- A chair can be used for someone who is semi-conscious and has some degree of upper body strength (see figures 17.26 a – c).
- A stretcher attachment should be used for an unconscious person or someone with no upper body strength (see figures 17.26 d – f)
- The unconscious person's airway should be maintained throughout the manoeuvre.

SKILL LEVEL

The handler must have received training in this manoeuvre.

DANGERS/ PRECAUTIONS

- The handler needs to be aware that, in the event of a person having a seizure, there are likely to be unpredictable movements.
- The safe working load of the hoist should be checked, to ensure that the weight of the person does not exceed it.

FURTHER OPTIONS

Option 1
Using an evacuation board

- A minimum of five handlers are required to undertake this manoeuvre – three in the pool and two pool side.
- The handlers must move the person to one side of the pool, parallel to the side, which allows easy egress.
- One handler supports the person's head, while the other two support the body (see figure 17.27a).
- An evacuation board is placed in the pool, between the person and the poolside (see figure 17.27a).
- The board is tilted and pushed into the water and allowed to float up under the person (see figure 17.27b).
- The person is then secured to the board, using the straps provided (see figure 17.27c).
- The board is rotated so that the head end is towards the side of the pool

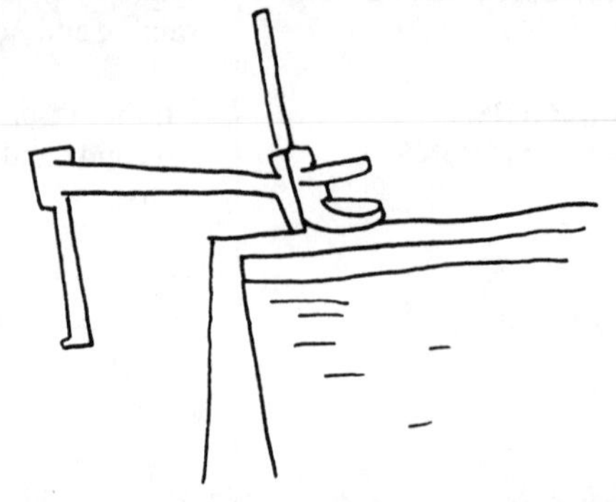

FIG 17.26a

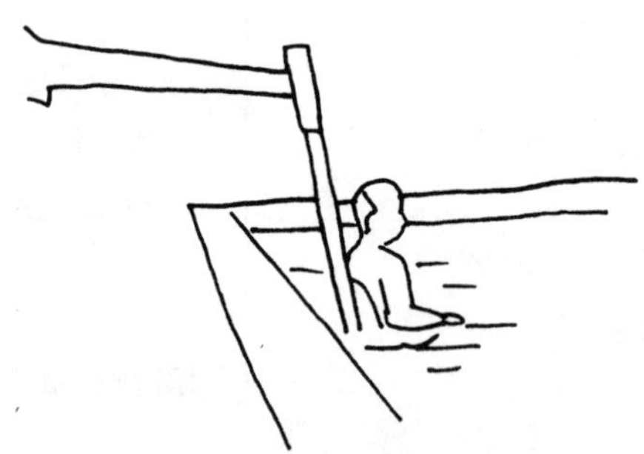

FIG 17.26b

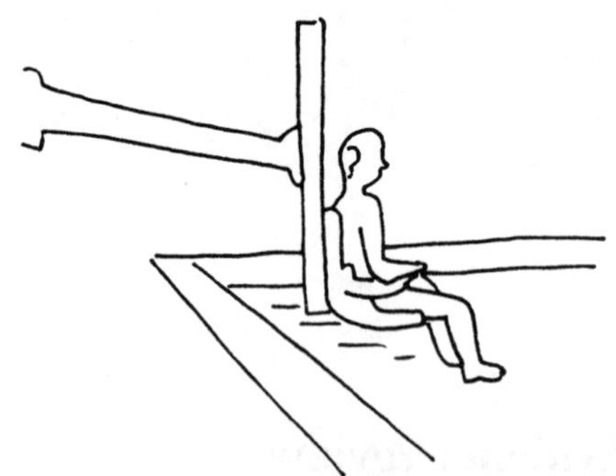

FIG 17.26c

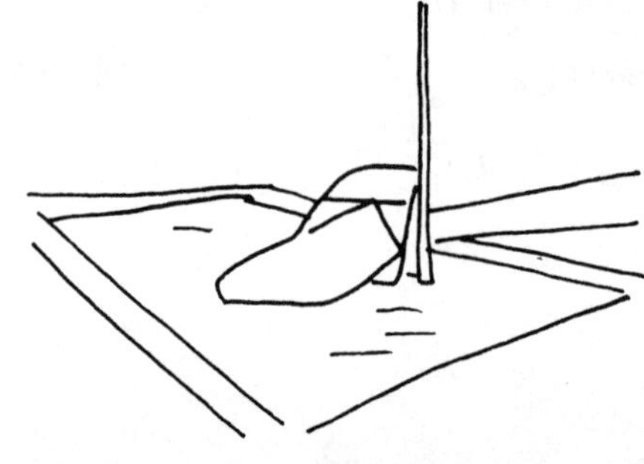

FIG 17.26d

(see figure 17.27d).

- One person continues to support the person's head whilst the other two push down on the foot end of the board, raising the head end high enough to rest on the side of the pool. At the same time, the two handlers on the pool side pull the head end of the board (see figure 17.27e).
- The person is slid out of the pool, either onto the poolside or directly onto a trolley.
- Once the person is stabilised, they are raised using an appropriate manoeuvre (see tasks 8 and 12).

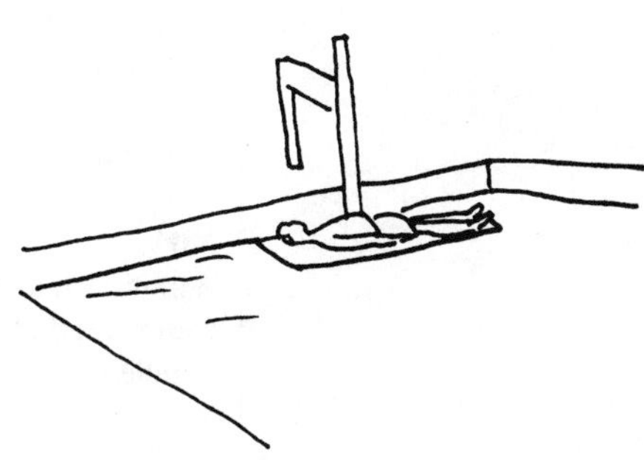
FIG 17.26e

SKILL LEVEL

The handler must have received training in this manoeuvre. A high level of skill and physical fitness of the handler is required.

EVIDENCE AVAILABLE

(Resuscitation Council (UK) 2001). Guidance for safer handling during resuscitation in hospitals, Resuscitation Council (UK).

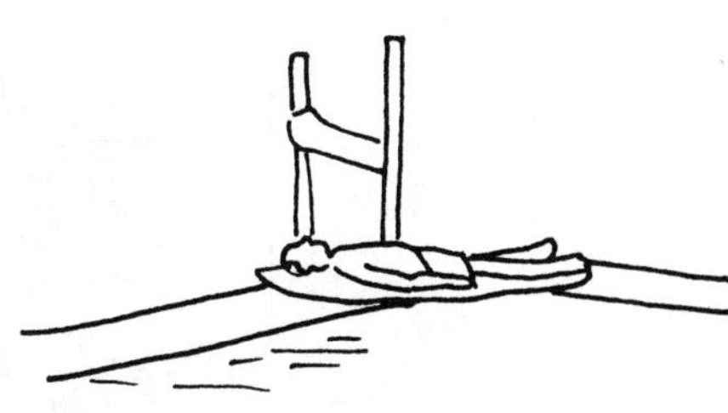
FIG 17.26f

DANGERS/ PRECAUTIONS

- The safe working load of the board should be checked, to ensure that the weight of the person does not exceed it.
- The handler supporting the person's head must ensure that the head and neck are maintained in neutral alignment.
- The handlers at pool side are required to adopt an awkward posture in order to reach the board in the water (see figure 17.27e). This can be improved by the use of extension straps attached to the head end of the board.

FURTHER OPTION

Option 2
Use of a handling net

- A handling net could be used in place of a board for evacuation, particularly for children and out of hydrotherapy pools, if no hoist is available.
- The net is placed underneath the person, ensuring that the whole body is supported.
- The handlers must move the person to one side of the pool, which allows easy egress.
- A minimum of two handlers are required, one in the pool and one at the pool side.
- The child is then lifted out of the pool (see figure 17.27g).
- The use of a handling net, as opposed to directly holding the child, will minimise injury to the child and allows the handlers to adopt a better position.

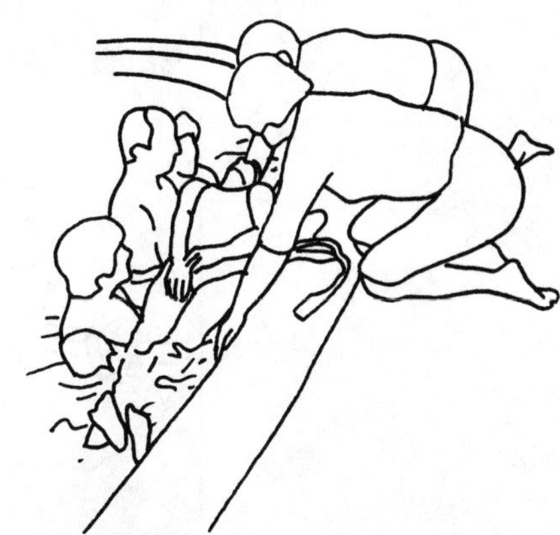
FIG 17.27a

SKILL LEVEL

The handler must have received training in this manoeuvre.

DANGERS/ PRECAUTIONS

- The safe working load of the net should be checked, to ensure that the weight of the person does not exceed it.
- The handlers will be taking all of the

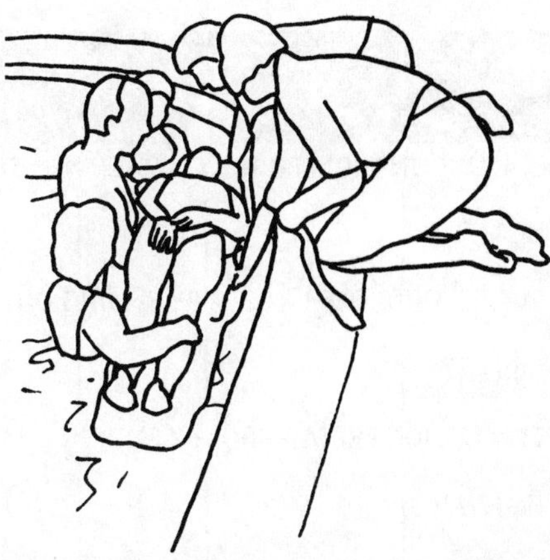
FIG 17.27b

person's body weight, increasing the risk of injury to the handlers. The handlers may also be lifting from below mid lower leg height.

NB

A manual handling risk assessment must be completed that is specific to the person and handlers.

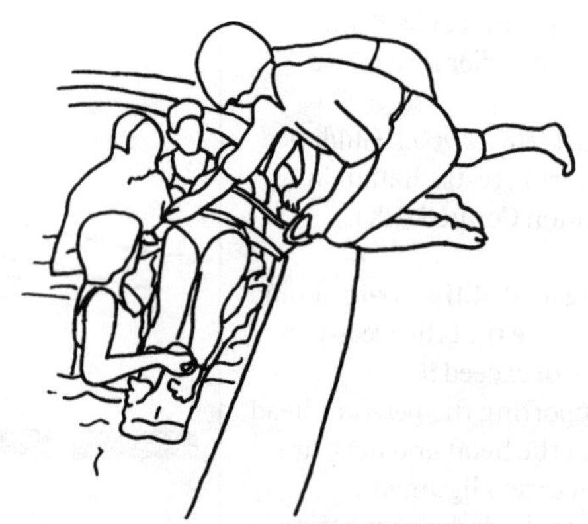
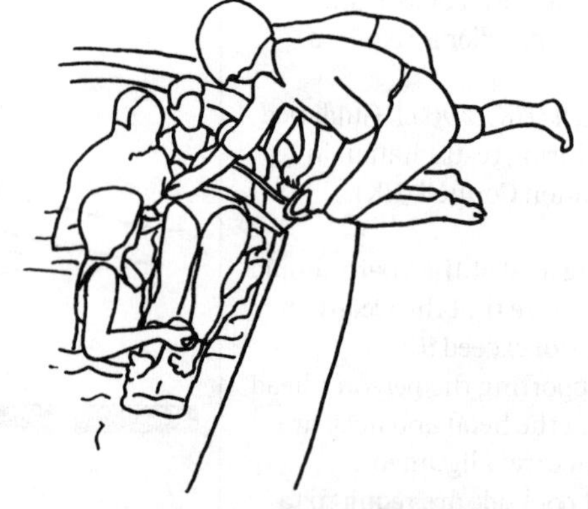

FIG 17.27c

FIG 17.27d

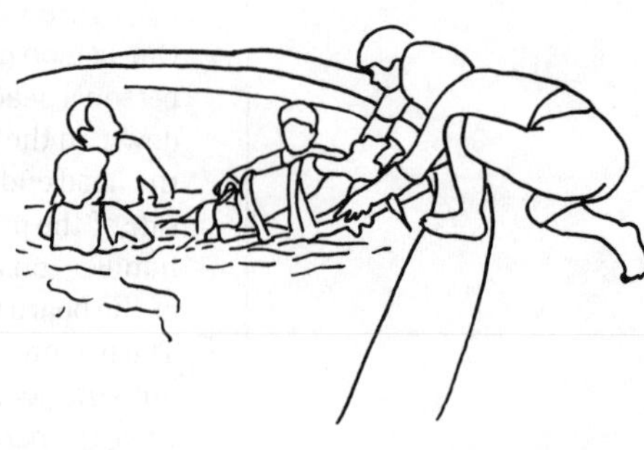

FIG 17.27e

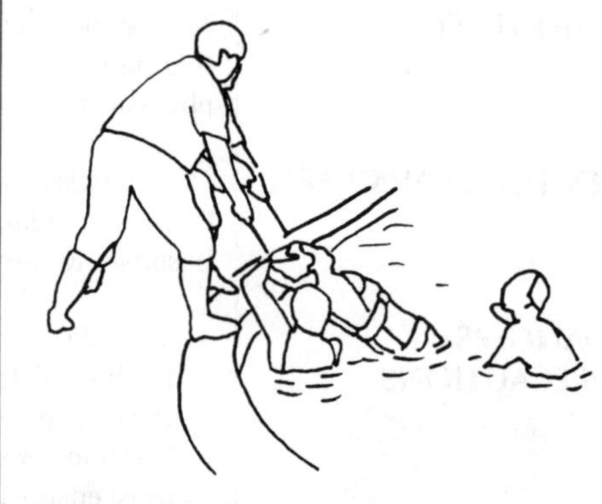

FIG 17.27f

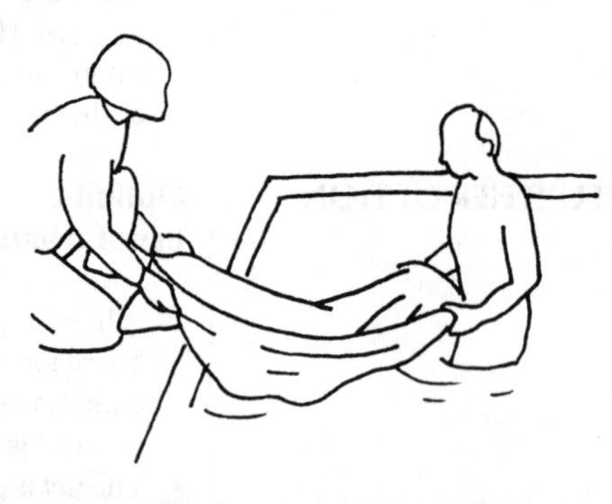

FIG 17.27g

Evidence review

Technique	REBA	Activity	Comfort	FIM	Mobility gallery	Skill level	Comment
EVACUATION FROM POOL BY ATTACHING STRAPS							
Fig 17.27c	11	1	5	1	E	Proficient	Postural risk attaching straps
EVACUATION FROM A POOL BY SLIDING OUT WITHOUT EXTENSION STRAPS							
Fig 17.27a	11	1	3	1	E	Proficient	
EVACUATION FROM A POOL BY SLIDING OUT WITH STRAPS							
Fig 17.27f	9	1	7	1	E	Proficient	More comfortable with straps as smoother and less noise, less frightening

Task Sixteen

Lowering a patient from a complete/incomplete strangulation

co-written with Emily Millar, Homefirst Community Trust

DESCRIPTION

This is a high risk activity. Where the risk to the handlers is considered too great, it may be appropriate to cut the ligature, preserving the knot, and allow the person to fall unhindered to the ground.

Suspended Strangulation

- Staff attending the scene will hold the person's thighs and raise them slightly, to reduce tension on the ligature (see figure 17.28a).
- If the person is at a height that the staff find difficult to reach, tension on the ligature can be reduced by placing a table / chair underneath the person.
- One handler will cut the ligature from the point of suspension, preserving the knot (see figure 17.28b).
- Another handler will support the person's head, while other staff lower the person into a supine position onto the floor/ground.
- Remove the ligature from the neck, using a ligature cutter if required.
- Assess vital signs and commence resuscitation, if appropriate.
- When ready, raise the person from the floor, using an appropriate manoeuvre (see tasks eight and twelve).

Incomplete Strangulation

Kneeling, semi-seated, and lying.

- Staff attending the scene will hold the person's thighs, hips, or the person's belt or clothes, and raise them slightly, to reduce tension on the ligature.
- One handler will cut the ligature from the point of suspension, preserving the knot.
- One handler must support the person's head as the person is lowered to the ground.

Lying Strangulation

- Staff will slide the patient up towards the point of suspension, to reduce the tension on the ligature before removal.

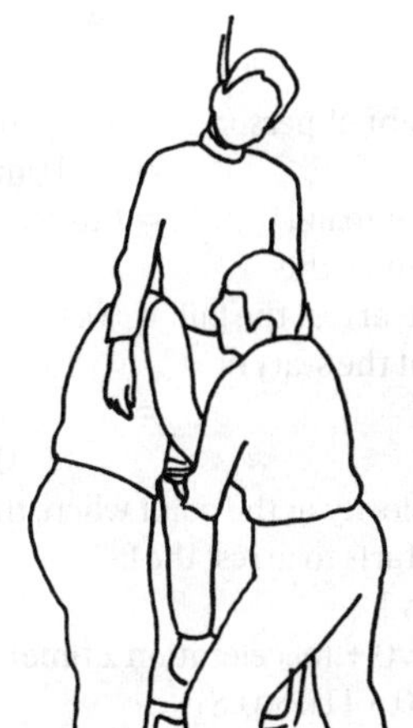

FIG 17.28a

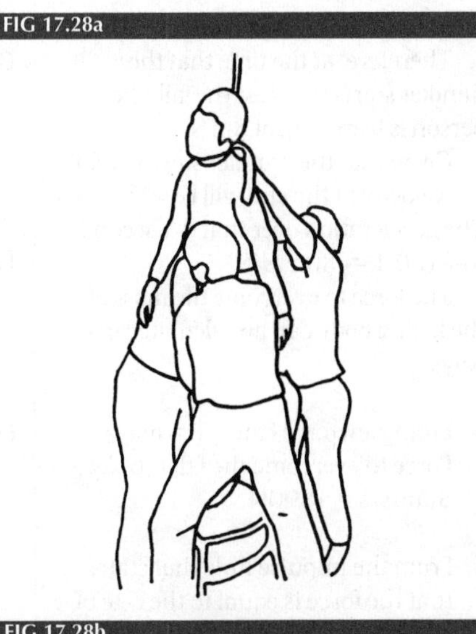

FIG 17.28b

SKILL LEVEL

The handler must have received training in this manoeuvre. The handler must be physically fit.

DANGERS/ PRECAUTIONS

- The handlers will be taking all of the person's body weight, increasing the risk of injury to the handlers.
- In a kneeling or semi-seated strangulation incident, the handlers may have to adopt an awkward position in order to elevate the person to reduce tension on the ligature.
- The handlers must be aware of their environment and of any possible danger to themselves.

NB

A manual handling risk assessment must be completed that is specific to the person and handlers.

Technique	REBA	Activity	Comfort	FIM	Mobility gallery	Skill level	Comment
LOWERING A PATIENT FROM A COMPLETE/INCOMPLETE STRANGULATION							
Fig 17.28b	11	1	1	1	E	Novice	

Force calculation

The force required to support a falling person (*Fray 2003*)

A handler is supporting a person during walking, when the person starts to fall. The handler manages to arrest the fall, before lowering the person to the floor. The force required can be calculated.

Body weight of person = 60kg
Gravity = 10m/s/s
Time taken to fall = 0.8 seconds
Time taken by the handler to arrest the fall = 0.1 second
Velocity at the start of the fall = v0 = 0m/s

The velocity at the point where the handler starts to arrest the fall
= v1
= v0 + (acceleration x time)
= 0 + (10 x 0.8)
= 8 m/s

Therefore, at the time that the handler starts to arrest the fall, the person is travelling at 8m/s.

Given that the handler stops the fall, the velocity at the end will be v2 = 0m/s. The deceleration over that 0.1 second = (0-8) / 0.1 = -80m/s/s.

The force to overcome the mass of the falling body can be calculated in two ways.

a From Newton's Law: F = ma
Force to overcome the fall = 60kg x 80m/s/s = 4800N

b From the Impulse Rule that states that the force is equal to the rate of change in momentum

Force to overcome the fall = (m2v2 – m1v1) / Time taken
= (0 – 60kg x 8m/s) / 0.1 seconds
= – 480 / 0.1= 4800N

Using both methods, the force to overcome the falling person is equal to 4800N or 480kg.

Acknowledgements

The authors of this chapter would like to thank the following for their assistance.

Sally Williams, Jenny Horwood, Peter Wilson, Paul Meek, Emily Millar.

References

Adams J, Tyson S (2000). The effectiveness of physiotherapy to enable an elderly person to get up from the floor, Physiotherapy, April 2000, 86, 4, 185-189

BackCare (1999). Safer handling of people in the community, National Back Pain Association

Cryer and Patel (2001). Falls, fragility and fractures, National Service Framework for older people: The case for and strategies to implement joint health improvement and modernisation plans for falls and osteoporosis.

Fray M (2003). (unpublished) Worked example for catching a falling body, Module 4, Postgraduate Diploma in Back Care Management, Loughborough University.

Fray M, Ratcliffe I, Jones B, Parker A, Booker J, Warren C, Rollinson G (2001). Care handling for people in hospitals, community and educational settings – A code of practice. Derbyshire Inter-Agency Group.

Health and Safety Executive (2004). Manual Handling Operations Regulations – as amended. HMSO, London

Health and Safety Executive (2004). (unpublished). Data abstracted from RIDDOR database.

McCarthy L (1998). Safe handling of persons on cervical traction. Nursing Times, 94:14 p57-58.

Meek P (2004). Manual Handling. Solutions, Training and Advisory Ltd, 2004.

Morton H, Parry JA (2001). Transfer to the floor. Paper presented at National Back Exchange Conference, by Hilary Morton, North East Wales NHS Trust, (2001).

National Back Exchange, Oxford Region Group (1999). Generic safe systems of work for person handling and inanimate load management, Version 8.

National Back Pain Association/Royal College of Nursing (1997/8). The guide to the handling of persons: Introducing a safer handling policy, 4th Edition, National Back Pain Association.

Reece AC, Simpson JM (1996). Preparing older people to cope after a fall, Physiotherapy April 1996, 82. 4. 227-235.

Resuscitation Council (UK) (2001). Guidance for safer handling during resuscitation in hospitals, Resuscitation Council (UK).

Tinetti ME et al. (1988). Risk factors for falls among elderly persons living in the community, New England Journal of Medicine 1988; 319: 1701-7.

Tinetti ME, Liu WL, Claus EB (1993). Predictors and prognosis of inability to get up after falls among elderly persons, Journal of the American Medical Association, 269, 1, 65-70

Watson JE, Royle JR (1987). Watson's Medical-Surgical Nursing and Related Physiology, p817, Balliere Tindall.

18 Controversial techniques

Sue Ruszala MSc MCSP DipTP SRP
Manual Handling and Ergonomics Adviser
United Bristol Healthcare Trust

Over the years techniques have been developed to enable people to be moved, or assisted to move, and transferred as comfortably and safely as possible. Most of the early methods involved handlers lifting all or most of the person's weight. However, evidence now available suggests that these practices present a high risk of musculoskeletal injury to handlers. Discomfort and injury to the person being lifted have also been identified. More suitable aids, equipment and furniture are now available to facilitate improved handling practices, such that the manual lifting of people should no longer be necessary except in exceptional circumstances. It must be questioned, therefore, whether it is acceptable to continue with lifting techniques where and if alternative and safer methods are available. This chapter will review the people handling techniques that have previously been described as "condemned", "unsafe" *(NBPA, 1981,1987, 1992, 1998; BackCare, 1999)* or "controversial" *(Hignett et al, 2003)* and discuss the evidence to support their risk status and recommendation for removal from routine practice.

1 Introduction

All manual techniques that involve lifting all or most of the person's weight will be reviewed. This includes assisted transfer and assisted standing methods where the handler may take the person's weight due to the nature of the task and environment, the characteristics of the person or the skill needs of the technique. Single hug transfers and repositioning activities have been shown to be most widely associated with low back pain in handlers *(Marras et al, 1999; Knibbe and Friele, 1996; Smedley et al, 1995)*. Both the handler and person are at risk of injury during these activities, the results of which will impact on the effectiveness of the organisation as well as those injured and their families.

Moving people is a complex procedural task that may involve a number of associated tasks and /or sub tasks. For example, if a person is to be manually lifted from a bed to chair using a Hammock lift (figure 18.3d) the sub tasks may include:

- Clearing the area around the bed.
- Positioning the chair by the bed.
- Managing any attachments to the person.
- Lifting the person into an upright sitting position.
- Removing pillows.
- Lowering the back rest.
- Lifting the person to side of bed.
- Lifting person from bed to chair.
- Lifting the person again into a more suitable comfortable final position.
- Lifting the person to rearrange clothing.
- Lifting feet onto footrests or footstool.
- Rechecking of attachments.
- Arranging the area to suit the person's needs.

The risk of handler injury is further compounded by factors inherent in the required task, including: asymmetrical lifting, stooping, leaning sideways, and twisting *(Hye-Knudson et al, 2004; Hignett, 1996; Owen et al, 1992)*, also sudden trunk loading if a person collapses (*Essendrop et al, 2004*–see also chapter 17). Awkward postures are difficult to avoid, especially in areas where access to the person is restricted. The risk of cumulative strain injury to the handler is further increased by the number of times per shift the lifts are repeated, the duration of the lifting component of the task, the weight of the person and the postures adopted during the whole task *(Garg et al, 1992)*. Some examples of activities with hazardous postures are identified later in the chapter under factors predisposing to injury. Sadly however, backache is still often considered to be just part of the job *(Owen, 1999)*.

Whilst modern training programmes aim to promote non lifting methods (see chapter 12–18), in practice the transference of these skills from the classroom to the clinical area can be difficult to achieve. A literature review produced a strong evidence statement that training interventions predominantly based on training or education alone have no impact on working practices *(Hignett et al, 2003)*. In hurried and awkward situations handlers may revert to methods they are familiar and comfortable with, despite knowing that they are not recommended practice. Some handlers prefer to rely on these familiar techniques, or they may believe them to be best practice for the person with handling needs. Handlers who use lifting techniques in the work environment often expect and encourage new staff to use them as well and thus these potentially damaging techniques are perpetuated *(Green, 1996)*. Changing this 'custom and practice' approach to the continued use of easy to apply techniques in preference to evidence-based, safer methods will need a combination of change management strategies and ergonomic improvements (see chapters 3 and 4). Managers need to use risk assessment (see chapter 9) to ensure adequate equipment, documented protocols, relevant training and sufficient workplace supervision are provided in order to facilitate the transference of safer handling practices to the workplace *(HSC, 1998)*.

2 Methodology

This chapter reviews the techniques identified as controversial from the four editions of the "*Guide to the Handling of Patients*" *(NPBA, 1981, 1987, 1992, 1998)*, and "*Safer Handling in the Community*" *(BackCare, 1999)*. The key features of the techniques and their known modifications will be identified, although readers will need to refer to the previous editions, or *Hollis (1991)*, for a full description of each lift. Each of the methods will be supported with the available evidence to underpin the high-risk status, including:

- Research findings in studies which examine named manual lifting or transfer techniques.
- Recommended techniques agreed through a consensus of Back Care Advisors – *the Derbyshire Inter-Agency Group* (*DIAG, 2001*).

- Published professional opinion in the "*The Guide to the Handling of Patients*" (*NPBA, 1981, 1987, 1992, 1997/8*), and "*Safer Handling in the Community*" (*BackCare, 1999*).

3 Risks to the handler

Handlers are known to be at risk of back pain and other musculoskeletal injuries during person lifting activities due to the following:

- **Biomechanics:** (see chapters 5 and 6) lifting techniques may result in handlers at some stage being required to adopt an asymmetrical, awkward, stooped and unstable posture and to hold the weight of the person away from the body. These can increase the forces on the handler's spine and shoulder as follows:
  - Lifting at arms length induces a major flexion and compression strain on the spine, and stress on the shoulder and arm joints.
  - Stooping or lifting in a forward lean position increases the flexion and compression strain on the spine.
  - Sideways lifting adds a lateral twisting movement to the compression strain.
  - Lifting outside of the handler's base of support results in a potentially unstable lift with an increased risk of loss of balance, for example, should the person move unexpectedly.
  - Lifting beyond the distance recommended in the technique may result in a twisting movement, for example, when using the through-arm lift to move a person up the bed handlers may opt for one long move rather than two or three shorter moves, which can result in twisting during the extended aspects of the move.

- **Handler characteristics:** (see chapters 1, 7 and 9) the average weight of a person is likely to exceed the guidance on safe working loads in the *Manual Handling Operations Regulations* (*HSE, 1992*) and the lifting ability of most handlers *(Garg et al, 1992)*. Whilst it has previously been suggested that two handlers may be able to lift up to 8 stones in ideal situations *(RCN, 1993)*, in reality the environment usually falls short of the ideal. A risk assessment process is now recommended *(RCN, 1996)*, even for babies and small toddlers in awkward handling situations. Handlers with musculoskeletal problems cannot be expected to lift manually, nor can any handler if pregnant, in poor health, recovering from illness, or fatigued. Many handlers have been found unable to perform manual lifts on low beds, as the leg or hip movement required of them may be restricted or painful. All lifting techniques become more complex when handlers of different heights are working together as either the taller person amends their technique and posture in an attempt to share the load more evenly, or the shorter handler takes the greater part of the load.

- **Handler risk perception:** each handler will have their own perception of risk in handling based on their training and previous experiences, however colleagues and techniques may influence their behaviour *(Green, 1996)*. Many new handlers will conform to the social norm and copy practices of others with whom they work. Poor techniques then become accepted practice. Handlers need to be aware that inappropriate or rough handling techniques could be construed as physical abuse or negligent practice, especially with vulnerable adults *(NMC, 2002, sections 13 and 18)*.

- **Physical and behavioural characteristics of the person:** people are difficult to move as they are not of uniform shape or size, have no handles, may be attached to equipment such as pumps, orthopaedic appliances and urinary devices, and may perceive and react to situations in different and sometimes unpredictable ways. They may have varying levels of balance and mobility; contracted, spastic or flaccid muscles; or involuntary movement of their limbs. In addition they may be unco-operative, confused, aggressive, agitated, resist movement or move unexpectedly during the technique. These characteristics may also be influenced by other factors such as pain, fear, anxiety, medication, drowsiness or even the suitability of the clothes or shoes they are wearing for the task. Suitable and sufficient risk assessment prior to movement must include all these factors, as they will influence the selection of the technique. Care plans must reflect an up-to-date assessment of the handling needs of the person and be readily accessible to all relevant handlers.

- **Level of person cooperation:** people are not always able to consistently cooperate with the instructions they have been given. It may result, for example, in a person not actively contributing enough in a bed to chair transfer and therefore leaving the handler to take more of the weight than expected. This may be due to a variety of causes including poor communication; misunderstanding or an aspect of their medical condition, and relevant details will need to be documented in the care plan.

- **Workload pressures:** may encourage handlers to take short cuts and revert to manual lifting techniques as a means of getting the work done. Equipment may not be easily available or shared between too many people. Staffing levels at night are usually lower and assistance may not always be available or easily accessible thus encouraging handlers to manage as best they can which may include manual lifting. Those assigning workload must have a thorough appreciation of the handling and mobility needs of individual persons, and of the overall workload of the handlers involved. These are both an integral part of good risk management practice (see chapter 9).

- **Environmental characteristics:** (see chapter 4) creating suitable and sufficient space by the person is essential to safe practice. It is not always possible to achieve this due to environmental constraints especially when working in poorly designed wards and departments, in a person's own home, or in the wider community. An unsuitable environment may result in handlers adapting their body postures or amending the techniques to enable the task to be done, but at the expense of increasing injury risk levels.

- **Equipment and furniture provision:** (see chapters 4, 9, 12–18) manufacturers are continuously developing products to improve compatibility with other equipment and furniture. In the meantime some handlers are still required to work in areas where beds, commodes and chairs are of a fixed height, chair arms are not removable and equipment is unusable. For example hoists which are incompatible with beds due to inadequate space underneath, chairs with bases too wide for hoists, or sliding boards which cannot be used due to different seat heights. Adequate provision of suitable equipment and/or furniture may avoid the need for handlers to manually lift in these mismatch situations.

- **Person expectations of handling:** (see chapters 2 and 9) some people may have expectations of how they wish to be handled, including manual lifting. It is not uncommon for this issue to arise, maybe by way of misinformed preconceptions as to what might be involved in using equipment, or because of anxieties about 'the unknown'. The relevant manager should address these issues as part of the risk assessment. An integral part of this decision making process is the documentation detail which should reflect the person's request including the options tried and rationale supporting the agreed outcome. Managers and those involved in devising handling plans should have change management and negotiation skills, enabling them to understand the various perspectives of the person, their relatives and the handlers expected to carry out the tasks. All handlers should have an appreciation of how it feels, personally, to be moved using equipment such as a hoist, be appropriately skilled with the model used and feel adequately supported by their line managers and supervisors to use the documented safer handling methods. They also need to be able to clearly explain the benefits of non-manual lifting methods. Handlers may otherwise feel compelled to comply with the wishes of the person or run the risk of complaints.

- **Linking the person to the handler:** techniques where the person is encouraged to hold on to the handler should be avoided, as injury could occur to either or both of them. The person could suddenly pull on the handlers as a result of becoming agitated, or move unpredictably and the transfer may then become unstable. Such methods include placing the person's arms round the handlers' neck or trunk (figure 18.5e), or holding onto handling belts fitted to the handler. Handholds that encourage a person to grasp the handlers' thumbs can also cause damage if the person does not, or cannot, let go. Similarly, linking arms (figure 18.1h) with a person during assisted walking may encourage the person to lean on handlers and take their weight should they become less steady, or even collapse.

4 Risks to the person

During manual lifting techniques a person is at risk due to the following:

- **Discomfort:** the physical contact required to hold the person can cause discomfort or pain both during the lift and for a time after the move has been completed. This is not surprising for example, with the through-arm lift between bed and chair (figure 18.3d) where one handler lifts most of the weight by embracing the person's trunk and grasping the forearms. Handlers may also be positioned where they are unable to observe the person's face and notice any discomfort created by the lift.

- **Injury:** most of the lifting methods involve holding the person manually or using equipment such as a handling sling in order to physically lift and carry them. Whilst positioning the handlers' arms or introducing handling slings, shearing on the person's skin may occur which can result in pain or tearing of the skin. Grasping of a person's wrists, arms or legs can also cause pain, bruising and skin tears. In the drag lift (figure 18.1e) the person's weight is taken on the bony area of the handler's forearm, which can cause discomfort, damage to soft tissue around the shoulder, glenohumeral dislocation and even fracture of the humerus. The buttocks and heels are often not lifted high enough and therefore subjected to unnecessary and unacceptable levels of friction and shear that may contribute to the development of pressure sores.

- **Impact on medical condition:** the medical condition of the person also needs to be taken into consideration. Those with arthritic or painful joints may find the pressures of a drag, shoulder or through-arm lift (figures 18.1e, 18.4a, 18.3a) painful. People with hip problems, abdominal complaints or post-surgery may not be able to sit forward enough for lifts to be performed without increasing pain. Some people have found the pressure on the chest wall during the through-arm and shoulder lifts can cause breathing difficulties or increased pain, for example, after thoracic surgery.

- **Mobility goals:** all people should be encouraged to move independently where assessment indicates that they are able to do so, and where this is a reasonable care or rehabilitation aim. Individual care plans need to document realistic mobility goals. Some techniques where the handler stands directly in front of the person when assisting standing, sitting and chair transfers (figure 18.5b) restrict the essential forward movement of the person, therefore impeding rather than assisting the person's ability to perform the move.

- **Person experience:** some people may perceive that techniques such as the shoulder lift (figure 18.4a), assisted stand or transfer (figure 18.5b) techniques where the handler stands in front invade their personal space. Others may sense a lack of control during the move, or feel 'bundled up' by the handler, or may find a particular method degrading. Alternatively some people can find it daunting to have open spaces in front of them and a strategically placed chair or similar device in front of them may be reassuring. Additional risk assessment is necessary if a patient is anxious or fearful as an alternative handling method may be indicated.

5 Manual lifting, standing and transfer techniques

Task One

Drag lift – (axilla, auxiliary, underarm, *shoulder, *through-arm lift, hook and toss)

* names duplicated in other techniques

DEPENDENCY LEVEL

Mobility Gallery B, C, D
FIM 1, 2, 3

KEY FEATURE

To lift a person up the bed (see figure 18.1a). A person is lifted with the handlers' hands or arms positioned under the person's axilla or upper arm. Whilst usually carried out from the front, it can be performed from the back.

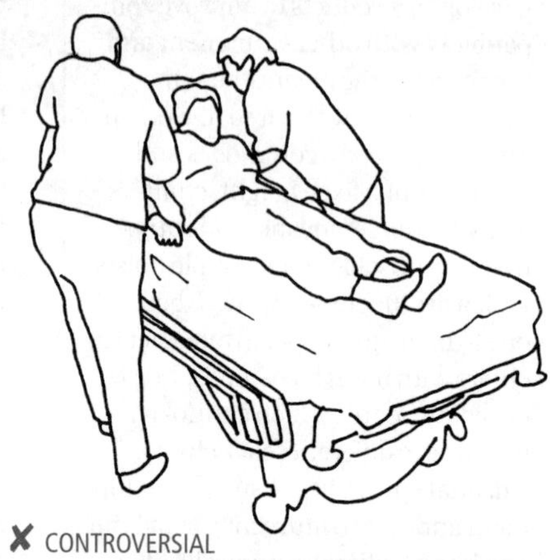

✗ CONTROVERSIAL

FIG 18.1a

DANGERS/ PRECAUTIONS

Person's weight is taken on the relatively narrow and less fleshy areas of the handlers' arms, and may cause pain, soft tissue injury, gleno-humeral dislocation and even fracture of the humerus. The sacrum, buttocks and heels can drag on the bed or chair and contribute to the development of pressure sores. A person may offer their abducted arms as a natural "handle" and, when used to assist standing, prevents the person from using the chair arms. The feeling of security may encourage the person to lean on the handlers and the passive nature of the technique may encourage a feeling of helplessness. The drag lift discourages normal movement and therefore restricts independence and impedes rehabilitation.

Handlers are lifting in an asymmetrical, stooped, twisted and side flexed posture and are therefore prone to moving outside of their base of support. A person may be asked to assist the handlers by pushing with their legs, however compliance cannot be assured and can result in no assistance, pushing at the wrong time or pushing excessively, which can unbalance the handlers. The handlers may not be able to see the person's face and observe any adverse effects. Whilst the drag hold may not always appear to be a lifting activity, the person can unexpectedly collapse putting all the weight on the handlers, which significantly increases the risk of injury.

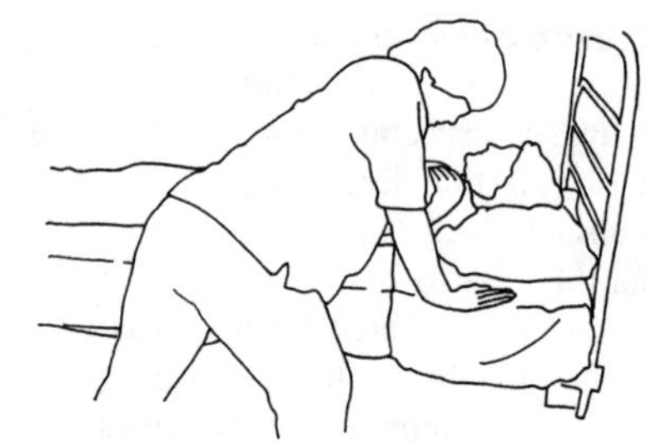

✗ CONTROVERSIAL

FIG 18.1b

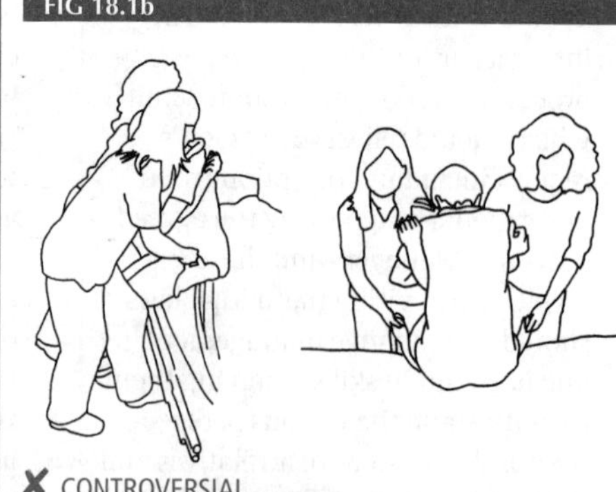

✗ CONTROVERSIAL

FIG 18.1c

MODIFICATIONS

- **Sitting person up from supine in bed** (figure 18.1b) handlers are required to lift over half of the weight of the dependent person, they are difficult to grasp and may be unpredictable during movement. The person's head may also need support.
- **Cross-arm lift** (figure 18.1c) handlers lift between bed and chair with a handling sling positioned under the upper thighs, whilst their nearside arms hold the person's bodyweight forward over the sling.
- **Leg and arm lift** (figure 18.1d) handlers

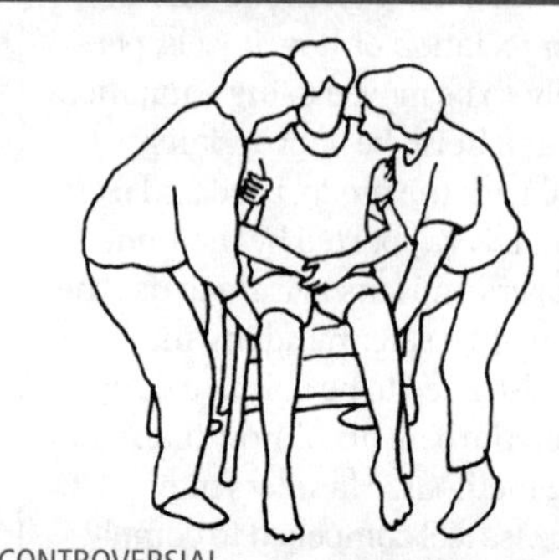

✗ CONTROVERSIAL

FIG 18.1d

hold the person's upper arms and thighs to lift which increases the stoop and twist of the handlers' postures and may also cause discomfort and bruising on the person's thigh.

- **Assisting person between sitting and standing** (figure 18.1e, below) handlers hold the person's upper arm which may feel secure, however this can encourage a person to expect to be lifted onto their feet. A handling sling is sometimes used (figure 18.1f).
- **Assisting person during standing and walking** (figure 18.1g, 18.1h) the handlers' hold feels secure, however this can encourage a person to lean on them or expect the handlers to hold them up. In confined spaces the "shuffling round" transfer action of feet predisposes both the person and handlers to become unstable. It is almost impossible to lower a collapsed person safely as handlers cannot release themselves and have to stoop to lower the person to the floor or lift to carry to a chair.
- **Lifting person from floor** (figure 18.1i) lifting from floor level is more awkward and difficult and therefore increases the risk of injury. Even when the person's feet are blocked, handlers are still required to lift the full bodyweight of the person.

EVIDENCE AVAILABLE

Research: drag lift exceeds safe lifting limits *(Essendrop et al, 2004: Marras et al, 1999; Laflin and Aja, 1995; Winkelmolen et al, 1994; Khalil et al, 1987)*; demonstrates high risk of injury to handlers *(Pheasant and Stubbs, 1992)*.
Consensus: high risk based on MHOR weight thresholds *(DIAG, 2001)*.
Professional opinion: lifting technique poses a high risk of injury to handler therefore classified as unsafe *(NBPA, 1981, 1987, 1992 & 1998; BackCare, 1999)*.

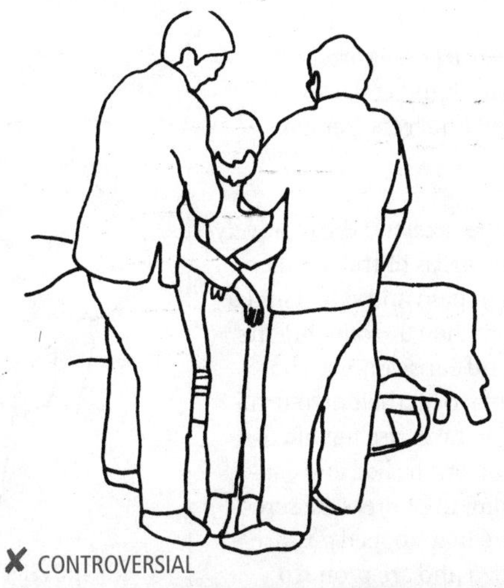

✘ CONTROVERSIAL

FIG 18.1e

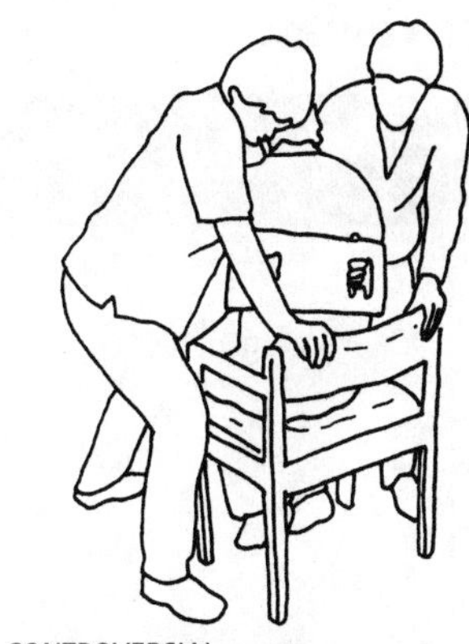

✘ CONTROVERSIAL

FIG 18.1f

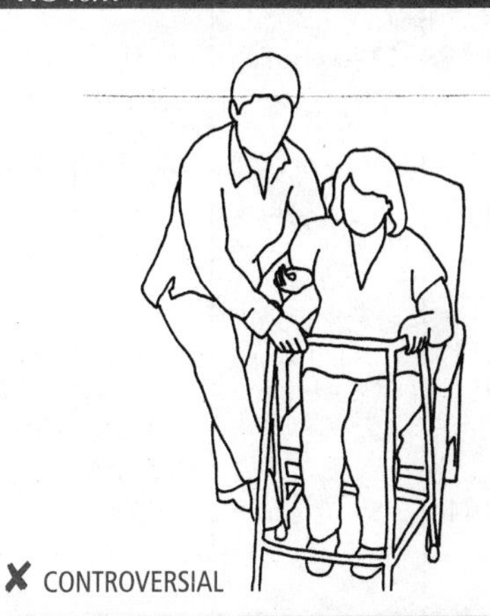

✘ CONTROVERSIAL

FIG 18.1g

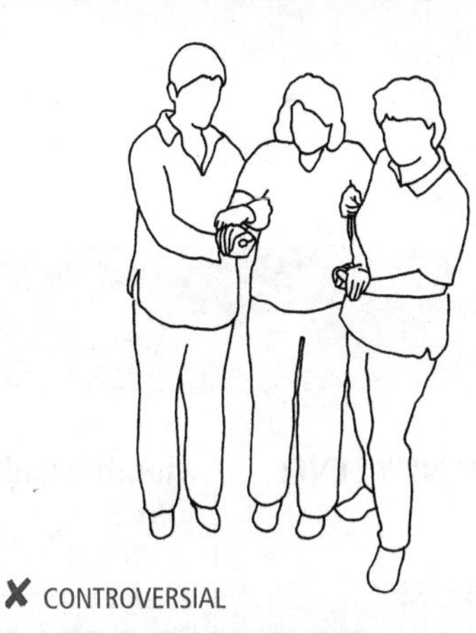

✘ CONTROVERSIAL

FIG 18.1h

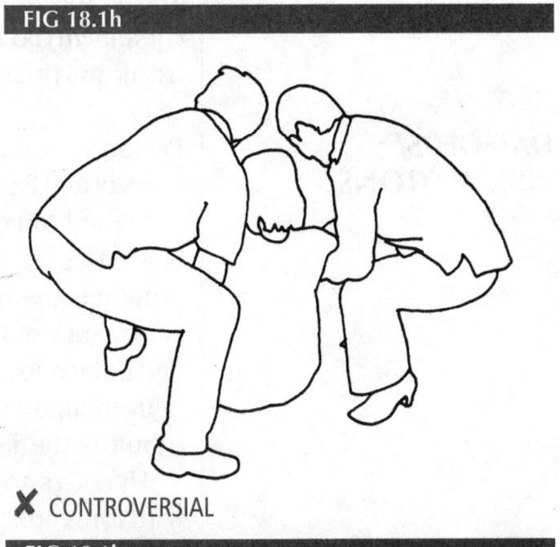

✘ CONTROVERSIAL

FIG 18.1i

Evidence review

Technique	REBA	Activity	Comfort	FIM	Mobility gallery	Skill level	Comment
DRAG LIFT							
Fig 18.1a	13 – Very high	1	1	1	D	Novice	Very high risk to handler, but no activity required from person
Fig 18.1b	14 – Very high	7	3	1	D	Novice	Requires high level of activity from a low ability person. Very high postural risk
Fig 18.1c	14 – Very high	1	2	1	D	Advanced beginner	For less able person, very high risk
Fig 18.1d	12 – Very high	5	1	3	C	Novice	For more able person, less comfortable but slightly lower risk. Can be performed by a novice.
Fig 18.1e	14 – Very high	5	4	3	C	Advanced beginner	Slightly higher risk that previous technique, a harder technique since not for a novice
Fig 18.1f	8 – High	6	6	3	C	Novice	Lower postural risk to handlers, activity level matches persons ability level
Fig 18.1g-h	11 – Very high	7	5	3	B	Novice	Able person able to contribute to manouvre, but high risk level to handler
Fig 18.1i	14 – Very high	3	1	2	D	Novice	

Task Two

Orthodox lift – (cradle, traditional, armchair, curl, barrow)

DEPENDENCY LEVEL

Mobility Gallery E
FIM 1

KEY FEATURE

To lift a person up the bed (see figure 18.2a). The person is lifted with handlers' arms (or equipment) positioned under the person's trunk and thighs.

DANGERS/ PRECAUTIONS

Person's weight may be taken on the relatively narrow and less fleshy areas of the handlers' arms, and can result in pain and skin damage. Skin shear may occur when introducing the arms or equipment and cause injury. The person may not be able to lift their own head and if the buttocks and heels are not lifted high enough may drag on the bed and contribute to the development of pressure sores.

Handlers are lifting in a stooped posture with arms outstretched and are prone to twisting and moving outside of their base of

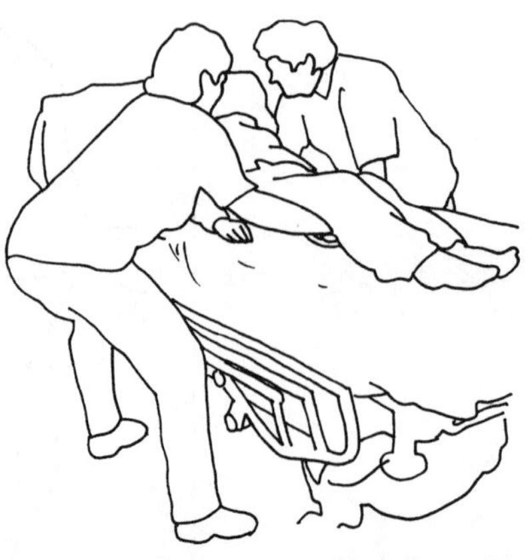

✘ CONTROVERSIAL

FIG 18.2a

support in the final stages of the lift. With a more dependent person the handlers may spread their arms, however, this increases the postural stresses and the person will sag in the middle. The orthodox lift was also used to lift a person to the side of the bed, introduce or remove a bedpan and transfer to a chair.

MODIFICATIONS

- **Flip turn** (figure 18.2b, below) requires one or two handlers to lift and turn the person in one move onto their side and presents a risk of back and arm injury to the handler and skin shear on the buttocks of the person.
- **Two sling lift** (figure 18.2c) encourages a twisted stance, as although it avoids reaching under the person to lift, it does not reduce the distance of the load from the handlers' spines.
- **Draw sheet lift** (figure 18.2d) lifting a person with bed linen is no longer accepted practice, as draw sheets are not designed as lifting aids. There is a risk of ripping which results in unexpected movement to the handler and risk of injury from the sudden movement.
- **Two poles and canvas lift** (figure 18.2e) two or more handlers lift and transfer a person using the arms and shoulders mainly due to environment constraints preventing the knees from being used, often resulting in awkward, stooped and twisted movements.
- **Three person lift** (figure 18.2f) needs three or more handlers to be of compatible height, and results in stooping to lift if the bed or trolley is too low.

EVIDENCE AVAILABLE

Research: orthodox lift demonstrates high risk of injury to handlers *(Marras et al, 2000; Pheasant and Stubbs, 1992)*; exceeds safe lifting limits *(Schibye and Skotte, 2000; Winkelmolen, 1994; McGill et al, 1990, Torma-Krajewski, 1987)*.
Consensus: high risk based on MOHR weight thresholds *(DIAG 2001)*.
Professional opinion: lifting techniques pose high risk of injury therefore classified as unsafe *(NBPA, 1992 & 1998; BackCare, 1999)*.

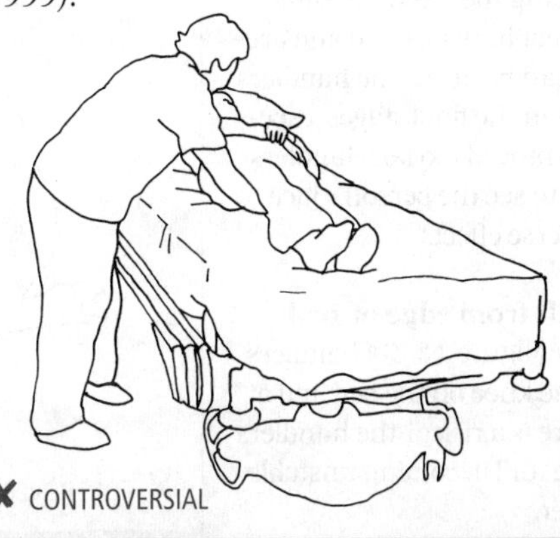

✗ CONTROVERSIAL

FIG 18.2b

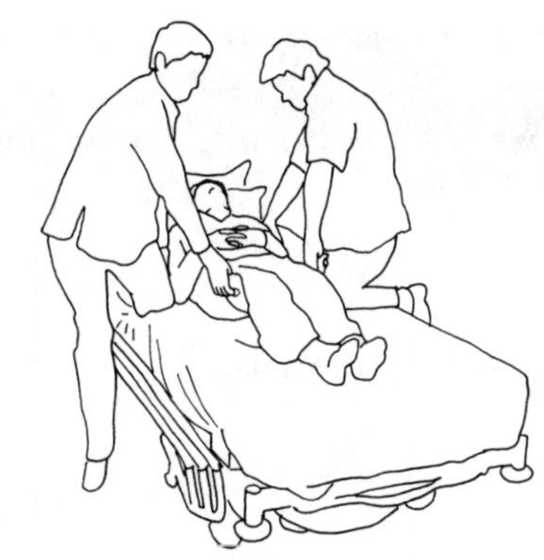

✗ CONTROVERSIAL

FIG 18.2c

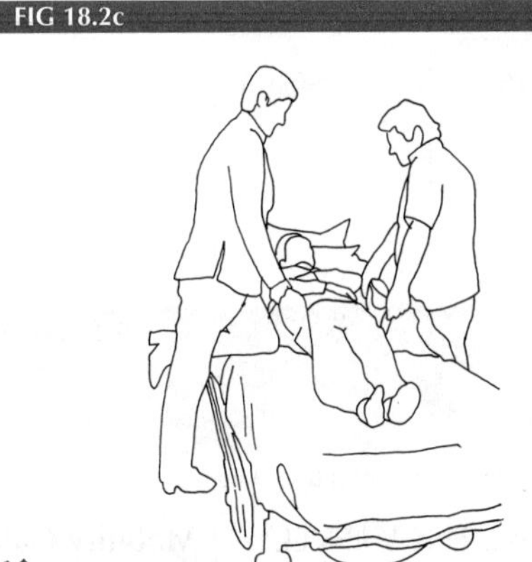

✗ CONTROVERSIAL

FIG 18.2d

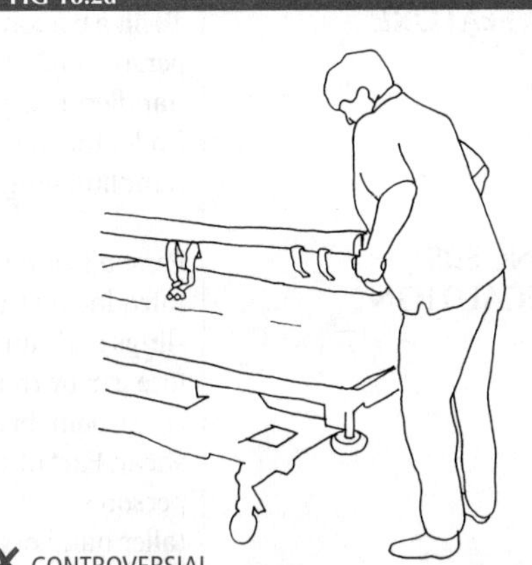

✗ CONTROVERSIAL

FIG 18.2e

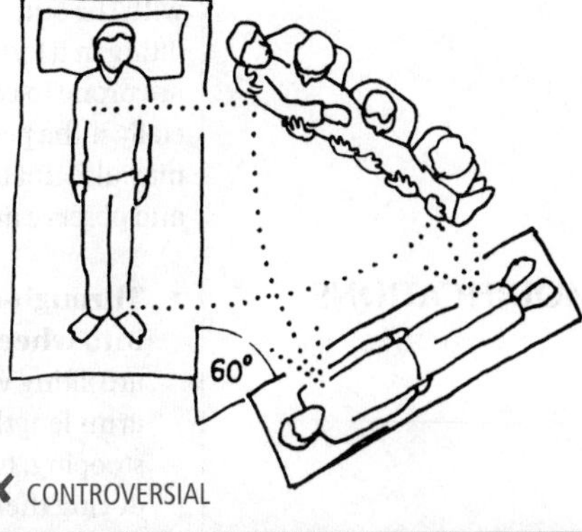

✗ CONTROVERSIAL

FIG 18.2f

Evidence review

Technique	REBA	Activity	Comfort	FIM	Mobility gallery	Skill level	Comment
ORTHODOX LIFT							
Fig 18.2a	12 – Very high	1	1	1	E	Novice	Very high risk, very uncomfortable and no activity from the person
Fig 18.2b	11 – Very high	1	3	1	E	Novice	Very high risk, low level of comfort and no activity from the person
Fig 18.2c	10 – High	1	4	1	E	Novice	High postural risk, low level of comfort and no activity from the person
Fig 18.2d	11 – Very high	1	7	1	E	Novice	Very high risk, but good level of comfort, no activity from the person
Fig 18.2e	8 – High	1	7	1	E	Novice	A high risk level, but on edge of medium, comfortable for person being moved. No activity from the person
Fig 18.2f	NO EVIDENCE						

Task Three

Through-arm* (hammock, top and tail, hump and dump)

* names duplicated in other techniques

DEPENDENCY LEVEL

Mobility Gallery C, D
FIM 1, 2

KEY FEATURE

To lift a person up the bed (figure 18.3a). The person is lifted in a slumped sitting position by handlers grasping the person's forearms and under the upper thighs (manually or using a handling sling).

DANGERS/ PRECAUTIONS

Person's skin may be subject to shear when introducing the handlers' arms or handling slings and can cause injury. The grasp on the forearm by the handler during lifting may also cause pain, bruising and injury due to skin shear. Part of the pull may be under the person's axilla, especially when applied by taller handlers. If not lifted high enough, the buttocks and heels drag on the bed and contribute to the development of pressure sores.

Handlers are holding the handling sling with the outer arm reaching forward and are lifting in a forward lean posture. The handlers are prone to twisting in the final stages, especially if the person is moved too far. Handlers may also not be able to see the person's face and observe any adverse effects.

MODIFICATIONS

- **Through-arm lift from edge of bed into wheelchair** (figure 18.3b) handlers are lifting with one knee on the bed and at arms length. There is a risk of the handlers stooping, twisting and becoming unstable during the transfer.
- **Through-arm lift up a low bed with**

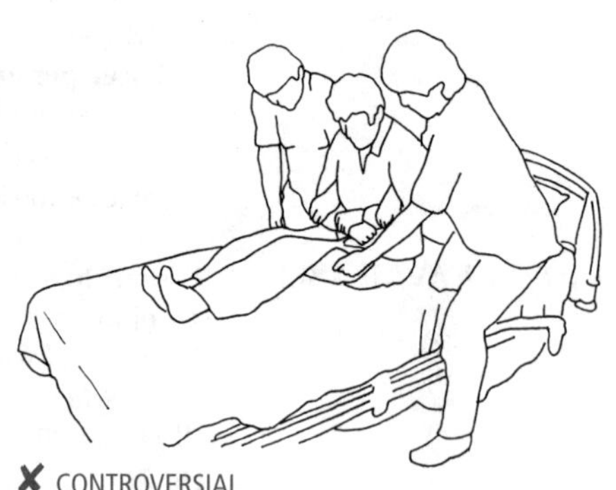

✘ CONTROVERSIAL

FIG 18.3a

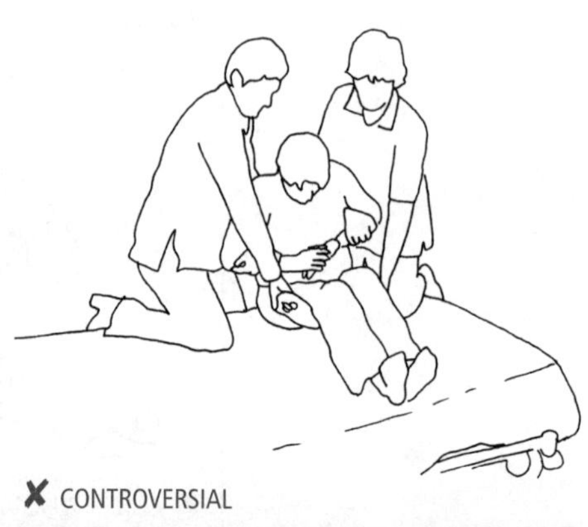

✘ CONTROVERSIAL

FIG 18.3b

one handler with person helping (figure 18.3c, below) handler is at risk of lifting in an awkward position due to restricted environment or unpredictable movement of the person.

- **Hammock lift** (figure 18.3d) top handler takes most of the person's weight and must stoop to lift/lower the person into the chair as the seat back prevents the knees from bending. However, both the handlers are at risk of twisting and holding the load away from them during the transfer, especially if there are obstructions such as chair backs, chair arms or differences in seat height.
- **Leg and arm/Through-arm lift up the chair with two handlers** (figure 18.3e, 18.3f) to reposition a slumped person back in the chair with two handlers either using a handling sling under the thighs or, if the person's legs are grasped manually, results in an even more stooped and twisted posture.
- **Through-arm lift up the chair with one handler** (figure 18.3g) repositioning the person in this manner requires the handler to lift in a stooped position due to the chair back restricting knee flexion. The lift may need to be prolonged whilst clothing is rearranged.

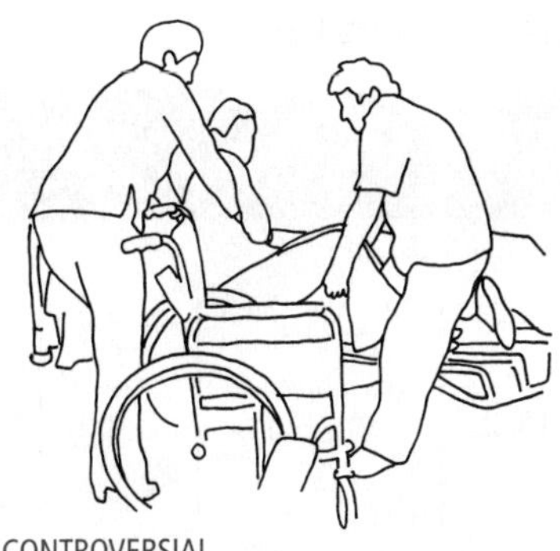
✘ CONTROVERSIAL
FIG 18.3d

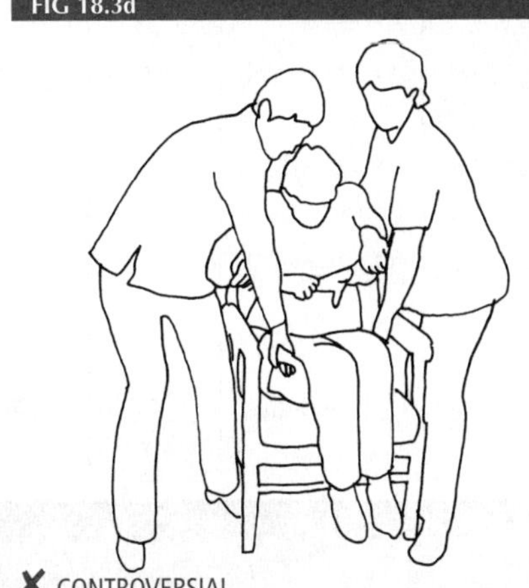
✘ CONTROVERSIAL
FIG 18.3e

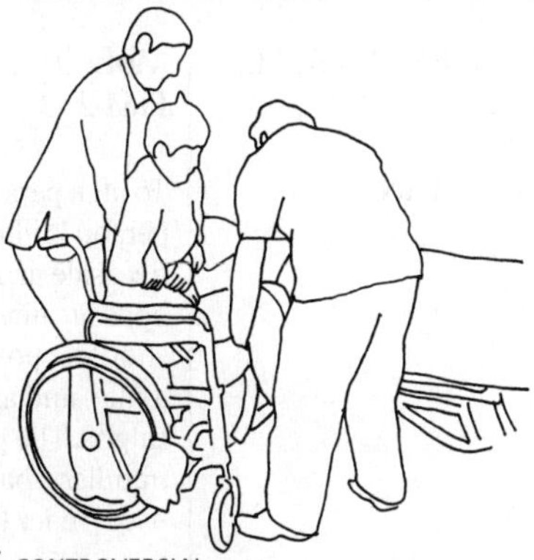

EVIDENCE AVAILABLE

Research: through-arm lift exceeds safe lifting limits *(Varcin-Coad and Barrett, 1998; Laflin and Aja, 1995; Winkelmolen et al, 1994)*. Demonstrates high risk of injury to handlers *(Pheasant and Stubbs, 1992)*.
Consensus: high risk based on MOHR weight thresholds *(DIAG, 2001)*.
Professional opinion: lifting techniques pose high risk of injury therefore classified as unsafe. *(NBPA, 1992 & 1998; BackCare, 1999)*.

✘ CONTROVERSIAL
FIG 18.3f

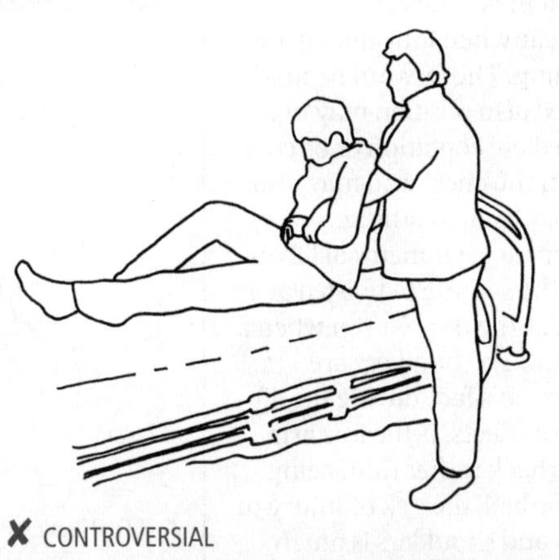
✘ CONTROVERSIAL
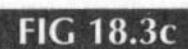
FIG 18.3c

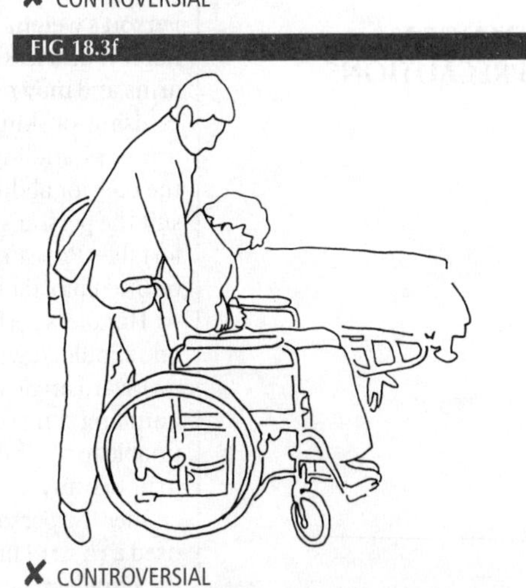
✘ CONTROVERSIAL
FIG 18.3g

Evidence review

Technique	REBA	Activity	Comfort	FIM	Mobility gallery	Skill level	Comment
THROUGH ARM LIFT							
Fig 18.3a	11 – Very high	3	3	1	C	Advanced beginner	Very high risk, very little activity from the person, low level of comfort
Fig 18.3b	10 – High	4	2	2	C	Advanced beginner	High risk, little activity from a reasonably able person, low level of comfort
Fig 18.3c	13 – Very high	1	3	1	D	Advanced beginner	Very high risk with negligible activity from the person, low comfort level
Fig 18.3d	12 – Very high	3	1	1	C	Advanced beginner	Very high risk, very little activity from the person, very low level of comfort
Fig 18.3e	11 – Very high	1	4	1	D	Advanced beginner	Very high risk with negligible activity from the person, low comfort level.
Fig 18.3f	11 – Very high	1	3	1	D	Novice	No handling sling is very slightly less comfortable, but can be performed by a less skilled handler
Fig 18.3g	10 – High	1	1	1	D	Advanced beginner	High risk with very low comfort and activity levels

Task Four

Shoulder lift * (Australian)

* names duplicated in other techniques

DEPENDENCY LEVEL

Mobility Gallery C, D
FIM 2, 3

KEY FEATURE

To lift a person up the bed (figure 18.4a). The person is lifted in a sitting position using the nearside arms of two handlers facing the opposite direction to the person with their shoulder positioned close to the person's axilla, and arms clasped under the upper thighs. The person rests their arms on the handlers' backs, and a handling sling may be used under the thighs.

DANGERS/ PRECAUTIONS

Person's weight is taken on the relatively narrow and less fleshy areas of the handlers' arms and may result in discomfort or bruising, or skin shear when introducing the arms or handling sling. The forward bend of the body or abducted arm position may not suit the person's medical condition or be comfortable. Pressure on the chest wall may also be uncomfortable or affect breathing.

Handlers perform an asymmetrical lift on one shoulder, with the same arm twisted at an awkward angle under the thighs even when a handling sling is used. The handlers are unable to see the person's face during the lift to notice any adverse effects. If the free arm cradles the person's back rather than being used as a strut on the bed, the risk of injury to the handlers' backs and shoulders is much higher as they are lifting in a forward bend

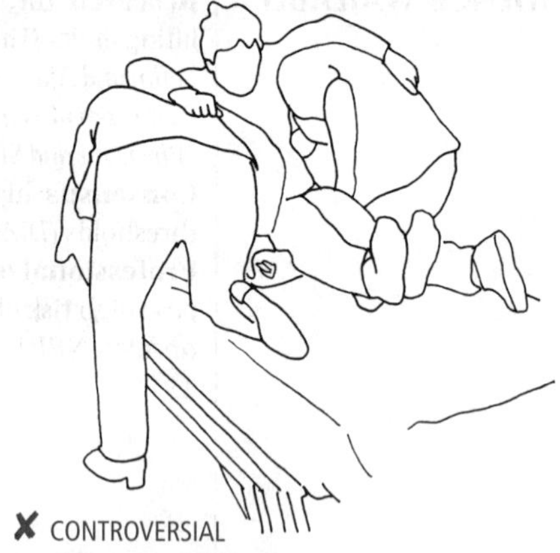

✘ CONTROVERSIAL

FIG 18.4a

✘ CONTROVERSIAL

FIG 18.4b

position. A person may try and help by push unexpectedly with their legs during the lift and pushing the handlers off balance, or they may suddenly decide to lift themselves up by pressing down on the handler's backs. A person may need to be lifted into the sitting position before applying the shoulder lift.

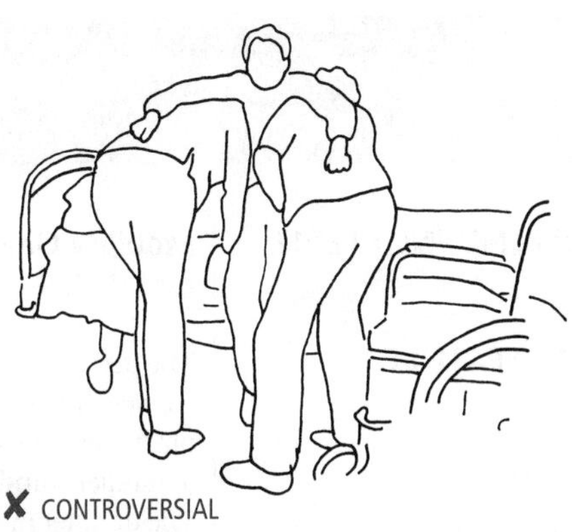

✘ CONTROVERSIAL

FIG 18.4c

MODIFICATIONS

- **Shoulder slide** – as shoulder lift (figure 18.4a) using a slide sheet under the person's buttocks and legs to avoid lifting.
- **Combined lift** (orthodox and shoulder lift) (figure 18.4b, previous page) both of these lifts are classified as high risk.
- **Shoulder lift to transfer between edge of bed and chair** (figure 18.4c) the additional task of carrying the person and poor stability during the transfer stage add to the risks. Also the free arm can no longer act as a strut to reduce the load on the spine.
- **Reverse shoulder lift from edge of bed onto wheelchair or commode** (figure 18.4d) handlers are required to stoop, lift the person at arms length, and twist to move the person into the chair. The handlers' base with one knee on the bed mattress is unstable.
- **Shoulder lift on a low or double bed, or floor** – (figure 18.4e) lifting a person from a crouched kneeling position is awkward and encourages the handlers to lift at arms length. Many handlers may find the position impossible to adopt due to individual physical capability.

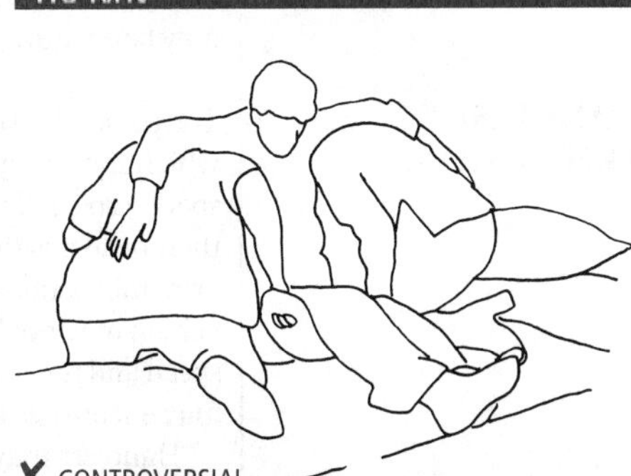

✘ CONTROVERSIAL

FIG 18.4d

EVIDENCE AVAILABLE

Research: shoulder lift exceeds safe lifting limits (*Winkelmolen et al, 1994*); high risk of back injury to handlers (*Gabbett, 1998*); low risk of injury to handlers (*Pheasant and Stubbs, 1992*); least stress on handlers when free arm is used as a strut and most when used to cradle person's back (*Scholey, 1982; Stubbs and Osborne, 1979*).
Consensus: high risk based on MHOR weight thresholds (*DIAG, 2001*).
Professional opinion: lifting techniques pose high risk of injury, therefore classified as unsafe (*NBPA, 1998; BackCare, 1999*).

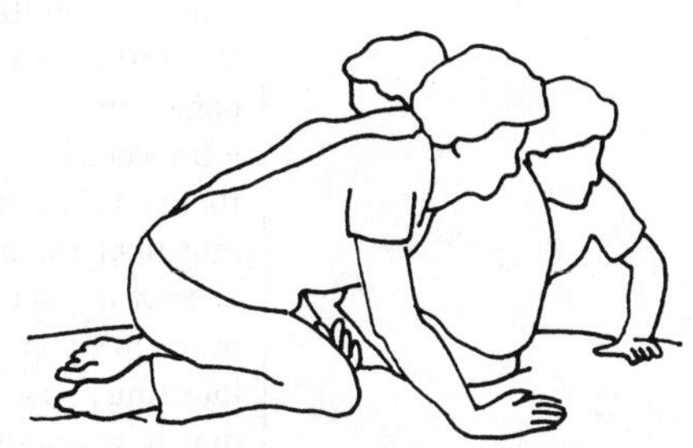

✘ CONTROVERSIAL

FIG 18.4e

Evidence review

Technique	REBA	Activity	Comfort	FIM	Mobility gallery	Skill level	Comment
SHOULDER LIFT							
Fig 18.4a	13 – Very high	2	6	2	C	Advanced beginner	Very high postural risk, low activity and adequate comfort levels
Fig 18.4b	12 – Very high	1	4	2	D	Competent	Very high postural risk, low activity and low comfort levels
Fig 18.4c	12 – Very high	3	5	3	C	Competent	Very high postural risk, low activity and adequate comfort levels
Fig 18.4d	12 – Very high	3	6	3	C	Competent	Very high postural risk, low activity and reasonable comfort levels

Task Five

Front assisted stand and pivot transfers (axillary, bear hug, hug, clinging Ivy, rocking-lift, elbow-lift, belt holds from front, face to face)

DEPENDENCY LEVEL

Mobility Gallery B
FIM 2, 3, 4

KEY FEATURE

The person in a seated position is either assisted into standing, or transferred using a pivot movement to another seated position by a handler standing directly in front of them. The handler may use a variety of holds, a knee or foot block may be applied, and the person may be encouraged to hold onto the handler.

DANGERS/ PRECAUTIONS

The person is firmly held for these transfers, which some may find invades their personal space, especially when hugged or when the their head positioned under the handler's arm. Independent movement is restricted, the person may not be moved at their preferred speed and the passive nature of the transfer may encourage a feeling of helplessness.

Handlers may use a rocking movement to build up momentum for these transfers. This increases the risk of becoming unstable due to the difficulty in controlling the amount of effort required to stand and turn in the restricted space. In some cases a second handler may stand behind the person to assist the transfer. To stand independently the person needs to lean forward, and this action is impeded by a handler standing in front of them and is therefore dysfunctional. Handlers may not be able to see the person's face and observe any adverse effects. Handlers are prone to stooping in both the lifting and lowering phases, and their base of support may be restricted if a knee or foot block is applied. The person may be linked to the handler and if either should become unstable during the movement one may pull the other down when collapsing, or the handler may try to carry the person round to complete the transfer. Handler injuries occur as they may take a considerably larger part of the person's weight than anticipated due to poor application of this complex technique or unpredictable movement of the person. Because a large part of the person's weight may potentially be taken during the assisted stand or transfer, these techniques are seen as controversial.

MODIFICATIONS

- **Assisted stand by holding hands** (figure 18.5a)
- **Assisted stand or transfer using a handling sling** (figure 18.5b)
- **Bear hug assisted stand or transfer** (figure 18.5c)
- **Bear hug hold with person's arms**

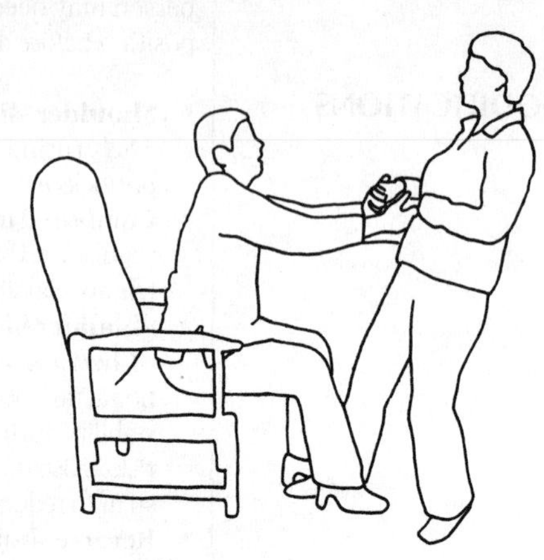

✗ CONTROVERSIAL

FIG 18.5a

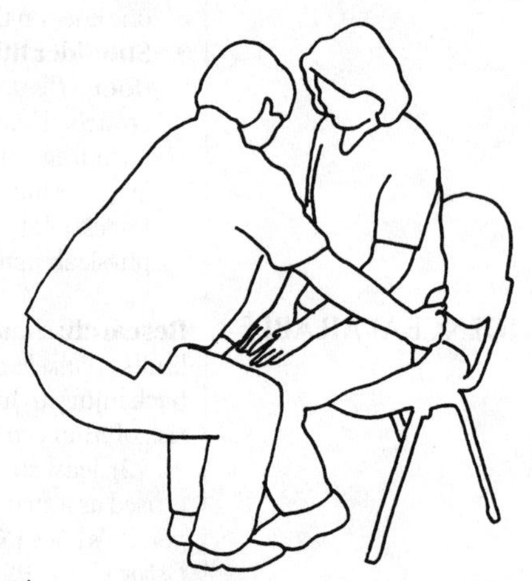

✗ CONTROVERSIAL

FIG 18.5b

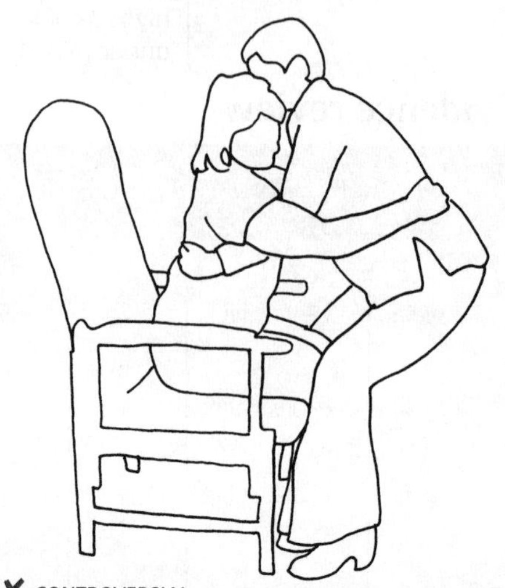

✗ CONTROVERSIAL

FIG 18.5c

Controversial techniques

around handler's neck (figure 18.5d, below)
- **Rocking-lift or belt hold from front assisted stand or transfer with one handler** (figure 18.5e, below)
- **Rocking-lift or belt hold from front assisted stand or transfer with two handlers** (figure18.5f-g)
- **Elbow-lift transfer through 90° or 180°** (figure18.5h)
- **Axillary hold for assisted stand or transfer** (figure 18.5i)

EVIDENCE AVAILABLE

Research: methods exceed safe lifting limits *(Schibye and Skotte, 2000; Zhuang et al, 2000; Marras et al, 1999; Ulin et al, 1997; Winkelmolen, 1994; Benevolo et al, 1993; Garg and Owen, 1992; Gagnon and Lortie, 1987)*; axillary hold pivot through 90° performed by one person moderate risk, using elbow hold through 180° moderate to high risk *(Pheasant and Stubbs, 1992)*.
Consensus: high risk based on MHOR weight thresholds *(DIAG, 2001)*.
Professional opinion: technique potentially unstable, person compliance unpredictable, and lifting techniques pose high risk of injury, therefore classified as unsafe *(NBPA, 1992 & 1998; BackCare, 1999)*.

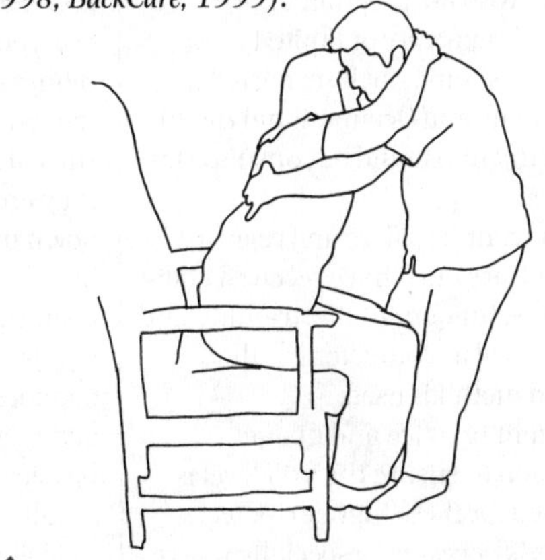

✗ CONTROVERSIAL
FIG 18.5d

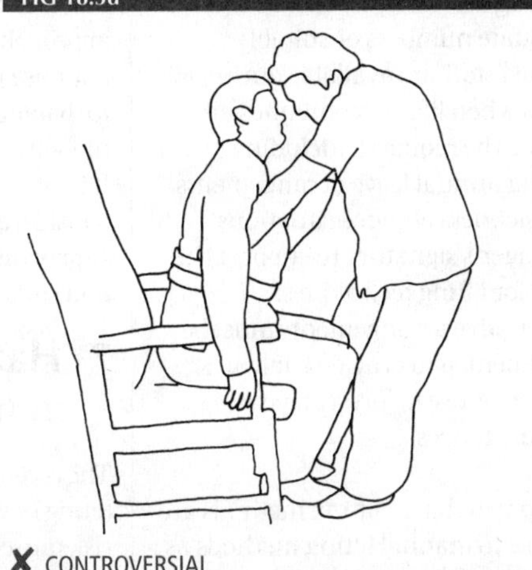

✗ CONTROVERSIAL
FIG 18.5e

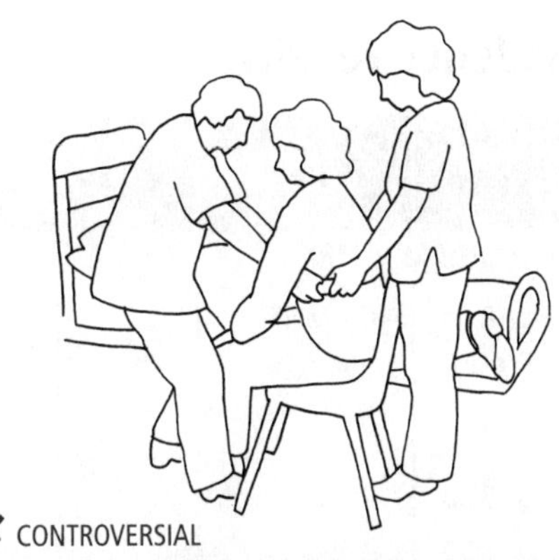

✗ CONTROVERSIAL
FIG 18.5f

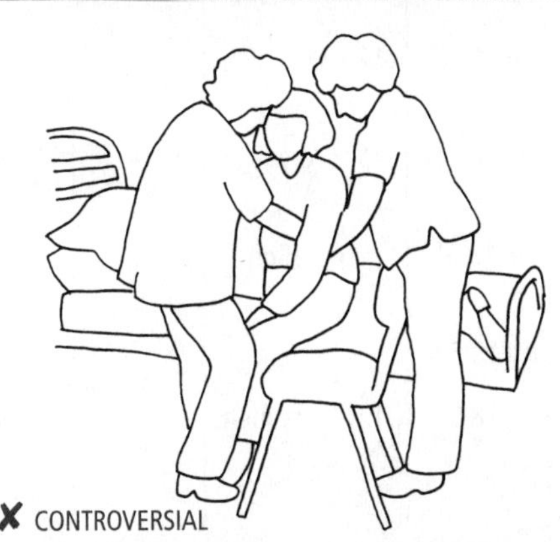

✗ CONTROVERSIAL
FIG 18.5g

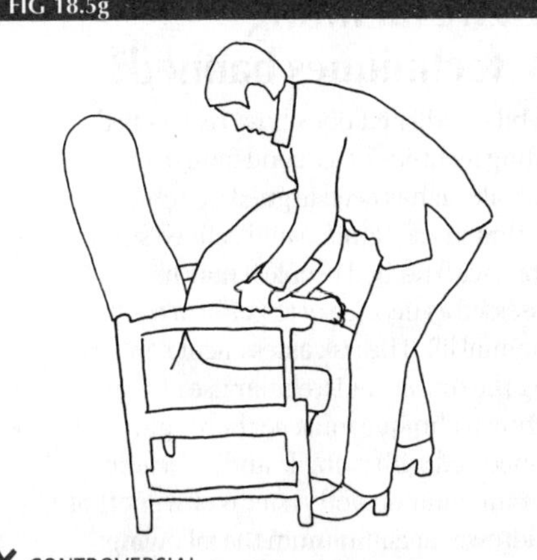

✗ CONTROVERSIAL
FIG 18.5h

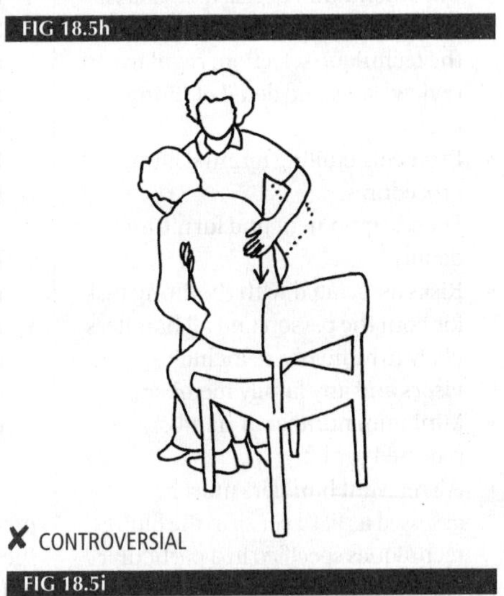

✗ CONTROVERSIAL
FIG 18.5i

Evidence review

Technique	REBA	Activity	Comfort	FIM	Mobility gallery	Skill level	Comment
THROUGH ARM LIFT							
Fig 18.5a	6 – Medium			3	B	Novice	Medium postural risk, can be done by a novice activity and comfort not scored, but person appears to be active, matching their ability
Fig 18.5b	12 – Very high	8	8	4	B	Advanced beginner	Very high risk activity, the person is very active, and is comfortable
Fig 18.5c	NO EVIDENCE						
Fig 18.5d	12 – Very high	7	8	4	B		Very high risk activity, the person is active, and is comfortable
Fig 18.5e	11 – Very high	8	8	4	B	Novice	Very high risk activity, the person is very active, and is comfortable.
Fig 18.5f	10 – High	8	8	4	B	Novice	Very high risk activity, for novice. the person is very active, and comfortable.
Fig 18.5g							Not assessed
Fig 18.5h	12 – Very high	2	4	2	B	Proficient	Very high risk, the person is neither very active or comfortable – for a less able person

6 Are all lifting techniques banned?

Whilst earlier editions have reclassified lifting techniques as 'condemned' or 'unsafe', it has been argued (see chapter 2) that in very limited and defined situations with named people it may be assessed as necessary to perform a manual lift. The risk assessment supporting the routine or irregular use of any lifting technique must be thorough, supported with suitable and sufficient documentation and systems of work that addresses at a minimum the following:

- Documentation of risk assessment with clinical reasoning supporting the technique selection, regular review dates and detail of lifting needs.
- Protocol detailing manual lifting procedures.
- Space, equipment and furniture details.
- Risks associated with the lifting task for both the person and all handlers likely to be involved, including supervisors and any family members.
- Minimum number of handlers required per lift.
- All relevant handlers must be assessed as fit to perform the lifting techniques specified in a particular care plan. Handlers of incompatible height, who are pregnant, have reduced capability or limited mobility, should not be expected to participate and Occupational Health Departments should be consulted for advice.
- All relevant handlers and relevant supervisors must have received additional technique specific training and be assessed as competent in the named methods used.
- Sufficient practice and update provision to ensure the skill level is retained for these higher risk techniques is necessary, especially where they are only performed occasionally.
- Staffing rosters must ensure adequate numbers of suitably trained staff are available during all times when lifting techniques are likely to be required, including during annual leave arrangements and sickness absence situations.
- Manager's signature to support the need for lifting techniques.
- Alternative arrangements must be documented to provide a fallback option for use in foreseeable circumstances.

Equipment based lifting methods are preferable to manual lifting methods as the person is fully supported throughout the technique and the transfer is therefore more controlled and safer for everyone. During manual lifting techniques however there may be a tendency for handlers to follow an "I've started so I must finish" approach as they are often not able to set the patient down mid-transfer. One "no strenuous lifting" programme, which combined training with assured availability of equipment was found to improve the comfort of the person during handling activities, and also to decrease the physical demands and fatigue of the handlers (*Yassi et al, 2001*).

Policies that incorporate a blanket ban on all lifting techniques should be modified to adopt a risk management approach. The aim of this should be to optimise person and handler safety, and to 'balance' this with the person's mobility needs and broader care needs. It is essential that all relevant factors are considered in the assessment, and the supporting documentation is suitable and sufficient for the given situation.

7 Hazardous postural activities

The risks to handlers through manual lifting have been explored, however these risks are compounded by activities that also require twisting, stooping, and prolonged maintenance of poor postures.

Examples include:

- washing people in low baths (figure 18.6a).
- putting on footwear (figure 18.6b).
- lifting immobile legs onto foot rests or foot stools (figure 18.6c).
- applying bandages or elastic stockings (figure 18.6d).
- providing care on low beds (figure 18.6e) or mattresses on the floor.
- stooping to help a person drink or eat (figure 18.6f).
- holding flaccid limbs in theatre situations for prepping.
- any hygiene and clinical procedures where leaning, twisting and sustained poor postures are unavoidable.

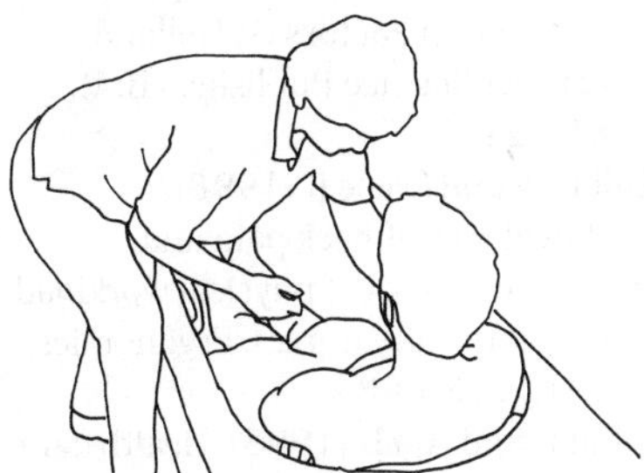

✗ HAZARDOUS POSTURE

FIG 18.6a

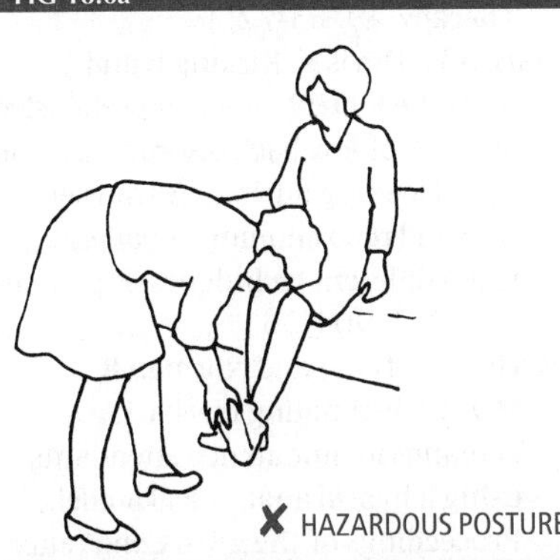

✗ HAZARDOUS POSTURE

FIG 18.6b

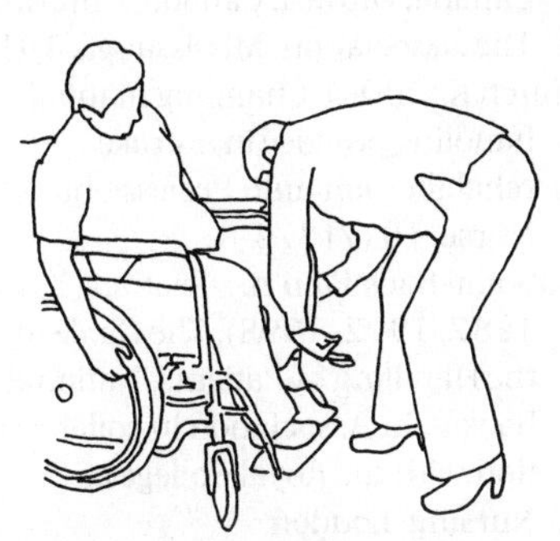

✗ HAZARDOUS POSTURE

FIG 18.6c

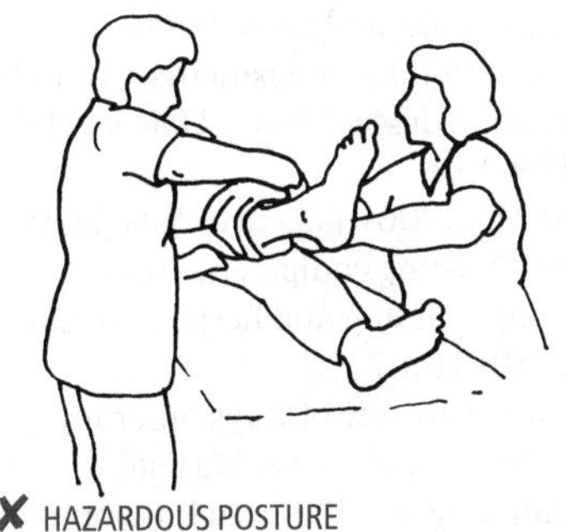

✗ HAZARDOUS POSTURE

FIG 18.6d

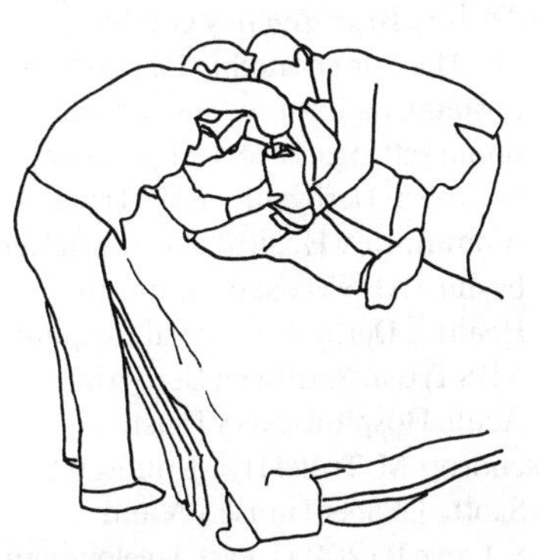

✗ HAZARDOUS POSTURE

FIG 18.6e

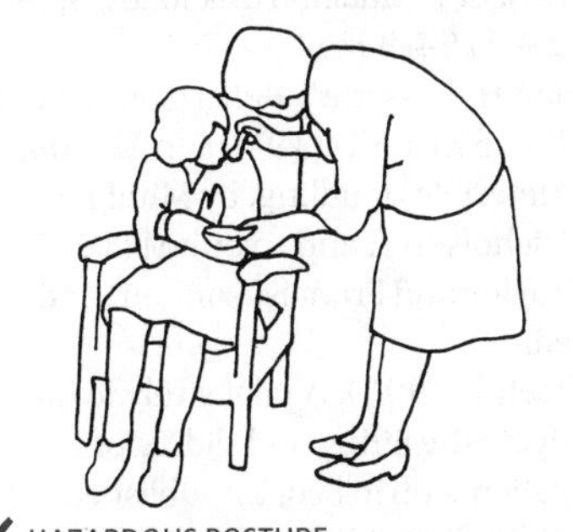

✗ HAZARDOUS POSTURE

FIG 18.6f

Taking the time to adequately plan and prepare the environment prior to undertaking manual handling tasks will minimise the postural risk. Introducing regular stretching activities and rest breaks will reduce the risk of cumulative strain.

8 Rehabilitation handling

Rehabilitation handling differs from care handling in that its central premise is the promotion or maintenance of mobility and functional independence in accordance with individual person treatment goals *(CSP, 2002)*. Whilst the whole multi-disciplinary team may contribute to the achievement of this aim, experienced or specialist therapists usually lead it.

The individual risk assessment should meet the identified needs without endangering the person, handlers or others. Equipment should be used to complement handling techniques during rehabilitation in both the acute and functional stages where appropriate *(Ruszala and Musa 2004; Mutch 2004; ACPIN 2001; Busse 2000)*. Treatment goals must be documented and supported with the relevant clinical reasoning. All handling methods should be realistic and achievable for both the person and those delivering the service. This may result in experienced or specialist therapists providing more advanced mobility techniques during treatment activities than less experienced therapists and handlers on the ward, and recommending the use of assisted devices such as standing aids and hoists for certain tasks.

Mutch (*2004*) suggests the main difference between therapists and handlers performing specialist techniques is that whilst therapists receive specialist training, handlers learn by watching the therapists and following their example, and this results in inconsistent methods. Any handler who has not been assessed as competent in any relevant handling technique should always feel empowered to say "no" and use agreed safer handing alternatives. Similarly, if a handler is concerned that a person may not be able to contribute adequately to the movement, they should use a documented safer method.

Where handling techniques are delegated to other handlers or family members, care must be taken to ensure that it is in accordance with agreed local protocols and adequately supported through risk assessment, training, competency assessment and supervision. These requirements are integral to standards of professional practice and the professional duty of care.

9 Summary

People should be encouraged and allowed to move independently and contribute to the move where assessed as able, or moved using methods that minimise the risk of injury to the person and handler. Manual lifting methods do not support either of the above and as a result of the evidence provided they should be considered as posing a high risk of musculoskeletal injury to handlers, and potential risk to people. In almost all situations manual people lifting can be replaced with safer alternatives and therefore it is appropriate for these to be implemented as a matter of priority.

10 Key points

Moving a person is a complex task that requires more handling activities than the individual lifting techniques described.

- Most people are too heavy, large, unwieldy or unpredictable to justify being lifted manually.
- Serious injury to the person and the handlers can result from manual lifting.
- Equipment based lifting methods are available and should be used subject to adequate risk assessment.
- Appropriate equipment and furniture should be easily available to avoid the need for handlers to use manual lifting methods.
- Poor working positions and static postures can accentuate strain on handlers and increase the risk of injury, including that from cumulative strain.
- Rehabilitation handling risk assessment must take into account the safety of handlers as well as the potential benefit for the person.
- Risk assessments should be based on a balanced decision making process rather than on blanket policies which may proscribe certain manual techniques.

Acknowledgements

I would especially like to thank Heather Kirton, Melanie Fewkes and colleagues at the United Bristol Healthcare NHS Trust for their valued contributions and memorable photographic sessions.

References

The Association of Chartered Physiotherapists Interested in Neurology (ACPIN) Manual Handling Working Party (2002). Guidance on Manual Handling in Treatment, Barnwell's Print Ltd, Aylesham

BackCare (1999). Safer Handling in the Community, Backare, London

Benevolo E, Sessarego P, Zelaschi G, and Franchignoni F (1993). An ergonomic analysis of five techniques for moving patients, Giornale Italiano di Medicina del Lavoro, 15: 139-144

Busse M (2000). Effective rehabilitation and hoisting equipment: a case study, Nursing and Residential Care, 2 (40) 168-73

Chartered Society of Physiotherapy (2002). Guidance in Manual Handling for Chartered Physiotherapists, Professional Development Department, CSP, London

Derbyshire Inter-Agency Group (2001). Care handling for people in hospital, community and educational settings. A code of practice. Southern Derbyshire NHS Trust (Community Health), Northern Derbyshire NHS Trust (Community Health), Derbyshire Royal Hospital NHS Trust, Southern Derbyshire Acute Hospitals NHS Trust.

Essendrop M, Trojel Hye-Knudsen C, Skotte J, Faber Hansen A and Schibye B (2004). Fast development of high intra-abdominal pressure when a trained participant is exposed to heavy, sudden trunk loads, Spine 29 (1) 94-99

Farfan H, Cossette J, Robertson G, Wells R and Kraus H (1970). In Manual Materials Handling, by Mital A, Nicholson A and Ayoub M (1997). Taylor and Francis: London, 2nd edn

Gabbett J (1998). A pilot study to investigate the lifting and sliding of patients up in bed, unpublished M.Sc. dissertation, University of Surrey

Garg A, Owen B and Carlson B (1992). An ergonomic evaluation of nursing assistants' job in a nursing home, Ergonomics, 35 (9) 979-95

Gagnon M and Lortie M (1987). A biomechanical approach to low-back problems in nursing aides, in Asfour, S. (ed) Trends in Ergonomic / Human Factors IV, Holland: Elsevier Science Publications BV, 795-802

Green C (1996). Study of the moving and handling practices on two medical wards British Journal of Nursing, 5 (5) 303-11

Health and Safety Executive (1992). Manual Handling Operations Regulations – Guidance on Regulations, HMSO, Norwich

Health and Safety Commission (1998). Manual Handling in the Health Services, HMSO, Norwich

Hignett S (1996). Work-related back pain in nurses, Journal of Advanced Nursing, 23: 1238-1246

Hignett S, Crumpton E, Ruszala S, Alexander P, Fray M and Fletcher B (2003). Evidence-Based Patient Handling, Routledge, London

Hollis M (1991). Safer Lifting for Patient Care, Blackwell Scientific Publications, London, 3rd edn.

Hye-Knudson C, Schibye B, Hjortskov N and Fallen N (2004). Trunk motion characteristics during different patient handling tasks International Journal of Industrial Ergonomics, 33 (4) 327-337

Khalil T, Asfour S, Marchette B and Omachonu V (1987). Lower back injuries in nursing: a biomechanical analysis and intervention strategy in Asfour S (ed) Trends in Ergonomics/Human Factors IV, Holland: Elsevier Science Publishers B. V., 811-21

Knibbe J and Friele R (1996). Prevalence of back pain and characteristics of physical workload of community nurses, Ergonomics, 39 (2): 186-98

Laflin K and Aja D (1995). Health care concerns relating to lifting: an inside look at intervention strategies, American Journal of Occupational Therapy, 49: 63-72

Marras W, Davis K, Kirking B and Bertsche P (1999). A comprehensive analysis of low back disorder risk and spinal loading during the transferring and repositioning of patients using different techniques, Ergonomics, 42, 7, 904-26

McGill S, Potvin J and Norman R (1990). Estimating low back demands in ambulance attendants using a hybrid anatomical model, Proceedings of the 23rd Conference of human Factors Association of Canada, Ottowa, Canada, Ontario: The Association, Mississauga, 191-5

Mutch K (2004). Changing manual-handling practice in a stroke rehabilitation unit, Professional Nurse, 19 (7) 374-8

National Back Pain Association (1981, 1987, 1992, 1998). The Guide to the Handling of Patients, National Back Pain Association in collaboration with the Royal College of Nursing, London

Nursing and Midwifery Council (2002). Practitioner-Client relationships and the prevention of abuse, sections 13 and 18, Nursing and Midwifery Council, London, 2nd edn

Owen B, Garg A and Jensen R (1992). Four methods for identification of most back-stressing tasks performed by nursing assistants in nursing homes, International Journal of Industrial Ergonomics, 9: 213-20

Owen B (1999). Decreasing the back injury problem in nursing personnel, Surgical Services Management, 5 (7) 15-21

Pheasant S and Stubbs D (1992). Back pain in nurses: epidemiology and risk assessment, Applied ergonomics, 23 (4) 226-232

Royal College of Nursing Advisory Panel (1993). Code of Practice for the Handling of Patients, London, 3rd edn

Royal College of Nursing (1996) Code of Practice for the Handling of Patients, London, 4th edn

Ruszala S and Musa I (2005). An evaluation of equipment to assist patient sit to stand activities in physiotherapy, Physiotherapy, (in press)

Scholey M (1982). The shoulder lift, Nursing Times, March 24: 506-7

Schibye M and Skotte J (2000). The mechanical loads on the low back during different patient handling tasks, Proceedings of the IEA2000/HFES 2000 Congress, The Human Factors and Ergonomics Society, California: Santa Monica, 5: 785-8

Smedley J, Egger P, Cooper C and Coggon D (1995). Manual handling activities and risk of low back pain in nurses, Occupational & Environmental Medicine, 52: 160-3

Stubbs D and Osborne C (1979). How to save your back. A comparison between the nursing profession and the construction industry Nursing, 3: 116-24

Torma-Krajewski J (1987). Analysis of lifting tasks in the health care industry, in Occupational Hazards to Health Care Workers, American Conference of Governmental Industrial Hygienists, 51-68

Ulin S, Chaffin D, Patellos C, Blitz S, Emerick C, Lundy F and Misher L (1997). A Biomechanical Analysis of Methods Used for Transferring Totally Dependent Patients, SCINURSING, 14 (1) 19-27

Varcin-Coad L and Barrett R (1998). Repositioning a slumped patient in a wheelchair. A biomechanical analysis of three transfer techniques AAOHN Journal, 46 (11) 530-6

Winkelmolen G, Landeweerd J and Drost M (1994). An evaluation of patient lifting techniques, Ergonomics, 37 (5): 921-32

Yassi A, Cooper J, Tate R, Gerlach S, Muir M, Trottier J and Massey K (2001). A randomised controlled trial to prevent patient lift and transfer injuries of health care workers Spine, 26 (16): 1739-1746

Zhuang Z, Stobbe T, Hsiao H, Collins J and Hobbs G (2000). Biomechanical evaluation of assistive devices for transferring residents, Applied Ergonomics, 30: 285-94

Appendix 1

Rapid Entire Body Assessment (REBA)

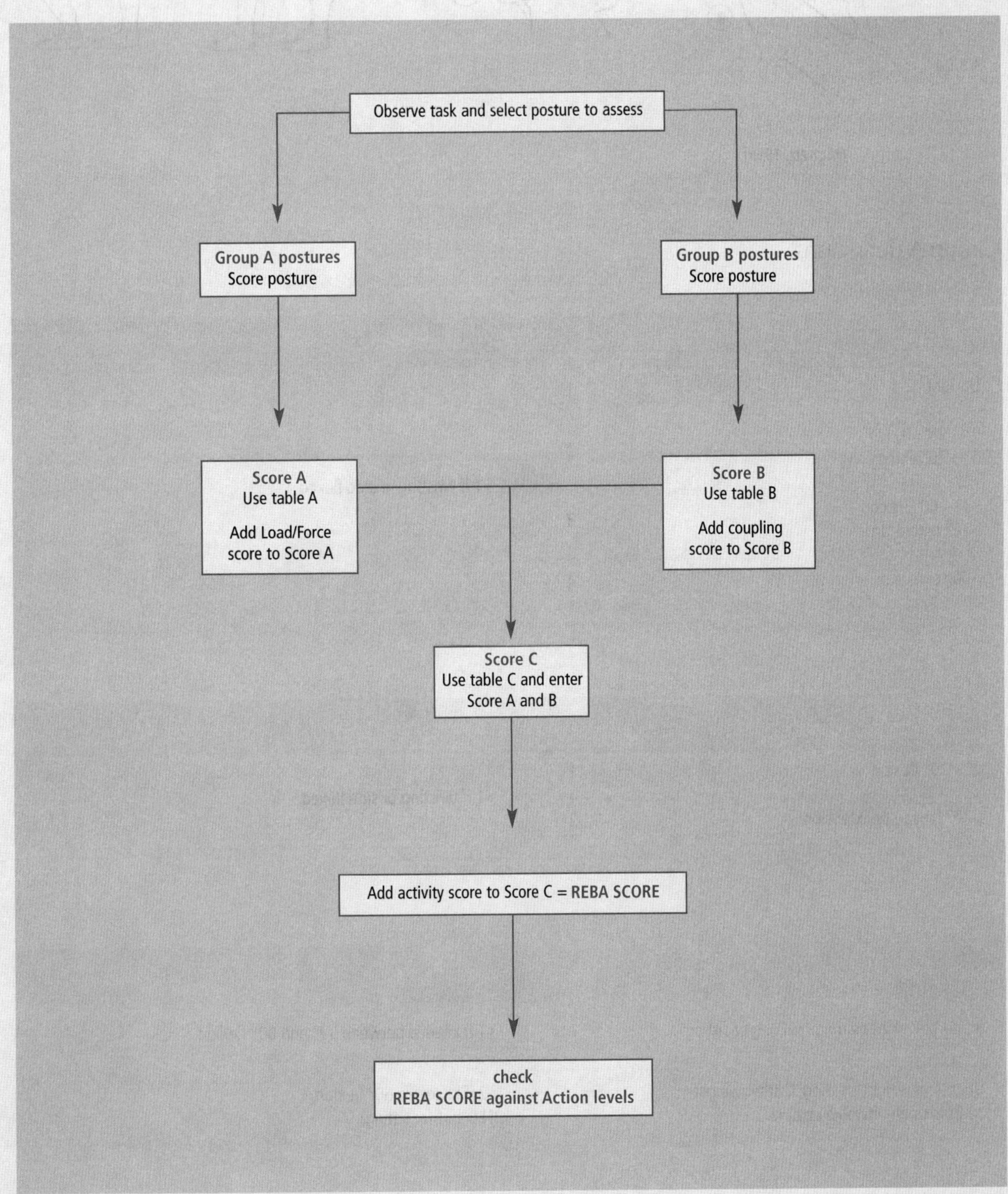

Using REBA *(Hignett and McAtamney, 2005)*

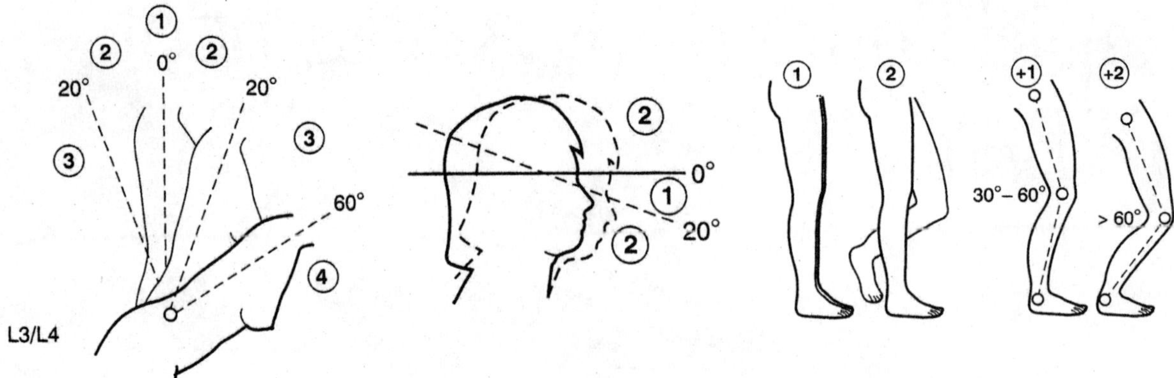

Group A postures *(Hignett, 1998)*

Group A definitions

Trunk postures

Movement	Score	Change score
Upright	1	+1 if twisting or side flexed
0° – 20° flexion 0° – 20° extension	2	
20° – 60° flexion >20° extension	3	
>60° extension	4	

Neck postures

Movement	Score	Change score
0° – 20° flexion	1	+1 if twisting or side flexed
>20° flexion or extension	2	

Leg postures

Position	Score	Change score
Bilateral weight bearing, walking or sitting	1	+1 if knee(s) between 30° and 60° flexion
Unilateral weight-bearing, feather weight-bearing or an unstable posture	2	+2 if knee(s) >60° flexion (N.B. not for sitting)

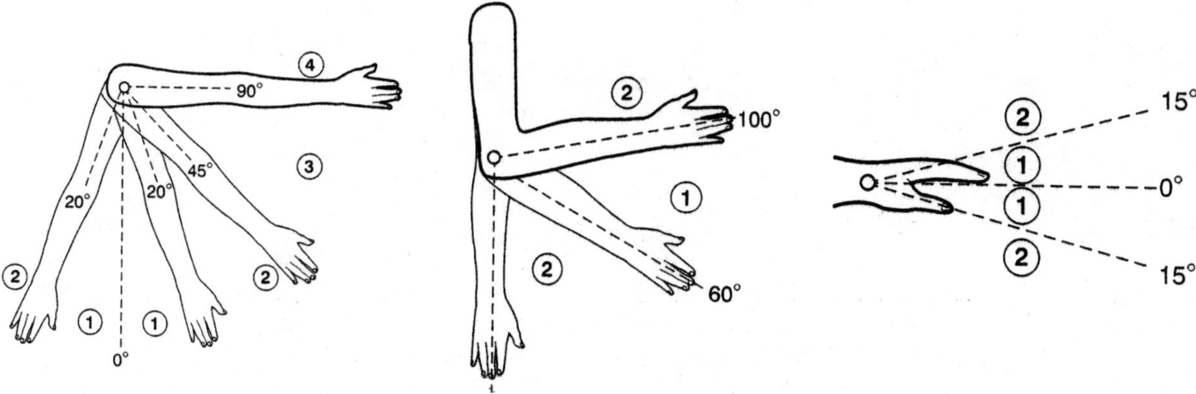

Group B postures *(Hignett, 1998)*

Group B definitions

Upper arms

Position	Score	Change score
20° extension to 20° flexion	1	+1 if arm is: abducted and/or rotated +1 if shoulder is raised -1 if leaning, supporting weight of arm or if posture is gravity-assisted
>20° extension 20° – 45° flexion	2	
45° – 90° flexion	3	
>90° extension	4	

Lower arms

Movement	Score
60° – 100° flexion	1
<60° flexion >100° flexion	2

Wrist

Movement	Score	Change score
0° – 15° flexion/extension	1	+1 if wrist is deviated or twisted
>15° flexion/extension	2	

REBA score sheet

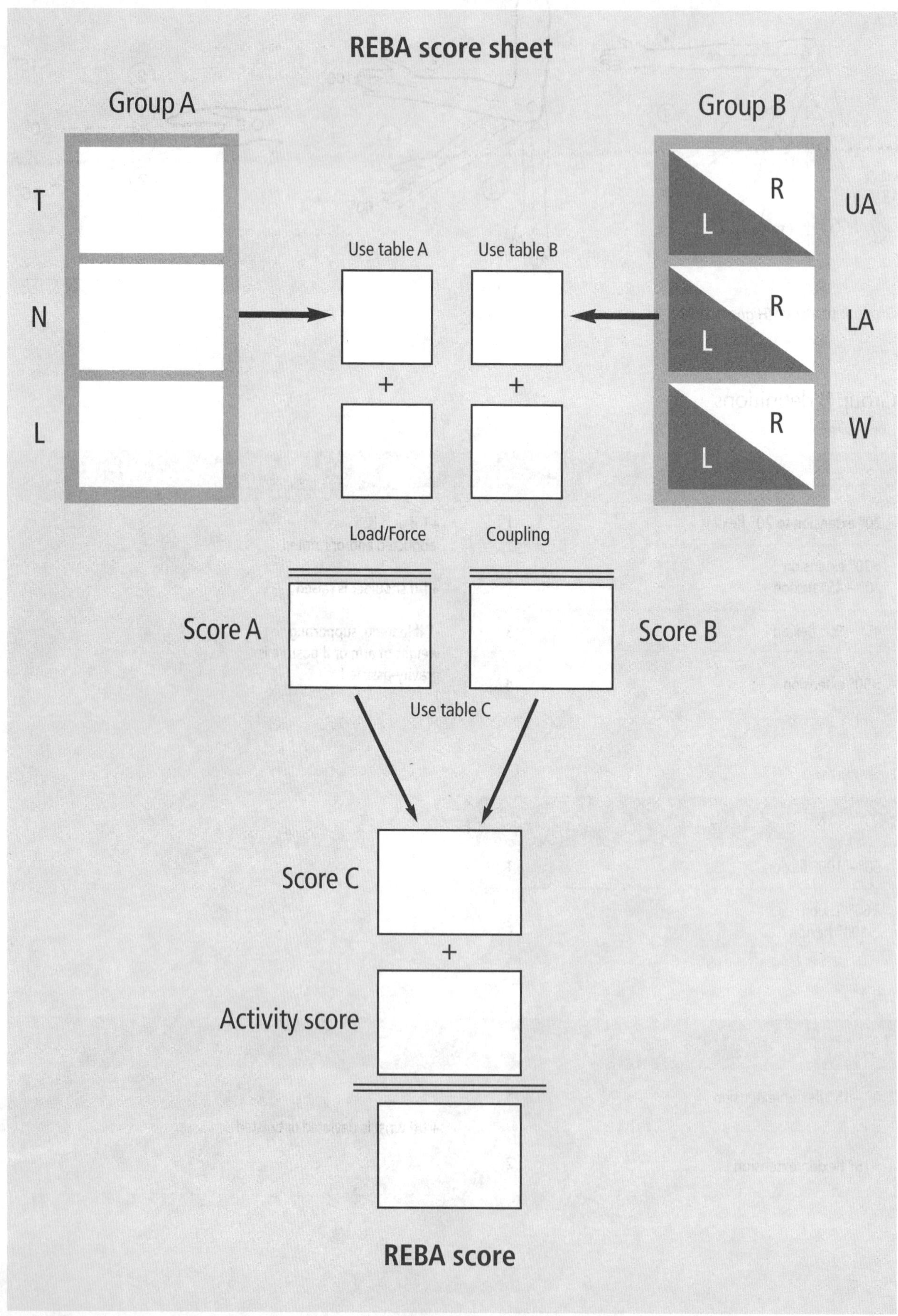

Table A

Trunk	Neck											
	1				2				3			
Legs	1	2	3	4	1	2	3	4	1	2	3	4
1	1	2	3	4	1	2	3	4	3	3	5	6
2	2	3	4	5	3	4	5	6	4	5	6	7
3	2	4	5	6	4	5	6	7	5	6	7	8
4	3	5	6	7	5	6	7	8	6	7	8	9
5	4	6	7	8	6	7	8	9	7	8	9	9

Load/Force

0	1	2	+1
<5kg	5 – 10 kg	>10kg	Shock or rapid build up of force

Table B and coupling

Table B

	Lower arm					
Upper Arm	1			2		
Wrist	1	2	3	1	2	3
1	1	2	2	1	2	3
2	1	2	3	2	3	4
3	3	4	5	4	5	5
4	4	5	5	5	6	7
5	6	7	8	7	8	8
6	7	8	8	8	9	9

Coupling

0 GOOD	1 FAIR	2 POOR	3 UNACCEPTABLE
Well fitting handle and a mid-range power grip	Hand hold is acceptable but not ideal or coupling is acceptable via another part of the body	Hand hold is not acceptable although possible	Awkward, unsafe grip, no handles. Coupling is unacceptable using other parts of the body

Table C and activity score

Table C

SCORE A	SCORE B 1	2	3	4	5	6	7	8	9	10	11	2
1	1	1	1	2	3	3	4	5	6	7	7	7
2	1	2	2	3	4	4	5	6	6	7	7	8
3	2	3	3	3	4	5	6	7	7	8	8	8
4	3	4	4	4	5	6	7	8	8	9	9	9
5	4	4	4	5	6	7	8	8	9	9	9	9
6	6	6	6	7	8	8	9	9	10	10	10	10
7	7	7	7	8	9	9	9	10	10	11	11	11
8	8	8	8	9	10	10	10	10	10	11	11	11
9	9	9	9	10	10	10	11	11	11	12	12	12
10	10	10	10	11	11	11	11	12	12	12	12	12
11	11	11	11	11	12	12	12	12	12	12	12	12
12	12	12	12	12	12	12	12	12	12	12	12	12

Activity score

+1	1 or more body parts are static e.g. held for longer than 1 minute
+1	Repeated small range actions e.g. repeated more than 4 times per minute (not including walking)
+1	Action causes rapid large range changes in posture or an unstable base

Action levels

Action level	REBA score	Risk level	Action including further assessements
0	1	Negligible	None necessary
1	2 – 3	Low	May be necessary
2	4 – 7	Medium	Necessary
3	8 – 10	High	Necessary soon
4	11 – 15	Very high	Necessary NOW

Appendix 2

Risk assessment filter

Reproduced from the **Guidance (L23) to the Manual Handling Operations Regulations 1992** (as amended) with the permission of the Controller of Her Majesty's Stationery Office

Risk assessment filter

1 The filter described in this Appendix is relevant to:
   a lifting and lowering;
   b carrying for short distances;
   c pushing and pulling; and
   d handling while seated.

2 It is most likely to be useful if you think that the activity to be assessed is low risk – the filter should quickly and easily confirm (or deny) this. If using the filter shows the risk is within the guidelines, you do not normally have to do any other form of risk assessment unless you have individual employees who may be at significant risk, for example pregnant workers, young workers, those with a significant health problem or a recent manual handling injury.

However these filter guidelines only apply when the load is easy to grasp and held in a good working environment.

3 However, the filter is less likely to be useful if:
   a there is a strong chance the work activities to be assessed involve significant risks from manual handling; or
   b the activities are complex. The use of the filter will only be worthwhile if it is possible to quickly (say within ten minutes) assess whether the guidelines in it are exceeded.

4 In either of these cases using the filter may not save any time or effort, so it may be better to opt immediately for the more detailed risk assessment in Appendix 4*.

5 The filter is based partly on data in published scientific literature and partly on accumulated practical experience of assessing risks from manual handling. Its guideline figures are pragmatic, tried and tested; they are not based on any precise scientific formulae. The intention is to set out an approximate boundary within which the load is unlikely to create a risk of injury sufficient to warrant a detailed assessment.

6 Application of the guidelines will provide a reasonable level of protection to around 95% of working men and women. However, the guidelines should not be regarded as safe weight limits for lifting. There is no threshold below which manual handling operations may be regarded as 'safe'. Even operations lying within the boundary mapped out by the guidelines should be avoided or made less demanding wherever it is reasonably practicable to do so.

Using the filter

7 The filter is in several parts, covering lifting and lowering, frequent lifting, carrying, twisting, carrying, pushing and pulling and handling when seated. Use the guideline figures in each part to help you assess the task.

8 You will need to carry out a more detailed assessment (see Appendix 4*) if:
   a using the filter shows the activity exceeds the guideline figures;
   b the activities do not come within the guidelines, eg if lifting and lowering unavoidably takes place beyond the box zones in Figure 23;
   c there are other considerations to take into account;
   d the assumptions made in the filter are not applicable, for example when carrying the load it is not held against the body;
   e for each task the assessment cannot be done quickly.

9 Paragraphs 28-29 and Table 3 provide an aide memoire for recording the findings from using the filter and reaching a judgement whether or not a full assessment is required.

Lifting and lowering

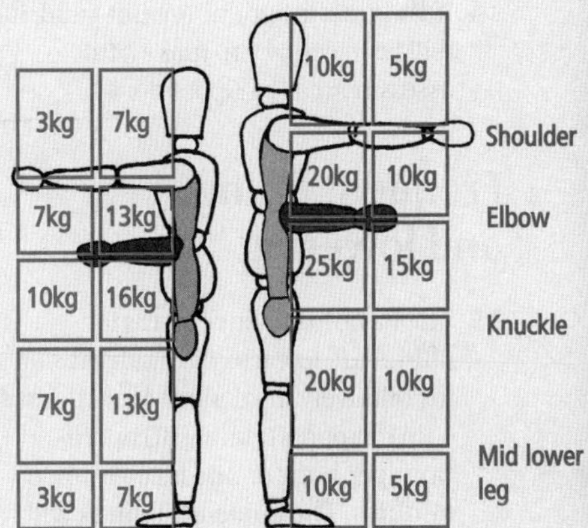

Figure 23 Lifiting and lowering

10 Each box in the diagram contains a guideline weight for lifting and lowering in that zone. Using the diagram enables the assessor to take into account the vertical and horizontal position of the hands as they move the load, the height of the individual handler and the reach of the individual handler.

As can be seen from the diagram, the guideline weights are reduced if handling is done with arms extended, or at high or low levels, as that is where injuries are most likely.

11 Observe the work activity being assessed and compare it to the diagram. First decide which box or boxes the lifter's hands pass

through when moving the load. Then assess the maximum weight being handled. If it is less than the figure given in the box, the operation is within the guidelines.

12 If the lifter's hands enter more than one box during the operation, then the smallest weight figure applies. An intermediate weight can be chosen if the hands are close to a boundary between boxes.

13 The guideline figures for lifting and lowering assume:

a the load is easy to grasp with both hands;
b the operation takes place in reasonable working conditions; and
c the handler is in a stable body position.

14 If these assumptions are not valid, it will be necessary to make a full assessment as in Appendix 4*.

Frequent lifting and lowering

15 The basic guideline figures for lifting and lowering in Figure 23 are for relatively infrequent operations – up to approximately 30 operations per hour or one lift every two minutes. The guideline figures will have to be reduced if the operation is repeated more often. As a rough guide:

Where operations are repeated	Figures should be reduced by
Once or twice per min	30%
Five to eight times per min	50%
More than 12 times per min	80%

16 Even if the above conditions are satisfied, a more detailed risk assessment should be made where:

a the worker does not control the pace of work;
b pauses for rest are inadequate or there is no change of activity which provides an opportunity to use different muscles; or
c the handler must support the load for any length of time.

Twisting

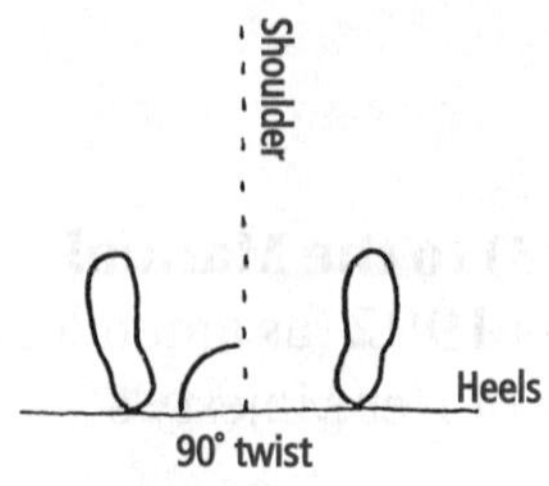

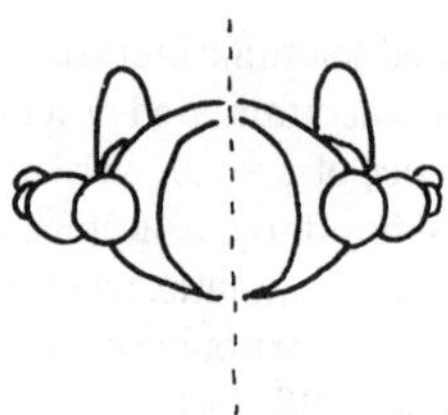

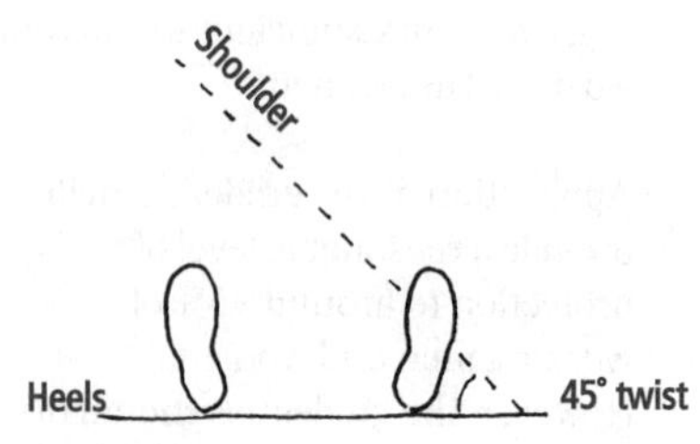

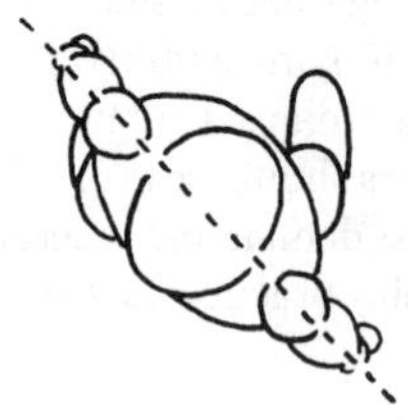

Figure 24 Assessing twist

17 In many cases manual handling operations will involve some twisting, ie moving the upper body while keeping the feet static (see Figure 24). The combination of twisting and lifting and twisting, stooping and lifting are particularly stressful on the back. Therefore where the handling involves twisting and turning then a detailed assessment should normally be made.

18 However if the operation is:

a relatively infrequent (up to approximately 30 operations per hour or one lift every two minutes); and
b there are no other posture problems,

then the guideline figures in the relevant part of this filter can be used, but with a suitable reduction according to the amount the handler twists to the side during the operation. As a rough guide:

If handler twists through (from front)	Guideline figures (Figure 24) should be reduced
45°	10%
90°	20%

19 Where the handling involves turning, ie moving in another direction as the lift is in progress and twisting, then a detailed assessment should normally be made.

Guidelines for carrying

20 The guideline figures for lifting and lowering (Figure 23) apply to carrying operations where the load is:

a held against the body;
b carried no further than about 10 m without resting.

21 Where the load can be carried securely on the shoulder without first having to be lifted (as, for example when unloading sacks from a lorry) the guideline figures can be applied to carrying distances in excess of 10 m.

22 A more detailed assessment should be made for all carrying operations if:

a the load is carried over a longer distance without resting; or
b the hands are below knuckle height or above elbow height (due to static loading on arm muscles).

Guidelines for pushing and pulling

23 For pushing and pulling operations (whether the load is slid, rolled or supported on wheels) the guideline figures assume the force is applied with the hands, between knuckle and shoulder height. It is also assumed that the distance involved is no more than about 20 m. If these assumptions are not met, a more detailed risk assessment is required (see the push/pull checklist in Appendix 4*).

Guidelines figure for stopping or starting a load	
Men	20kg (ie about 200 newtons)
Women	15kg (ie about 150 newtons)

Guidelines figure for keeping the load in motion	
Men	10kg (ie about 100 newtons)
Women	7kg (ie about 70 newtons)

24 As a rough guide the amount of force that needs to be applied to move a load over a flat, level surface using a well-maintained handling aid is at least 2% of the load weight. For example, if the load weight is 400 kg, then the force needed to move the load is 8 kg. The force needed will be larger, perhaps a lot larger, if conditions are not perfect (eg wheels not in the right position or a device that is poorly maintained). Moving an object over soft or uneven surfaces also requires higher forces. On an uneven surface, the force needed to start the load moving could increase to 10% of the load weight, although this might be offset to some extent by using larger wheels. Pushing and pulling forces will also be increased if workers have to negotiate a slope or ramp (see paragraph 164 in the main document). Even where the guideline figures in paragraph 23 are met, a detailed risk assessment will be necessary if risk factors such as uneven floors, confined spaces, or trapping hazards are present.

25 There is no specific limit to the distance over which the load is pushed or pulled as long as there are adequate opportunities for rest or recovery. Refer to the push/pull checklist (see Appendix 4*) if you are unsure and carry out a detailed risk assessment.

Guidelines for handling while seated

26 The basic guideline figures for handling operations carried out while seated, shown in Figure 25, are:

Men	Women
5 kg	3 kg

Figure 25

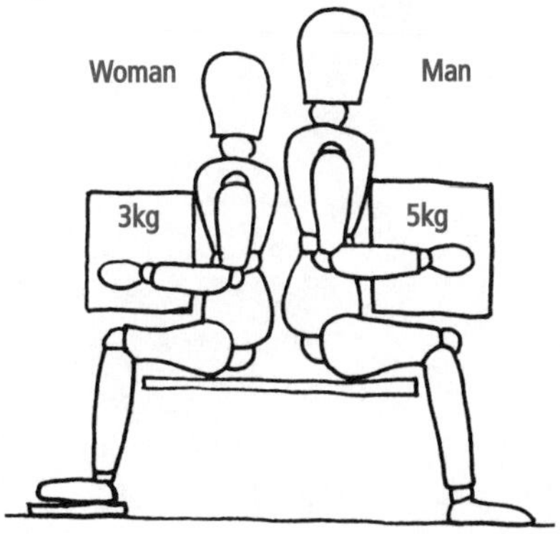

27 These guidelines only apply when the hands are within the box zone indicated. If handling beyond the box zone is unavoidable, a more detailed assessment should be made.

Recording findings and reaching a decision

28 For each task, use the filter to assess each of the activities involved (some tasks may only involve one activity, eg lifting and lowering, while others may involve several). Table 3 can be used to record the results; this is not a legal requirement but may be useful if problems later on are associated with the task.

29 Identify if each activity being performed comes within the guidelines and if there are other considerations to take into account (it may be helpful to make a note of these). Then make a final judgement of whether the task needs a full risk assessment. Remember you should be able to do this quickly – if not then a full risk assessment is required (see Appendix 4*).

Table 3 Application of guidelines

Task			
Activity	For each activity, does the task fall outside the guidelines YES/NO	Are there any other considerations which indicate a problem YES/NO (indicate what the problem is, if desired.)	Is a more detailed assessment required? YES/NO
Lifting and lowering			
Carrying			
Pushing and pulling			
Handing while seated			

Limitations of the filter

30 Remember: The use of these guidelines does not affect the employer's duty to avoid or reduce the risk of injury where this is reasonably practicable. The guideline figures, therefore, should not be regarded as weight limits or approved figures for safe lifting. They are an aid to highlight where detailed risk assessments are most needed. Where doubt remains, a more detailed risk assessment should always be made.

31 The employer's primary duty is to avoid operations which involve a risk of injury or, where it is not practicable to do so, to assess each such operation and reduce the risk of injury to the lowest level reasonably practicable. As the probability of injury rises, the employer must scrutinise the operation increasingly closely with a view to a proper assessment and the reduction of the risk of injury to the lowest level reasonably practicable. Even for a minority of fit, well-trained individuals working under favourable conditions, operations which exceed the guideline figures by more than a factor of about two may represent a serious risk of injury.

* **Reference to Appendix 4 relates to Appendix 4 of the guidance on the regulations and not this publication**

Appendix 3

Training guidance and competencies

Royal College of Nursing
Produced as part of the RCN Working Well Initative

1 Introduction

The Royal College of Nursing gets lots of request for information about manual handling training. The College's Back in Work project (RCN 2000) shows that achieving real improvements in staff health calls for an integrated approach. Management issues, staff issues, problem solving, change management, equipment provision and training must all be taken into account.

Often, though, providing training is the first – and sometimes the only – action employers take in attempting to comply with the manual handling legislation.

According to UK health and safety law, this is unacceptable. This guidance puts manual handling training in the context of a fully integrated risk management system that meets all the legal requirements.

Policy

The RCN has worked alongside Liko (UK) Ltd to produce this guidance, which is underpinned by our Safer Handling Policy:

"The aim is to eliminate hazardous manual handling in all but the most exceptional of life-threatening situations. Patients should be encouraged to assist in their own transfers and handling aids must be used whenever they can reduce the risk of injury. Handling patients manually may continue only if it does not involve lifting most or all of a patient's weight. Care must also be taken when supporting a patient and pushing and pulling should be kept to a minimum. Staff should assess the capabilities and rehabilitation needs of a patient to decide on which, if any handling aids are suitable." *(Royal College of Nursing 2000).*

2 Why do we need more guidance?

There has long been a need for definitive standards in manual handling training, and many authorities have issued training guidance in the past. However, much of this focuses on the content, length and duration of training, and adopts a prescriptive, didactic approach.

This guidance aims to reflect the diverse opinions and working practices of a range of professionals in different areas. It draws on research based evidence of what works, and seeks to promote excellence in practice by setting the guidance within the framework of clinical governance.

It therefore focuses on the competencies staff need to achieve safer patient handling. The guidance aims to bridge the gap between theory and practice by changing attitude and behaviour to managing manual handling risks in a variety of workplace settings.

Clinical Governance

Clinical governance is "A framework (or system) through which NHS organisations are accountable for continuously improving the quality of their services and safeguarding high standards of care by creating an environment in which excellence in clinical care can flourish" *(Department of Health 1998).* To make sure the guidance complies with the existing clinical governance framework, we used a practice development model which takes into account the fact that manual handling activities also take place in non-clinical or social care settings.

Practice Development

This guidance is set in the context of practice development: how health care professionals can continue to develop their knowledge and skills in order to provide better patient care.

Practice development must be enabled and supported by facilitators who are committed to systematic, rigorous and continuous processes of change. These processes will free practitioners to work in ways that better reflect the perspectives of both service users and providers. There are three essential elements for successful implementation *(Manley K 1992).*

1 The nature of the evidence
2 The context or environment
3 The method of facilitation.

1 The nature of the evidence

Evidence should be scientifically robust. It should reflect the professional consensus and meet patient needs. There is a large body of evidence around the area of manual handling. This guidance incorporates information form relevant literature, particularly on manual handling as a solution to the problem of musculo-skeletal pain and injury.

2 The context or environment

The work environment should be receptive to change, with a culture that prioritises health and safety. Organisations must identify who is responsible for manual handling and give them the resources, time and knowledge they need to carry out the necessary tasks *(Health and Safety Executive 1999).*

3 Method of facilitation

Organisations should use skilled external clinical facilitators to bring about changes in the work environment. Practice development theories identify two forms of facilitation.

Task facilitation – where facilitators enable individuals or groups to carry out a specific task.

Holistic facilitation – a complex, systemic process, enabling and empowering individuals or groups to analyse, reflect and change their own attitudes, behaviours and ways of working. Holistic facilitators help people use new theoretical insights to transform themselves and change the systems that hinder improvements in practice.

According to our focus groups, task facilitation is the most common type.

However, the literature states that "holistic facilitation" is necessary to achieve excellence in practice. Clinical supervision is one potential model of a holistic facilitation style.

Clinical supervision

Clinical supervision describes the formal process of professional support and learning which helps individual practitioners to develop knowledge and competence, assume responsibility of their own practise and safeguard patients in complex clinical situations. Clinical supervision can take place individually or in groups. The exact model to be followed will vary according to the organisational context *(Royal College of Nursing 1999)*.

A new approach

The principles of change management and participative ergonomics underpin this guidance. The terminology used should reflect the move towards a new model. Instead of "training" we will use "education" when talking about formal updates and achieving core competencies, "supervision" when discussing line management and "facilitation" to refer to refresher or problem-solving sessions, and to co-ordinating supervision activities.

This guidance promotes a patient-centred approach and excellence in care. Staff health and patient care should no longer be viewed as two separate issues (Royal College of Nursing (2001) *Changing practice – improving health: an integrated back injury prevention programme for nursing and care homes.* London: RCN (publication code 001 255).); excellence in manual handling is part of achieving excellence in care. The aim is to change practice and staff behaviour by creating a good manual handling culture based on a sound education process with adequate supervision.

3 The guidance – what to do

This guidance covers:

- Creating the right context among both staff and clients for a successful manual handling culture, including an organisational flowchart and details of responsibility, accountability and delegation
- Facilitating change, including the personnel needed
- Practical steps towards achieving the competencies needed
- The documentation needed to audit and review the change process
- Patient/client needs
- A list of competencies required for back care advisers (BCAs), supervisors and other staff

The right context

The right organisational context is one that helps staff achieve the competencies they need. It should include the following (see flow chart below).

Responsibility

The employer/chief executive has ultimate responsibility under the law, which cannot be delegated. If the employer delegates the operational aspects of ensuring safer manual handling, they must ensure the person responsible has adequate time, resources and knowledge (see under "Delegation" below) *(Health and Safety Executive 1999)*.

Accountability

In order to optimise staff health and patient care the "risk management" audit process should stipulate adherence to the manual handling policy. This will allow staff to give manual handling risk feedback to their employer, in turn helping employers to meet their statutory responsibilities.

Delegation

Delegation must be handled through the line management chain, starting with a nominated board member with overall responsibility for managing manual handling risks. Roles and responsibilities should be clearly stated in job descriptions and monitored through regular appraisal. The first frontline level of management will be the clinical manager.

Good management practice within an agreed system of manual handling supervision is essential. Manual handling is a core competency for many staff caring for patients, and managers are responsible for assessing and assuring the clinical effectiveness and competence of their staff in this as well as all other clinical areas.

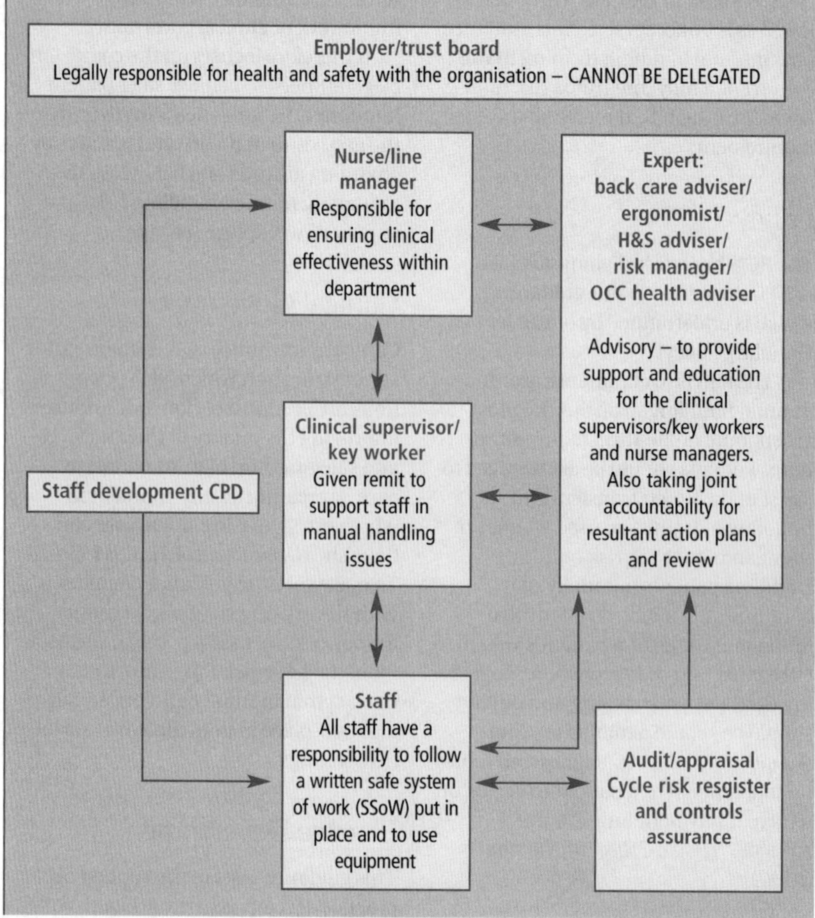

Facilitating change

As well as the right organisational context, the right personnel are essential to facilitate change, ensure that staff get the training they need, and provide ongoing clinical support and supervision.

Personnel

The manager is responsible for making sure good manual handling practice is followed in all care settings. Managers can delegate this task to any competent person, provided they have adequate, time, resources, knowledge and competence (Health and Safety Executive (1999) *The Management of Health and Safety at Work Regulations.* Sudbury: HSE.) – a clinical supervision model (Royal College of Nursing (1999) *Look back, move on: clinical supervision for nurses.* London: RCN) may help managers assess and enhance staff competence.

This person – the manual handling supervisor or key/link worker – is responsible for supervising manual handling in their work area. They must have all the necessary competencies to fulfil the role and meet the standards set by organisational policy and legislation (see below, under "The competencies").

Whoever is responsible for managing manual handling should have access to competent advice and the expertise of a back care adviser (BCA)/manual handling expert, who should also provide the necessary education. Risk managers, ergonomists, occupational health advisers and health and safety advisers can also be education providers. Throughout the rest of this guidance we will use the abbreviation "BCA" to refer to all such experts/competent persons.

Employers also need competent help for a BCA to apply the provisions of health and safety law, including the law relating to manual handling (Health and Safety Executive (1999) *The Management of Health and Safety at Work Regulations.* Sudbury: HSE). Employers should consider appointing one or more employees to provide this help. If there is no competent person within the organisation, employers will need to look outside.

The BCA should be given adequate information and support, and must have all the competencies outlined in this document. The role of the BCA is mainly advisory, and should include facilitating a holistic approach to safer patient handling and manual handling in the organisation. The BCA should also be involved in formulating strategy.

A safe manual handling system is a legal as well as a professional requirement. The BCA should set up systems to ensure that all staff have adequate knowledge of manual handling issues, and that they achieve the competencies set out in this guidance before handling patients. The BCA should also help whoever is managing manual handling to achieve effective clinical supervision and keep their knowledge up to date.

Facilitation techniques

The BCA should help and enable, rather than tell or persuade. The content and duration of training or practice development should be tailored to the specific needs of the trainees and to the context in which they work.

For example, a one-on-one supervision session with a competent staff nurse working with patients who have complex needs may take the form of a detailed individual risk assessment for each patient.

By contrast, a community-based nurse supervising a small group of carers with a stable group of clients may choose a more prescriptive documented manual handling plan based on the needs of individual clients. Carers will normally be asked to tell managers about any changes in patient/client needs, so that care plans can be reviewed. This may in turn trigger a review of the skills staff need.

Achieving the necessary competencies

BCAs must update their knowledge regularly so that they can advise at both strategic and organisational levels as well as facilitating the educational needs of manual handling supervisors.

Appointed manual handling supervisors must achieve and build upon their competencies so that they can advise line managers and staff.

Managers are responsible for the clinical competence of their staff and for ensuring that competencies are kept up to date. Managers can delegate this responsibility to a manual handling supervisor (see above under "Delegation").

All staff should achieve the competence requirements listed in this guidance before handling patients. They should be given adequate supervision and opportunity to update the skills needed for their particular work area. Updates should take the form of both formal and informal clinical problem solving, supervision and feedback on the job.

Students of placement must achieve the required competencies before handling patients. There should be a clear agreement on who is responsible for the assessment, supervision and support of students or cadets working in clinical areas.

Documentation

All education and supervision sessions, whether formal (usually a classroom based planned session) or informal (planned or unplanned, often "on the job") should be documented. This can be done in various ways.

Documentation for formal sessions should cover content and duration, and include a list of attendees. Informal problem-solving sessions will often be documented in patient notes. Individual competence and progress should be documented in a personal development plan, to be reviewed and discussed with the line manger on a regular basis. Individuals can choose how frequently these reviews take place, although managers remain responsible for ensuring that individual staff contribute to the clinical effectiveness of the whole department.

Patient/client needs

Manual handling is often carried out by family members and social care staff, who do not have access to a full-time expert. Care in a client's home, for example, can present particular difficulties. Clinical supervision modes, though, will work in any context, and managers are responsible for ensuring good practice.

BCAs can be brought in to provide specialist advice, and will need to develop an understanding of the specific therapeutic, clinical, organisational and client needs in each case. As in any other situation, the BCA must take joint responsibility for following up and reviewing any actions taken as part of their service to the employer.

This guidance does not affect the relationship between a disabled person and their personal assistant, who is employed by the disabled person to provide support in personal, domestic, social and employment activities. Training/clinical supervision should be set up following discussion and negotiation between the disabled person and their PA: the disabled person is an expert on their own handling needs, but not necessarily on biomechanics and safer handling practices.

Disabled people have a duty of care in common law to ensure the safety of their employees, and may need to get advice from a BCA.

4 Competencies for manual handling

In this section we look at the competencies needed by:

- BCAs
- Manual handling supervisors
- Anyone handling patients/clients

The competencies:

- Should be used to underpin education plans and supervision sessions, to identify educational needs or skills gaps and to assess competence.
- Can by used to establish the curriculum and learning outcomes for formal and informal education or training sessions.

Staff can use the competencies to record achievements and to reflect on their practice development needs. Competencies can also be turned into audit standards.

The required competencies

In the next section we look in detail at the competencies required by people involved in handling patients or clients.

The three domains

The competencies fit into three domains of practice development needs.

1. Management of risk.
2. Creating safe systems of work.
3. Professional effectiveness and maintaining standards.

Each domain contains written competencies to be achieved by the three staff groups. This guidance specifies both the competency to be achieved and the performance criteria necessary to demonstrate it.

Domain 1: Management of risk

Competencies for back care advisers

1 Identify, assess and reduce risk at organisational and departmental level

Performance criteria

A Evidence of the development and implementation of a system for monitoring and analysing safe systems of work, including the upkeep of detailed records.

B Evidence of the development and implementation of a communications strategy throughout the organisation, including feedback to and liaison with clinical managers, the board and individuals.

C Attendance at relevant strategic/operational organisational and departmental meetings. There should be evidence of written reports and feedback to appropriate staff.

D Evidence of facilitating appointed manual handling supervisors and others where appropriate to ensure safer manual handling.

E Evidence of a rigorous audit trail to demonstrate effectiveness.

F Evidence that effective risk assessments have been completed – with review dates- and that they have been followed up.

Competencies for line managers/appointed manual handling supervisors/key workers

1 Identify, assess and reduce risk at departmental level

Performance criteria

A Evidence implementing an organisational system for monitoring and analysing safe systems of work in local areas.

B Evidence of maintaining and supporting the communications strategy throughout the organisation.

C Attendance at relevant organisational and departmental meetings and dissemination of information to staff. There should be evidence of effective communication among departmental staff, for example documentation showing effective handovers, care planning and problem solving.

D Evidence of facilitating staff to ensure safer manual handling within the department.

E Evidence of compliance with and completion of the organisation's audit trail to demonstrate effectiveness.

F Evidence that effective departmental risk assessments have been completed – with review dates and that they have been followed up.
G Evidence of compliance with all manual handling policies and procedures by all staff within the department.
H Evidence of supervision of all staff, including completion of records and competence in manual handling for each staff member.

Competencies for all patient/client handlers

1 Work within agreed framework to minimise risk to self and to patient

Performance criteria

A Evidence of compliance with safer patient handling techniques and organisational and local safe systems of work. Recorded in competency record.
B Evidence of the ability to select and use appropriate equipment for client needs and safer patient handling. Recorded in competency record.
C Evidence of attendance at handover and contribution to care planning and problem solving. Recorded in notes/minutes of meetings and personal development plan/competency record.
D Evidence of implementation of care plans and understanding/reporting of problems or changes in risk assessment using the "Task, Individual, Load, Environment" (TILE) format. Recorded in competency record and personal development plan.
E Evidence of taking up opportunities for formal and informal education and discussing manual handling training needs with line manager. Recorded in teaching session registers of notes/minutes of meetings.
F Evidence of knowing when to stop and ask for help or guidance, including knowing the risk to self of unsafe manual handling practices. Recorded in competency record.
G Evidence of understanding body dynamics and safer patient handling principles using reflective practice skills. Recorded in competency record and personal development plan.

Domain 2: Creating safe systems of work

Competencies for back care advisers

1 Enable individuals and groups within the organisation or carry out manual handling activities safely, with minimal threat to their musculoskeletal health

Performance criteria

A Evidence of facilitating others and supervising organisational success in the risk assessment process. Line managers should be able to understand and evaluate TILE assessments.
B Evidence of the development and implementation of a strategy to ensure organisational success in equipment provision, selection and usage. This includes facilitating and supervising manual handling supervisors and line managers so they understand the needs of their departments and how to meet them.
C Evidence of facilitation of manual handling supervisors and line mangers to ensure that the organisation encourages staff to care for their own musculoskeletal health. This involves formally and informally supervising the education of line managers to ensure that they understand the manual handling needs of their client group.
D Evidence of development and implementation of a strategy to ensure that the organisation evaluates client needs in the context of safer handling practice. This will involve care planning and facilitating and supervising the education of line managers to ensure that they understand the manual handling needs of their client group.
E Evidence of advocacy between (a) staff and clients, (b) staff and the organisation, and (c) other staff.
F Evidence of advice to the organisation on appropriate equipment purchase strategy based on proactive audit, evaluation (including user trials) and selection to enable each department to meet its clients' needs.

2 Working with others to create and sustain a culture which promotes health in the workplace with respect to musculoskeletal injury issues

Performance criteria

A Evidence of influencing organisational change by providing evidence at strategic and operational levels of the implementation of actions identified following risk assessment, including review and evaluation of success.

B Evidence of influencing and directing policy and practice including dynamic/changing (according to evidence) manual handling policy and procedures. This should be reviewed regularly.

C Evidence of collaboration with all other key stakeholders, user groups and other staff. This includes networking links to groups within and without the organisation.

Competencies for line managers/appointed manual handling supervisors/key workers

1 Enable individuals and groups within the organisation or carry out manual handling activities safely, with minimal threat to their musculoskeletal health

Performance criteria

A Evidence of facilitating staff and supervising local performance in the risk assessment process. This includes ensuring that all staff can understand, evaluate and follow a basic TILE assessment.

B Evidence and facilitating staff and supervising local performance in equipment provision, selection and usage. This involves documented discussion with staff about equipment problems and shortfalls in order to ensure that appropriate equipment provision is requested via the channels set out by the BCA.

C Evidence of working with staff and the BCA to ensure that equipment meets the needs of the client group.

D Evidence of facilitating staff and supervising local performance in encouraging staff to care for their own musculoskeletal health. This involves giving all staff the opportunity to be educated in understanding musculoskeletal risk and self help.

E Evidence of facilitating staff and supervising local performance in evaluating client needs in the context of safer handling practice. This involves ensuring that care plans and individual client assessments are carried out and documented, that these are appropriate and that recommendations are implemented by all staff. This can be documented at staff meetings and handovers.

F Evidence of advocacy between staff and clients, and other staff.

G Evidence of supervision and problem solving with individuals and groups within the department. This will include identifying needs and shortfalls with staff and providing supplementary input where necessary. Completion of staff competency records and informal training sessions, including patient notes and handovers, will provide this documentation.

2 Working with others to create and sustain a culture which promotes health in the workplace with respect to musculo-skeletal injury issues

Performance criteria

A Evidence that actions identified following risk assessment have been implemented, including review and evaluation of performance within the local area.

B Evidence that organisational policy and practice has been implemented within the local area and that results are regularly reviewed.

C Evidence of collaboration with all other staff and clients in implementing policy and procedures.

Competencies for all patient/client handlers – minimum requirements

1 Comply with departmental and organisational policies and procedures to carry out manual handling activities safely, with minimal threat to their musculoskeletal health

Performance criteria

A Evidence of contributing to the risk assessment process within the local area including the ability to understand, evaluate, and to follow a basic TILE assessment. Recorded in competency and development.

B Evidence of contributing to departmental decision-making in equipment provision, selection and usage to meet client needs. Recorded in meeting records and then in competency record and personal development plan.

C Evidence of maintaining self-care in relation to musculoskeletal health. Recorded in competency record and personal development plan, and attendance at the relevant education sessions where appropriate.

D Evidence of ability to act as an advocate for clients; that is, of understanding client needs. This will be reflected in their contribution to problem solving and care planning.

E Evidence of participation in problem-solving sessions and care planning for safer patient handling. Recorded in competency record and personal development plan.

F Evidence that they recognise their own limitations. All requests for help should be documented.

G Evidence of supporting co-workers to ensure that policy, procedures and departmental risk assessments are followed. Recorded in competency record and personal development plan.

2 Working with others to create and sustain a culture which promotes health in the workplace with respect to musculoskeletal injury issues

Performance criteria

A Evidence of collaboration with other staff and clients in implementing policy and procedures. Recorded in competency record and personal development plan.

Domain 3: Professional effectiveness and maintaining standards

Competencies for back care advisers

1 Maintain accurate records and documentation that comply with professional, legal and administrative requirements.

Performance criteria

A Evidence of a system for ensuring clear, legible, confidential records of risk assessment process throughout the organisation, including evaluation dates, follow-up and outcome information.

B Evidence of a comprehensive system for staff education which meets the legal standard and includes the achievement of competencies by managers or appointed manual handling supervisors. Both formal and informal teaching should be recorded.

2 Promote improved standards of quality of care of clients/patients.

Performance criteria

A Evidence of evaluation of research, expert opinion and other evidence and the integration of new ideas into existing policies and procedures for continuous improvement in client./patient care.

3 Practice and promote continuing professional development (CPD)

Performance criteria

A Evidence of taking responsibility to enhance, update and develop appropriate knowledge and skills.

Competencies for line managers/appointed manual handling supervisors/key workers

1 Maintain accurate records and documentation which comply with professional, legal and administrative requirements

Performance criteria

A Evidence of clear, legible, confidential records of risk assessments within the department, including evaluation dates, follow-up and outcome information.

B Evidence of up-to-date care plans for all patients with risk assessment integrated into the process.

C Evidence of both formal and informal teaching and problem solving in order to achieve and build upon the minimum standard competencies for all staff.

2 Promote improved quality of patient care

Performance criteria

A Evidence of the integration of new, evidence based ideas into existing departmental procedures for continuous improvement in patient/client care.

3 Practice and promote continuing professional development (CPD)

Performance criteria

A Evidence of taking responsibility to enhance, update and develop appropriate knowledge and skills.

Competencies for line managers/appointed manual handling supervisors/key workers

1 Maintain accurate records and documentation which comply with professional, legal and administrative requirements

Performance criteria

A Evidence of clear, legible, confidential records of risk assessments within the department, including evaluation dates, follow-up and outcome information.

B Evidence of up-to-date care plans for all patients with risk assessment integrated into the process.

C Evidence of both formal and informal teaching and problem solving in order to achieve and build upon the minimum standard competencies for all staff.

2 Promote improved quality of patient care

Performance criteria

A Evidence of the integration of new, evidence based ideas into existing departmental procedures for continuous improvement in patient/client care.

3 Practice and promote continuing professional development (CPD)

Performance criteria

A Evidence of taking responsibility to enhance, update and develop appropriate knowledge and skills.

Competencies for all patient/client handlers – minimum requirements

1 Maintain accurate records and documentation which comply with professional, legal and administrative requirements

Performance criteria

A Evidence of working with line manager to keep clear, legible, confidential records of risk assessments within the department. These should include evaluation dates, follow-up and outcome information. Recorded in competency record and personal development plan.

B Evidence of contributing to the maintenance of up-to-date care plans that reflect risk assessments. Recorded in competency record and personal development plan.

C Evidence of receipt of formal and informal education and problem solving, including identification of education needs in collaboration with line manager.

2 Promote improved standards of quality of care of clients/patients

Performance criteria

A Evidence of working with colleagues to ensure that all staff work within policies and procedures. Recorded in competency record and personal development plan.

B Evidence of feeding back on the effects of the integration of evidence based new ideas into practice for continuous improvement in client care. Recorded in staff meeting minutes and handovers, and in competency records.

3 Practice and promote continuing professional development (CPD)

Performance criteria

A Evidence of taking responsibility to enhance, update and develop appropriate knowledge and skills.

5 Case studies

The evaluated projects outlined below provide two examples of how the competency approach to manual handling training works effectively in practice.

Case study 1

When electric beds were introduced at Kings College Hospital, the hospital devised a comprehensive training programme for staff including:

- Specific training sessions organised and held centrally
- Provision of one bed on the receiving ward prior to full equipping to allow staff to familiarise themselves with the equipment
- On-ward training during delivery and over the next three days
- Repeat training during monitoring visits throughout the first month following installation

Six months later, the effectiveness of the training was audited along with the staff's ability to use the beds. The audit showed that despite the training programme, 25 % of the staff still felt that their training had been inadequate. Tests showed that only 50 % of staff knew how to convert the bed into the chair position, while only 25 % knew about the lockout controls and how to locate and use the egress handle.

The company that supplied the beds has now built training into the service support it provides. Key performance targets, including the provision of direct local training and problem solving, have been incorporated into nurse advisers' objectives. These targets are monitored quarterly and have financial penalties attached to them to ensure compliance.

Manual handling refresher training and ward based problem solving sessions have focused on helping staff understand the key functions of the electric beds and get the maximum benefit from them. As a result, over 65 % of staff now have the knowledge they need. This work based approach has also led to improved standards of practice.

Case study 2

Nottingham City Hospital is a 1,200–bed specialist teaching hospital. It employs approximately 5,000 staff, of whom 50 % are nurses. Since 1994 Dr Sue Hignett has been leading a project to incorporate ergonomic principles into the trust's strategies for managing manual handling risks.

The ergonomic strategy includes both top-down and bottom-up approaches. In the six years since the strategy was implemented, the number of manual handling incidents and days lost due to musculoskeletal sickness has consistently gone down. A simple calculation carried out by the HSE (based on the Wigan and Leigh model) suggests that the strategy has led to savings of more than £3,690,000 over the three-year period between 1996 and 1999.

The standard for back care training states that all staff should attend a back care session within a month of starting work. New starters should not be asked to carry our patient handling tasks until they have attended a training session. Updates are required every two years for patient handling staff and every three years for other staff. *(Hignett S 2001).*

6 Getting RCN approval for your training programme

RCN accreditation assures the quality of a product, person or place, and means that it is fit for purpose and for practice. Our professional accreditation differs from academic validation in that it examines the impact that the person being accredited or the product being approved can have on nurses, nursing or the environment or culture of care.

Our purpose is to improve for patients and clients, our ultimate beneficiaries. By approving educational initiatives such as moving and handling initiatives, both nurses and their employers can be assured of the quality of the training that nurses have undertaken and the care that they can deliver.

How to gain accreditation

Contact the RCN Accreditation Unit (RCN AU) (see the bottom of this section for contact details). If your initiative is a study day, workshop, seminar, training course or similar initiative that lasts for between one and five days and does not lead to a formal award, please ask for an approval of events pack.

If your initiative includes a range of content and teaching strategies on a coherent theme and there will be a clinical assessment of the course material, possibly including the development of a personal portfolio which could be submitted for APL/APEL at a recognisable level, please request a pack for the approval of short professional courses. Initiatives in this category will normally last for over five days.

Once you have received your pack, please complete the application form and send it to the RCH AU with the appropriate fee and a rationale stating how your initiative addresses each of the competencies.

All applications are sent to a subject reviewer and educational reviewer whose job is to decide whether the application meets the standards for RCN approval. They will also write a report justifying their decision. If the reviewers have any concerns about you application we will help you address these, shaping your initiative so that it gets approval and meets the latest government recommendations, offering the best service to nurses and their employers.

Certificates

All nurses attending RCN AU approved initiatives are issued with a certificate from the RCH AU showing either the number of hours attended or the number of CEPs awarded.

The RCN developed CEPs as a form of "professional currency" to help nurses keep track of their own CPD. CEPs are available wherever active learning can be demonstrated – this might mean asking nurses to complete a reflective practice profile, or developing an action plan for putting learning outcomes into practice.

If you would like your attendees to gain CEPs, this should be built into the original application for approval. You should also indicate who will be assessing this active learning, and explain why they are qualified to do this.

Certificates can be kept in the individual nurse's portfolio, showing the number of hours of CPD undertaken. They can also help nurses meet PREP requirements for the Nursing and Midwifery Council (NMC).

Competency and criteria achievement

The competencies in this document will enable your organisation to improve is manual handling systems. They can be achieved only in the context of a positive health and safety culture. If you would like to get your training programme approved by the RCN, please complete the grid below to show that you have met the initial criteria for approval and send it to the RCN AU along with your other application forms.

Contact details

If you have any enquiries about RCN approval please contact:

RCN Accreditation Unit
20 Cavendish Square
London
W1G 0RN

Tel: 020 7647 3824/3716/3647
E Mail: accreditation@rcn.org.uk

	Criteria	Yes/No
A	The programme meets the appropriate competency levels outlined in the guidance	
B	The programme shows the link between training for manual handling and supervision of staff in the workplace and also shows how trainers manage this link	
C	The assessment of practice is linked to environmental management, risk management and care planning in the workplace	
D	The trainers used in the programme meet eth competencies listed in this guidance for a BCA or key worker	
E	The programme shows how supervision of practice in the workplace is used as part of the training process	
F	The programme includes a communication strategy for promoting best practice in manual handling within the workplace	

References

Department of Health (1998). A First Class Service: quality in the new NHS. London: DH (available from www.doh.gov.uk)

Health and Safety Executive (1999). The Management of Health and Safety at Work Regulations. Sudbury: HSE.

Hignett S (2001). Embedding ergonomics in hospital culture: top-down and bottom-up strategies. Applied Ergonomics 32, 61-69.

Manley K (1992). 'Quality assurance: the pathway to excellence in nursing', Chapter 7 in Bryzinska G and Jolley M (eds) Nursing Care: the challenge to change. London: Edward Arnold.

Royal College of Nursing (1999). Look back, move on: clinical supervision for nurses. London: RCN

Royal College of Nursing (2000). Introducing a safer patient handling policy. London: RCN (publication code 000 603)

Royal College of Nursing (2001). Changing practice – improving health: an integrated back injury prevention programme for nursing and care homes. London: RCN (publication code 001 255).

Appendix 4

ARJO
Mobility Gallery

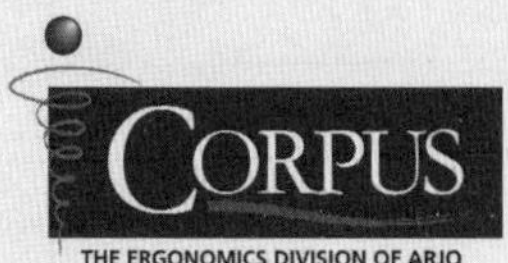

What is the ARJO Mobility Gallery

The ARJO Mobility Gallery is a classification system based on five people. Each person has different personal characteristics and background details. The people are classified according to their degree of functional mobility.

For classification purposes, we have decided to focus on functional mobility, not specific diseases and related diagnoses. People live with the consequences of diseases, which affect their capacity to carry out daily activities, and this fact is at the heart of the classification system. It is therefore the consequences of a disease and the resulting level of functional mobility, rather than the disease itself, which largely determines dependency on care.

People with a similar medical condition do not necessarily have the same capacity for performing daily activities. The spectrum of capacity among those with a common condition is very broad. Some people may be as active as before, others may be severely impaired in their daily life. A number of factors other than medical conditions affect a persons' actual capacity to perform daily tasks. The result, their functional capacity, determines what they need and also how we can provide optimum care. This makes it essential not only to be aware of the medical side, but also to make a detailed assessment of a persons' functional capacity.

Dementia and other factors

The ARJO Mobility Gallery illustrates five degrees of functional mobility and indicates the relative dependence on care in each case. There are, of course other factors besides mobility that affect dependence on care. In elderly care, one of the major factors is Alzheimer's dementia. It should be emphasised that all of the people in the gallery – from Albert to Emma – can be envisaged with different degrees of dementia, ranging from symptom-free to advanced stages.

Why do we need classification?

People in nursing homes and other care facilities are individuals with different diseases, problems, backgrounds and wishes for the future. We want to offer them all a standard of care that will allow them to maintain an optimum quality of life.

But, from a handler's perspective, we want to achieve this without compromising our own health. Quality of care and optimum working conditions are complementary. This is demonstrated by the ARJO Positive Eight concept. This concept shows that if the right choices are made, quality of care and optimum working conditions reinforce each other in a positive way.

But, this positive reinforcement only occurs if the right choices are made. In elderly care, these choices are made on the basis of our individual assessments. We make choices tailored to their needs and desires. It is important to recognise that there is no such thing as a "typical" person. In everyday care, these assessments are the basis for millions of choices. These choices are often made unconsciously. In order to plan care for our people, we need to make conscious, well-balanced choices. Therefore, some sort of standardisation and classification is needed in combination with tailoring care to the individual person. This will lead to clear care plans and monitoring of care plan suitability, which in turn makes it possible to plan the policy of a health care organisation.

The aim of the ARJO Mobility Gallery

The need for standardisation and classification is one of the reasons why ARJO developed the Mobility Gallery – a classification system that involves five people. The ARJO Mobility Gallery will promote the development of a high standard of care by providing insight on care requirements, monitoring changing needs and protecting the health of handlers (training, equipment and working environment).

Clinicians recognise that comprehensive functional assessment of elderly people is central to maximising their physical and cognitive functioning and quality of life *(Hawes et al 1997)*. Studies have confirmed that introducing the RAI (Resident Assessment Instrument) significantly improved a person's outcome in four crucial areas (ADL function, cognitive function, urinary continence and social engagement) *(Philips et al 1996)*.

There was also an increase in the assessment of potential for improving a person's' functional capacity *(Hawes et al 1997)*.

The Gallery's links with existing systems

The development of the Mobility Gallery by ARJO is partly based on the RAI, but also on studies made in Holland. *(Knibbe, JJ, NA Hulshof, AP Stoop, RD Friele, Kleine hulpmiddelen: hulp voor bewoners en zorgverleners?, NIVEL, Utrecht, 1998)*.

Its focus on the functional consequences of diseases links the ARJO

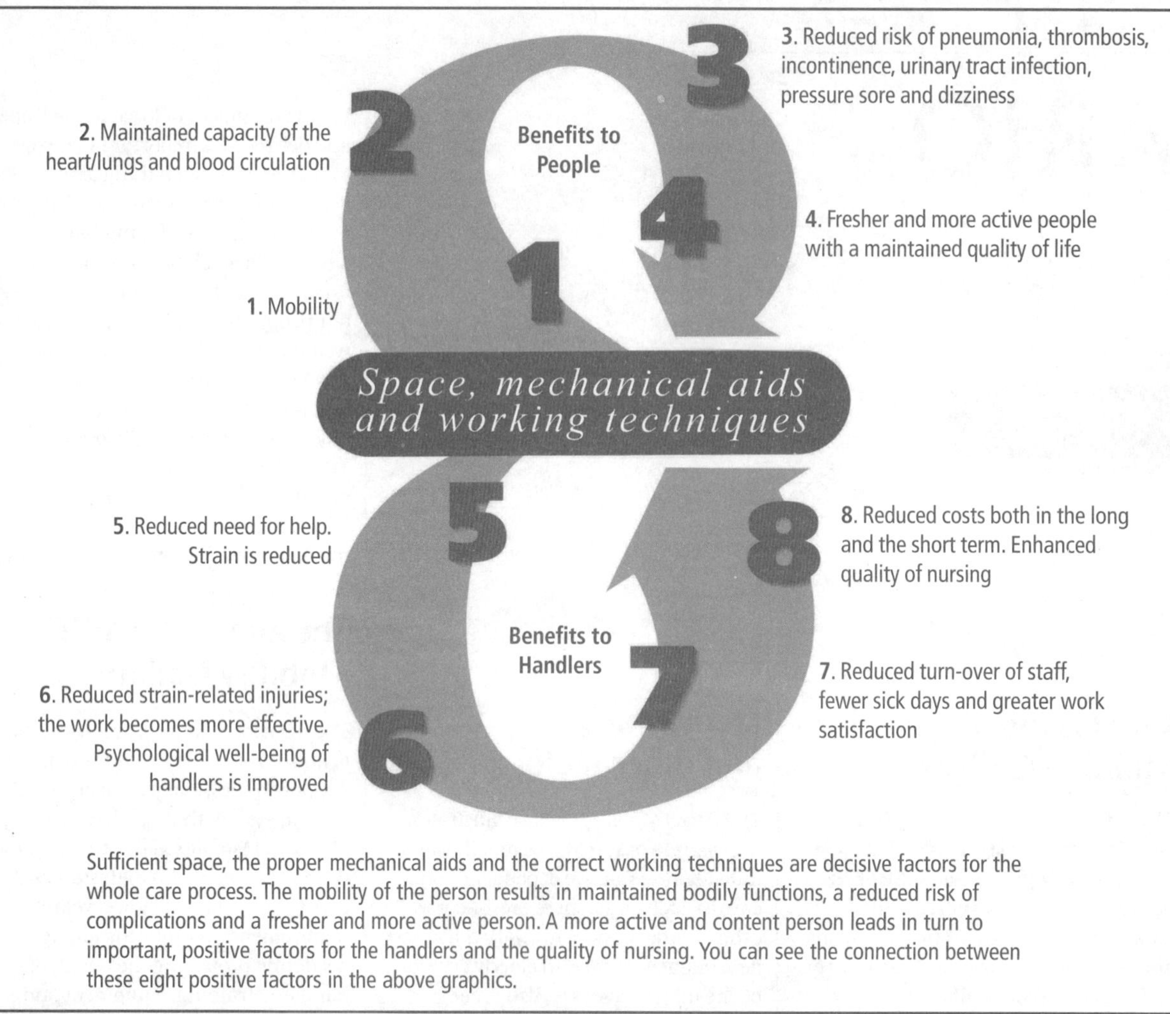

Sufficient space, the proper mechanical aids and the correct working techniques are decisive factors for the whole care process. The mobility of the person results in maintained bodily functions, a reduced risk of complications and a fresher and more active person. A more active and content person leads in turn to important, positive factors for the handlers and the quality of nursing. You can see the connection between these eight positive factors in the above graphics.

Mobility Gallery with existing international classification and assessment systems such as the ICIDH and RAI.

The ICIDH (International Classification of Impairments, Disabilities and Handicaps), developed by the WHO (World Health Organisation), is often used in rehabilitation and is familiar to most physiotherapists.

The RAI (Resident Assessment Instrument) was developed in the USA, but has been introduced in many European countries, Australia and Japan over the past five years, allowing international comparisons. Originally developed in the USA to improve the quality of care, RAI was also adopted for use by Medicare and Medicaid facilities in order to apply for funding.

The intention was that improved individual assessment would make care plans more comprehensive and person-specific, and thus enhance the quality of care. The RAI system promotes this by providing both the assessments (Minimum Data Set RAI-MDS) and care plan guidelines in the Resident Assessment Protocols (RAPs).

The assessment part of the RAI (MDS) may pinpoint important problem areas. These will, more or less automatically, trigger one or more of the Resident Assessment Protocols (RAPs). The protocols provide guidelines for specific problem areas such as incontinent or skin care. A study of facilities using the RAI showed that it enhanced the quality of care *(Philips et al 1996)*.

Individual Assessment

The ARJO Mobility Gallery differs from the RAI and ICIDH, but does not replace these standards. However, it is linked to them in terms of functional mobility. This enables rapid understanding, combining of data on care plans, a common language, and also links the ARJO Mobility Gallery to other relevant mobility-related care topics such as incontinence, skin problems and pressure sores.

The ARJO Mobility Gallery is far more than a classification system. The five people offer a personification of five degrees of functional mobility. They are based on the kind of people you meet in care facilities. With names, pictures and backgrounds, we have tried to give them a personal presence. Detailed images provide a basis for discussing care and rehabilitation choices with the advantages of classification and standardisation.

The Gallery's role in planning for tomorrow's care

The ARJO Mobility Gallery not only assists care planning and guides quality improvement processes, but also provides support for decision-makers at the facility level. For example, in the building or redesigning of elderly care facilities, it is crucial for architects and planners to grasp the exact functional demands of the home's residents, not only now, but in the years ahead. As a basis for this, ARJO developed the ARJO Guidebook for Architects and Planners. The ARJO Mobility Gallery takes the ARJO Guidebook one step further and makes communication easier between handlers and architects. It provides both a practical insight on the needs of present and future people as well as their aspirations for quality of life.

The ARJO Guidebook for Architects

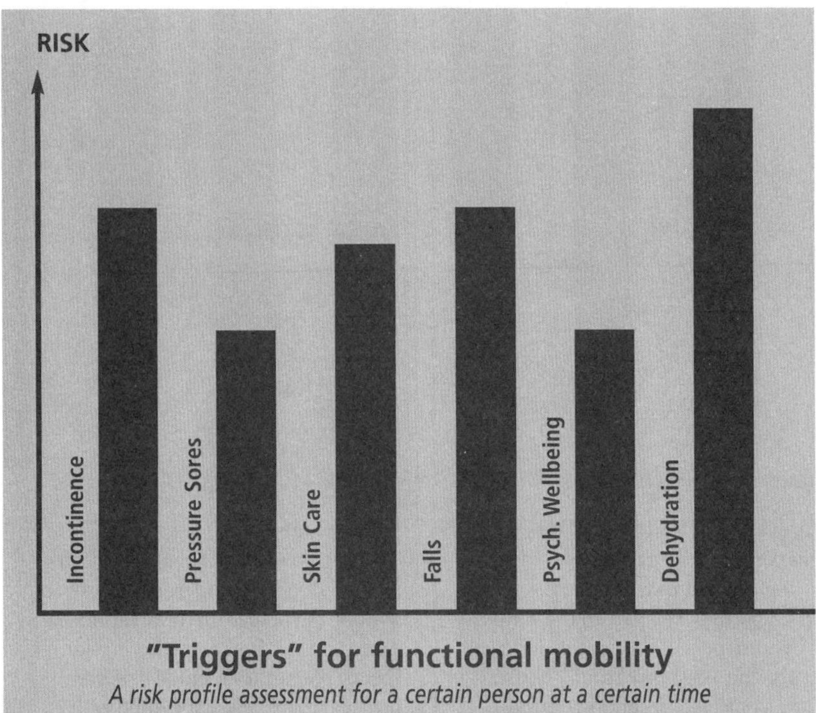

and Planners and the ARJO Mobility Gallery form a strong combination, creating a common language for the design of environments with people in mind.

Functional mobility: use it or lose it

Mobility is a fundamental part of people's lives. If mobility is reduced, the psychological and social consequences are far-reaching. People become isolated and often experience a loss of personal esteem. They may even become severely depressed. On the physical side, reduced mobility leads to a rapid decrease in muscle power, physical condition and general capacity. If this situation continues, problems such as immobile joints, pressure sores, osteoporosis and pneumonia often occur.

Loss of mobility can occur very rapidly if, for instance, a fall causes a fracture. Among the elderly, however, the process is usually slow and gradual. In the latter case, it often goes unnoticed, as people tend to adapt their lifestyles and daily habits accordingly. They go out less often, drink less to reduce bathroom visits, or simply take longer to get dressed in the morning. Other people, including handlers, may not notice these changes in time. When they do, it may be too late, as some physical changes are very difficult to reverse in the elderly. Spotting changes in time, making simple, accurate assessments and offering solutions may prevent the occurrence and increase of avoidable dependency.

Research shows that elderly people change their daily habits to a great extent before they ask for help. For these people, proper aids and equipment may postpone or eliminate these changes and allow them to maintain their toileting habits and social life. In this case, the aim is to prevent avoidable dependency.

Albert, the first person in the gallery, is a good example of this often forgotten category of people. Providing him with adequate aids tailored to his needs at the right time may prevent him from declining unnecessarily fast.

It is just as important to stimulate, maintain and even increase the mobility of other people, including many of those who receive assistance with daily activities. The spectrum of functional mobility can be divided into the five classifications of the ARJO Mobility Gallery.

"Use it or lose it" – when people use their functional capacity, it will have a positive effect on health and wellbeing. Even minor movements and activities can have a positive effect. For example, rising to a standing position a few times a day maintains co-ordination as well as preventing the loss of muscle and bone tissue. The ARJO Positive Eight maps out the beneficial effects of maintaining mobility.

On the other hand, there are people for whom it is no longer relevant or desirable to stimulate mobility or activity. It is important, for example, to provide those in the last phase of life with the best care we can offer and prevent complications caused by immobility such as pressure sores. Stimulating their mobility may become an impossibility. For these people, a correct assessment may also point to the use of certain types of equipment to make their lives easier and make it possible for handlers to provide optimum care without compromising their own health. Emma is an example of a person entering that final stage. Between Albert and Emma are three other people, all with different degrees of functional mobility. You can recognise them by their alphabetical names: Albert, Barbara, Carl, Doris and Emma, which are also used in the mobility scheme.

The people

Albert

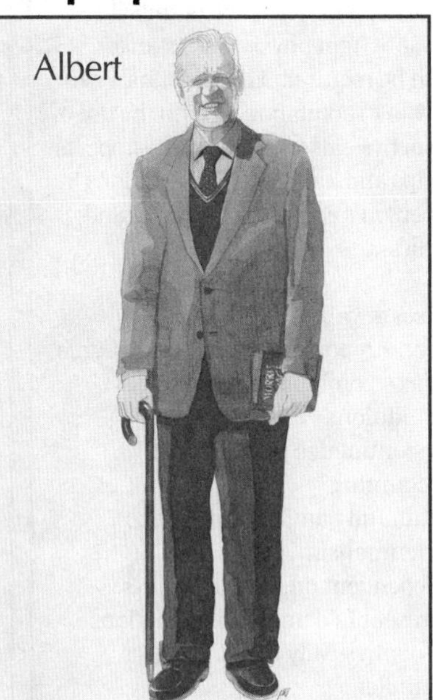

Male, age 75, 82 kg/1180 lbs
This person is able to perform daily activities independently. Special aids or appliances may be needed.

- Ambulatory, but uses a cane for support
- Independent, he can clean and dress himself
- Physically and mentally active
- Tires quickly
- Continent
- Requires careful monitoring

Barbara

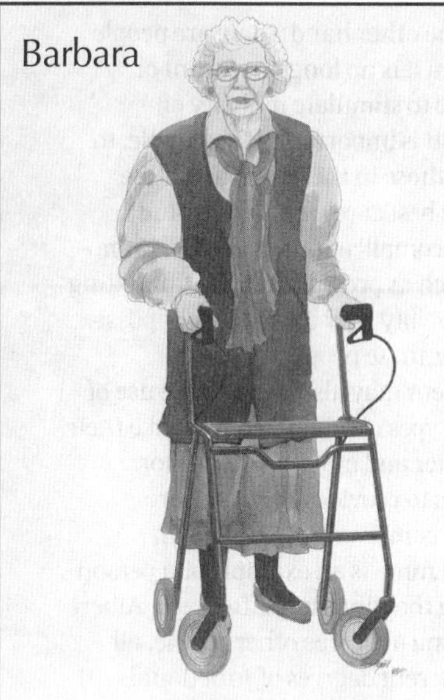

Female, age 82, 61 kg/134 lbs
This person is not capable of performing daily activities without help. However, the assistance required is not physically demanding for handler. Assistance may consist of verbal support, feedback or indications, but light physical assistance might be required. This assistance can be given in combination with the use of supportive aids (walking aids, supports or grips and handles) or adaptations in the person's environment (grips and handles).

- Uses a walker
- Can support herself to some degree
- Has a combination of medical conditions
- Incontinence problems are beginning
- Stiff and painful joints due to rheumatism
- Dependent on handler who is present in demanding situations
- Not physically demanding for handler
- Remaining capacity should be stimulated

Carl

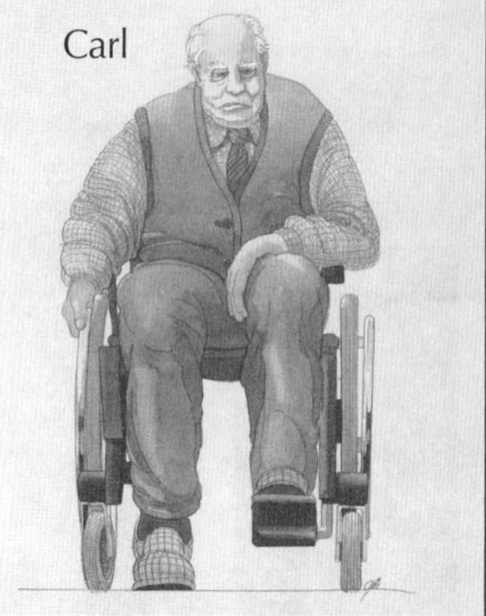

Male, age 80, 95 kg/ 208 lbs
This person is not capable of performing daily activities without assistance, but is able to participate in the activity or perform part of the routine independently. The assistance would, if given without special precautions, entail a risk of physical overload for the handler. The resulting load would be in excess of safe limits relating to manual handling or static loads. In these cases, it is necessary to use equipment that will reduce risk for the handler to safe levels. At the same time, these people are able to actively participate in movements and it is important for the person to maintain or improve this capacity as much as possible. Assistance given in these instances is, for example, transfer using an active lift.

- Sits in wheelchair
- Left-side hemiplegic
- Some capacity to support himself
- Can stand for short periods
- Mentally capable of decision-making
- Urine incontinent
- Dependent on handler
- Physically demanding for handler
- Needs equipment to cope with loss of mobility and to protect his handler from transfer-related injuries
- Important to stimulate remaining capacity and slow down deterioration of mobility

Doris

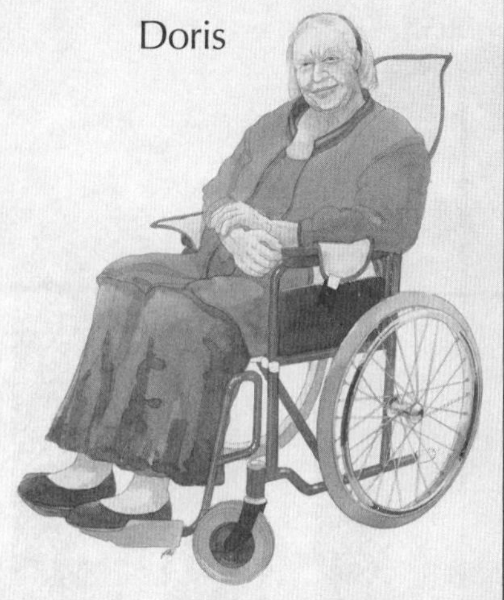

Female, age 80, 90 kg/198 lbs
This person is not capable of performing daily activities independently or to actively participate in these routines. Assistance in this case will, without special precautions, entail a risk of physical overload for the handler. It is necessary to use equipment that eliminates the risk of overloading. The person can, in this case, not participate actively in the movement. In spite of this, wherever and whenever possible, it remains important to activate the person. The assistance provided in this case, for example, transfer using a passive lift. An extra point to note in this case is the prevention of conditions associated with immobility.

- Sits in wheelchair
- No capacity to support herself
- Cannot stand unsupported
- Increasing dementia
- Doubly incontinent
- Dependent on handler
- Physically demanding for handler
- Needs equipment such as passive lift to cope with loss of function and to protect her handlers
- Important to slow down deterioration of mobility

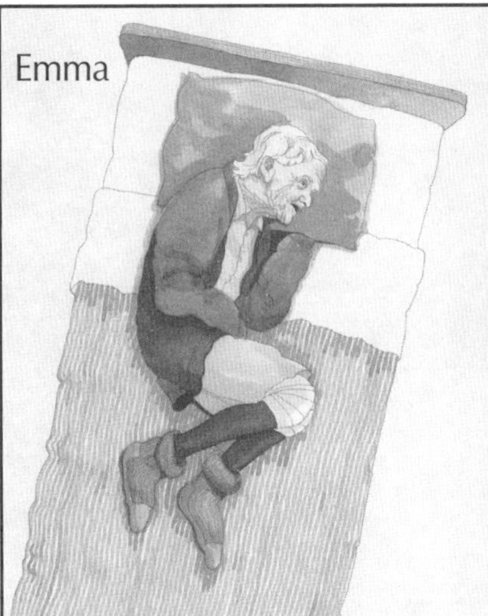

Female, age 86, 42 kg/ 92 lbs
This person is not capable of performing daily activities independently or to actively participate in these routines. The assistance given in this case will, without special precautions, entail a risk of physical overload for the handler. It is necessary to use equipment that eliminates this risk of overloading. The person can, in this case, not participate actively in this movement. In some cases active participation may have to be avoided. Promoting or stimulating mobility and activating the person is no longer an aim of the care plan. Priority is given to providing optimum care and prevention of complications caused by immobility. Transfers in this case are carried out using a passive lift.

- Passive person
- Almost completely bedridden
- In later stages of dementia
- Decreasing in weight
- Doubly incontinent
- Totally dependent
- Physically demanding for handler
- Mechanical aids should always be used to transfer
- Aim is to avoid complications caused by long-term confinement to bed and make her as comfortable as possible

ARJO is dedicated to delivering quality products, solutions and programmes that enhance the daily living of the elderly, infirm and sick, and provide a safe and healthy working environment for the people who care for them. ARJO has gained unrivalled knowledge on the day-to-day practicalities of geriatric and hospital care from over 40 years of contact with all aspect of nursing worldwide. Our expertise spans four core competencies: Injury Prevention, Care of People, Infection Control and Facility Planning.

Our aim is to promote positive outcomes in the world of health care through optimum hardware and enhanced awareness.

ARJO

ARJO, St Catherine Street, Gloucester GL1 2SL
Tel: 08702 430 430 Fax: 01452 428 344
Email: uksales@arjo.co.uk or ukservice@arjo.co.uk
www.arjo.com

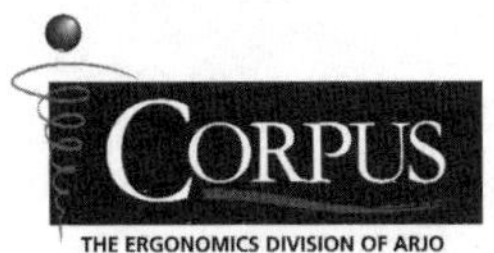

CORPUS
The holistic approach to safer handling through tailored assessments, interventions, and support programmes.
Tel: 01452 428700 Fax: 01452 428329
Email: info@corpusinfo.co.uk

Index

A

B

C

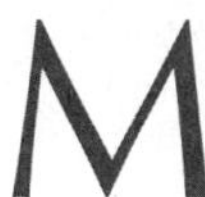

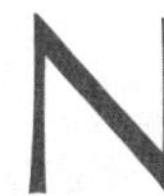

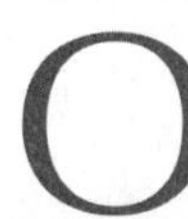

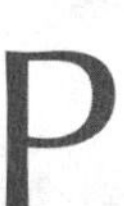

Q

R

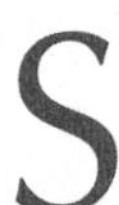

T

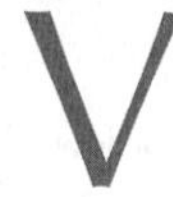

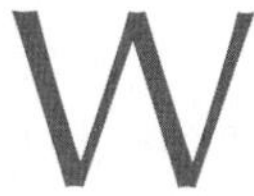

W

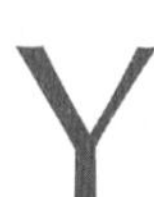

Disabled Living Centres

Aylesbury (Southern)
Independent Living Exhibition
Brookside Centre
Station Way
AYLESBURY
Buckinghamshire HP20 2SQ
Tel: 01296 398 616
Fax: 01296 435110 needs to specify recipient.
E-mail: ile_aylesbury@hotmail.com

Beckenham (Southern)
Lewis House Independent Living Centre
Lewis House
30 Beckenham Road
BECKENHAM
Kent BR3 4LS
Tel: 0208 663 3345
Fax: 0208 663 1442
E-mail: trevor-bath@freeola.com

Belfast (N. Ireland)
Independent Living Centre
Regional Disablement Services
Musgrave Park Hospital
Stockmans Lane
BELFAST
Northern Ireland BT9 7JB
Tel: 028 9066 9501 Ext. 2708
Fax: 028 9068 3662
Mini-com: 028 9066 3008
E-mail: ilc.mph@greenpark.n-i.nhs.uk

Birmingham (Central)
Birmingham Centre For Independent Living
St Marks Street
Springhill
BIRMINGHAM
West Midlands B1 2HU
Tel: 0121 464 4942
Fax: 0121 464 4944
Mini-com: 0121 464 7565
E-mail: heather_coleman@birmingham.gov.uk

Boston (Central)
Disabled Living Centre
British Red Cross
Scott House
BOSTON
Lincolnshire PE21 6DG
Tel: 01205 367 597
Fax: 01205 367597
E-mail: sara_lou9@hotmail.com

Brighton (Southern)
Daily Living Centre
Unit 1
Hove Business Centre
Off Fonthill Road
Hove
BRIGHTON
East Sussex BN3 6HA
Tel: 01273 731 208
Fax: 01273 726820
Mini-com: 01273 725421
E-mail: bhdlc@bhdlc.fsnet.co.uk

Bristol (Southern)
Disabled Living Centre (West of England)
The Vassall Centre
Gill Avenue
Fishponds
BRISTOL
Avon BS16 2QQ
Tel: 0117 965 3651
Fax: 0117 965 3652
Mini-com: 0117 965 3651
E-mail: info@dlcbristol.org
Web: www.dlcbristol.org

Bury St. Edmunds (Central)
West Suffolk Disability Resource Centre
Papworth House
4 Bunting Road
BURY ST. EDMUNDS
Suffolk IP32 7BX
Tel: 01284 748888
Fax: 01284 748889
Mini-com: 01284 748881
E-mail: WSDRC@papworth.org.uk
Web: www.papworth.org.uk

Caerphilly (Wales)
Centre for Help and Advice for the Disabled
Ty Clyd Bungalow
Heol Fargoed
Bargoed
CAERPHILLY
Wales CF81 8PP
Tel: 01443 822 262
Fax: 01443 822 286
E-mail: info@chad-ilc.co.uk
Web: www.chad-ilc.co.uk

Cardiff (Wales)
Disabled Living Centre (Rookwood Lodge)
Rookwood Hospital
Fairwater Road
Llandaff
CARDIFF
Wales CF5 2YN
Tel: 029 20560704/02920313751
Fax: 029 20 578509
E-mail: DLC.enquiries@CardiffandVale.wales.nhs.uk

Castleford (Northern)
Ability Centre
Highfield
Love Lane
CASTLEFORD
West Yorkshire WF10 5RT
Tel: 01977 724 012
Fax: 01977 727095
E-mail: SC_CCabilitycentre@wakefield.gov.uk

Crewe (Northern)
Crewe Independent Living Centre
O.T Department
Leighton Hospital
Middlewich Road
CREWE
Cheshire CW1 4QJ
Tel: 01270 612 343
Fax: 01606 79260

Dewsbury (Northern)
Social Services Information Point
Walsh Building
Town Hall Way
DEWSBURY
West Yorkshire WF12 8EQ
Tel: 01924 325 070
Fax: 01924 325077
E-mail: ssip.dewsbury@kirklees.gov.uk

Doncaster (Northern)
South Yorkshire Centre for Independent Living
Disability Resource Centre
Sovereign House
Heavens Walk
DONCASTER
South Yorkshire DN4 5HZ
Tel: 01302 769 219
Fax: 01302 327778
Mini-com: 01302 329788
E-mail: admin@sycil.org.uk
Web: www.sycil.org.uk

Dudley (Central)
Disabled Living Centre
1 St. Giles Street
Netherton
DUDLEY
West Midlands DY2 0PR
Tel: 01384 813 695
Fax: 01384 813 696

Dundee (Scotland)
Ability Centre
The MacKinnon Centre
491 Brook Street
Broughty Ferry
DUNDEE
Scotland DD5 2DZ
Tel: 01382 431990

Fax: 01382 431989
Mini-com: None
E-mail: ability.centre@
dundeecity.gov.uk

Dunstable (Central)
The Disability Resource Centre
Poynters House
Poynters Road
DUNSTABLE
Bedfordshire LU5 4TP
Tel: 01582 470900
Fax: 01582 470959
Mini-com: 01582 470968
E-mail: information@drcbeds.org.uk
Web: www.drcbeds.co.uk

Eastbourne (Southern)
East Sussex Disability Association
1 Faraday Close
Hampden Park
EASTBOURNE
East Sussex BN22 9BH
Tel: 01323 514 500
Fax: 01323 514 501
Mini-com: 01323 514 502
E-mail: info@esda.org.uk
Web: www.esda.org.uk

Edinburgh (Scotland)
Lothian Disabled Living Centre
Astley Ainslie Hospital
Grange Loan
EDINBURGH
Scotland EH9 2HL
Tel: 0131 537 9190
Fax: 0131 537 9190
Mini-com: 0131 537 9190
E-mail: lothiandlc@O2.co.uk

Elgin (Scotland)
Moray Resource Centre
Maisondieu Road
ELGIN
Scotland IV30 1RX
Tel: 01343 551 339
Fax: 01343 542014
Mini-com: 01343 551376
E-mail: info.dlc@comm.moray.gov.uk

Exeter (Southern)
Independent Living Centre
14 Marsh Green Road North
Marsh Barton
EXETER
Devon EX2 8LT
Tel: 01392 687 276
Fax: 01392 687277

Grangemouth (Scotland)
Dundas Resource Centre
Oxgang Road
GRANGEMOUTH
Scotland FK3 9EF
Tel: 01324 504 311
Fax: 01324 504312
E-mail: lindsay.russell@falkirk.gov.uk

Halton & Chester (Northern)
Halton Independent Living Centre
Collier Street
Runcorn
HALTON
Cheshire WA7 1HB
Tel: 01928 563 340
Fax: 01928 582950
E-mail: jean.hutfield@
cahc-tr.nwest.nhs.uk

Hillingdon (Southern)
Hillingdon Independent Living Centre
Wood End Centre
Judge Heath Lane
HILLINGDON
Middlesex UB3 2PB
Tel: 0208 848 8260
Fax: 0208 8488 262
Mini-com: 0208 848 8323 (DASH)
E-mail: Heather.Russell@
hillingdon.nhs.uk

Ipswich (Central)
Ipswich & East Suffolk Independent
Living Centre
7 Wren Avenue
IPSWICH
Suffolk IP2 0TJ
Tel: 01473 686804

Leeds (Northern)
The William Merritt Disabled Living
Centre
St Mary's Hospital
Green Hill Road
Armley
LEEDS
West Yorkshire LS12 3QE
Tel: 0113 305 5332
Fax: 0113 231 9291
Mini-com: 0113 3055332
E-mail: thewilliammerritt.dlc@nhs.net
Web: www.williammerrittleeds.org

Leicester (Central)
Leicester Disabled Living Centre
Red Cross Medical Aid Dept.
76 Clarendon Park Road
LEICESTER
Leicestershire LE2 3AD
Tel: 0116 270 0515
Fax: 0116 244 8625
E-mail: dlcinfo@redcross.org.uk

Lincoln (Central)
Disabled Living Centre
Ancaster Day Centre
Boundary Street
LINCOLN
Lincolnshire LN5 8NJ
Tel: 01522 545111
Fax: 01522 545 111

Liverpool (Northern)
Liverpool Disabled Living Centre
101–103 Kempston Street
LIVERPOOL
Merseyside L3 8HE
Tel: 0151 298 2055
Fax: 0151 298 2952
Mini-com: 0151 298 2055
E-mail: disabled.living.centre@
liverpool.gov.uk
Web: www.liverpooldisabledliving
centre.com

London (Southern)
Disabled Living Foundation
380–384 Harrow Road
LONDON
London W9 2HU
Tel: Helpline: 0845 130 9177
Fax: 0207 266 2922
Mini-com: 0870 603 9176
E-mail: advice@dlf.org.uk
Web: www.dlf.org.uk

Lowestoft (Central)
Waveney Centre for Independent Living
161 Rotterdam Road
LOWESTOFT
Suffolk NR32 2EZ
Tel: 01502 405 454
Fax: 01502 405452
Mini-com: 01502 405454
E-mail: WCIL@socserv.suffolkcc.gov.uk

Macclesfield (Northern)
Independent Living Centre
Macclesfield District General Hospital
Gawsworth Building
Victoria Road
MACCLESFIELD
Cheshire SK10 3BL
Tel: 01625 661 740
Fax: 01625 661245 (c/o Wheelchair
Services

Manchester (Northern)
Regional Disabled Living Centre
Disabled Living
Redbank House
4 St Chad's Street
MANCHESTER
Gtr. Manchester M8 8QA

Tel: 0161 214 5959
Fax: 0161 835 3591
Mini-com: None
E-mail: info@disabledliving.co.uk
Web: www.disabledliving.co.uk

Middlesbrough (Northern)
Independent Living Centre
c/o Lansdowne Centre
Lansdowne Road
MIDDLESBROUGH
Cleveland TS4 2QT
Tel: 01642 250749
Fax: 01642 250749

Milton Keynes (Southern)
Milton Keynes Centre for Integrated Living
330 Saxon Gate West
Central Milton Keynes
MILTON KEYNES
Buckinghamshire MK9 2ES
Tel: 01908 231 344
Fax: 01908 231335
Mini-com: 01908 231505
E-mail: maggiemkcil@aol.com

Newcastle (Northern)
Disability North
The Dene Centre
Castle Farm Road
NEWCASTLE UPON TYNE
Tyne & Wear NE3 1PH
Tel: 0191 284 0480
Fax: 0191 213 0910
Mini-com: 0191 285 7261
E-mail: reception@disabilitynorth.org.uk
Web: www.disabilitynorth.org.uk

Newton Aycliffe (Northern)
Home Independence Service
Abbey Day Centre
Abbey Road
Pity Me
DURHAM
County Durham DH1 5DQ
Tel: 0191 384 9590
Fax: 0191 375 0801
E-mail: christine.tarling@durham.gov.uk

Northwich (Northern)
Northwich Independent Living Centre
Victoria Infirmary
Winnington Hill
NORTHWICH
Cheshire CW8 1AW
Tel: 01606 79260
Fax: 01606 79260

Norwich (Central)
Disablity Resource Centre
County Hall
Mautineau Lane
NORWICH
Norfolk

Nottingham (Central)
Disabilities Living Centre
Middleton Court
Glaisdale Parkway
Off Glaisdale Drive
Bilborough
NOTTINGHAM
Nottinghamshire NG8 4GP
Tel: 0115 985 5780
Fax: 0115 928 4914
E-mail: info@dlcnotts.co.uk
Web: www.dlcnotts.co.uk

Oxford (Southern)
Dialability
The Oxford Centre for Enablement
Windmill Road
Headington
OXFORD
Oxfordshire OX3 7LD
Tel: 01865 763 600
Fax: 01865 764 730
Mini-com: 01865 764 729
E-mail: helpline@dialability.org.uk
Web: www.dialability.org.uk

Paisley (Scotland)
Disability Centre for Independent Living
30 Seedhill Road
PAISLEY
Scotland PA1 1SA
Tel: 0141 847 4959
Fax: 0141 847 4956

Papworth (Central)
Cambridgeshire Disabled Living Centre
Pendrill Court
PAPWORTH EVERARD
Cambridgeshire CB3 8UY
Tel: 01480 830 495
Fax: 01480 830495
Mini-com: 01480 839 154

Semington (Southern)
Wiltshire & Bath Independent Living Trust
Independent Living Centre
St George's Road
SEMINGTON
Wiltshire BA14 6JQ
Tel: 01380 871 007
Fax: 01380 871113
E-mail: info@ilc-semington.freeserve.co.uk
Web: www.ilc.org.uk

Shipley (Northern)
Disability Equipment Bradford
103 Dockfield Rd
SHIPLEY
West Yorkshire BD17 7AR
Tel: 01274 589162
Fax: 01274 530432
E-mail: equipment@disabilityadvice.org.uk

Shrewsbury (Central)
Shropshire Disability Resource Centre
Lancaster Road
Harlescott
SHREWSBURY
Shropshire SY1 3NJ
Tel: 01743 444 599
Fax: 01743 461349
Mini-com: 01743 444569
E-mail: Jhall@shropshiredisability.org
Web: www.shropshiredisability.org

Southampton (Southern)
Southampton Aid & Equipment Centre
Royal South Hants Hospital
Brintons Terrace
SOUTHAMPTON
Hampshire SO14 0YG
Tel: 02380 825 288
Fax: 02380 825254
E-mail: steve.slater@scpct.nhs.uk

Stamford (Central)
Disability Living Centre (Lincolnshire)
33 Ryhall Road
STAMFORD
Lincolnshire PE9 1UF
Tel: 01780 480 599
Fax: 01780 480603
E-mail: brcdlc@ukonline.co.uk

Stockport (Northern)
The Independent Living Centre
St Thomas's Hospital
Shawheath
STOCKPORT
Cheshire SK3 8BL
Tel: 0161 419 4476
Fax: 0161 419 4480
E-mail: Lindsey.Edwards@stockport-tr.nwest.nhs.uk

Swindon (Southern)
Options Plus
The Independent Living Centre
Stratton Road
SWINDON
Wiltshire SN1 2PN
Tel: 01793 643 966
E-mail: info@optionsplus.co.uk
Web: www.optionsplus.co.uk

Tower Hamlets (Southern)
Equipment Demonstration Centre
Resource Centre
40–60 Southern Grove
TOWER HAMLETS
London E3 4PX
Tel: 020 7364 5957
Fax: 020 7364 5655

Truro (Southern)
Cornwall Mobility Centre Ltd
Tehidy House
Royal Cornwall Hospital
TRURO
Cornwall TR1 3LJ
Tel: 01872 254 920
Fax: 01872 254 921
E-mail: mobility@rcht.swest.nhs.co.uk

Warrington (Northern)
Warrington Centre for Independent Living
Beaufort Street
Old Liverpool Road
WARRINGTON
Cheshire WA5 1BA
Tel: 01925 638 867
Fax: 01925 241852
E-mail: cilteam@disabilitypartnership.org.uk
Web: www.disabilitypartnership.org.uk

Welling (Central)
Head of Physical Disabilities & Specialist Service
Bexley Council
Hillview
Hill View Drive
WELLING
Kent DA16 3RY
Tel: 020 8303 7777
Fax: 020 83084997
E-mail: vinod.kumar@bexley.gov.uk
Web: www.bexley.gov.uk

Welwyn Garden City (Southern)
Hertfordshire Action on Disability
The Woodside Centre
The Commons
WELWYN GARDEN CITY
Hertfordshire AL7 4DD
Tel: 01707 384 260
Fax: 01707 371 297
Mini-com: 01707 324581
E-mail: sue@hadnet.org.uk
Web: www.hadnet.co.uk

Wolverhampton (Central)
The Neville Garratt Centre for Independent Living
Wolverhampton Social Services
Bell Street
WOLVERHAMPTON
West Midlands WV1 3PR
Tel: 01902 553 666
Fax: 01902 553643
Mini-com: 01902 553677
E-mail: elizabeth.hollins@wolverhampton.gov.uk

BackCare

The Charity for Healthier Backs

BackCare, registered as the National Back Pain Association, is a national registered medical charity, founded in 1968, dedicated to educating people on how to manage and avoid back pain and to supporting those living with back pain.

The Objects for which the Association is established are:

- To carry out and promote research into the causes, cure and prevention of illness, complaints and disorders in or associated with the back of the body and other allied conditions and to publish and make available the results of such research; and
- The relief of persons who suffer such conditions; and
- The advancement of education of the public concerning such conditions

BackCare provides information and support through its publications, website, telephone helpline and local self-help groups.

The charity also funds research and campaigns to raise the profile of issues surrounding back pain.

Through bringing together a membership of medical and clinical professionals, therapists, employers and people with back pain, BackCare's vision is to have a significant impact on reducing the number of people experiencing preventable back pain, and to ensure that appropriate support is available to those living with back pain.

BackCare, registered charity number 256751, www.backcare.org.uk

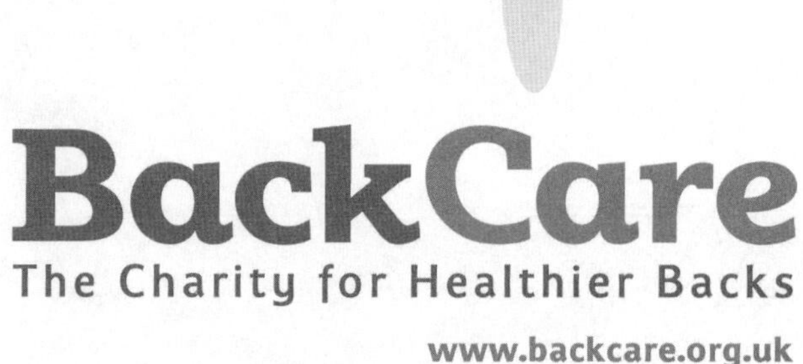